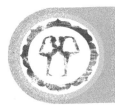

APPLIED ANATOMY & PHYSIOLOGY OF
YOGA

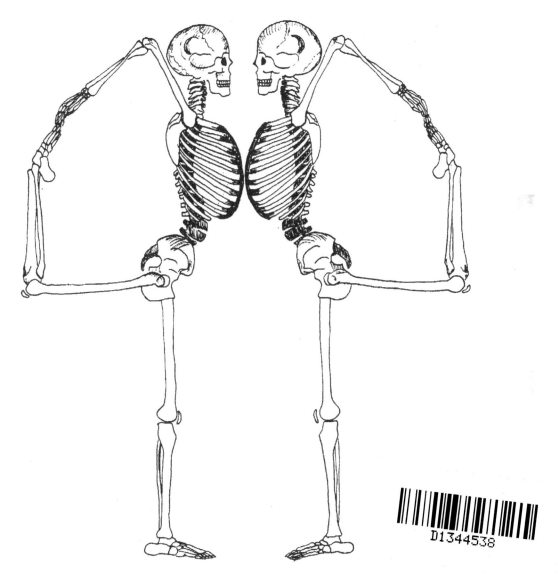

Simon Borg-Olivier
MSc BAppSc (Physiotherapy)

Bianca Machliss
BSc BAppSc (Physiotherapy)

©**Yoga**Synergy Pty Limited 1995-2013

ISBN 1-921080-00-0

This edition first printed August 2005

Reprinted with amendments April 2006

Reprinted with amendments November 2007

Reprinted with amendments and additions May 2010

Reprinted with amendments and additions January 2011

Reprinted with amendments October 2013

Important note to readers

Every effort has been made to ensure that the information in this publication is as up to date and accurate as possible. However, the subject matter is complex and readers are advised to seek expert advice when faced with specific problems. This work is intended as a guide to the subject and should not be used as a substitute for professional advice and treatment.

Reviews and Comments on 'Applied Anatomy and Physiology of *Yoga*'

Drawing on their physiotherapy training and in-depth knowledge of western anatomy and physiology, along with their profound understanding of yoga asanas and experience as yoga teachers, authors Simon Borg-Olivier and Bianca Machliss have produced a text that provides an in-depth exploration of the functional anatomy and physiology of yoga. This text presents a wealth of knowledge for yoga practitioners and teachers as well as anyone interested in understanding the impact of yoga on the physical body and is now a prescribed text for the course on 'Applied Anatomy and Physiology of Yoga' within the online Master of Wellness Program at RMIT University.

Professor Marc Cohen, Professor of Complementary Medicine, RMIT University

'Applied Anatomy and Physiology of Yoga' is highly recommended to yoga teachers, physical therapists, occupational therapists and yoga practitioners. As a physical therapist and a long time Iyengar yoga practitioner myself, I searched for a book that would help me analyse yoga postures anatomically, biomechanically and therapeutically. When I was introduced to an earlier version of this book I was amazed at its accuracy and application to therapy; but the improvements made in this current edition make it an even more effective reference book. As a physical therapist I own many other anatomy and physiology books, which I use when researching a topic. When cross-referencing information in 'Applied Anatomy and Physiology of Yoga' I found the accuracy and comprehensiveness to be excellent compared with other yoga anatomy books currently on the market, which include many inaccuracies. The book is also a great reference source for physical therapists and others that have an interest in yoga.

Dalia Zwick PT PhD Physical Therapy Supervisor, The Women's Center, Premier HealthCare, New York, NY

'Applied Anatomy & Physiology of Yoga' is a stunning Achievement and is the finest book I have encountered on the subject. My Jaw-dropped as I perused it last night and I am amazed at the clever correlations you have put together. Simon and Bianca deserve every success and should be very proud of themselves – the work is an magnum opus and awesome in it's completeness and depth.I am particularly impressed by their insights into Mudras, Bandhas, Nadi's and Pranayama. The book is full of pearls never before delineated. A true conjunction of East and West.

Dr Jonn Mumford (Swami Anandakapila Saraswati); Therapist and Multiple Author including 'Ecstasy Through Tantra' and 'A Chakra & Kundalini Workbook: Psycho-Spiritual Techniques for Health, Rejuvenation, Psychic Powers & Spiritual Realization'

The depth of information and knowledge in 'Applied Anatomy and Physiology of Yoga' is breath taking. This book explores the effects of yoga on each part of the body through the use of asanas, bandhas, mudras and kriyas while minimising the risk of injury. This book explores the ability of hatha yoga to develop both strength and flexibility and at the same time to use yoga as a therapy for healing musculoskeletal injuries. If detail and knowledge is your thing, you will not be able to go past this text. Rarely has the use of bandhas integrated with the asanas been so well explained and with such detail and clarity. Highly recommended.

International Yoga Teachers Association Journal: International Light, October – December 2005

'Applied Anatomy and Physiology of Yoga' is an invaluable resource for both teachers and students wanting to take more responsibility for their own practice. In reading the text, it seems obvious that the authors are expert yoga practitioners and teachers, not just proficient in anatomy and physiology. Most injuries in yoga did not occur because a posture or movement was inappropriate for a student, but rather because a teacher did not understand the body well enough to teach the exercise safely. This book provides yoga teachers and students with clear explanations and instructions which they can use in their own teaching and practice. The information comes in a clear well-illustrated and engaging way that does not overcomplicate and succeeds in making anatomy and physiology relevant to the actual practice of yoga.

Liz Bennett BAppSc(Physiotherapy) (University of South Australia), Yoga Teacher and Physiotherapist

'Applied Anatomy and Physiology of Yoga' makes a unique contribution to the yoga community. The anatomy and physiology of the human body is presented in a way that is accessible to all and the application of this to the practice of yoga is clearly defined. For yoga practitioners, the book provides clear explanations of why the positioning in each asana and the use of *bandhas* and *mudras* are important in ensuring a safe and effective practice. It will help yoga teachers to understand the technical aspect of yoga from a western scientific point of view as well as from a yoga physiology point of view, and help them to give clear explanations to their students. For those interested in yoga therapy, this book serves as a valuable resource which demonstrates how, with knowledge of applied anatomy, yoga can be used effectively as a therapy.

Melanie Gallagher BSc(Physiotherapy) (Curtin University, Western Australia), Physiotherapist

This book is a highly valuable resource to anyone interested in learning more about the workings of the body - particularly students of yoga, teachers in training and experienced teachers! The book elucidates the principles of yoga developed over the ages, in a methodical and easy to understand way, by translating them into scientifically-based and relevant concepts for readers in the modern world. The authors sift through the enormous, sometimes esoteric, wealth of Eastern knowledge and bring together the most important ideas for modern yoga practitioners and students of the body. Each chapter logically integrates yogic understanding with anatomical and physiological theory - pinpointing essential information and providing in-depth explanation where appropriate, assisted by the very handy use of applicable photos throughout. Through the filter of their own accomplished understanding and experience, the authors help readers differentiate between the anatomical and physiological effects of postures, and to identify and distinguish between relative differences in subtle movements. Those seeking to inspire and cultivate their yoga practice, or deepen their understanding of the body, should read this book from cover to cover!

Piotr Bozym B.A. LL.B. (Hons), Lawyer, Editor, Yoga Teacher

A must read for all yogi's who wish to understand the science and improve their ability to practise our beautiful art! This book explains how traditional yoga has to be approached with an understanding of the anatomy and physiology of the 'modern' body. Bianca and Simon detail how to safely apply logical principles to physical yoga and conventional exercise. The application of these principles maximises the circulation of energy (prana) and information (citta) within our bodies to establish yoga (union) with improved health and longevity while protecting the body and avoiding injuries. This is a big 'textbook', but it is delivered in an easy to read format which is well worth getting by everyone who is interested in practicing effective yoga in a safe environment.

Emily Odillo Maher, Yoga Teacher

In an industry overrun with books that are not worth the paper they are written on, Yoga Synergy's Applied Anatomy and Physiology of Yoga is the 'real deal'. It distils a huge amount of complex information into easily digestible chapters. For those daunted by the mountain of dry, textbook theory surrounding this subject, this book is a breath of fresh air. It is the perfect balance between theory and practice, to ensure complex concepts are transferred to the student in a way that is easy to understand and apply. I learned things on a very practical level which I could apply to my clients straight away, rather than just leaving with my brain full of jumbled facts.

John Fell, C.H.E.K Practitioner

If you choose to pursue more serious study and practice of both *hatha* yoga and meditation, you might find it helpful to include a standard reference manual in your quest. For anyone seeking an authoritative and comprehensive correlation of hatha yoga with both anatomy and physiology, the manual, 'Applied Anatomy & Physiology of Yoga' satisfies. It has detailed analysis of postures, breathing, and other practices. This complete guide, which includes many photos and illustrations, a full glossary and anatomical index, is both an easy read and a source of reliable information, and one you will not want to be without!

Rev Donna Ferri, Spiritual Counsellor and Healer, Meditation Teacher

'Applied Anatomy and Physiology of *Yoga'* provides the missing link between east and west. You can't learn *yoga* without doing it, and you can't do *yoga* without learning it. If you are going to put your body on the line to explore *yoga*, then you had better learn how to protect it if you are going to survive the journey. This book teaches the *yogi's* 'suit-of-armour', the nine *bandhas* or body locks that take the danger out of *yoga*. Once you are so aligned it is safe and effective to apply seven powerful pumps described in the book for moving energy around your body. Then hang on for the ride of your life!

Jon Gould, Yoga teacher and Director, Yoga Alchemy

'Applied Anatomy and Physiology of Yoga' is an invaluable book for anyone wishing to deepen their knowledge and understanding of the body. Simon and Bianca are clear in their teaching, and present the content in an easy to understand manner. The science of yoga is presented in a way which can be applied by everyone very practically both in their own practice and in the teaching of others. It has made a huge difference in my own personal practice giving me a greater strength and flexibility and a deeper awareness of my body both internally and externally.

Steven Harris, Yoga Teacher

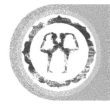
Contents

List of main figures
(Only the main figures are listed here. Many other diagrams and photographs have been woven into the text and have no numbers)

List of main tables

List of applications of anatomy and physiology theory to *yoga*

Foreword

Applied Anatomy & Physiology of *Yoga* is intended to be used by *yoga* teachers, *yoga* practitioners and others who use stretching, strengthening, breathing and other *yoga*-like exercises as part of their health regime.

This book was designed as the main text for our course **YogaSynergy Applied Anatomy & Physiology of *Hatha Yoga*: Course for Teachers & Students**. Our full course is run annually in Sydney from May to August. Shorter forms of the course are run throughout the year in other cities and overseas on the invitation of other yoga schools. There is also now an online version of the course for those who cannot get to a live course (http://anatomy.yogasynergy.com). While attendance at the course is encouraged for those who can do it, this book stands alone as a valuable reference tool. Many additional articles on the **Applied Anatomy and Physiology of *Yoga*** and related topics are also available from our internet blog site (http://blog.yogasynergy.com).

This book and its related course include a study of the basic anatomy and physiology required to understand *yoga*, but the main emphasis is on the practical or applied aspects of anatomy and physiology theory. The main purpose of this book is to use an understanding of basic anatomy and physiology to:

- enhance one's yoga practice
- improve one's ability to increase strength, flexibility, cardiovascular fitness and inner wellbeing
- minimise the risk of injuries as a result of *yoga* practice
- help to use *hatha yoga* to recover from a variety of musculoskeletal injuries and medical conditions.

Applied Anatomy & Physiology of *Yoga* has three main components spread throughout the book. The first component is theoretical (non-applied) anatomy and physiology. This information is mainly presented in the first half of each chapter. Those who have already studied basic anatomy and physiology may not need to read these sections fully or may wish to use these sections of the book as a reference only. Although this theoretical information is important and will be new for some readers, it will be revision for other readers, and has therfore been presented in a slightly smaller font to delineate it from the applied information. Some of the tables and diagrams have been compiled from a variety of difficult-to-access material and are therefore useful references.

For those wishing to gain further understanding of basic anatomy or physiology, we recommend *The Anatomy Colouring Book* (3rd Ed. by Kapit, W. and Elson, L.M. (2001) New York: Addison Wesley) (ACB) and *Bodyworks* (by Francine St George. (1999) Sydney: ABC Books).

The second component of this book is the practical application of the anatomy and physiology theory to the practice of *yoga* or, more specifically, *hatha yoga* (physical *yoga*). This subject is mainly discussed in the introductions and in the second half of each of the chapters of this book. In these applied sections the various aspects of *hatha yoga* are demonstrated and discussed in relation to the theoretical component. The aspects of *hatha yoga* examined include *asanas* (static postures) and *vinyasas* (dynamic exercises), *pranayama* (breath-control) and *dhyana* (meditation). Much emphasis is also placed on the role of *bandhas* [Section 1.7.3], which are discussed on a physical level as the co-activation or simultaneous tensing of opposing muscles around joint complexes [Section 1.5.3]; and *mudras* [Section 1.7.2], which are muscle control exercises or gestures that effect the flow of energy within the body and can tension (stretch) nerves and acupuncture meridians. Throughout the book there are also special shaded boxes entitled APPLICATION TO YOGA, which come directly after the basic statements on anatomy and physiology and help to make these statements relevant to the *yoga* practitioner. Intelligent use of anatomy and physiology theory can enhance all aspects of *hatha yoga* as well as other exercise forms. Readers are invited to attempt the various postures and exercises using this information but all caution must be taken. **Please note that all care must be taken if attempting any of the exercises discussed in this book, as not every exercise will be safe for everyone in its full form. In addition, it is sometimes useful while learning theory and exercise together to carefully attempt a less safe or less correct version of a pose to see its effects in a controlled situation. People should not make such attempts if they have specific problems in related parts of the body.**

The third component is concerned with safety in *yoga* classes and practice. This involves learning how to appropriately adapt the *yoga* to suit individual students. By knowing the anatomical and physiological limitations that the human body has, one has tools to safely modify *hatha yoga* exercises for individuals with musculoskeletal problems or those with special medical conditions. This also serves as an introduction to the concept of *yoga cikitsa* (*yoga* therapy) [Section 1.8], in which a teacher may use *hatha yoga* to facilitate and perhaps assist in the recovery from an illness or heal a musculoskeletal injury or may, instead, see the wisdom of referring students with difficult problems to other health practitioners. By appreciating the anatomical and physiological potential that the human body has, one can safely take each student to their personal maximum in order to challenge their mind while further improving their levels of strength, flexibility and cardiovascular fitness.

The traditional way to impart the teaching of *hatha yoga* has been for teachers to teach individuals on a one-to-one basis. Today, however, the most common method of teaching yoga is in large group situations. Therefore, an anatomical and physiological understanding of potential benefits or risks of each *yoga* exercise allows one to more safely teach a large class of heterogeneous students. With such an understanding, a good teacher can give one set of instructions to everyone in a large mixed class in such a way that each student is directed along a systematically arranged and anatomically safe pathway to arrive at their own safe yet effective versions of each posture.

In this book we have endeavoured to help readers understand *yogic* applied anatomy and physiology by simplifying the material in several ways. Common everyday words are usually included in brackets adjacent to technical and *Sanskrit* terms. Technical terms are usually underlined to help the reader mentally note that it is a technical term and, if necessary, to check the meaning of the word in the glossary [Appendix E] or index (for clarity, words are not underlined in titles and tables). *Sanskrit words are kept in italics* to help the reader mentally note that it is a *Sanskrit* term and, if necessary, to check the meaning of the word in the glossary [Appendix F] or index. Where possible concepts and terms are cross-referenced to other Sections, Figures or Tables using small font and square brackets, eg *bandhas* [Section 1.7.3]. Abbreviated references to other texts and source material are also noted in the text using small font and square brackets, eg [Iyengar, 1966], with the full references shown where possible in the Reference list [Appendix G].

In this book there are a series of small photos of *yoga* postures and body parts that are not included in the list of Figures but are placed within the text to help clarify the *Sanskrit* names of poses used and their many variations. An asterix (*) next to a pose in this book denotes the pose as being a more complex or difficult version of the pose. Note also the naming of postures is generally along the lines of B.K.S. Iyengar's *Light on Yoga* [Iyengar, 1966], with the exclusion of the numbering of postures with the same name and the inclusion of descriptive *Sanskrit* terms, eg *virabhadrasana II* in *Light on Yoga* is written here as *parsva virabhadrasana*.

This book describes some practical applications of anatomy and physiology theory to hatha yoga that are unique to the YogaSynergy style. This is the case especially in relation to bandhas and mudras. Bandhas [Section 1.7.3], which are often thought of as internal locks, are described in this book as co-activations (simultaneous tensing) of antagonistic (opposing) muscle groups around the nine main joint complexes. In this book we have described nine bandhas in their locked (ha-bandha) forms and their unlocked (tha-bandha) forms. Most texts only refer to the three central bandhas: mula uddiyana and jalandhara. B.K.S. Iyengar [1966] describes these as 'the three main bandhas', thus implying the existence of other bandhas without actually naming them. Our understanding of how to generate the six peripheral bandhas is based on the teaching and inspiration of B.K.S. Iyengar. Mudras [Section 1.7.3] are usually described in this book as the tensioning (stretching) of nerves and acupuncture meridians and their associated nadis (subtle channels). Much of the information in this book regarding the bandhas and mudras is previously unpublished and is derived from the personal research of the authors. If intelligently applied this information can be a useful addition that can enhance the safety and effectiveness of all forms of hatha yoga.

Yoga is an ancient science and art that is continually evolving as we are, but it is also probable that much information has been lost in time. With the current interest in yoga, this lost information is being slowly rediscovered. Hence, we consider this book to be a work in progress. Should you wish to provide any feedback or point out mistakes that may not yet have been picked up, please email us at yoga@yogasynergy.com.

Acknowledgements

We would like to acknowledge the following people as being instrumental to our learning of Yoga, Anatomy and Physiology. Firstly, we would like to thank all of the great yoga teachers we have had. In particular we would like to thank Sri B.K.S. Iyengar, Sri K. Pattabhi Jois, and Sri T.V.K. Desikachar for their teaching and for their immense contribution to the knowledge and understanding of yoga. We especially thank our main yoga teachers Natanaga Zhander (Shandor Remete), Professor Bhim Dev and Master Zen Hua Yang for the inspiration and insight into yoga that they have so generously shared with us. We are also grateful to the Schools of Biology and Physiotherapy at the University of Sydney. In particular, we would like to thank Dr Keith Brown, Professor Roberta Shepherd, Professor Janet Carr, Karen Ginn and Rob Herbert. Special thanks to physiotherapist Francine St George for her invaluable teachings, and physiotherapists Natasha Rai and Joelene Murdoch for their help with information and real time ultrasound of trunk and spinal muscles.

Thanks are also due to Alejandro Rolandi who has helped us with many of the diagrams and figures and also with many photo sessions over the last few years. Alejandro took most of the photos included with our photographs in this book. It is fair to note that the photos in these notes that are out of focus are not those taken by Alejandro!

Special thanks also go to Rachel Buchan and Vitoria Borg-Olivier, both experienced yoga practitioners, who allowed themselves to be photographed in the 39th week of their pregnancies and who – one week later – gave birth to beautiful baby girls, Natasha and Amaliah.

Special thanks to Mark Lee and Low Jun Kit and Usha Nair for their work in reformatting and publishing this book. Thank you to Anne Lawson who gave invaluable help and advice on typesetting and formatting. Thanks to Verity Gill for her cover design. Thanks to Ric Allport and Suzi Borg-Olivier for their expertise in computing and other areas. Thanks to the following people who generously gave their time to read various chapters and make corrections and suggestions: Alex Armstrong, Anne Lawson, Birgit Venetz, Dalia Zwick, Jamie Mackenzie, Jon Gould, Liz Bennett, Ngaio Richards, Prudence Murphy, Rosemarie Stabback, Ruth Dentice, Sam Bettison and Steven Hinchliffe. Also thanks to the following students of YogaSynergy who read various chapters and pointed out spelling mistakes and other inaccuracies: Amber Shuhyta, Anita Ullmann, Annie Tennant, Barbara Page, Bernard Harris, Carolyn Bowra, Chris Muir, Clayton Janes, Daniella Solomon, Deborah Hennessey, Deborah Vaughan, Elizabeth Pulie, Florence Kolb, Francesco Santangelo, Genevieve Moran, Helen Mamas, Jacasta Berry, Jo Blackman, John Hazlewood, Julie Hare, Julie Wilcox, Karen Horne, Ken Latta, Kristen Clarke, Madeleine Marty, Mallory Grill, Mark Robberds, Maree Thomas, Martyn Wilson, Nadine Campbell, Nick Bowd, Nicky Baruch, Oliver Granger, Paul Doney, Paula Shaw, Penny Gill, Peter Chwal, Rachel Ward, Rebecca Shaw, Robert Callan, Ruby Grennan, Sally Tsoutas, Sam Burshtein, Sarah Downs, Sean Mullin, Sevadevi Glover, Sonia Groen, Sonja Faulkner, Stacy Wright, Steve Bohill, Vallie Mullins, Vanessa Rigley, Verity Gill, Xanthe Heubel and Zoe Braithwaite. Thanks also to all the people who generously gave their time to read various chapters and make corrections and suggestions in particular Jon Gould, Daniella Solomon and Mark Robberds. Thanks to Danielle Ryan, Laura Bruce and Yasmin Schubach for proof reading and entering corrections into the manuscript. Special thanks to Anne-Louise Dadak, Leo Bonne and Verity Gill for compiling this updated 2011 edition of the book.

Many thanks go to Vitoria, Amaliah and Eric Borg-Olivier, and Juliano Pereira de Sa and Lorenzo Machliss de Sa who were very supportive throughout the writing of this book. Also special thanks to our parents Marie Borg-Olivier, George Borg-Olivier, Margot Machliss and Bernard Machliss for their ongoing support, inspiration and encouragement.

Simon Borg-Olivier & Bianca Machliss, 1 January 2011.

Figure 1.1 Skeletal system: bones and joints in anatomical position

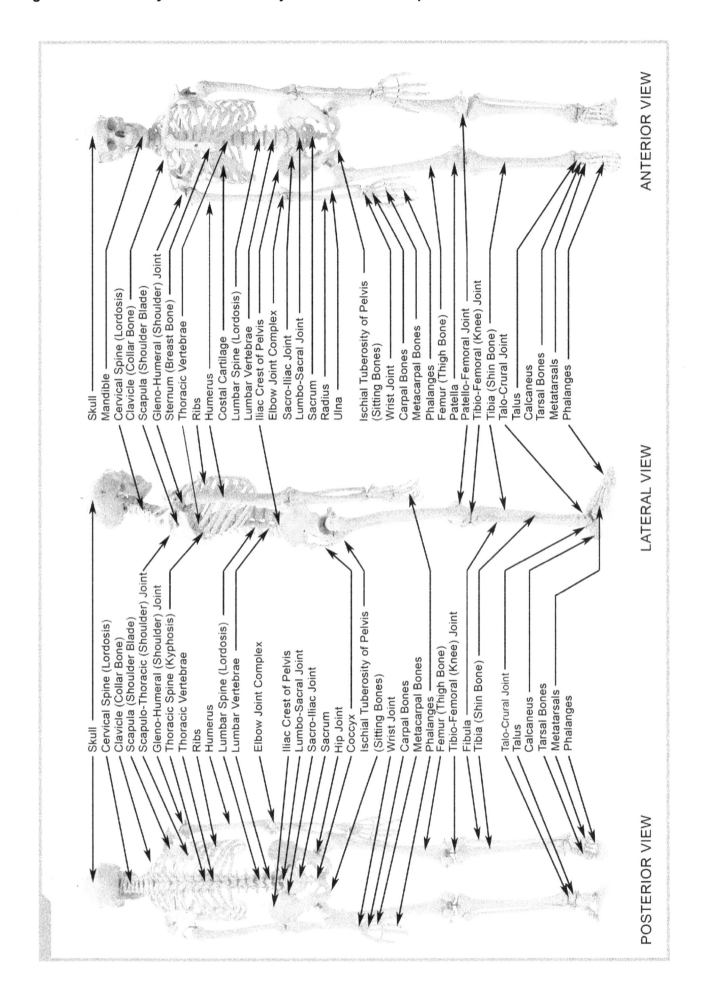

Figure 1.2 Main muscles of the body as seen in anatomical position

Drawings adapted from 'BodyWorks' courtesy Francine St George

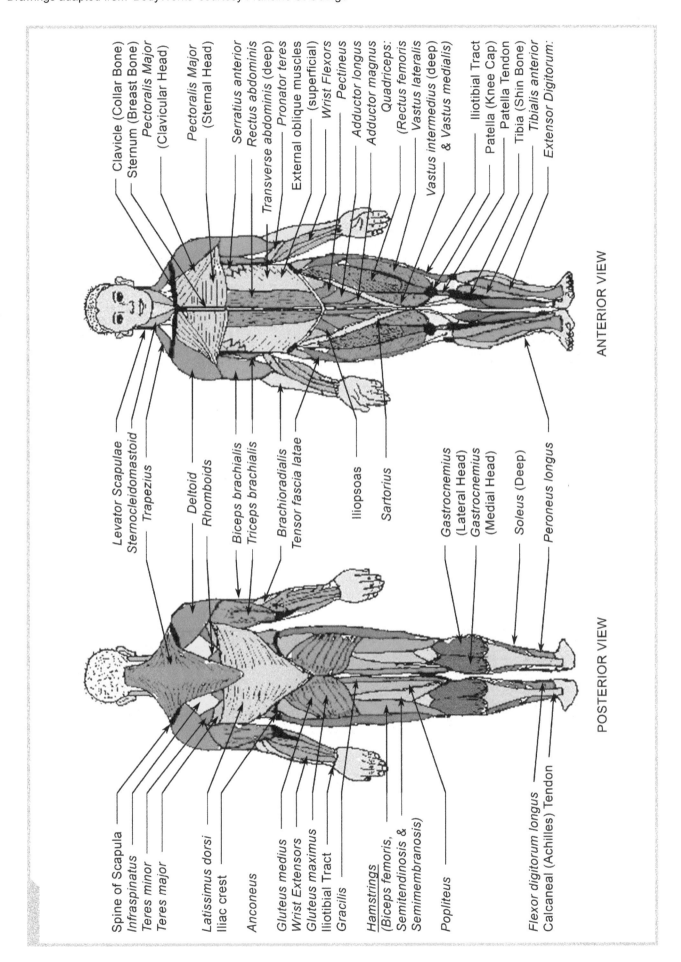

ANTERIOR VIEW

Clavicle (Collar Bone)
Sternum (Breast Bone)
Pectoralis Major (Clavicular Head)
Pectoralis Major (Sternal Head)
Serratius anterior
Rectus abdominis
Transverse abdominis (deep)
Pronator teres
External oblique muscles (superficial)
Wrist Flexors
Pectineus
Adductor longus
Adductor magnus
Quadriceps:
(Rectus femoris
Vastus lateralis
Vastus intermedius (deep)
& Vastus medialis)
Iliotibial Tract
Patella (Knee Cap)
Patella Tendon
Tibia (Shin Bone)
Tibialis anterior
Extensor Digitorum:

Levator Scapulae
Sternocleidomastoid
Trapezius
Deltoid
Rhomboids
Biceps brachialis
Triceps brachialis
Brachioradialis
Tensor fascia latae
Iliopsoas
Sartorius
Gastrocnemius (Lateral Head)
Gastrocnemius (Medial Head)
Soleus (Deep)
Peroneus longus

POSTERIOR VIEW

Spine of Scapula
Infraspinatus
Teres minor
Teres major
Latissimus dorsi
Iliac crest
Anconeus
Gluteus medius
Wrist Extensors
Gluteus maximus
Iliotibial Tract
Gracilis
Hamstrings
(Biceps femoris,
Semitendinosis &
Semimembranosis)
Popliteus
Flexor digitorum longus
Calcaneal (Achilles) Tendon

15

Figure 1.3 Surface anatomy: main muscles of the body & surface markings

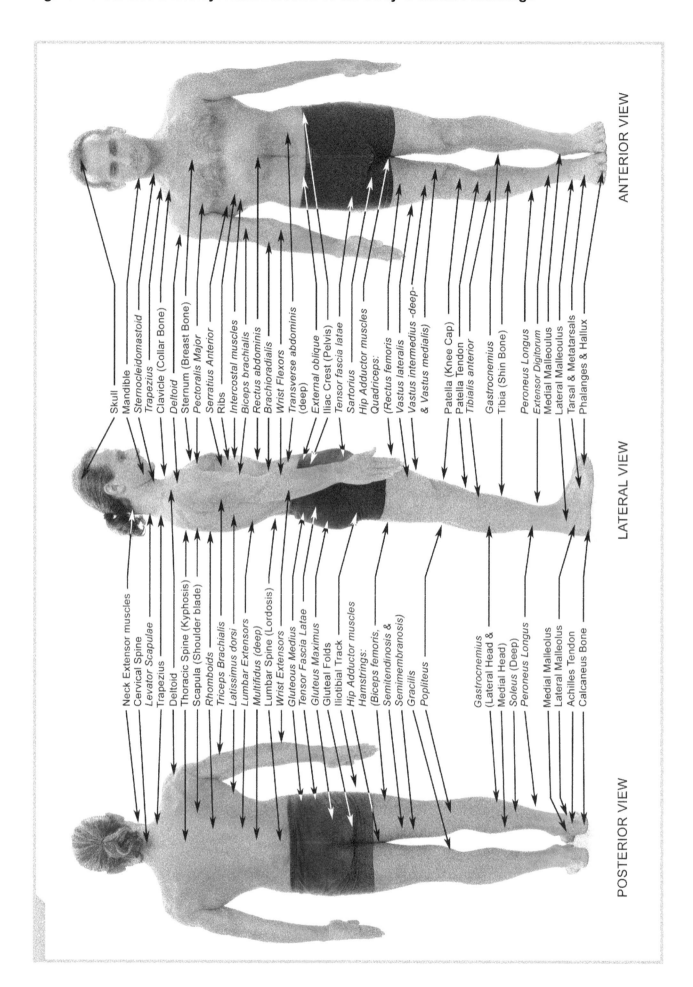

ANTERIOR VIEW

LATERAL VIEW

POSTERIOR VIEW

Skull
Mandible
Sternocleidomastoid
Trapezius
Clavicle (Collar Bone)
Deltoid
Sternum (Breast Bone)
Pectoralis Major
Serratus Anterior
Ribs
Intercostal muscles
Biceps brachialis
Rectus abdominis
Brachioradialis
Wrist Flexors
Transverse abdominis (deep)
External oblique
Iliac Crest (Pelvis)
Tensor fascia latae
Sartorius
Hip Adductor muscles
Quadriceps:
(Rectus femoris
Vastus lateralis
Vastus intermedius -deep-
& Vastus medialis)
Patella (Knee Cap)
Patella Tendon
Tibialis anterior
Gastrocnemius
Tibia (Shin Bone)
Peroneus Longus
Extensor Digitorum
Medial Malleoulus
Lateral Malleolus
Tarsal & Metatarsals
Phalanges & Hallux

Neck Extensor muscles
Cervical Spine
Levator Scapulae
Trapezius
Deltoid
Thoracic Spine (Kyphosis)
Scapula (Shoulder blade)
Rhomboids
Triceps Brachialis
Latissimus dorsi
Lumbar Extensors
Multifidus (deep)
Lumbar Spine (Lordosis)
Wrist Extensors
Gluteous Medius
Tensor Fascia Latae
Gluteus Maximus
Gluteal Folds
Iliotibial Track
Hip Adductor muscles
Hamstrings:
(Biceps femoris,
Semitendinosis &
Semimembranosis)
Gracilis
Popliteus

Gastrocnemius
(Lateral Head &
Medial Head)
Soleus (Deep)
Peroneus Longus
Medial Malleolus
Lateral Malleolus
Achilles Tendon
Calcaneus Bone

Figure 1.4 Surface anatomy: main muscle groups of the body

(The approximate region of each muscle group is indicated. See Figures 1.2 and 1.3 for individual muscles.
Abbreviations: ST = Scapulothoracic Joint; GH = Glenohumeral Joint)

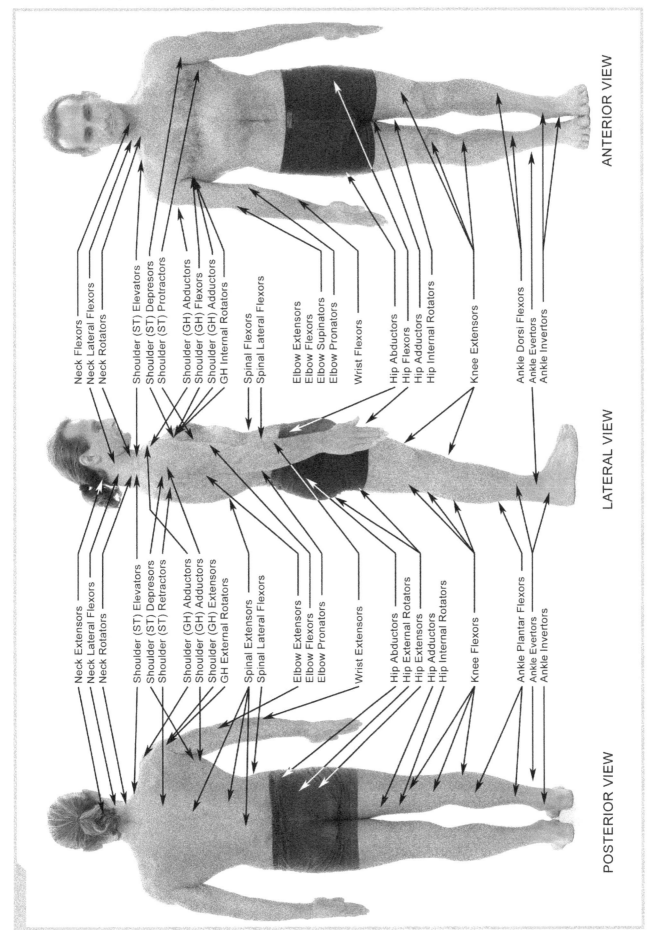

ANTERIOR VIEW

LATERAL VIEW

POSTERIOR VIEW

Chapter Breakdown

****

The word *yoga* means union, joining, or to link together as one whole. *Yoga* is the art and science of resolving the inherent opposition in all things to create a union of body, mind and soul. Meditation is an integral component and the essence of *yoga*.

Yoga is literally a holistic system. Iyengar [2001] describes *yoga* as **"...the path, which integrates the body, senses, mind and the intelligence with the self"**. Feuerstein [1996] describes the *yoga* approach as simplifying one's consciousness and energy to the point where we no longer experience any inner conflict and are able to live in harmony with the world. In India, *yoga* is traditionally thought of as a means to understanding the relationship between one's individual self (*jivatma*) and the universal self (*Paramatman*). In the dualist *Samkhya* philosophy, on which classical *yoga* was originally based, *yoga* is the result of joining *jivatma* with *Paramatman*. In the non-dualist *Vedanta* and *Tantric* philosophies, which modern *yoga* has absorbed, *yoga* is the process of realising that the *jivatma* and the *Paramatman* are in fact the one same entity.

The paths to achieve *yoga*, or to realise *yoga,* are many. Hence, there are many types of *yoga* and each type of *yoga* has many styles. Essentially all the activities of *yoga* can be divided into two parts that can be referred to as physical *yoga* and non-physical *yoga*. Physical *yoga*, which consists of physical exercises (*Asana*) and breath-control (*Pranayama*), is often thought of as a static or slow-moving type of stretching and relaxation. However, it can also include strenuous exercises that tone muscles, tension (stretch) nerves and stimulate the cardiovascular system [Raju et al., 1994]. Physical *yoga* can be very fast and may include repetitive exercises that resemble Western style callisthenics and gymnastics. Physical *yoga* can manipulate internal organs [Kuvalayananda, 1925] and modify blood chemistry [Miyamura et al., 2002]. Non-physical *yoga*, which consists of ethical disciplines and meditative practices, can help to expand one's mind, explore one's emotions, and develop the relationships between oneself and the rest of the world.

Classifying the systems of *yoga* is problematic as there is considerable overlap between the various types of *yoga*. Table 1.0 shows the relationship between the traditional eight limbs of *astanga yoga* and the functional divisions of *yoga*. All eight limbs can be applied to most types of *yoga* including *hatha yoga* and *raja yoga*.

Table 1.0 Practical divisions of *yoga* based on the *astanga yoga* system

FUNCTIONAL DIVISIONS OF THE ACTIVITIES OF *YOGA*	EIGHT LIMBS OF ASTANGA YOGA	FUNCTIONAL DIVISIONS OF THE ACTIVITIES OF *YOGA*
Non-physical *yoga*	1. **Yama** (our attitudes towards our environment) 2. **Niyama** (our attitudes towards ourselves)	**Ethical disciplines** (which include the essence of *jnana yoga*, *bhakti yoga* and *karma yoga*)
Physical *yoga*	3. **Asana**	**Physical exercises** (which include *asanas*, *vinyasas*, *bandhas*, *kriyas* and *mudras*)
	4. **Pranayama**	**Breath-control**
Non-physical *yoga*	5. **Pratyahara** (meditative sense-control) 6. **Dharana** (meditative concentration) 7. **Dhyana** (meditative contemplation) 8. **Samadhi** (meditative absorption)	**Meditative practices** (which include techniques of *raja yoga*, *mantra yoga*, *yantra yoga* and *laya yoga*)

1.0.1 The History of *Yoga*

The history of *yoga* and meditation is the subject of much controversy. Conventional belief is that *yoga* originated in India at least 5,000 years ago [Feurestein, 1996; Ghosh, 1999], but traditional Indian belief is that *yoga* itself is far older and was practised all over the world. Artwork depicting images of people or gods in advanced *yoga* postures are dated at 2,700 BCE [Desikachar, 1998]. *Buddhist yoga* arose out of Indian *yoga* in about the fifth century BCE and slowly spread into the rest of Asia. Indian *yoga* came to China around 500 CE and developed into *Taoist yoga*. Modern *yoga* has evolved and blended from two distinct and possibly unrelated sources, *Vedic yoga* and *Tantric yoga*.

1.0.1.1 *Vedic yoga*

Vedic yoga is one of the six interrelated systems of classical Indian philosophical thought that draws on interpretations of reality based on the *Vedas*, which most authors believe are India's most ancient texts. *Vedic yoga*, formalised in the *Patanjali yoga sutra*, is based on the dualist Samkhya school that teaches all things arise from two ultimate realities, spirit (*purusa*) and matter (*prakrti*).

Vedic yoga includes *jnana yoga* (*yoga* of self-knowledge), based on the non-dualist Vedanta school, which says there is only one ultimate reality (*Brahman*) making its appearance to our senses as an illusion (*maya*), and that all things are one, only appearing to be separate.

1.0.1.2 *Tantric yoga*

Tantric yoga is based on an important non-classical school of Indian philosophy called *Tantra*. *Tantric* texts (*Tantras*) are based on ancient texts called *Agamas*, which may pre-date the *Vedas* [Shah, 2001]. *Tantra* is non-dualist like *Vedanta,* but is polarity based. In *Tantra*, everything consists of opposite and attracting forces, such as male and female. *Tantra* is the base for most *yoga* and meditation practised today. *Tantric yoga* embraces all aspects of life. *Tantric yoga* is often misunderstood and misrepresented and thought to deal only with sexual activity and black magic. However, *hatha yoga, Buddhist yoga* and *Taoist yoga* all have significant *Tantric* influences.

1.0.1.3 *Karma yoga, jnana yoga* and *bhakti yoga*

The first main written mention of *yoga* is in the *Bhagavad Gita*, which was written in the fifth century BCE, and which extols the virtues of *yoga* [Desikachar, 1998]. The *Bhagavad Gita* discusses the three great paths (*margas*) of action (*karma marga*), knowledge (*jnana marga*) and devotion (*bhakti marga*) [Iyengar, 1993]. *Karma yoga* is the *yogic* path of action or the *yoga* of work. *Jnana yoga* is the *yogic* path of self-knowledge. *Bhakti yoga* is the *yogic* path of devotion.

1.0.1.4 *Astanga yoga*

The second major extant text on *yoga* is the *Patanjali-yoga-sutra*, which was written in the second century BCE. The *Patanjali-yoga-sutra* explains that the means to achieve *yoga* are by following an eight-limbed (*asta-anga*) path to the ultimate state of meditative absorption (*Samadhi*). Most *yoga* can be classified in the terms of *astanga yoga*.

The eight limbs (*angas*) of *astanga yoga* [Iyengar, 1988; 1993] are:
*   *Yama* (our attitudes towards our environment)
*   *Niyama* (our attitudes towards ourselves)
*   *Asana* (physical exercises)
*   *Pranayama* (breath-control)
*   *Pratyahara* (meditative sense-control)
*   *Dharana* (meditative concentration)
*   *Dhyana* (meditative contemplation)
*   *Samadhi* (meditative absorption).

The first two limbs of *astanga yoga*, *Yama* and *Niyama*, are the *yogic* ethical disciplines; a set of universal truths about one's attitude to oneself and to one's environment. Encompassed in these two limbs is the essence of *karma yoga, jnana yoga* and *bhakti yoga* [Iyengar, 1993].

The second two limbs of *astanga yoga*, *Asana* and *Pranayama*, can be termed physical yoga. In its most basic form, physical yoga is simply sitting in a comfortable posture (*Asana*) and being aware of one's breathing (*Pranayama*).

The last four limbs of *astanga yoga*, *Pratayahara, Dharana, Dhyana* and *Samadhi,* are the meditative practices. These meditative practices are equivalent to the generic term meditation as it is used in Western literature.

The main types of *astanga yoga* are *mantra yoga, hatha yoga, laya yoga* and *raja yoga* [Pranavananda, 1992]. Each of these *yogas* involves the application of ethical disciplines (*Yama* and *Niyama*), physical exercises (*Asana*), breath-control (*Pranayama*), and meditative practices (*Pratayahara, Dharana, Dhyana* and *Samadhi*).

1.0.1.5 *Mantra yoga*

Mantra yoga uses chanting of sounds and phrases (usually in *Sanskrit*) to induce a meditative state. Chanting can be audible or mental, and with or without breath-control. *Mantra yoga* techniques are used in traditional *hatha yoga*, Transcendental Meditation (TM) and many *Buddhist* meditative practices.

1.0.1.6 *Hatha yoga*

Hatha yoga (*yoga* of physical forces) is what most people in the Western world think of as *yoga* as it contains physical exercises (*Asana*), breath-control (*Pranayama*) and meditative practices. *Hatha yoga* was first described in the 2000-year-old text *Yoga yajnavalkya samhita*. Better known texts on *hatha yoga* include *Siva-samhita, Gheranda-samhita* and *hatha pradipika*, which are relatively recent writings of between 400 and 900 years old. The *hatha yoga* texts appear to be copies of earlier works of *Tantric* origin. *Hatha yoga* is in essence a type of *Tantric yoga* with four physical stages, namely *Sat-kriya* (cleansing processes), *Asana* (physical exercises), *Mudra* (energy-control), and *Pranayama* (breath-control); and three non-physical or meditative stages, namely *Pratyahara* (meditative sense-control), *Dhyana* (meditative contemplation or visualisation) and *Samadhi* (meditative absorption). Although *hatha yoga* is typified by a series of exercises that are used to generate and manipulate physical and subtle forces in the body, its main aim is the same as every other form of genuine *yoga*, namely self-realisation. The *Gheranda samhita* states that the sole reason to learn *hatha yoga* is as a path to *raja yoga* [Pranavananda, 1992].

Iyengar [2001], a foremost modern exponent of *hatha yoga*, describes *hatha yoga* as sighting the soul through the restraint of energy. *Hatha yoga* is a physical method that uses an awareness of the breath to link then unify the various aspects of the body and mind, allowing them to behave as one functional unit.

In practice, some, or all, of the elements of *hatha yoga* listed below may be performed concurrently. For example, a *yogin* can do any exercise with an ongoing meditative awareness and concentrated control of the body. Some muscles may be stretching, some tensing, and others relaxing; one part of the body kept static and another part moving; while at the same time there is an ongoing meditative contemplation (*Dhyana*) and meditative absorption (*Samadhi*) on breath-control (*Pranayama*) and meditative sense-control (*Pratyahara*).

1.0.1.7 *Laya yoga*

Laya yoga is a type of *astanga yoga* that involves deep absorptive concentration. *Laya yoga* has assumed an intermediate position between *hatha yoga* and *raja yoga*. The complicated processes of *hatha yoga* posture and breathing, and the advanced and difficult *raja yogic* processes of concentration are simplified in *laya yoga* [Goswami, 1979]. *Laya yoga* also includes the essence of *mantra yoga*. The final stage of *laya yoga* involves an advanced stage of visualisation (*yantra yoga*) that stimulates the flow of energy through the body in a profound way. This final stage is termed *kundalini yoga*.

1.0.1.8 *Raja yoga*

Raja yoga, the royal path to the ultimate meditative state (*Samadhi*), is what most people think of as meditation and is considered the most difficult type of *astanga yoga* [Pranavananda, 1992]. *Raja yoga* is considered the non-physical approach to achieve *yoga*. *Raja yoga* is essentially about controlling the mind and unifying one's intelligence with one's consciousness [Ghosh, 1999]. The main emphasis of *raja yoga* is the <u>meditative practices</u>, which are advanced techniques of <u>meditative sense-control</u> (*Pratayahara*), <u>meditative concentration</u> (*Dharana*), <u>meditative contemplation</u> or visualisation (*Dhyana*), and <u>meditative absorption</u> (*Samadhi*). *Raja yoga* has little emphasis on physical work beyond sitting in a stable posture (*Asana*) with an erect <u>spine</u>. However, the <u>physical exercises</u> (*Asana*) of *hatha yoga* can help prepare one for the challenge of sitting comfortably for a long time in the *raja yoga* <u>meditative state</u>.

1.0.1.9 *Buddhism*

Buddhism arose out of *yoga* in the fifth century BCE and slowly spread across Asia. The Buddha was a dedicated *yogin* (*yoga* practitioner) with a passion for meditative absorption [Feuerstein, 1996]. *Buddhist yoga* includes the use of such techniques as posture (*Asana*) and control of the life force (*Pranayama*). *Buddhist* texts, as in Hindu schools of *yoga,* emphasise erect body posture. However, in constrast to the Hindu schools of *yoga*, *Buddhist yoga* does not advocate breath retentions. Instead practitioners follow the breath with the mind. *Buddhist yoga* often incorporates *mantra yoga*, *yantra yoga* and *mudras* (energy-control gestures) in order to facilitate <u>meditative practices</u>. *Buddhist yoga* was derived from *Vedic yoga* in India, but is now prevalent throughout Asia.

1.0.1.10 *Taoist yoga*

Yoga was introduced to China about 500 CE and developed into *Taoist yoga*. Qi-gong is the main type of *Taoist yoga*. *Taoist yoga* is used by Shaolin monks to tone and flex their bodies, to gather *chi* energy (*chi* in *Taoist yoga* is the equivalent of *prana* in *hatha yoga*), and to prepare for meditation. In *Taoist* training, breath has four levels. Windy-breath is noisy and usually present upon physical exertion. Raspy-breath can be heard by others and is usually due to disturbed emotions or sickness. Qi-breath is so quiet that one cannot even hear one's own breath. Resting-breath is the ultimate Qi-gong state of breathing when one cannot tell whether one is breathing or not [Liu, 1991]. The contemporary Qi-gong master Sat Chuen Hon [2002] writes of breathing in *Taoist yoga* in exactly the same terms that breathing is described in the ancient Indian texts.

> **"It is only when one achieves the level of breathing of total smoothness of resting-breath that one can consider to have really attained the beginning level of Qi-gong practice ...very few practitioners can practice with Qi-breath and only a few great masters have demonstrated the ability to maintain a flowing state of Resting-breath while practising Tai-ji or Qi-gong forms. One experiences Resting-breath more readily when doing seated meditation. Once one has reached the level of deep theta brain-waves or the deep *Samadhi* state, the sound of one's own breathing disappears and one no longer notices whether one is breathing or not."**

1.0.1.11 History of *yoga* as a therapy

In the twenty-first century, *yoga* is used to develop and maintain physical and mental health. The concept of using *yoga* as a therapy for the body and the mind is not new. *Yoga* as a therapy had its first probable mention in the *Yoga yajnavalkya samhita*, which dates to the second century BCE. More recent *hatha yoga* texts such as the *Hatha pradipika* also mention the various therapeutic benefits of *yoga*.

Yoga made its first main impact on the West when **Swami Vivekananda** (1863–1902) spoke on *jnana yoga* at the Parliament of Religions held in Chicago in 1893. In 1920, **Paramahansa Yogananda** (1893–1952), who wrote *Autobiography of a Yogi* [1946], arrived in Boston and established the Self-Realisation Fellowship. In 1924, **Swami Kuvalayananda** (1883–1966), founded the *Kaivalyadhama Yoga* Research Institution in Lonavala India, which contributed greatly to modern scientific studies of *yoga* in India, and which are mostly published in the quarterly journal *Yoga Mimamsa* from 1924.

In the same period, **Swami Sivananda** (1887–1963), an Indian medical doctor, studied, practised, and taught *yoga* in its many forms. Sivananda authored over 200 books including *Kundalini Yoga* [1994] and founded the Divine Life Society, an *ayurvedic* pharmacy, the *Yoga Vedanta* Forest Academy, and an eye hospital.

Another great yogi of this era was **Swami Yogeshwarananda** (1887–1985), who founded the *Yoga Niketan* Trust, and travelled the world extensively. Yogeshwarananda wrote an important book on the deepest states of meditation called *Atma Vijnana* – Science of Soul [1959], and he wrote a definitive early book on *hatha yoga* called *Bahiranga Yoga – First Steps to Higher Yoga* [1970].

Shyam Sundar Goswami (1891–1979) was a pioneer of the scientific exposition of *yoga* in the West. He was a master of *hatha yoga* and his treatise on *laya yoga* [Goswami, 1980] is regarded as the best on this subject.

Probably the finest *hatha yogi* and *Astanga yogi* of the twentieth century was **Sri Tirumalai Krishnamacharya** (1888–1989). As a youth, Krishnamacharya studied for seven years with Sri Ramamohan Brahmachari, who was one of last great Himalayan *yoga* masters. Krishnamacharya travelled extensively throughout India in the 1930s lecturing on *yoga* and demonstrating *yoga-siddhis*, (*yogic* special powers) in order to create a resurgence of the dying *yoga* tradition. These demonstrations included suspending his pulse, stopping cars with his bare hands, performing difficult *asanas*, and lifting heavy objects with his teeth [Ruiz, 2001]. Krishnamacharya was a great scholar with seven PhDs, who used his vast knowledge of the ancient texts to synthesise an excellent system of *yoga* therapy. Krishnamacharya was the teacher of the four most influential *yoga* masters of the modern age, namely Indra Devi, K. Patabhi Jois, B.K.S. Iyengar, and T.V.K. Desikachar.

Indra Devi (1899–2002), author of the first bestseller on *yoga* called *Forever Young, Forever Healthy* [1953], was Krishnamacharya's first western student, and first female student, in 1937. She founded the first modern school of *yoga* in Shanghai China, where she taught Madame Chiang Kai-Shek. In China, she also taught Russian-born Michael Volin, who subsequently took over Devi's school, then came to introduce *yoga* to Australia in the 1950s. Devi convinced Soviet leaders that *yoga* was not a religion and brought her *yoga* to the Kremlin in her native Russia, where it had been illegal. In 1947, she opened a school in Hollywood and became known as the 'First Lady of *Yoga*', and taught actresses like Marilyn Monroe, Greta Garbo, Elizabeth Arden and Gloria Swanson, and also taught Richard Hittleman who presented *yoga* to a large audience in his long-running television show in the United States during the 1970s [Ruiz, 2001].

Sri K. Patabhi Jois (1915–), author of *Yoga Mala* [1953], was instructed by Krishnamacharya from age twelve to teach what is now referred to as *Astanga-vinyasa*. *Astanga-vinyasa-yoga* includes five physically demanding sequences of postures that have become very popular in the west in the past ten years. While these sequences can be effective for some people, they are quite inaccessible for many, and even dangerous for untrained people who have predisposing medical conditions or musculoskeletal problems. This smooth flowing practice emphasises a type of dynamic meditation with focus on breathing in a particular fashion, gazing at particular spots (*dristhis*), while maintaining firmness in the <u>abdomen</u> (*bandha*). The continual flow of this practice develops a tremendous amount of heat that tends to allow an increase in flexibility but does not allow much time to adjust body alignment or consider all issues of safety. While the *Astanga-vinyasa* system can be a therapy for those who are already reasonably healthy, it does not generally allow enough modification of the exercises to allow a broad range of people to take up the practice.

Sri B.K.S. Iyengar (1918–), author of *Light on Yoga* [1966], teaches a very exacting and methodological style of *yoga*, referred to by his students as *Iyengar yoga*, which often modifies postures with the use of props such as chairs, blankets, belts and blocks. Iyengar has researched and experimented with *yoga*-therapy for over 50 years with tens of thousands of students. He has successfully applied *yoga* to a large variety of musculoskeletal injuries and medical conditions. Iyengar has regularly used *yoga* to help people with problems such as knee ligament ruptures, shoulder and hip pain, wrist and ankle sprains, paraesthesia, paralysis, intervertebral disc bulges and other spinal injuries. He has used *yoga* to treat people with conditions such as asthma and bronchitis, constipation and diarrhoea, epilepsy, polio, muscular dystrophy and AIDS [Raman, 1998]. Postures taught in Iyengar-style classes are fundamentally the same as those taught in *Astanga-vinyasa-yoga* classes, but they are usually held for a longer time, and often a rest period is given, during which time various aspects of the posture are intellectually examined and safety issues are discussed. Specific guidance on how to effectively do each posture are given throughout most classes. However, while being a demanding yet relatively safe approach to <u>physical yoga</u>, this style of teaching may be perceived by some yoga practitioners to compromise the meditative flow of the practice, and can cool the body down.

T.V.K. Desikachar (1938–), author of *The Heart of Yoga* [1995], is the son of Krishnamacharya. The teaching of Desikachar, termed *vini yoga*, is more congruent with the evolved way that Krishnamacharya was teaching in the later half of his life. Students are usually taught on an individual basis, with each student being prescribed specific sequences of postures, with specific breath-control (*Pranayama*) for each.

Modern *yoga* has also been influenced by the teaching and writing of several other important teachers. Three prominent students of Sivananda were Swami Vishnu Devananda (1917–1993), who wrote *The Complete Illustrated Book of Yoga* and translated the *Hatha Yoga Pradipika* [1987]; Swami Satyananda (1923–), who wrote *Kundalini Tantra* and *Asana Pranayama Mudra Bandha* [1966]; and Swami Satchidananda (1914–2002), who founded Integral *Yoga*, which has been adapted successfully by Dr Dean Ornish to treat heart patients [Ornish et al., 1990].

Many of the world's alternative therapies and physical therapies are *yoga*-based. Techniques resembling *yoga* and often derived from *yoga* are often used for therapy in the world today. Many people who teach and practise these techniques may not realise they are *yoga*-based. Physical and psychological therapists often use relaxation and meditation techniques derived from *yoga*. Many of the exercises that are taught as exercise based physiotherapy are derived from *yoga*. Pilates is a *yoga*-based form of physical training that is especially popular as a therapy in the dance community. Pilates instructors and exercise-based physiotherapists even teach some concepts that are directly from the heart of traditional *yoga*. One example is the concept of core stabilisation, which is described in *yoga* texts as *bandha*, but which is often neglected or not known by many modern *yoga* teachers.

1.0.2 The Scientific Validity of *Yoga*

A MEDLINE literature search on *yoga* reveals that there are 726 scientific articles relating to *yoga* written from 1965 to March 2005. These articles claim the benefits of *yoga* range from improvements in strength [Madanmohan et al., 1992], flexibility [Ray et al., 2001], aerobic ability [Balasubramanian & Pansare, 1991], to improvements in muscle tone, rheumatoid arthritis, lung function, concentration, poor eyesight, obesity, indigestion, back pain, hypertension, various respiratory diseases, sinusitis, arthritis, diabetes (I and II), as well as anxiety, nervousness, attention deficit and memory loss. Many of these articles make interesting reading and may be perfectly correct in their claims regarding *yoga*, but very few present valid scientific proof of the benefits of *yoga*. Only 54 articles were based on randomised, controlled trials on *yoga,* and some of these report that either *yoga* has no effect [eg Kroner-Herwig et al., 1995] or that the effect is not significant [Shaffer et al., 1997].

Similarly, a MEDLINE search on meditation reveals that there are 1031 scientific articles regarding meditation written from 1965 to March 2005. Of these, only 63 were based on randomised, controlled trials.

Randomised, controlled trials of *yoga* have shown that *yoga* is effective in increasing joint flexibility [Ray et al., 2001], management of coronary artery disease [Manchanda et al., 1980], increasing regression of coronary atherosclerosis [Manchanda et al., 2000], coping with exam stress [Malathi & Damodaran, 1999] management of hypertension [Patel & North, 1975], management of stress in epilepsy [Panjwani et al., 1995], relief in hand osteoarthritis [Garfinkel et al., 1994], the ability to perform complex tasks [Manjunath & Telles, 2001], long-term management of bronchial asthma [Nagarathna & Nagendra, 1985], and reduction of medication in asthma [Singh et al., 1990]. A randomised controlled trial of specialised breath-control (unilateral nostril breathing) was found to increase spatial memory [Naveen et al., 1997].
While there is not much valid scientific research published on *yoga*, there are many well researched papers on the scientific elements of yoga. The main scientific components or the elements of yoga are:

* Stretching
* Isometric strengthening
* Isotonic strengthening
* Isokinetic strengthening
* Joint range of movement exercises
* One-legged exercises
* Cardiovascular (aerobic) conditioning
* Breathing
* Unilateral nostril breathing
* Sense control

- Concentration
- Relaxation
- Visualisation
- Meditation.

MEDLINE searches on the topics such as those following can reveal many research articles or papers, which provide tangible evidence regarding the benefits of *yoga*: <u>isometric exercise</u> [eg Monteiro Pedro *et al.*, 1999], breathing exercise [eg Yan & Sun, 1996], stretching [eg Herbert & Gabriel, 2002], relaxation [eg Weber, 1996], posture [eg Cholewicki et al., 1997], one-legged exercises [eg Kannus et al., 1992], <u>antagonistic muscle co-activation</u> [eg Glasscock et al., 1999], aerobic conditioning, unilateral forced nostril breathing [Naveen et al., 1997], Valsalva [Bazak , 1990] and Mueller manoeuvres [Gioia et al., 1995], visualisation [Kominars et al., 1997], and mental imagery [eg Hudetz et al., 2000].

However, to justify the validity of *yoga* with such a reductionist approach goes against the very nature of *yoga* as a time-honoured holistic science. The best evidence available in support of *yoga* comes from the millions of people around the world who have practised *hatha yoga* throughout the ages, and who continue to practice because of the positive benefits that can be obtained.

1.0.3 Why Study the Anatomy and Physiology of *Yoga*?

Hatha yoga may be learnt by practising *yoga* postures and exercises until they are perfected, without having any knowledge of anatomy and physiology. However, in some cases, incorrect practice or unsafe technique can aggravate a practitioner's pre-existing medical problems or it can actually create new problems. A practitioner who learns *yoga* without an understanding of anatomy and physiology may become very adept at understanding their own body, but may not be able to relate to the individual differences in other peoples bodies.

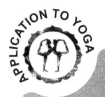

No 1.1 Apply the principles of anatomy and physiology to improve your *yoga*, your health and your ability to communicate with or teach others

A sound understanding of human anatomy and physiology and how it is applied to the *hatha yoga* postures and exercises can help to:
- Improve levels of cardiovascular fitness, strength and flexibility
- Minimise the risk of exercise-related (or *yoga*-related) injuries
- Improve ability to recover after injury or a medical condition
- Deepen understanding of other people's bodies and help improve their bodies with a safe and effective teaching style
- Liaise and communicate with other medical practitioners.

The *hatha yoga* described in this book is based on the style developed and taught at the Sydney-based school, *YogaSynergy*. The teaching at *YogaSynergy* represents a synthesis between traditional *hatha yoga* as passed down from Sri T. Krishnamacharya and his main teachers and exercise-based physiotherapy. Although aspects of *Synergy-style yoga* are rarely used in other yoga styles, it is not our aim to develop a new style of *yoga*. We see *Synergy-style yoga* as traditional *hatha yoga* adapted for the Western body by the systematic applications of the principles of anatomy and physiology.

The three most important, and relatively novel, aspects of the *Synergy-style yoga* and the contents of this book, which have all been developed through a thorough examination of both traditional *hatha yoga* teaching and scientific research, are:
- A gradual build-up for each *asana* (static posture) or *vinyasa* (dynamic exercise), from the simplest or easiest first stage version of a posture to the most complex or hardest version of a posture. Each stage incorporates various amounts and intensities of the main elements of each pose, but always with an inherent balance between strength and flexibility.

- The incorporation of the nine main *bandhas* of *bandha-hatha yoga* [Section 1.7.3, Appendix C] as a means for generating and moving energy through the body as well as stabilising each of the nine major joint complexes [Section 1.5.3].
- The emphasis on *mudras* and *nadi-hatha yoga* [Section1.7.2] as a means of taking full advantage of nerve reflexes [Section 1.7.2.2.1], fascial connections between tissues [Section 1.3.2.1.3], as well as tensioning (stretching) nerves [Section 1.7.2.1], *nadis* (subtle channels) [Section 1.7.2] and acupuncture meridians [Figures 9.1 – 9.7].

1.0.4 A Working Model for Why and How *Hatha Yoga* Actually Works

Beneficial side effects of practising *hatha yoga* may include increases in strength, flexibility and the ability to relax [Section 1.0.2]. However, one of the main physiological purposes of *hatha yoga* is to improve the circulation of information, energy and matter throughout the body. Stimulation of body circulation is one of the main ways *hatha yoga* actually works [Section 8.4].

Hatha yoga stimulates circulation by creating regions of differential pressure throughout the body. Energy and matter always tend to move from regions of high pressure to regions of low pressure [Resnick & Halliday, 1977]. The word **Hatha** is Sanskrit for force [Kapp, 2001], and can also represent pressure. Pressure is defined as 'force per unit area' [Resnick & Halliday, 1977]. According to Woodroffe [1922], Iyengar [1966] and Devananda [1987], the sounds **Ha** and **Tha** are Sanskrit for sun and moon respectively. The sound **Ha** represents or implies heat, which is created by high pressure. The sound **Tha** represents or implies coolness or cold, which is created by low pressure [Borg-Olivier & Machliss, 1997] [Figure 1.5].

Therefore, **hatha yoga**, which means literally **a force union or forced union**, works by setting up regions of relative high pressure and low pressure (forces) throughout the body, which help stimulate the circulation or flow of information, energy and matter, in a manner similar to the way that the heart works [Section 8.1.3.2]. As soon as a relative difference in pressure comes into existence within the body, there is a physiological tendency for **energy** (eg heat)**, matter** (eg blood and intracellular fluid), and **information** in the form of neurotransmitters, hormones, immunotransmitters and other more subtle agents, to **move from the region of higher pressure towards the region of lower pressure** [Borg-Olivier & Machliss, 1997] [Figure 1.5].

When the pressure in one part of the body is increased, this pushes energy and matter away from that region in a manner similar to squeezing the water out of a sponge. In other parts of the body the pressure is reduced and this pulls energy and matter towards that region, in a manner similar to putting a squashed sponge in water and letting it expand or stretch, drawing water into it.

Hatha yoga sets up differential pressures (relatively high and low pressures) within the body in six main ways using:
- Muscle activation (increasing local pressure) and muscle relaxation (decreasing local pressure) in certain *asanas* (static postures) and *vinyasas* (dynamic exercises and linking movements between *asanas*), which engage the musculoskeletal pump [Section 8.1.2.3.1]
- Specific *pranayamas* (breath-control exercises) which change the pressures in the thorax and abdomen, as well as the normal actions of the respiratory pump [Section 8.1.2.3.2], where a reduction in abdominal and thoracic pressure causes inhalation while an increase in pressure causes exhalation
- The effects of the force of gravity [Section 12.7.1.3.3.2], especially noticeable in the inverted and semi-inverted postures the *yoga* system offers
- The effects of the *asanas* (static postures), which physically compress some parts of the body (ie increasing local pressure), while stretching other parts of the body (ie decreasing local pressure)
- The effects of the *bandhas* [Section 1.7.3], which usually involve co-activation of opposing muscles across joints and can either increase (*ha-bandhas*) or decrease (*tha-bandhas*) local pressure [Section 1.7.3.4 & Appendix C]
- The effects of movement of the body and movement of the body parts to initiate centripetal, centrifugal and inertial forces around the body that can affect circulation. This is especially noticeable when the movements are fast and sharp in turning.

Figure 1.5: The Mechanism of *Hatha Yoga* [Borg-Olivier & Machliss, 1997]

> ## *HATHA* = force   *YOGA* = union
> ## PRESSURE = Force / Area
> ## (i.e. pressure is force per unit of area)
> ## *HA* = Sun => Heat => *High Pressure*
> ## *THA* = Moon => Cool => *Low Pressure*
> ## *HATHA* = Force => Forces of high & low pressure
> ## *HATHA-YOGA* => A union (*YOGA*) in the body resulting from movement (circulation) of energy from regions of
> ## *High Pressure* (= *HA* force) to *Low Pressure* (= *THA* force)

The circulation of body substances, through blood vessels and intracellular spaces, between two different body parts, increases proportionally as the relative **difference** in pressure between the two body parts increases. Therefore, to achieve maximum stimulation of circulation with a minimum of effort, it is important that one part of the body is kept at a very low pressure. This is one reason why the face and neck are usually kept completely relaxed (ie at a low pressure) while doing *yoga*. If this is not ensured, then blood pressure [Section 8.4.2] and stress levels can increase significantly.

The movement of energy, matter and information in the body is promoted and pumped through the body by six (6) pumps other than the heart, which is the cardiovascular pump [Section 8.1.3.2]. These other pumps are referred to as the musculoskeletal pump [Section 8.1.2.3.1], the respiratory pump [Section 8.1.2.3.2], the gravitational pump, the postural pump, the muscle co-activation pump [Section 1.7.3] and the centripetal pump [Section 12.7.2.2.1].

Yoga utilises the musculoskeletal pump of circulation [Orsted et al., 2001] during *vinyasa* when one changes from one posture to the next. As muscles tense, they increase local pressure in the veins and push blood and intracellular fluid in the direction of the heart. One-way back-flow valves in the veins prevent movement of blood away from the heart in the veins. When a muscle relaxes, it decreases local venous pressure and pulls blood from regions more distal to the heart to that region.

Yoga utilises the respiratory pump of circulation [Hillman & Finucane, 1987] with *Pranayama*. Breath-control can affect the pre-load of the blood into the heart, which can alter heart rate depending on whether the inhalation is directed to the thorax, which increases heart rate, or the abdominal region, which decreases heart rate.

Yoga utilises a gravitational pump of circulation using *viparita-karani* [Section 12.7.1.3.3.2]. *Viparita karani* represents all the inverted or semi-inverted postures. Simple postures such as lying supine and resting the

legs vertically up a wall 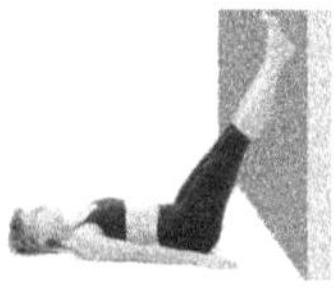 and more advanced poses like *sirsasana* 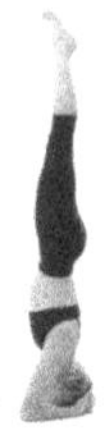 (head stand), reverse the natural flow of gravity and can offer the same benefits as the technique referred to as postural drainage used in physiotherapy [Fink, 2002].

Yoga utilises a postural pump of circulation using *asanas*. *Asanas* are generally thought of as static

postures. Relative to normal postures, such as anatomical position (*savasana* 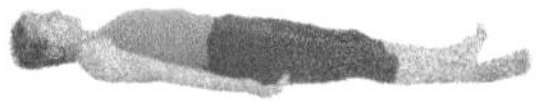), *asanas* can physically compress (increase the pressure) at one region of the body while expanding or stretching (decreasing the pressure) in another region of the body.

Yoga utilises a muscle co-activation pump of circulation using *bandhas*. A *bandha* involves co-activation to create regions of high pressure (*ha bandhas*) or regions of low pressure (*tha bandhas*). Energy, in the form of blood and heat (among other things), will try to move from the regions of high pressure to the regions of low pressure. Intelligent control of the formation of these *bandhas* during a *yoga* practice can regulate the circulation in any part of the body.

Yoga utilises a centripetal pump (or inertial pump) of circulation during *vinyasa*. While the body, or parts of the body, moves through space, in its everyday activities and especially during a dynamic *yoga* practice, the blood and intracellular fluids move along with the body at a constant velocity. However, when the body, or a body part, changes its velocity by accelerating, or changing its direction of movement, the blood will initially keep moving with the same velocity and direction. Intelligent control of movement during a *yoga* practice allows the centripetal pump to significantly affect the flow of blood through the body, and allows energy to be gathered and moved through the body as required.

Circulation through the body is further discussed in terms of these six pumps and this model for how *hatha yoga* works is in Section 8.4.

1.1 ANATOMICAL TERMINOLOGY

The following simple anatomical terms can greatly facilitate an understanding of the body and communication between health practitioners:

- **Anterior**: relatively closer to the front of the body
- **Posterior**: relatively closer to the back of the body
- **Medial**: relatively closer to midline of the body
- **Lateral**: relatively further from the midline of the body
- **Proximal**: relatively closer to the attachment of a limb, or the point of origin
- **Distal**: relatively further from the attachment of a limb, or the point of origin
- **Superior**: relatively closer to the head
- **Inferior**: relatively further from the head.

1.1.1 Anatomical Position:

Anatomical position is the standard position which most anatomical terminology relates to. It is standing erect with the arms placed by the side of the body and with the palms facing forward (like a standing version of *savasana,* the *yoga* relaxation posture) [Figure 1.3 Anterior View].

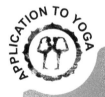

No 1.2 Observation of body symmetry and asymmetry in *yoga* postures can help identify problems

By understanding the symmetry inherent in the ideal, healthy body in the anatomical position (*savasana*) one can compare and contrast the joint positions in various postures, which are also symmetrical and also those postures which are not symmetrical and look for regions of asymmetry, which may be the cause of musculoskeletal or physiological discomfort [Appendix B].

1.2 ORGANISATION OF THE BODY

For the purposes of study, the human body can be thought of as consisting of several levels of organisation:

- **Chemical level**: At the atomic level, atoms such as carbon (C), hydrogen (H), oxygen (O), nitrogen (N), calcium (Ca), potassium (K), phosphorous (P) and sodium (Na) are the most important for maintenance of life. At the molecular level, atoms combine to make simple molecules such as water (H_2O), carbon dioxide (CO_2) and phosphate (PO_4), which then combine to form large complex molecules such as proteins, carbohydrates, fats, vitamins and DNA (deoxyribonucleic acid).

- **Cellular level**: Cells are made of complex molecules and generally consist of a central nucleus (containing the DNA or genetic material), surrounded by a peripheral cytoplasm. Cells are the basic structural and functional units of an organism.
- **Tissue level**: Tissues are groups of similar cells and the substances surrounding them, which work together to perform a particular function. The four basic tissue types are epithelial, connective, muscular and nervous tissue.
- **Organ level**: Organs are structures which are composed of two or more types of tissues and which have specific functions, eg heart, lungs, liver, kidney, brain.
- **Body system level**: A body system is loosely defined as a collection of related organs, tissues, and structures sharing a common function. The concept of a body system is a useful tool in the study of human biology. Important body systems include the:

  - **Skeletal system**, which consists of bones and the ligaments joining the bones.
  - **Articular system**, which consists of joints, joint capsules and articular discs.
  - **Muscular system**, which consists of muscles and tendons, which join muscles to bones.
  - **Nervous system**, which consists of the brain, nerves and neurotransmitters, which control the body and communicate via electrochemical signals.
  - **Respiratory system**, which consists of lungs, windpipe (trachea) and nasal cavity.
  - **Cardiovascular system**, which consists of the heart, blood vessels and the blood flowing through the system.
  - **Digestive system**, which consists of the digestive tract from the mouth to the anus and the associated digestive glands and organs that break down and assimilate food.
  - **Lymphatic system**, which consists of the lymph glands, lymph ducts and the lymph flowing through the system, and is concerned with the recovery of tissue fluid.
  - **Immune system**, which consists of immune system cells and body defence mechanisms.
  - **Endocrine system**, which consists of the endocrine glands and the hormones they secrete, and is concerned with control and communication throughout the body by chemical signals.
  - **Urinary system**, which consists of the kidneys and ureters, and is concerned with water and acid-alkali balance, and the elimination of wastes from the body.
  - **Reproductive system**, which consists of the sexual organs and their associated glands.

It must be understood however that these commonly used divisions are quite arbitrary and all have overlapping functions and locations. Often it is more useful to talk about combined systems such as the musculoskeletal system (muscular system and skeletal systems), and the cardiopulmonary system (cardiovascular system and respiratory system).

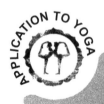

No 1.3 Yoga aimed at one body system can also affect other systems

Yoga is a holistic system and so is the human body. By working on one body system such as the musculoskeletal system, all the other body systems are also significantly affected. The yoga practitioner and yoga teacher must be aware that simple hatha yoga , while at first glance only works on the muscles and joints, can actually have a profound effect on the cardiopulmonary system and the nervous system and can be shown to affect the other body systems.

1.3 BODY TISSUE TYPES [Table 1.1]

The four main tissue types of the body are described in Table 1.1. These tissues are:
1. Epithelial tissue [Section 1.3.1]
2. Connective tissue [Section 1.3.2]
3. Muscle tissue [Section 1.6 & Chapters 2-7]
4. Nervous tissue [Section 1.3.4 & Chapter 9]

Table 1.1 Four main tissues of the body [Section 1.3]

1. EPITHELIAL TISSUE [Section 1.3.1]	2. CONNECTIVE TISSUE [Section 1.3.2]	3. MUSCLE TISSUE [Section 1.3.3]	4. NERVOUS TISSUE [Sections 1.3.4, Chapter 9]
1. Skin Epithelium	1. FIBROUS CT • Loose CT • Dense regular CT (tendons and ligaments) • Dense irregular CT (Joint capsules)	1. VOLUNTARY MUSCLE • Skeletal muscle	1. Central nervous system (CNS) • Brain • Spinal cord 2. Peripheral nervous system (PNS): • Cranial nerves • Spinal nerves
2. Visceral (Organ) Epithelium	2. CARTILAGE • Hyaline • Elastic • Fibrocartilaginous	2. INVOLUNTARY MUSCLE • Cardiac (heart) muscle • Smooth muscle	PNS DIVISIONS: a) Somatic nervous system (voluntary) b) Autonomic nervous system (involuntary) • Sympathetic nervous system • Parasympathetic nervous system
3. Blood vessel Epithelium	3. BONE • Compact bone • Spongy bone		
4. Glandular Epithelium	4. BLOOD • Red blood cells • White blood cells • Platelets • Plasma		

1.3.1 Epithelial Tissues
1.3.1.1 Functions of epithelial tissues
The many various epithelial tissues have roles in:
* Lining every surface of the body
* Protection
* Absorption
* Synthesis and secretion
* Temperature regulation
* Fluid regulation
* Excretion

1.3.2 Connective tissues (CT)
Connective tissue (CT) contains a very wide variety of specialised cells. Many different types of cells perform the functions of binding, general support, connection, protection, storage, transportation, defence and repair. The state of a persons connective tissue plays a significant role in determining that persons range of joint motion (ROM).

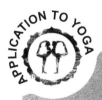

No 1.4 Condition of one's connective tissue affects one's flexibility

To a large extent the degree of flexibility a person has is dependent on the condition of the connective tissue [Alter, 1996].

Types of connective tissues (CT)
1.   Fibrous Connective tissue [Section 1.3.2.1]
2.   Cartilage [Section 1.3.2.2]
3.   Bone [Section 1.3.2.3]
4.   Blood [Chapter 8]

Functions of connective tissues (CT)
1.   Support
2.   Packing
3.   Storage
4.   Transport
5.   Defence
6.   Repair

1.3.2.3 Structure of connective tissues (CT)

Connective tissue consists of connective tissue cells in an intracellular matrix.

> ### Connective tissue (CT) = CT Cells + Intracellular Matrix

- **Connective tissue cells** specialised for fibrous CT, cartilage and bone are described below [Sections 1.3.2.1, 1.3.2.2 & 1.3.2.3]; and later [Section 8.1.1] for blood.
- **The intracellular matrix** that CT cells are in varies immensely for each of the four types of CT. The intracellular matrix of fibrous CT has varying levels of flexibility and strength, while that of cartilage and especially bone are quite rigid. Conversely, the intracellular matrix of blood is like a soupy liquid.
- The intracellular matrix consists of a number of different types of fibres of different relative amounts for each of the four CT tissue types, and a ground substance, which is the binding agent that holds the matrix and cells together.
    - **Intracellular Matrix = CT Fibres + Ground Substance**
    - *CT* **Fibres** include:
        - **Collagen fibres**, which are strong and relatively non-elastic fibres making up about one third of all body protein
        - **Elastin fibres**, which have physiological and biochemical elastic properties
        - **Reticulin fibres**.
    - **Ground substance** mainly consists of:
        - **Water**, at different relative amounts for each of the four CT types, and
        - **Glycosaminoglycans (GAGs)** which are hydrating agents – molecules that can absorb and bind water to a high degree.

1.3.2.1 Fibrous connective tissue

There are four main types of connective tissue:
1.   **Loose Areolar CT** is found deep in the skin and other epithelial tissues
2.   **Dense Regular CT** is found in ligaments and tendons
3.   **Dense Irregular CT** is found in the fascia, joint capsules and in the dermis of the skin. Dense irregular CT is omni-directional
4.   **Fat cells** are specialised loose CT designed for the storage of fat.

The human body contains many structures that are composed of connective tissue. The most important to understand for *yoga* are ligaments, tendons and fascia.

1.3.2.1.1 Ligaments

> Ligaments are dense regular connective tissue structures that **join bone to bone**.

Ligaments function as mechanical restraints, keeping bones joined together. They:
- Contain proprioceptive sensory organs
- Cannot stretch much
- Do not regenerate or repair easily
- Only function to restrain a joint at the end of the range of movement (ROM) of the joint.

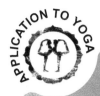

No 1.5 Protect ligaments from overstretching

Ligaments should not be overstretched. Therefore, at the extremes of joint movement the muscles crossing that joint may be kept gently tensed to avoid an over-stretch of the ligaments.

1.3.2.1.2 Tendons

Tendons are dense regular connective tissue structures that **join muscle to bone.**

Tendons have characteristics similar to that of ligaments, with the exception that:
- Tendons are slightly less elastic than ligaments, in order to transfer energy directly from the muscle to the bone
- Tendons have better healing power than ligaments.

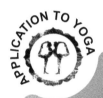

No 1.6 Increase tendon stretching with muscle tension

The stretch on a tendon may be significantly increased if the attached muscle is gently and carefully tensed. For example, in *supta virasana* the stretch on the quadriceps tendon and the patella tendon [Section 5.2.2] may be increased by pressing the feet into the floor in order to activate the knee extensors.

1.3.2.1.3 Fascia

Fascia is the thin, strong and extensible connective tissue that **surrounds and separates individual muscle fibres, bundles of fibres and entire muscles** [St George, 1999].

Fascia surrounds and is contiguous (merges) with the tendons of the muscles. Fascia helps muscles move more easily and helps muscles keep their shape and form. Fascia is therefore sometimes referred to as the glad wrap of the muscles [St George, 1999].

Fascia also exists around nerves, and certain organs. The outer layer of fascia provides muscles with their shape and form.

Fascial connections join one muscle to another and essentially connect the entire body. It is through fascial connections that movement of the toes can be felt in the scalp [Alter, 1986].

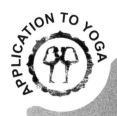

No 1.7 Use fascial connections between muscles and the stretch reflex to enhance muscle activations

It is because of <u>fascial connections</u> throughout the musculoskeletal system and by virtue of the <u>myotatic (stretch) reflex</u> [Section 1.7.2.2] that <u>activation</u> (or stretch) of one muscle can trigger the <u>activation</u> of another muscle at a distant part of the body that is not directly joined to the first muscle. For example, it is much easier to tighten the abdominal muscle <u>transversus abdominis</u> [Section 7.2.3] if the shoulders are pulled towards the hips by activating the underarm muscle <u>latissimus dorsi</u> [Section 2.3]. This is because these two muscles are joined by <u>fascial connections</u>. Hence <u>activation</u> (or stretch) of <u>latissimus dorsi</u> <u>tensions</u> (stretches and pulls on) <u>transversus abdominis</u> [Section 7.2.3] which then responds with <u>myotatic (stretch) reflex</u> <u>activation</u>.

There is a thin layer of fluid that lies between the <u>fascia</u> and the muscle or tissue it covers. This fluid, which helps the tissues glide and move more easily around and over each other, is <u>thixotropic</u>, like the <u>synovial fluid</u> in joints [Section 1.5.2.3]. Therefore, this fluid will become less viscous (more runny) in an environment that is relatively warmer and/or more <u>alkaline</u>.

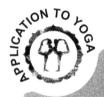

No 1.8 Enhance muscle stretching and nerve tensioning with movement and muscle activation to increase body heat

As the body gets warmer, through the movements from one *yoga* posture to the next, and through the application of the nine major joint *bandhas* or muscle <u>co-activations</u> [Section 1.7.3], the fluid layer between the <u>fascia</u> and the tissues that the <u>fascia</u> covers (e.g. muscles and nerves) becomes more lubricated and the muscles and nerves can move more freely.

1.3.2.1.4 Joint flexibility
The <u>range of motion</u> (ROM) of a joint and its ability to move is restricted 47% by the <u>ligaments</u> and <u>joint capsule</u>, 41% by the <u>fascia</u>, 10% by the <u>tendons</u> and 2% by the skin [Alter, 1996].

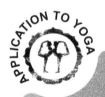

No 1.9 Aim to stretch the fascia not the ligaments or joint capsule

A joint flexibility program should be targeted at stretching the <u>fascia</u>. One should not aim to stretch the <u>ligaments</u> and <u>joint capsule</u> as this may lead to instability of the <u>joint complex</u>. One way of doing this in exercises that may risk over-stretching ligaments or joint capsule is to keep the muscles around a joint gently activated (tensed) while they are being stretched. Since muscles are directly joined to fascia but are not directly joined to ligaments or joint capsules muscle tension during stretching exercises will target the fascia over the ligaments or joint capsule.

1.3.2.2 Cartilage
<u>Cartilage</u> is a tough, rubbery tissue that covers and cushions the ends of the bones and absorbs shock. It is also one of the materials out of which the ears, the nose and the trachea are made.

1.3.2.2.1 Functions of cartilage
The main function of <u>cartilage</u> is to strengthen and support areas requiring varying degrees of flexibility.
<u>Cartilage</u> also assists in movement over <u>articular (joint) surfaces</u> and allows the joint to move easily without pain.

No 1.10 Protect cartilage with some muscle tension while stretching

While stretching take care to protect the <u>cartilage</u> that lines all the major joints, the <u>cartilaginous discs</u> that rest between each <u>spinal vertebra</u> (<u>intervertebral discs</u>), and the <u>cartilaginous discs</u> that reside inside the knee joints (<u>menisci</u>). This is done by applying the *bandha* principle [Section 1.7.3] of creating and maintaining a gentle muscular firmness around a joint before trying to bend or stretch a joint. Bending or stretching a joint may result in the joint space being compressed to the point that the <u>cartilage</u> becomes damaged.

1.3.2.2.2 Types of cartilage

1.3.2.2.2.1 Hyaline cartilage (*Hylos* = glass)
- Most common type of <u>cartilage</u>
- Found over <u>articular surfaces</u>, respiratory rings in windpipe
- Aids joint movement.
- Frictionless (100 times as slippery as ice skates on ice).

1.3.2.2.2.2 Elastic cartilage
- Hyaline <u>cartilage</u> + elastic fibres
- Flexible supportive <u>cartilage</u>
- Found in external ear, epiglottis.

1.3.2.2.2.3 Fibrocartilage
- Contains large amounts of collagen.
- Found in intervertebral discs, articular discs (eg the <u>menisci</u> of the knee joint), and <u>pubic symphysis</u>.
- Resists <u>tension</u> and absorbs shock.

1.3.2.2.3 Characteristics of cartilage
There is an absence of <u>blood vessels</u> in <u>cartilage</u>. Therefore, this tissue relies heavily on diffusion for access to nutrients. Consequently, <u>cartilage</u> has a poor ability to heal or regenerate.

<u>Cartilage</u> has no nerve supply and therefore one cannot actually feel pain from cartilage damage. Hence, injures in <u>cartilage</u> will not immediately be felt. Usually one only feels the <u>effect</u> of the injury to <u>cartilage</u>, which may be a loss of function in a joint, at some later time when the damage to the <u>cartilage</u> has gone too far to be repaired.

With age and/or excessively acidic diet, insoluble mineral salts deposit in <u>cartilage</u> [Section 10.3] leading to stiffness, brittleness and <u>osteochondritis</u> (inflammation or defective growth of part of a bone or cartilage).

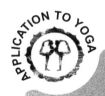

No 1.11 Regulate and reduce the amount of air you breathe and modify your diet to improve joint flexibility

Pranayama practice (breath-control) both during and separate to *Asana* practice (physical *yoga*) can help to protect the health of your <u>cartilage</u> and improve joint flexibility by reducing the amount of insoluble mineral salts in your body. If you practise *pranayama* that eventually leads to a reduction in <u>minute ventilation</u> (the amount of air breathed each minute), then this causes a build-up of <u>carbon dioxide</u> in the blood and a mild <u>respiratory acidosis</u> due to <u>carbonic acid</u> is created [Section 8.4]. This may be altered by a diet high in fresh vegetables, salad and fruit thus allowing a metabolic alkalosis which leaves low levels of mineral salts in the body and reduces the tendency to deplete minerals from the bones [Section 10.3].

1.3.2.3 Bone

Bone tissue is rigid living connective tissue that makes up bones. There are 206 bones in the skeleton of the human body

1.3.2.3.1 Functions of bone

- Protects and supports the body and its internal structures
- Withstands and recovers from mechanical forces (Wolffs Law)
- Provides the body with efficient mechanical performance in terms of being lightweight with ease and freedom of movement
- Responds to external stimuli
- Produces blood cells
- Stores minerals, including Calcium (Ca+) Phosphorous (P) in the form of hydroxyapatite crystals $(Ca_{10}(PO_4)_6(OH)_2)$.

1.3.2.3.2 Characteristics of bone:

- Bone tissue consists of widely separated cells surrounded by large amounts of matrix
- The matrix of compact bone contains by weight approximately:
  - 70% mineral salts (mostly hydroxyapatite)
  - Fibres (mostly collagen fibres)
  - Ground substance (extracellular fluid + proteoglycans),
- Bone is more rigid and stronger than cartilage and can thus withstand compression,
- Bone is metabolically active
- Bone is highly structured to achieve maximum support.

1.3.2.3.3 Types of bone

1.3.2.3.3.1. Compact bone tissue

- Compact bone consists of osteons (Haversian systems), which are dense concentric-ringed units that are well supplied with blood and nerves.
- Compact bone lies over spongy bone and composes most of the diaphysis (shaft of a long bone).

1.3.2.3.3.2. Spongy bone tissue

- Spongy bone consists of a thin latticework of plates called trabeculae that are arranged according to mechanical stresses applied to bone.
- Spongy bone forms most of the structure of short, flat and irregular bones, and the epiphyses (ends) of long bones.

1.3.2.3.4 Bone re-modelling

Living bones are plastic tissues [Moore 1992]. They are very responsive to the forces in their external environment.

> **Wolffs Law**
>
> "The form of a bone being given, bone elements will place or displace themselves in the direction of the functional stress, and will increase or decrease their mass to reflect the amount of the functional stress."

First stated in 1892 by Wolff, this very profound and important law describes the nature of the effect of the external environment and therefore the choice and will of an individual to affect the growth and development of a bone. Evidence that is more recent suggests that other tissues may also be subject to this law.

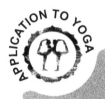

No 1.12 Bone density and bone shape can change with regular *yoga*

Wolffs Law implies that if one has a mal-aligned or mal-formed bony structure, then with repeated correcting exercises or *yoga* postures that put specific forces on that bone region, there is the possibility of re-aligning the bones.

Similarly, Wolffs Law implies that if one works incorrectly or with mal-alignment during repetitive daily activities or exercise, or while performing *hatha yoga* postures, then bone growth may be adversely affected.

1.3.3 Muscle Tissue

Muscle is a tissue type composed mainly of contractile cells that effects movement in the body. The human body has over 650 individual muscles [Sections 1.6, 2.3. 3.3, 3.6, 4.4, 5.3, 6.3 & 7.2].

1.3.3.1 Types of muscle tissue

There are three (3) types of muscle tissue:

1.3.3.1.1 Skeletal muscle
- Skeletal muscle is voluntary in its control,
- Skeletal muscle attaches to, and exerts a force on, the bones.

1.3.3.1.2 Smooth muscle
- Smooth muscle is autonomous (involuntary in its control)
- Smooth muscle is located in walls of hollow structures eg blood vessels, walls of the gastrointestinal tract and most abdominal organs, and in skin attached to hair follicles.

1.3.3.1.3 Cardiac muscle
- Cardiac muscle is the autonomous muscle of the heart.

1.3.3.2 Characteristics of muscle tissue

Muscle tissue:
- Joins body parts, via tendons, to attachments (places where muscle tendons attach)
- Conducts electrical signals from the nervous system (action potentials)
- Contains contractile proteins (muscle filaments)
- Generates tension
- When stimulated by nervous impulses attempts to pull the proximal & distal attachments of a muscle towards each other
- Requires calcium and ATP (major energy carrying molecule of all living cells) to start the contractile process

1.3.3.3 Functions of muscle tissue

Through sustained activation (generation of tension) or by alternating between activation and relaxation, muscle tissue is able to function in four ways:

1. **The production of body motion,** or motion of parts of the body.
2. **Stabilisation** of joints, body positions and regulation of organ volume.
3. **The generation of heat (thermogenesis).** Approximately 85% of all body heat is generated by muscle activations.
4. **The generation of pressure gradients** (high pressure when a muscle shortens as a result of tension, and low pressure when a muscle stretches), which result in the movement of energy (in the form of heat, and bio-electrical energy), blood, intracellular fluid, energy carrying molecules such as ATP and glucose; and information-carrying molecules such as DNA, RNA, neurotransmitters and hormones.

1.3.3.4 How muscles generate tension – sliding filament mechanism

Muscle tension or activation is stimulated by an electrochemical signal propagated through the nervous tissue of a nerve [Section 1.3.4 & 9.1]. The mechanism by which muscles are activated is believed to be by an (ATP driven) inter digitation (overlapping) of small muscle filaments (actin & myosin), which leads to a decrease in length of each basic muscle unit (sarcomere) [Figure 1.6].

Figure 1.6 How muscles are activated at the molecular level:

Contractile protein muscle filaments (horizontal lines) pulled together after the application of an electrical nerve signal and energy in the form of ATP overlapping in the process of <u>muscle activation</u>

Proximal
Attachment

Distal
Attachment

Contractile protein muscle filaments with slight overlap before <u>muscle activation</u>

⇓

- **Nerve impulse (electrical signal)**
- **ATP (energy source) + calcium**

⇓

Proximal   ⇓   ⇓   *Distal*
Attachment   *Attachment*

1.3.4 Nervous Tissue

<u>Neurons</u> or nerve cells, the main cells of the <u>nervous system</u> [Section 1.8.1 & Chapter 9], are able to conduct electrochemical impulses. They have a <u>cell body</u> (which contains the nucleus) and an <u>axon</u> (long-branched processes), which are usually enveloped in an insulating <u>phospholipid</u> called the <u>myelin sheath</u>.

1.3.5 Tissue Injury and Inflammation

When there is an injury in the body, tissues initially become inflamed. <u>Inflammation</u> [Sections 1.8.1 & 10.2] is a localised, protective response to tissue injury designed to destroy, dilute, or wall off the infecting agent or injured tissue. <u>Inflammation</u> is characterised by five cardinal signs:

(i)   Redness
(ii)   Pain
(iii)   Heat
(iv)   Swelling
(v)   Loss of function (sometimes).

1.4 THE SKELETAL SYSTEM

A general overview of the <u>skeletal system</u> can be seen at the start of this chapter [Figure 1.1]. More detailed information about specific joints is also available for the shoulder [Figures 2.1-2.4], the elbow [Figures 3.1–3.5], the wrist [Figures 3.1 & 3.7], the pelvis and hip [Figures 4.1–4.3], the knee [Figures 5.1–5.6], the ankle and foot [Figures 6.1–6.4], and the spine [Figures 7.2–7.7].

1.4.1 Classification of Bones

Bones are classified as long, short, flat, irregular, or sesamoid.

Bone markings provide landmarks for study, and are used to further classify and characterise bones. They include:
* <u>Projections in bones</u>: <u>spine</u>, crest, line, trochanter, tubercle, tuberosity, head, condyle, epicondyle, ramus.
* <u>Depressions in bones</u>: facet, fossa, fovea, groove/sulcus, foramen, canal/meatus, fissure, sinus, notch.

<u>Functions of Bone Markings</u>
* Strengthen bone
* Provide passages for nerves and <u>blood vessels</u>
* Promote bone to bone <u>articulation</u>
* Provide attachment sites for muscles

1.4.2 Axial Skeleton [Figures 1.1, 7.2–7.7]

The <u>axial skeleton</u> consists of 80 bones that lie around the central axis of the body: the <u>skull</u> bones (22), auditory ossicles (6), <u>hyoid bone</u> (1), ribs (24), <u>sternum</u> (breastbone) (1), and the <u>spinal vertebrae</u> (26).

1.4.3 Appendicular Skeleton [Figures 1.1, 2.1–2.4, 3.1–3.5, 4.1–4.3, 5.1–5.6, 6.1–6.4, 7.2–7.7]

The <u>appendicular skeleton</u> consists of the 126 bones contained in the upper (60) *and* lower (60) limbs and the <u>pectoral (shoulder) girdle</u> (4) and <u>pelvic (hip) girdle</u> (2).

1.5 THE ARTICULAR (JOINT) SYSTEM

A joint (= <u>articulation</u>) is defined as the point of contact between bones, between <u>cartilage</u> and bones, or between teeth and bones [Figure 1.7].

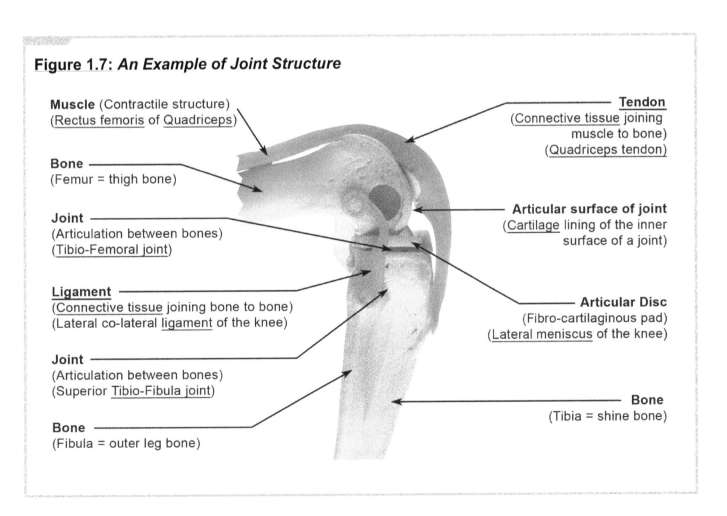

Figure 1.7: *An Example of Joint Structure*

Muscle (Contractile structure)
(<u>Rectus femoris</u> of <u>Quadriceps</u>)

Bone ——
(Femur = thigh bone)

Joint ——
(Articulation between bones)
(<u>Tibio-Femoral joint</u>)

Ligament ——
(<u>Connective tissue</u> joining bone to bone)
(Lateral co-lateral <u>ligament</u> of the knee)

Joint ——
(Articulation between bones)
(Superior <u>Tibio-Fibula joint</u>)

Bone ——
(Fibula = outer leg bone)

Tendon
(<u>Connective tissue</u> joining
muscle to bone)
(<u>Quadriceps tendon</u>)

Articular surface of joint
(<u>Cartilage</u> lining of the inner
surface of a joint)

Articular Disc
(Fibro-cartilaginous pad)
(<u>Lateral meniscus</u> of the knee)

Bone
(Tibia = shine bone)

Table 1.2 Types of joints and their features [Section 1.5]

FIBROUS JOINTS [Section 1.5.1]	CARTILAGINOUS JOINTS [Section 1.5.1]	SYNOVIAL JOINTS [Section 1.5.2]
Characteristics: • No joint cavity • Joint **held together by fibrous connective tissue** **Types of Fibrous Joints:** **1. Sutures** • **No significant movement** • Strong connective tissues binding • **Found only in the skull** **2. Syndesmosis** • **Small amount of movement** proportional to distance between bones & flexibility of fibrous tissue • Consisting of a ligament or fibrous membrane • **eg Interosseus membrane between radius & ulna; Distal ends of tibia & fibula** **3. Gomphosis** • **No significant movement normally** • **Joints between the teeth & jaw sockets**	**Characteristics:** • No joint cavity • **Joint held together by cartilage** **Types of Cartilaginous Joints:** **1. Synchondrosis** • **Slightly movable joints** • Hyaline cartilaginous joints. • Union between bone & cartilage. • **eg Costochondral (rib to cartilage) joint.** **2. Symphysis:** • **Slightly movable joints** • Fibrocartilaginous in structure. • Bones covered with hyaline articular cartilage & joined by strong fibrous tissue. • **eg Intervertebral discs, & pubic symphysis**	**Characteristics:** **Easily moveable joints** Synovial joints always have: • Joint cavity • Articular cartilage • Articular capsule • Fibrous capsule • Synovial membrane • Synovial fluid. Synovial joints usually have: • Accessory Ligaments Synovial joints sometimes have: • Articular discs • Labrum • Bursae **Types of Synovial Joints:** 1. **Ball & socket joint** 2. **Hinge joint** 3. **Saddle joint** 4. **Ellipsoid / condylar joint** 5. **Pivot joint** 6. **Plane/gliding joint**

1.5.1 Classification of Joints

There are three (3) main types of joints. Fibrous joints and cartilaginous joints are classified as immovable under normal conditions, while synovial joints are classified as freely moveable. Table 1.2 outlines the main features of each type of joint. Synovial joints are described in detail in the next section, as they are arguably the most important.

1.5.2 Synovial Joints

Synovial joints [Figure 1.7] are the most common and functionally important types of joints in the body, especially to do with movement, exercise and *yoga*.

1.5.2.1 Function of synovial joints

• Permit mobility of one bone against another
• Provide stability of the articulation between bones.

1.5.2.2 Important features of synovial joints

• Synovial joints always have:

  • A joint cavity between the articulating surfaces that is filled with synovial fluid [Section 1.5.2.3]
  • Articular cartilage, which covers and protects the surface of the articulating bones. Articular cartilage:
    • Is usually hyaline cartilage
    • Is deformable
    • Is permeable for nutrient diffusion
    • Allows for frictionless movement of joint
  • An articular capsule that consists of a
    • Fibrous joint capsule which is lined with a
    • Synovial membrane which secretes new synovial fluid, absorbs old synovial fluid, and is susceptible to inflammation

- Synovial joints usually have:
  - Accessory ligaments, which function in strengthening the articular capsules. They are either separate to the fibrous joint capsule (extrinsic ligaments) or part of the fibrous joint capsule (intrinsic ligaments).
- Synovial joints sometimes have:
  - Articular discs, which are usually fibrocartilaginous pads that protect and hold the bones together where joints are incongruous, eg the menisci of the knee.
  - **Labrum**: a fibrocartilaginous ring, which deepens the articular surface of one of the bones, eg the glenoid labrum of the shoulder joint complex.

1.5.2.3 Synovial fluid

The synovial fluid fills the joint or synovial cavity.

- Synovial fluid provides lubricant for joint motion
- Synovial fluid is a nutritive source for the articular cartilage
- Synovial fluid aids in removal of metabolic waste products from articular cartilage
- Synovial fluid is susceptible to inflammation [Section 1.3.3 & 10.2]
- The viscosity or thickness of the synovial fluid varies with environmental conditions (ie synovial fluid is thixotropic):
  - In conditions of heat or alkaline pH the synovial fluid becomes less viscous (more thin and runny), while in colder or more acidic conditions the synovial fluid becomes more viscous (thicker and less runny).

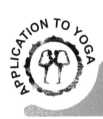

No 1.13 Joints are more flexible when they are warm and/or in an alkaline state

Synovial fluid is thixotropic (responds to the external environment). Therefore, joints will be more flexible, and better prepared for either a *yoga* practice or any exercise when they are warm and/or in an alkaline state.

Warming the body can either be achieved by placing the body in a warm environment (e.g. a hot room) or by engaging in muscular activity (i.e. either isotonic or isometric muscle activations). Most substances in the bloodstream easily enter the joint cavity [Moore, 1985]. Therefore, if the blood becomes more alkaline then so will the synovial fluid. Alkalising the blood can either be done temporarily with increased breathing (hyperventilation) [Section 8.2.9.4.1], or more permanently by adopting a more alkaline diet [Section 10.3].

Synovial fluid is also present in several other structures in the body, including bursae and synovial sheaths, which may be extensions of the joint capsule as in the shoulder joint [Moore, 1985], or may be seen independently of joint capsules. Bursae are closed flattened sacs filled with synovial fluid.

- Bursae:
  - Are found between the skin and the bone, or between muscle and bone
  - Are lined with a synovial-like membrane
  - Contain a capillary thin layer of synovial fluid
  - Are usually located in areas that are subject to friction eg, the ischial tuberosity (sitting bone) of the buttock
  - Function in reducing friction
- Synovial sheaths are tubular sheaths filled with synovial fluid surrounding tendons, acting as lubricating devices and permitting smooth gliding of the tendons.
- Bursae and synovial sheaths are filled with synovial fluid and so, like joint capsules, they are susceptible to swelling and inflammation.
- Synovial fluid is also present between muscles and the fascia encasing and surrounding muscles.
- A synovial-like fluid is also present between nerves and the connective tissue sheaths surrounding the nerves.

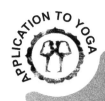

No 1.14 Muscles, tendons and ligaments are more flexible when they are warm and/or in an alkaline state

Synovial-like fluid is present around <u>tendons</u>, muscles and nerves, inside <u>bursae</u> and joints. Since this fluid is <u>thixotropic</u> (responds to the external environment) all these structures will be more flexible, and better prepared for either a *yoga* practice or any exercise when they are warm and/or in an <u>alkaline</u> state.

1.5.2.4 Classification of synovial joints
* **Number of axes of movement**:
    * Uni-axial joints cross and directly act on one joint only eg. hinge joints such as in the elbow
    * Bi-axial joints, eg. bi-condylar such as the knee
    * Multi-axial eg ball and socket joints such as the shoulder or hip
* **Shape of articular surface**: eg ovoid, sellar, concave, convex
* **Number of mating pairs**:
    * **Simple joint**: only one mating pair of bone surfaces eg <u>glenohumeral</u> (GH) joint of the shoulder [Section 2.2]
    * **Compound joint**: more than one pair of bone surfaces eg where the radius, ulna and humerus meet at the elbow joint [Section 3.2]
* **Complex joint**: contains an <u>articular disc</u> eg the <u>tibiofemoral joint</u> of the knee [Section 5.2]

1.5.2.5 Movements about a synovial joint

Following are definitions of the major actions or movements of <u>synovial joints</u> in the body. All movements are described from the <u>anatomical position</u> (which is like a standing version of *savasana* or the corpse posture). Movements about a <u>synovial joint</u> occur in pairs. Each movement has an opposing movement. For example, in a typical ball and socket joint like the <u>glenohumeral (GH) joint</u> of the shoulder [Section 2.2], or the <u>coxafemoral joint</u> of the hip [Section 4.2]:
* <u>Flexion</u> is the opposite of <u>extension</u>
* <u>Abduction</u> is the opposite of <u>adduction</u>
* <u>External rotation</u> is the opposite of <u>internal rotation</u>.

These six (6) primary movements (three (3) opposing pairs of movement), which can occur at a ball and socket-type <u>synovial joint</u> can be described as follows:

Flexion and Extension:
* <u>Flexion</u> involves bending or reducing the angle between the bones of a joint.
* <u>Extension</u> involves straightening or increasing the angle between the bones of a joint.

    One exception to this general rule is the shoulder. When taking the upper arm towards the head (not the body), it is <u>flexion.</u> When taking the arm towards the body from above the head while also moving it behind the body, it is called <u>extension</u>.

Abduction and Adduction:
* <u>Adduction</u> involves movement towards the midline of the body.
* <u>Abduction</u> involves movement away from the midline of the body.

External Rotation and Internal Rotation:
* <u>External rotation</u> (also called <u>lateral rotation</u>) involves rotation away from the midline of the body.
* <u>Internal rotation</u> (also called <u>medial rotation</u>) involves rotation toward the midline of the body.

Additional specialised movement pairs for the <u>scapula</u> (shoulder blade) are:
Elevation and depression: [Chapter 2]
* <u>Elevation</u> involves movement of <u>scapula</u> superiorly (ie movement of the shoulder blade towards the head).
* <u>Depression</u> involves movement of the <u>scapula</u> inferiorly (ie movement of the shoulder blade away from the head).

Protraction and retraction [Chapter 2]
* <u>Protraction</u> involves movement of the <u>scapula</u> anteriorly (ie movement of the shoulder blade away from the spine).
* <u>Retraction</u> involves movement of the <u>scapula</u> posteriorly (ie movement of the shoulder blade towards the spine).

Additional specialised movement pairs for the ankle and foot are:
Plantarflexion and dorsiflexion [Chapter 6]
- Plantarflexion: moving the foot away from the body. Plantarflexion at the ankle joint is analogous to flexion at the wrist.
- Dorsiflexion: moving the foot towards the body. Dorsiflexion at the ankle joint is analogous to extension at the wrist.

Additional specialised movement pairs for the elbow are:
Supination and pronation [Chapter 3]
- Supination involves turning the palm of the hand upwards (like external rotation of the forearm).
- Pronation involves turning the palm of the hand downwards (like internal rotation of the forearm).

Additional specialised movement pairs for the ankle and foot are:
Inversion and eversion [Chapter 6]
- Inversion involves turning the sole of the foot to face inwards (medial movement).
- Eversion involves turning the sole of the foot to face outwards (lateral movement).

Additional specialised movement pairs for the hip and pelvis are:
Anterior pelvic tilt and posterior pelvic tilt [Chapter 4]
- Anterior pelvic tilt is anterior movement of the superior pelvis (ie forward movement of the top of the hips, or pushing the coccyx or tailbone backwards).
- Posterior pelvic tilt is a posterior movement of the superior pelvis (backward movement of the top of the hips, equivalent to tucking the coccyx or tailbone anteriorly, ie forwards or under).

1.5.2.6 Closed-packed and loose-packed positions of a joint

The close-packed position of a joint is one in which the joint surfaces fit perfectly. Close-packed positions:
- have maximal joint surface contact area
- often occur at extreme of range of the most habitual movement
- have joint capsules and ligaments at maximal tension
- have their joint surfaces compressed
- have no further movement possible
- are susceptible to damage at the joint surfaces.

All other positions of a joint are referred to as loose-packed positions. Loose-packed positions:
- have articular surfaces that are not congruent
- have their joint capsule partly lax, allowing combinations of spin, roll and glide and permitting maximal joint range of motion (ROM)
- have reduced frictional and erosive effects
- maintain efficient joint lubrication and nutrition of articular cartilage.

1.5.3 Joint complexes

A joint complex is a group of joints that function essentially as a single unit. There are nine (9) important joint complexes in the body. These are the:

- Ankle joint complex [Section 6.2]
- Knee joint complex [Section 5.2]
- Hip joint complex [Section 4.2]
- Lumbar spine joint complex [Section 7.1]
- Thoracic spine joint complex [Section 7.1]
- Cervical spine joint complex [Section 7.1]
- Shoulder joint complex [Section 2.2]
- Elbow joint complex [Section 3.2]
- Wrist joint complex [Section 3.5].

Joint complexes are at the core of *hatha yoga bandhas* [Section 1.7.3]. Many of the muscles that act in joint complexes to assist in the formation of the *bandhas* are multi-articular muscles (ie they cross more than one joint) [Section 1.6.5.7].

1.5.4 Joint Diseases

1.5.4.1 Inflammatory joint diseases

Inflammatory joint diseases are conditions of the synovial membrane due to systemic diseases, infections, and or unknown causes.

Rheumatoid arthritis (RA) is a common inflammatory joint disease

- In RA the synovial membrane becomes more vascular, more permeable and accumulates inflammatory cells and debris.
- In RA, synovial fluid becomes thinner and increases in amount, causing the joint to swell and become painful with a loss of range of movement (ROM) and stability.
- In RA the articular cartilage may get completely eroded which is usually followed by fibrous connective tissues joining the bony ends together. The joint may then ossify and become immovable.

Causes of rheumatoid arthritis:

- Some authors have suggested that RA may be an autoimmune disease in which the body attacks itself.
- However, much evidence has now been accumulated that suggests that diet has an important role in the regulation of RA activity [Peltonen et al., 1997].
- It is well known that most substances in the bloodstream, whether normal or pathological, easily enter the joint cavity [Moore, 1985].
- Therefore it is suggested that inflammation of the joints resulting from an unknown substance that enters the joint cavity may in part result either directly from a dietary intake or indirectly from the substances produced by microbial degradation of dietary food (fermentation and putrefaction) in the gastrointestinal tract, which is then passed into the bloodstream and later into the joint cavities.

1.5.4.2 Degenerative joint diseases

Degenerative joint diseases involve localised wearing or deterioration of articular cartilage.

- **Osteoarthritis (OA)** is a common example of a degenerative joint disease.
    - OA results from a combination of aging, irritation of the joints, and wear and abrasion – commonly called wear and tear arthritis.
    - OA is a non-inflammatory progressive disorder of moveable joints especially those bearing weight.
    - OA is characterised by a slow degeneration of the cartilage, but rarely any change in the synovial membrane as in rheumatoid arthritis.
    - The bone ends gradually become exposed in OA and small bony bumps or spurs of new bony tissue are deposited on them, which reduces the size of the joint cavity and thus limits pain-free movement.

1.6 THE MUSCULAR SYSTEM

Muscles are contractile structures made up of muscle tissue [Section 1.3.3] and connective tissue [Section 1.3.2] that join different parts of the body together. When muscles are activating or generating tension, they appear to be trying to pull the body parts they are attached to closer towards each other. When muscles succeed in pulling their attachments closer together, this is called a concentric activation. When the attempt of a muscle to pull its attachments further apart is unsuccessful, if the attachments don't actually move at all then this is termed an isometric activation, or if the attachments are moved apart then this is termed an eccentric activation.

1.6.1 Skeletal Muscle Structure

The contractile elements of a muscle are formed from muscle tissue [Section 1.3.3]. Muscle tissue is arranged in bundles then wrapped in a thin strong, layer of connective tissue called fascia [Section 1.3.2.1.3]. The fascia wrapped muscle is attached to bones via tendons [Section 1.3.2.1.2] at their attachments.

- There are various types of skeletal muscle shape including parallel, fusiform, pennate, and circular.
- **Attachments** of muscles to bones by tendons are named the:
    - **Origin** (= the proximal attachment in muscle charts) of a muscle, which by definition remains stable and does not move during concentric muscle activation.
    - **Insertion** (= the distal attachment in muscle charts) of a muscle, which by definition moves during a concentric muscle activation.

Bones act as levers and the joints act as the fulcrums of these levers to produce movement in the body.

1.6.2 Mechanics of Movement

- A lever can be defined as a rigid rod that moves about some fixed point called a fulcrum.
- A fulcrum (F) is acted on at two different points on the lever called the effort (E) and the resistance (R).

First-class lever
- A first-class lever is the most efficient type of lever
- A first-class lever has the <u>fulcrum</u> (F) between the <u>effort</u> (E) and the <u>resistance</u> (R) (ie order is E-F-R)
- A mechanical example of a first-class lever is a seesaw
- A human example of a first-class lever is the head resting on the <u>spine</u>. When the head is raised the facial portion of the <u>skull</u> is the <u>resistance</u> (R), the atlanto-occipital joint between the <u>spine</u> and <u>skull</u> is the fixed point of the <u>fulcrum</u> (F) and the <u>activation</u> of the back muscles is the <u>effort</u> (E).

Second-class lever
- A second-class lever is the second most efficient type of lever
- F is at one end and R is between F and E (ie order is F-R-E)
- A mechanical example of a second-class lever is a wheelbarrow
- A human example of a second-class lever is the raising the heel off the ground so the body weight (R) is raised onto the ball of the foot (F) by <u>activation</u> of the calf muscles (E).

Third-class lever
- A third-class lever has the lowest efficiency
- F is at one end and E is between F and R (ie order is F-E-R)
- A mechanical example of a third-class lever is a crane
- Human examples of third-class levers are many and include the <u>adduction</u> of the thigh, and the flexing of the forearm at the elbow.

<u>Leverage</u>
- Mechanical advantage gained by a lever is largely responsible for a muscles strength, speed and joint <u>range of motion</u> (ROM)
- Consider two muscles of the same strength crossing and acting on the same joint. If one attaches close to the joint, and the second attaches far away from the joint, then the close attaching muscle will have a greater speed and ROM than the muscle attaching further away. The second further away muscle will have the greater strength and be able to produce the more powerful movement.

1.6.3 Types of Skeletal Muscle Activations

There are three (3) main types of skeletal <u>muscle activations</u>. These are <u>isotonic</u>, <u>isometric</u> and <u>isokinetic</u>.

1.6.3.1 Isotonic muscle activations

<u>Isotonic</u> <u>muscle activations</u> involve body movement and a change in muscle length. The muscle is said to be generating <u>tension</u> (activating) against a movable resistance. There are two types of <u>isotonic</u> activations – <u>concentric</u> and <u>eccentric</u>.

1.6.3.1.1 Concentric muscle activations

Concentric muscle activations are where the muscle shortens while working or generating an active <u>tension</u> eg the <u>quadriceps</u> when straightening the knee from a squat position.

1.6.3.1.2 Eccentric muscle activations

Eccentric muscle activations are where the muscle lengthens while working or generating an active <u>tension</u> eg the <u>quadriceps</u> when bending the knee to a squat position.

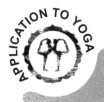

No 1.15 Use isometric and isotonic muscle strengthening in *yoga*

Basic practice of *hatha yoga asanas* (static postures) uses <u>isometric</u> activations when the body is kept still in postures and no movement about a particular joint is occurring. Basic practise of *hatha yoga vinyasas* (dynamic exercises) uses <u>isotonic</u> activations when the body is moving from one posture to the next and there is movement about a particular joint.

1.6.3.2 Isometric muscle activations

Isometric muscle activations involve no body movements and have no change in muscle length. Most static *yoga* postures have isometric muscle activations. The muscle is said to be generating tension against an immovable resistance.

1.6.3.3 Isokinetic muscle activation

Isokinetic muscle activations involve body movement and a change in muscle length. The muscle is said to be generating tension against a maximal resistance throughout full joint range of movement (ROM). Isometric and isotonic activations require no specialised equipment, but generally isokinetic exercises can only be performed with large and very expensive computer-backed machines.

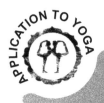

No 1.16 Use isokinetic muscle strengthening in *yoga*

Intelligent use of *hatha yoga asanas* (static postures) and *vinyasas* (dynamic exercises) enables one to work one limb or body part against another in such a way that a muscle can be made to generate tension against maximal resistance through its full joint range of motion (ROM), giving many of the same benefits that can be obtained from the large expensive computer-backed isokinetic exercise machines.

For example, *utthita pavanmuktasana*   (a one-legged standing pose with the non-weight-bearing knee flexed and hugged to the chest) becomes isokinetic in nature if one pulls the leg towards oneself with the arms (using elbow flexors, shoulder extensors and shoulder adductors) and resists this effort by pushing away the thigh (using the hip extensors), while moving back and forth between elbow extension and partial hip extension to elbow flexion and hip flexion.

The three main types of skeletal muscle activation are summarised in Table 1.3.

Table 1.3 Types of skeletal muscle activations and their characteristics [Section 1.6.3 & 1.6.5.5]

Isotonic	Isometric	Isokinetic
• Dynamic • Change in muscle length • Involves movement • Muscle generating tension against a moveable resistance **Two types of isotonic activations:** **(a) Concentric** • Muscle shortens while working/tensing **(b) Eccentric** • Muscle lengthens while working/tensing • Can be done in *yoga vinyasas*	• Static • **No** change in muscle length • **No** movement • Muscle generating tension against an immovable resistance • Can be done in *yoga asanas*	• Dynamic • Change in muscle length • Involves movement • Muscle generating tension against a maximal resistance throughout full range of movement (ROM) • Isokinetic activations require expensive computer rehabilitation equipment such as the CYBEX machine • Can be done in *yoga vinyasas*

1.6.4 Muscle Actions and Roles

Muscle actions and roles are often confused. Most tables of muscles only show muscle action. The muscles in these books also describe some muscle roles. For the study of applied anatomy, understanding the role of a muscle at any one time is very important.

1.6.4.1 Muscle action

Muscle action is the movement produced (eg flexion, extension) when a muscle activates concentrically (ie shortens due to its tension) in isolation. It is also defined as when a muscle pulls its insertion closer to its origin. The insertion of a muscle is defined to be the moving attachment. In applied anatomy, either or both ends of a muscle may actually move, but in anatomy tables, which were originally deduced from examining cadavers in the anatomical position or *Savasana*

(corpse posture) the insertion is always the distal attachment. By definition, a muscle action will always be the same for any given muscle.

1.6.4.2 Muscle role

The role of any muscle may vary with every movement that is made. The same muscle under different conditions may be working as an:

- **Agonist** if it is the principle muscle producing a movement,
- **Antagonist** if it must relax to allow the desired movement to occur, the antagonist opposes the agonist
- **Neutraliser** when it cancels out unwanted movements that would otherwise be produced by the agonist
- **Synergist** when it works with other muscles to produce a desired effect
- **Fixator** or **stabiliser** when it supports a body part so that another muscle may have a firm base to act on to produce the desired movement.

The balancing of the agonist muscle against its opposing antagonist is integral to the generation of *bandhas* [Section 1.7.3].

1.6.5 Factors Affecting Muscle Function

There are several factors that will alter a muscles function and its ability to perform certain tasks. Some of these factors are fixed for a particular muscle in every situation such as the type of joint [Section 1.6.5.1] or joints the muscle crosses, location of the muscle attachments [Section 1.6.5.2] and the type of muscle attachment [Section 1.6.5.3]. Other factors such as angle of muscle attachment [Section 1.6.5.4], type of muscle activation [Section 1.6.5.5], muscle role [Section 1.6.5.6], exercise type [Section 1.6.5.9] and muscle sufficiency [Section 1.6.5.8] will vary from one situation to the next and even vary through a joint range of movement (ROM).

1.6.5.1 Type of joint

Muscles will behave in different ways depending on what type of joint they are crossing (eg hinge, ball and socket, etc).

1.6.5.2 Location of the muscle attachments

The location of a muscle attachment relative to the joint will affect the lever-like quality of the muscle.
If the attachment is close to the joint then the muscle can act very quickly but it needs to be quite powerful to do so. Such a muscle is referred to as a spurt muscle. If a muscle is relatively distant from a joint then it will be able to move the joint with much greater ease because of the longer lever arm, but it will be slower in doing so. Such a muscle is referred to as a shunt muscle.

1.6.5.3 Type of muscle attachment

A muscle can be attached in many different ways. For example, there may only be one distal attachment or perhaps there are several attachments spread over a wide area.

1.6.5.4 Angle of muscle attachment

The angle of attachment of a muscle is the angle between the body of the muscle or the main line of force from which the muscle generates its contractile (pulling) force, and the central axis of the bone that the muscle is attached to. A change in the angle of attachment can significantly affect how effective the pulling power of that muscle is. If the angle of attachment (angle of pull) is close to 90^0, the pulling power of the muscle will be at its strongest. Conversely, if the angle of attachment (angle of pull) is close to 180^0 the pulling power of the muscle will be at its weakest.

1.6.5.5 Type of muscle activation [Section 1.6.3 & Table 1.3]

The type of muscle activation can either be:
- Isometric (static tension)
- Isotonic concentric (dynamically tensing or pulling while shortening)
- Isotonic eccentric (dynamically tensing or pulling while lengthening)
- Isokinetic (offering maximal resistance or pulling throughout the range of movement (ROM) whether the muscle is shortening, lengthening or staying the same length).

1.6.5.6 Role of a muscle [Section 1.6.4]

Each muscle always has a defined <u>action</u>, which does not change. However, at any one time a muscle will have a role for a particular situation (eg <u>stabiliser</u>, <u>neutraliser</u>, <u>agonist</u>, <u>antagonist</u>) which can vary from one situation to the next.

1.6.5.7 Number of joints crossed by the muscle

When a muscle is said to cross a joint it implies that it can exert a contractile force across that joint or move that joint.
- **<u>Single joint (uni-articular) muscles</u>** are muscles that cross only one joint, eg the elbow flexor <u>biceps brachii</u>.
- **<u>Two joint (bi-articular) muscles</u>** are muscles that cross two joints. For example, <u>biceps femoris</u> (the <u>lateral</u> hamstring muscle) crosses the knee joint and can flex the knee, but it also crosses the hip joint and can extend the hip. Another example is <u>rectus femoris</u> (the main <u>quadriceps</u> muscle), which crosses the knee joint and can extend the knee, but it also crosses the hip joint and can flex the hip.
- **<u>Multi-joint (multi-articular) muscles</u>** are muscles that cross more than one joint. They are economical since they are able to produce motion at more than one joint. Examples of <u>multi-joint muscles</u> are the extensors and flexors of the wrist, hand and fingers, and many of the spinal muscles.

1.6.5.8 Muscle sufficiency

The amount a muscle is lengthened (stretched) or shortened (not stretched) at the time it is <u>activated</u> (generates <u>tension</u>) is referred to as the <u>muscle sufficiency</u>. A muscle cannot adequately perform its role if it is <u>actively insufficient</u>, or if its <u>antagonist</u> is <u>passively insufficient</u>.

- **<u>Active insufficiency</u>** occurs when a muscle is in either a too shortened or too lengthened position to actively generate <u>tension</u>.
- **<u>Passive insufficiency</u>** occurs when a muscle (the <u>antagonist</u>) is to short (stiff) to allow the opposing muscle (the <u>agonist)</u> to act through its full <u>range of movement</u>.

For example, in a hamstring curl such as *niralamba natarajasana* movement may be restricted due to an inability for the shortened <u>hip extensors</u> and <u>knee flexors</u> (eg <u>hamstrings</u>) to generate sufficient <u>tension</u> (<u>active insufficiency</u>) while stiffness in <u>hip flexors</u> and <u>knee extensors</u> at the front of the thigh may prevent the <u>hip extensors</u> and <u>knee flexors</u> from taking the leg very far backwards into the air (<u>passive insufficiency</u>).

Similarly, in *niralamba padangusthasana* movement may be restricted due to <u>passive insufficiency</u> of <u>hip extensors</u> and <u>knee flexors</u> (eg <u>hamstrings</u>) and <u>active insufficiency</u> of <u>hip flexors</u> and <u>knee extensors</u>.

1.6.5.9 Type of joint movement or exercise

1.6.5.9.1 Open-chain (OC) movement or exercises

<u>Open-chain</u> (OC) movement or exercises are where the <u>distal</u> end of a limb is not fixed (ie free to move). Here the <u>origin</u> of a muscle (the part that does not move) is the <u>proximal attachment</u> and the <u>insertion</u> of a muscle (the part that moves) is the <u>distal attachment</u>. The limb is said to be acting in an <u>open kinetic chain</u>. Muscle actions in the tables in these notes (and in most anatomical texts) are described in terms of <u>open-chain</u> movements.

1.6.5.9.2 Closed-chain (CC) movement or exercises

<u>Closed-chain</u> (CC) movement or exercises are where the <u>distal</u> end of a limb or limb segment is fixed (ie attached to the floor or wall etc.). Here the <u>origin</u> of a muscle (the part that does not move) is the <u>distal attachment</u> and the <u>insertion</u> of a muscle (the part that moves) is the <u>proximal attachment</u>. The limb is said to be acting in a <u>closed kinetic chain</u>. Many of the movements in everyday life and during exercise are <u>closed-chain</u> movements or exercises.

1.6.5.9.3 Weight-bearing (WB) exercises

<u>Weight-bearing</u> (WB) exercises are static or dynamic exercises in which a particular limb or body part is taking part or all of the weight of the body and is said to be <u>loaded</u>.
Many but not all <u>weight-bearing</u> exercises are <u>closed-chain</u> exercises.

1.6.5.9.4 Non weight-bearing (NWB) exercises

Non weight-bearing (NWB) exercises are static or dynamic exercises in which a particular limb or body part is taking little or no body weight and is said to be unloaded.

Many but not all non-weight-bearing exercises are open-chain exercises.

1.6.6 Muscle Training

It has been shown that muscle training is quite specific [Carr & Shepherd, 1987]. In other words, a muscle will get good at doing precisely what it practises most. Table 1.4 describes three (3) main factors to consider in muscle training – muscle length, muscle activation type, and exercise type.

Table 1.4 Three different factors that lead to 16 possible states for each muscle [Section 1.6.6]

Muscle Length [Section 1.6.5.8]	Muscle activation type [Section 1.6.3 & 1.6.5.5]	Exercise type [Section 1.6.5.9]
	Relaxed (No muscle activation)	
Shortened (not stretched)	**Isometric** (Static muscle activation)	Open-chain exercise
	Isotonic concentric (Dynamic muscle activation)	
Lengthened (stretched)	**Isotonic eccentric** (Dynamic muscle activation)	Closed-chain exercise

Table 1.5 describes 16 different states of exercise and rest that any muscle may be in.
The most effective exercise includes muscle training in all these different states.

Table 1.5 Sixteen (16) different possible states for each muscle [Section 1.6.6]

	Muscle length	Muscle activation type	Exercise type
1.	Shortened (not stretched)	Relaxed	Closed-chain
2.	Shortened (not stretched)	Relaxed	Open-chain
3.	Shortened (not stretched)	Isometric	Closed-chain
4.	Shortened (not stretched)	Isometric	Open-chain
5.	Shortened (not stretched)	Concentric	Closed-chain
6.	Shortened (not stretched)	Concentric	Open-chain
7.	Shortened (not stretched)	Eccentric	Closed-chain
8.	Shortened (not stretched)	Eccentric	Open-chain
9.	Lengthened (stretched)	Relaxed	Closed-chain
10.	Lengthened (stretched)	Relaxed	Open-chain
11.	Lengthened (stretched)	Isometric	Closed-chain
12.	Lengthened (stretched)	Isometric	Open-chain
13.	Lengthened (stretched)	Concentric	Closed-chain
14.	Lengthened (stretched)	Concentric	Open-chain
15.	Lengthened (stretched)	Eccentric	Closed-chain
16.	Lengthened (stretched)	Eccentric	Open-chain

Additional notes for Tables 1.4 & 1.5

1. **Muscle length**: [Section 1.6.5.8] ie how lengthened (stretched) or shortened (not stretched) the muscle is. If the muscle is too long or too short, it becomes actively insufficient and not able to actively generate tension. For this table, it is assumed that the active muscle activation can only be performed before the muscle becomes actively insufficient. Only two lengths of the muscle (lengthened or shortened) are considered in these tables, but the number of possible lengths is obviously infinite.

2. **Muscle activation type**: [Section 1.6.3 & 1.6.5.5] Is the muscle relaxed (not activated and not generating tension) or activated? If activated, is the muscle tension isometric (static) or isotonic (dynamic/moving)? If isotonic, is the muscle activation concentric (associated with muscle shortening) or eccentric (associated with muscle lengthening)?

3. **Exercise type**:[Section 1.6.5.9], whether open or closed-chain. Hence, the total number of possible states of a muscle in this scenario is 16. (2 lengths states X 4 muscle activation types X 2 (OC or CC) exercise types = 16). Note that weight-bearing and non-weight-bearing [Section 1.6.5.9] are two more factors that could also be taken into account but have not been included here for simplicity.

Special Note: Muscle training is specific therefore yoga practice should be varied, ie muscles have been shown to get good at what they practice. Therefore, to be best trained one's *yoga* practice should include a variety of types of exercises for each muscle or muscle group.

Control over one's body in *hatha yoga* includes being able to bring each of the body's muscles into any of these states at will, as all these states are required to master the vast spectrum of *hatha yoga* postures and exercises.

A complete anatomical understanding of the body helps one to know when and why to exert such muscular control in order to prevent and treat injuries and give maximum benefit to the body.

A useful exercise is to pick a muscle or muscle group eg gluteus maximus (main buttocks muscle and hip extensor), then try and invent or describe and perhaps practice 16 different exercises which would represent the 16 different muscle states.

1.6.7 Working with Muscle Groups in *Hatha Yoga* Postures

IMPORTANT INFORMATION ON HOW TO SIMPLIFY THE APPLIED ANATOMY OF YOGA

Working with muscle groups rather than individual muscles simplifies the study of muscles and allows anatomical theory to be practically applied without having to learn hundreds of muscle names.

When working with musculoskeletal anatomy, it is ideal to know the exact locations and names of the muscles crossing a particular joint. This, however, takes most people hundreds of hours of study. Figures 1.2 and 1.3, at the start of this chapter, as well as the tables of muscle attachments throughout Chapters 2–7 serve as a reference to begin to learn where each muscle specifically attaches.

A simpler approach to learning about muscles considers all the muscles crossing a particular joint, that have the same function at that joint, to be one group. For example, all of the muscles that cross over the hip joint, and which cause hip flexion when they are activated, are called hip flexors. Similarly, all of the muscles which cross over the hip joint, and which cause hip extension when they are activated, are called hip extensors. Figure 1.4 at the start of this chapter shows the approximate regions of each of the bodys main muscle groups.

Since flexion and extension are antagonistic movements, it can therefore be seen that concentric muscle activation of a flexor muscle group, which takes a joint into flexion, will lengthen or stretch the antagonistic extensor muscle group. Similarly, concentric muscle activation of an extensor muscle group leading to joint extension will lengthen or stretch the antagonistic flexor muscle group.

Table A1 in Appendix A shows which muscle groups are actively tensing and which muscle groups are being lengthened or stretched in various *yoga* postures.

1.7 APPLIED ANATOMY & PHYSIOLOGY OF *HATHA YOGA*

Hatha yoga is commonly thought of as a series of static, passive, stretching and relaxation exercises that lead to meditation. It is not often realised that the flexibility *yoga* practitioners often obtain is balanced with musculoskeletal strength.

> In *hatha yoga*, the attributes of strength, flexibility and relaxation are developed concurrently through a practically-applied understanding of the principles of musculoskeletal anatomy and neurophysiology.

In other words, it is not sufficient to merely know how to passively stretch a muscle in a static posture, but one must have a practical understanding of how to activate or tense each muscle throughout its full range of joint motion, whether the muscle is stretched (i.e. in a lengthened state) or not stretched (i.e. in a shortened state). Furthermore, one must be able to control the tension of each muscle while its length is actually changing from short to long, and vice versa, at various speeds [Section 1.7.1].

In addition, the *yoga* practitioner should have a working knowledge of basic neurophysiology. One should have a practical understanding of nerve reflexes in order to be able to use this knowledge to help develop flexibility, strength and relaxation at the same time. Also, one should practically understand the concept of nerve tensioning and be able to safely tension (stretch) the nerves in order to further facilitate improvements in flexibility, strength and relaxation [Section 1.7.2].

When *hatha yoga* postures and exercises are correctly performed, the inherent balance between musculoskeletal strength and flexibility significantly affects the practitioner's neurophysiology. The balance between musculoskeletal strength and flexibility affects nerve reflexes and nerve tensioning (stretching) in a synergistic fashion to produce *bandhas* [Section 1.7.3].

> On a physical level, *hatha yoga bandhas* [Section 1.7.3] reflect the phenomenon of co-activation (simultaneous tensing) of antagonistic (opposing) muscle groups around a joint complex [Section 1.5.3].

1.7.1 *Hatha Yoga*: A Balance Between Strength, Flexibility and Relaxation

The union that is *hatha yoga* is partly in the balance between musculoskeletal strength and flexibility. A very flexible muscle or joint that has little strength may not be able to function properly in everyday life. Similarly, a very strong muscle or joint that is very stiff or immobile may also be unable to function properly in everyday life. If a joint or joint complex is forcibly stretched into an *asana* (*yoga* posture) while the muscles around the joint are passive, there is a risk that the joint may be damaged due to overstretch of the ligaments or joint capsule. If an inexperienced *yoga* practitioner tries to apply muscular tension around a joint after the joint has been placed in a stretched position, then they may have trouble activating either the agonist muscle due to active insufficiency or the antagonist muscle due to passive insufficiency. If a stretched muscle is activated or tensed then this may lead to an increase in the stretch of the muscle via nerve reflexes [Section 1.7.2]. However, there is a chance that tensing a stretched muscle may strain or tear muscle fibres which are trying to shorten while they are already under great tension.

The safest way to apply the principle of strength with flexibility is to commence a stretching posture with the muscles around the joint to be stretched already toned (i.e. in an active state). Although, a stretch initiated with muscular strength may not be as intense as a relaxed muscle stretch, the balance between strength and flexibility will be maintained, and the risk of over-stretching other structures such as ligaments [Section 1.3.2.1.1] and nerves [Section 1.7.2] will be avoided.

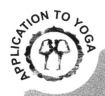

No 1.18 Use your own muscles to enter a posture

A general safety principle of *hatha yoga* is that one should only do the versions of postures that activation of your own muscles can achieve and maintain.

1.7.2 *Nadi Hatha yoga*: Nerve Tensioning and Stimulation of Nerve reflexes

When the practice of *hatha yoga* creates differential regions of pressure within the body [Section 1.0.4], *prana* (the vital force) is made to move along the *nadis*. A *nadi* is a subtle channel of energy found within the body along which moves *prana* and *citta* (consciousness) [Goswami, 1980]. When the body is stretched in a *yoga* practice, it is *nadis* as well as muscles that are stretched. <u>Blood vessels</u> and nerves are examples of gross manifestations of the *nadis* but are not actually the *nadis* themselves.

More subtle *nadis* include the so-called <u>acupuncture meridians</u> of eastern medicine [Motoyama 1993]. Western medicine acknowledges the existence of acupuncture or trigger points which are found along nerve pathways but it is reticent to acknowledge the existence of the acellular flows of energy that the meridians are supposed to represent.

The practice of *hatha yoga* must take into account the presence of *nadis* and in particular, on a gross level the presence of the nerves for two main reasons:

- Nerves have a profound effect on the body if they are impinged and also if they are tensioned (stretched).
- <u>Nerve reflexes</u> can affect the <u>activation</u> or <u>inhibition</u> of <u>muscle groups</u>.

1.7.2.1 Nerve-tensioning

When the *nadis* are stretched a significant proportion of the physical sensation that may be experienced results from nerves being tensioned (stretched). An increased sense of well-being can result if nerves are carefully tensioned. <u>Tensioning</u> (stretching) nerves mobilises and allows them to function more effectively as instigators of <u>muscle activation</u>. However, excessive <u>tensioning</u> or over-stretching may result in nerve damage, pain, or loss of muscle strength or control [Section 9.7.3].

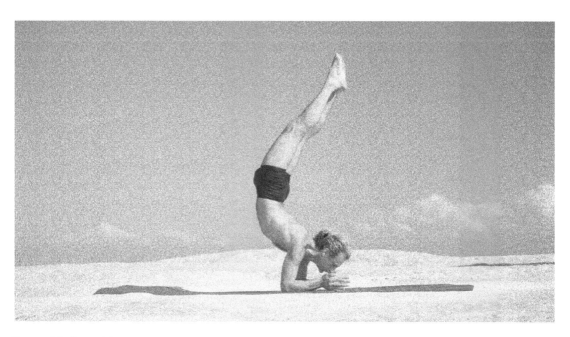

Simon Borg-Olivier with elbow flexion activating elbow extensors, shoulder flexion activating shoulder flexors, and tensioning the vagus nerve, in Sayanasana photo courtesy of Vitoria Borg-Olivier.

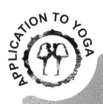

No 1.19 Be aware and apply caution when tensioning (stretching) nerves

Care must be taken when doing the following postures or stretches in order to take into account the possibility of nerves being over-tensioned or (over-stretched):

- *Halasana* (plough pose) may over-stretch and perhaps cause irritation to the nerve roots of the spinal cord.

- *Pascimottanasana* *uttanasana* and all straight-legged forward bends may cause an over-stretch of the <u>sciatic nerve</u> and possibly the <u>spinal cord</u> if the head and neck are in flexed position (i.e. chin brought to the chest) [Section 9.7.3].

- *Supta virasana* , *san calanasana* ,

  kulpha hanumanasana and all stretches of the front of the groin (<u>hip flexors</u>) may cause an over-stretch and perhaps damage to the <u>femoral nerve</u> [Section 9.7.3].

- All postures in which the arms are outstretched and the neck is being moved may cause an over-stretch and perhaps damage to the <u>brachial plexus</u>, the <u>median nerve</u>, <u>radial nerve</u> and <u>ulnar nerve</u> [Sections 3.8 & 9.7.3] [Figures 9.1-9.5].

  These include all postures that <u>tension</u> (stretch) nerves of the <u>brachial plexus</u> [Figures 9.1-9.5]. The <u>radial nerve</u> of the <u>brachial plexus</u> is <u>tensioned</u> in *atanu puritat mudra* [Figure 9.1] which also <u>tensions</u> the <u>large intestine meridian</u>. The <u>median nerve</u> of the <u>brachial plexus</u> is <u>tensioned</u> in *kloman mudra* [Figure 9.2] which also <u>tensions</u> the <u>lung meridian</u>.

  The <u>median nerve</u> is <u>tensioned</u> in *bukka puritat mudra* [Figure 9.3] which also <u>tensions</u> the <u>pericardium meridian</u>. The <u>ulnar nerve</u> of the <u>brachial plexus</u> is <u>tensioned</u> in *buddhizuddhi mudra* [Figure 9.4] which also <u>tensions</u> the <u>heart meridian</u>. The <u>ulnar nerve</u> also <u>tensions</u> *anumukha puritat mudra* [Figure 9.5] which also <u>tensions</u> the <u>small intestine meridian</u>. The names of these *mudras* [Appendix F: Glossary of Sanskrit Terms] relate to the <u>acupuncture meridians</u> which are being <u>tensioned</u> (stretched).

1.7.2.2 Stimulation of nerve reflexes

1.7.2.2.1 Nerve reflexes

A reflex is an automatic response to some types of stimulus. Three (3) reflexes or automatic responses of the nervous system are important to understand in *hatha yoga*.

1.7.2.2.1.1 The myotatic (stretch) reflex

Whenever a muscle is tensioned or stretched, the myotatic (stretch) reflex mechanism is initiated [Alter, 1996]. The myotatic (stretch) reflex can be thought of as a protective mechanism to maintain the homeostasis (the unchanging nature) of the body and prevent any sudden potentially damaging change that an extreme stretch could possibly incur. Stretching a muscle will result in the deformation of receptors called muscle spindles, which send a nerve impulse to the spinal cord. If the nerve impulse is strong enough it will trigger the nerve roots of the spinal cord to transmit an impulse to the stretched muscle that results in reflex muscle activation.

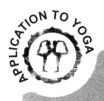

No 1.20 Inhibit the myotatic (stretch) reflex when stretching

The myotatic (stretch) reflex can be inhibited by:
- Moving slowly into a stretch
- Exhaling while moving into a stretch
- Concentrating on the muscle that is being stretched while it is being stretched
- Activating an antagonistic (opposing) muscle or muscle group (reciprocal innervation).

The myotatic (stretch) reflex can be taken advantage of by virtue of its ability to cause the recruitment of adjoining and distant muscles and muscle groups by virtue of the fascial (connective tissue) connections between muscles [Section 1.3.2.1.3].

1.7.2.2.1.2 Reciprocal innervation or reciprocal relaxation

Muscles usually operate as opposing pairs. Generally, when agonist muscles are activating, their opposing muscles, the antagonists, are relaxing. This organisation of co-ordinated and opposing agonist and antagonist muscles is called reciprocal innervation [Alter, 1996] or reciprocal relaxation. At the same time that a muscle receives excitatory impulses that cause it to be activated or tensed, the opposing muscles receive inhibitory impulses that cause it to relax. Reciprocal innervation also takes place when a muscle is stretched and the antagonistic (opposing) muscle is signalled to relax to allow the stretch to take place.

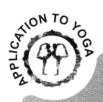

No 1.21 Use the reciprocal reflex to relax muscles being stretched

In order to help relax and stretch the knee flexors (such as the hamstrings at the rear of the thigh) it is useful to activate the knee extensors, by tensing the quadriceps at the front of the thigh.
In order to assist in the relaxation of the shoulder elevators (muscles between the neck and the shoulders), it is useful to activate the shoulder depressors, by tensing the muscles under the armpits.

1.7.2.2.1.3 Autogenic inhibition (inverse myotatic reflex)

When a muscle is stretched, it is initially subject to the myotatic (stretch) reflex [Section 1.7.2.2.1.1]. This will cause that muscle to become activated (i.e. it will generate tension in order to try and shorten as if trying to prevent the stretch). After a certain period of time (about 12-15 seconds) the muscle relaxes, usually before there is a risk of the muscle tearing if it were to remain active. Muscle activity is inhibited by a nervous system reflex signal from the spine (autogenic inhibition), which causes that muscle to subsequently relax. This phenomenon, known as a lengthening reaction is believed to occur after 12–15 seconds if the stretched muscle is initially in a relaxed state. The lengthening reaction is more noticeable however if a muscle is actively tensed while it is being stretched. After the active tension is released the muscle is usually seen to have stretched further.

1.7.2.2.2 Co-activation of muscles and its relationship to *nadis*, *bandhas* and *cakras*

Co-activation is when two antagonistic (opposing) muscle groups are simultaneously tensing and in some way working against each other. If the opposing muscles are activated with equal force, then the joint will be immobile but quite stable. If one muscle is activated more than the antagonistic (opposing) muscle then the joint will be able to move, but there will be some resistance to movement. Recent studies have demonstrated that co-activation is happening in most of the major joints in everyday life, but closed-chain exercises yield a higher incidence of co-activations than open-chain exercises [Hubley-Kozey & Earl, 2000].

Co-activation has a variable effect on the nervous system depending on the individual. In some cases it may result in the activation of all three nerve reflexes mentioned above [Section 1.7.2.2.1]. However, since co-activation is sometimes under voluntary control, all the nerve reflexes may be inhibited. Research studies have shown that during co-activation there is a significant interaction with the nervous system [Proske *et al.*, 2000; Aagaard *et al.*, 2000; Barbeau *et al.* 2000]. However, further research is needed to establish exactly what is taking place in the nervous system both in the co-activations that are generated by everyday life, and also with the voluntary co-activations generated as *bandhas* [Section 1.7.3] by the experienced *yoga* practitioner.

It may be suggested that the co-activations of opposing muscles across joint complexes that form *bandhas* [Section 1.7.3] generates heat energy (*prana*), which is then pushed and pulled along the *nadis* (subtle energy channels) by differential pressure gradients formed by the *bandhas*, to *marmas* (key places) where *cakras* (whirling energy centres) can be activated. Many authors say that *cakras* are related in some way to the nervous system and endocrine system [Saraswati, 1985; Motoyama, 1993]. The relationships between *nadis*, *bandhas* and *cakras* and how they relate to conventional western physiology are discussed in more detail in Section 12.7.

1.7.2.2.3 Stretching and its relation to the nervous system

Several methods of stretching have been described in the literature. Each may be used in a *yoga* practice and in other exercise but always with caution in mind.

- **Ballistic stretching** often involves dynamic bouncing in and out of stretches. It is considered to be dangerous by many authors as it is fast and this is generally not safe to teach in a *yoga* class as there is a risk of tearing muscles due to the myotatic (stretch) reflex activation. However, muscle training is very specific and it has been shown that ballistic stretching is important in the development of dynamic flexibility. An experienced *yoga* practitioner may have the skills to stretch safely with ballistic stretching but it is not recommended for most people.
- **Static stretching** is the opposite of ballistic stretching so the pros and cons of ballistic stretching are reversed here. In static stretches a stretch is moved into slowly and held for some time. Therefore the myotatic (stretch) reflex is inhibited and the inverse myotatic reflex comes into play. However, static stretching does not really prepare one for real life in which the activities tend to be ballistic in nature.
- **Passive stretching** is stretching where the individual makes no contribution to generating the stretching force beyond the weight of his or her own body. This type of stretching requires minimal effort but does not really have any training effect on the muscles, i.e. there is no motor learning effect.
- **Active stretching** [Figures 1.8-1.11] is accomplished by the voluntary use of one's muscles without external aid. Examples of comparisons between active and active-assisted stretches of the hips and spine can be seen in Figures 1.8-1.11.

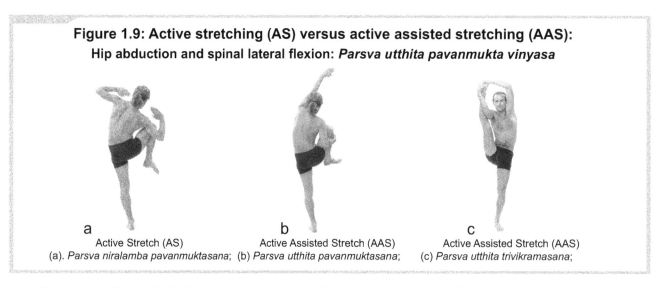

Figure 1.8: Active stretching (AS) versus active assisted stretching (AAS):

Hip flexion and spinal forward flexion: *Utthita pavanmukta vinyasa*

a
Active Stretch (AS)
(a). *Niralamba pavanmuktasana* (AS)

b
Active Assisted Stretch (AAS)
(b) *Utthita pavanmuktasana* (AAS)

c
Active Assisted Stretch (AAS)
(c) *Utthita trivikramasana* (AAS)

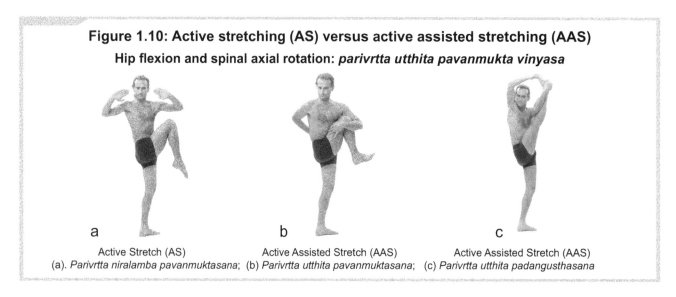

Figure 1.9: Active stretching (AS) versus active assisted stretching (AAS):

Hip abduction and spinal lateral flexion: *Parsva utthita pavanmukta vinyasa*

a
Active Stretch (AS)
(a). *Parsva niralamba pavanmuktasana*;

b
Active Assisted Stretch (AAS)
(b) *Parsva utthita pavanmuktasana*;

c
Active Assisted Stretch (AAS)
(c) *Parsva utthita trivikramasana*;

- **Passive-active stretching** starts as a passive stretch, and is followed by the individual trying to maintain the posture by activating the <u>agonist</u> muscles <u>isometrically</u> for a few seconds. This can strengthen the <u>agonist</u> as it works in a shortened range against a tight <u>antagonist</u>.

Figure 1.10: Active stretching (AS) versus active assisted stretching (AAS)

Hip flexion and spinal axial rotation: *parivrtta utthita pavanmukta vinyasa*

a
Active Stretch (AS)
(a). *Parivrtta niralamba pavanmuktasana*;

b
Active Assisted Stretch (AAS)
(b) *Parivrtta utthita pavanmuktasana*;

c
Active Assisted Stretch (AAS)
(c) *Parivrtta utthita padangusthasana*

- **Active assisted stretching** [Figures 1.8-1.11] is initiated by an individual's own muscle force then supplemented by an external force. This can help strengthen the <u>agonist</u> as it works in against a tight <u>antagonist</u>, and helps to establish a pattern for <u>motor control</u> (muscle control).

Figure 1.11 Active stretching (AS) versus active assisted stretching (AAS)
Hip flexion and spinal forward flexion: *Urdhva mukha pascima vinyasa*

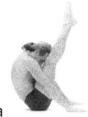 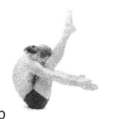 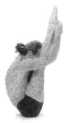

a — Active Stretch (AS)

b — Active Stretch (AS)

(a) & (b) *Niralamba urdhva mukha pascimottanasana (AS)*

c — Active Assisted Stretch (ASS)

(c) *Urdhva mukha pascimottanasana (ASS)*

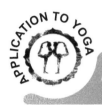

No 1.22 Active stretches are generally safer than passive stretches

Active stretches are a good way of preparing for active-assisted stretches, which are one of the most effective ways to safely develop a balance between strength and flexibility.

1.7.2.2.4 Proprioceptive neuromuscular facilitation (PNF)

Proprioceptive neuromuscular facilitation (PNF) is a method developed in the middle of the 20th Century to increase muscular strength, flexibility and coordination. PNF has been described as a method for promoting the neuromuscular mechanism by the stimulation of proprioceptors (receptors given information about body position). PNF techniques mimic techniques that advanced *yoga* practitioners have always used to increase strength, flexibility and relaxation. It is nevertheless useful to understand the technique and learn how to adapt it and safely teach it to beginner *yoga* students.

1.7.2.2.4.1 Neurological basis of PNF

PNF uses a variety of techniques, which include:

(i)   Facilitatory mechanisms to excite the motor neurons and cause a greater stimulation of muscle activity
(ii) Inhibitory techniques to reduce nervous excitability and muscle activation
(iii) Resistance techniques to get muscles to work effectively throughout their range of joint motion
(iv) Irradiation techniques which recruit synergistic muscles to assist the main muscles to accomplish their task
(v)   Nerve reflexes such as the myotatic (stretch) reflex, the reciprocal reflex and the inverse myotatic reflex [Sections 1.7.2.2.1.1-2]

The two most common techniques associated with the PNF system, and which are regularly used by the advanced *hatha yoga* practitioner (whether they know it or not) involve:

(i)   Activation of an agonist muscle during a stretch to elicit a reciprocal relaxation of the antagonist muscle, and increase the strength of the agonist in a shorted state [Section 1.7.2.2.1.2 Application to *yoga*].
(ii) Activation of an antagonist muscle during a stretch, which strengthens the antagonist in a lengthened state and which appears to increase the stretch of the antagonist muscle perhaps due to the effects of the inverse myotatic reflex [Section 1.7.2.2.1.3 Application to *yoga*] (although recent research makes the real cause as yet unclear).

1.7.3 *Bandha Hatha Yoga*: Co-activation of Opposing Muscle Groups Around Joint complexes

In traditional *hatha yoga*, a *bandha* (from the Sanskrit: meaning to bind or lock) is described as a subtle internal energy lock or grip. *Bandhas* are said to be used to control and guide the energy gathered and generated by the internal body pressures created during *hatha yoga* via the postures, the muscles and the breath [Sections 1.0.4 & 8.4.1].

On a more physical level a *bandha* is the co-activation of opposing muscles [Section 1.7.2.2] around a joint complex [Section 1.5.3] that helps stabilise, strengthen and energise that joint complex. Depending on the type of agonist-antagonist synergy that takes place, a joint will either be compressed or expanded [Section 1.7.3.4] by co-activated opposing muscles that form a *bandha*. Since one of the effects of co-activation and *bandhas* is to help circulate blood and energy around the body, it then follows that one may refer to the *bandha* system as a kind of muscle co-activation pump of blood around the body that is analogous to the musculoskeletal pump.

The formation of *bandhas* throughout the body depends on several important features of musculoskeletal structure and function.

- *Bandhas* are more easily created around joint complexes [Section 1.5.3] rather than simple joints.
- Muscles involved in the physical aspect of *bandhas* can be co-activated around joint complexes because of their tendency to be multi-joint muscles (i.e. they cross and have an effect over several joints) [Section 1.6.5.7].
- Co-activation of opposing muscles across a joint complex may also be promoted by the fascial connections between muscles and by virtue of the myotatic (stretch) reflex that can elicit the activation of muscles adjacent to muscles that have been voluntarily activated [Section 1.3.2.1.3].

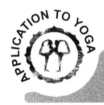

No 1.23 Use *bandhas* (co-activations) to stiffen weak flexible parts of the body in order to access stiff parts of the body

If the *bandhas* are not activated, then when a joint complex such as the lumbar spine joint complex [Section 7.1.5.3] is flexed or extended the stiffest part will be unlikely to bend, while the most flexible part will bend easily and may perhaps become unstable.

Example 1: Backward-bending (spinal extension) postures such as *bhujangasana* (cobra pose)

and *urdhva mukha svanasana* (upward-facing dog pose), tend to bend or stretch the weakest part of the lower back (lumbar spine) and often do not bend or stretch the upper back (thoracic spine). If the abdominal muscles and the deep muscles of the lower back (*mula bandha* [Section 1.7.3.1.1]) are tensed prior to coming into the pose by pulling with the armpit muscles (which tenses the back by activating spinal extensors) and pressing down from the sitting bones (which tenses the front of the body by activating spinal flexors), they can function to stabilise and protect the weakest parts of the lower back (which usually bend easily) and can prevent the lower back from over-stretching and risking possible injury. This allows the possibility for the stiffer parts of the spine to be mobilised (bent or stretched) instead.

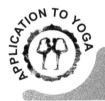

Example 2: Postures that simultaneously bend or stretch the knee and hip, such as *padmasana* (lotus pose), often tend to over-stretch the knee (which is a relatively weak and flexible joint) while often tending to only minimally bend or stretch the hip (which is a relatively stiff and strong joint). If the muscles around the knee (*anu bandha* [Section 1.7.3.2.5]) are tensed prior to coming into the pose, they can function to stabilise and protect the knee (which usually bends easily) and it can prevent the knee from over-stretching and risking possible injury. This allows the possibility for the hip (which tends to be stiffer) to be opened or stretched instead.

1.7.3.1 Central *bandhas*: co-activations of opposing muscles in spinal joint complexes

There are three (3) main or central bandhas. These are essentially co-activations of the opposing muscles of the lumbar, thoracic and cervical spine joint complexes.

In most of the texts on *yoga* only three main *bandhas* are described. These *bandhas* are intimately connected with the strength and stability of the lumbosacrococcygeal spinal joint complex of the lower back (*mula bandha*), the thoracic spine joint complex of the upper back (*uddiyana bandha*), and the cervical spine joint complex of the neck (*jalandhara bandha*). The formation of these three *bandhas* is also integral to the muscular sequence involved with deep or complete breathing [Sections 1.7.3.7, 8.2.8, 8.4.2].

1.7.3.1.1 Mula bandha [Figure 7.10c & Appendix C] [Figure 7.10b & Appendix C]

On a muscular level, *mula bandha* [Sections 7.1.5.3 & 7.5.1.1] is formed when the lumbosacrococcygeal spinal joint complex (lower back) is supported and stabilised by co-activation of antagonistic (opposing) muscle groups around the lumbar spine, sacrum and coccyx. The muscles involved with *mula bandha* include transversus abdominis, obliquus externus abdominis, obliquus internus abdominis and lumbar extensors such as multifidus. Co-activation of antagonistic muscle groups help stabilise and strengthen the lumbar spine in the same manner as that described by the system known as core stabilisation [Richardson & Jull, 1995].

A recent study [Cholewicki *et al.*, 1997] demonstrated that antagonistic trunk flexor-extensor muscle co-activation was present around the neutral spine posture in healthy individuals. This co-activation increased with added mass to the torso. Using a biomechanical model, the co-activation was explained entirely on the basis of the need for the neuromuscular system to provide the mechanical stability to the lumbar spine.

APPLICATION TO YOGA

No 1.24 A complete abdominal exhalation is only possible when the compressive *mula bandha* is firmly established

Mula bandha, in its compressive form, may be learnt by gently tensing the muscles of the perineum and lower abdomen and then making a complete exhalation by gently drawing the navel towards the spine without expanding the chest.

1.7.3.1.2 *Jalandhara bandha*

In a similar manner, *Jalandhara bandha* [Section 7.1.5.1 & 7.5.1.2] is formed when the cervical spine joint complex (neck) is supported and stabilised by co-activation of opposing muscles around these joints. *Jalandhara bandha* is generally formed by bringing the chin down towards the sternum (head flexion), while simultaneously moving the chin inwards towards the throat and the back of the neck (neck extension / retraction).

1.7.3.1.3 *Uddiyana bandha*

Uddiyana bandha [Sections 7.1.5.2 & 7.5.1.3] is formed when the <u>thoracic spine joint complex</u> (upper back) is supported and stabilised by <u>co-activation</u> of opposing muscles around these joints. *Uddiyana bandha* is essentially an expansion of the chest and rib cage due to the combined actions of the external and internal intercostal muscles. This leads to the creation of an expansive force or relatively low pressure that draws air into the <u>lungs</u> and blood up to the <u>heart</u> during an inhalation. *Uddiyana bandha* can also cause the abdominal region to appear to suck inwards when a false inspiration is made in which no air is allowed to enter the nose or mouth but the chest cavity nevertheless is made to expand via the intercostal muscles and also some of the accessory muscles of inspiration.

No 1.25 A complete thoracic inhalation is only possible when the expansive *uddiyana bandha* is firmly established

Uddiyana bandha may be initially learnt by expanding the chest and making a complete inhalation. Later the same muscles can be used to make the same expansion of the chest but without breathing. This generates the classical *uddiyana bandha* as shown above and in Figure 7.9.

1.7.3.2 Peripheral *bandhas*: co-activations of opposing muscles in upper and lower limb joint complexes

There are six (6) peripheral *bandhas*. These are co-activations of the opposing muscles of the main joint complexes of the upper and lower limbs

The concept that *bandhas* are <u>co-activations</u> of opposing muscles can be extended to the major joints of the upper and lower limbs. <u>Co-activation</u> of opposing muscles around <u>joint complexes</u> (*bandha*) provides the strength and stability to safely perform advanced *yoga* postures, and to assist in the flow of energy throughout the body.

Groups of people who practise extreme stretching exercises for a significant period of time without injury, all exhibit <u>co-activation</u> of opposing muscles around each of the major joints while they are stretching. Practitioners of the martial arts [Zehr et al., 1995], gymnastics and even classical ballet are all instructed to, and observed to, maintain <u>muscle tone</u> in their limbs (<u>co-activation</u>) when they perform extreme movements and stretches. This muscular <u>tone</u> is often also clearly visible in advanced *yoga* practitioners who can safely perform the more difficult *asanas*.

Studies on the stability of spinal <u>joint complexes</u>, such as the <u>lumbar spine joint complex</u> [Section 7.1.5.3], have demonstrated that a joint-stabilising effect from the <u>co-activation</u> of opposing muscles of the lower back and <u>abdomen</u> [Richardson & Jull, 1995] can reduce the risk of <u>lumbar</u> spinal injury and help minimise lower back pain. This concept of <u>co-activation</u> of opposing muscles can be expanded to other <u>joint complexes</u>. If a weak region of an upper or lower limb <u>joint complex</u> is not supported by some muscular <u>activation</u> or strength, then when that joint is moved to an extreme position (stretching), the weakest part of the joint will probably be the first part to move and may be the only part of the joint to be stretched at all. Hence, many stretching exercises which are extreme in nature, and which are not supported by some muscular <u>activation</u> or strength, are at risk of damaging joints.

There are numerous research studies available on the phenomenon of <u>co-activation</u> of opposing muscles. <u>Co-activation</u> of opposing muscles has been demonstrated in the <u>ankle joint complex</u> [Hubley-Kozey & Earl, 2000], knee joint complex [Aagaard et al., 2000], shoulder joint complex [Gribble & Ostry, 1998], elbow joint complex [Yamazaki et al., 1995], and wrist joint complex [Smith, 1981]. These studies support the basic concept that joint stabilisation is a result of co-activation of opposing muscles around these joint complexes.

Therefore, the concept or definition of a *bandha* as co-activation of opposing muscles around a joint complex can be extended to all major joint complexes in the body. In the various *yoga* postures and exercises joint *bandhas* are generated around the nine (9) major joint complexes.

> There are nine (9) major *bandhas* within the body. These are co-activations of antagonistic (opposing) muscles of the spine (3) and of the main joint complexes of the upper limb (3) and lower limb (3).

On one level, one can consider *bandhas* to be muscular stabilisers of the nine major joint complexes throughout the body. These nine *bandhas* in their various states and forms are the instigators of pressure gradients that assist in the flow of energy through the body.

The nine (9) types of major joint *bandhas* in the body considered in this book are:

- **Three (3) central or spinal *bandhas*** are related to the neck (cervical spine), upper back (thoracic spine) and lower back (lumbosacrococcygeal spine) regions of the spine respectively [Section 1.7.3.1].
    - *Jalandhara bandha* is formed when the neck joint complex [Section 7.1.5.1] is supported and stabilised by co-activation of opposing muscles around this joint complex.
    - *Uddiyana bandha* is formed when the upper back joint complex [Section 7.1.5.2] is supported and stabilised by co-activation of opposing muscles around this joint complex.
    - *Mula bandha* is formed when the lower back joint complex [Section 7.1.5.3] is supported and stabilised by co-activation of opposing muscles around this joint complex. (Note that here the lower back joint complex includes all the joints from the start of the lumbar spine (T12-L1) to the end of the coccyx including the sacrum and sacroiliac joints. The term lower back joint complex is used in these notes as an abbreviation for the lumbosacrococcygeal spinal joint complex).

- **Three (3) pairs of upper limb peripheral *bandhas*** related to the joint complexes of the shoulders, elbows and wrists respectively.
    1.7.3.2.1 *Amsa bandha*
    Amsa bandha is formed when the shoulder joint complex is supported and stabilised by co-activation of opposing muscles around this joint complex [Section 2.5.1, Figures 2.5, Table C1].
    1.7.3.2.2 *Kurpara bandha*
    Kurpara bandha is formed when the elbow joint complex is supported and stabilised by co-activation of opposing muscles around this joint complex [Section 3.9.1, Figure 3.8, Table C1].
    1.7.3.2.3 *Mani bandha*
    Mani bandha is formed when the wrist joint complex is supported and stabilised by co-activation of opposing muscles around this joint complex [Section 3.9.1, Figure 3.8, Table C1].

- **Three (3) pairs of lower limb peripheral *bandhas*** related to the joint complexes of the hips, knees and ankles respectively.
    1.7.3.2.4 *Kati bandha*
    Kati bandha is formed when the hip joint complex is supported and stabilised by co-activation of opposing muscles around this joint complex [Section 4.5.1, Figure 4.4, Table C1]
    1.7.3.2.5 *Janu bandha*
    Janu bandha is formed when the knee joint complex is supported and stabilised by co-activation of opposing muscles around this joint complex
    1.7.3.2.6 *Kulpha bandha*
    Kulpha bandha is formed when the ankle joint complex is supported and stabilised by co-activation of opposing muscles around this joint complex [Section 6.5.1, Figure 6.8, Table C1] .

The <u>tonic</u> (ongoing) <u>co-activation</u> of opposing muscles around nine major <u>joint complexes</u> can also be observed in the teaching and the advanced practice of other major physical disciplines involving movement and posture such as classical ballet and the martial arts [Alter, 1998]. Interestingly, <u>co-activation</u> has been observed more commonly in Type A personalities than in Type B personalities [Glasscock *et al,.* 1999].

In order to learn the *bandhas* for each joint, there are key *asanas* (*yoga* postures) *mudras* (yogic gestures), and *pranayamas* (*yoga* breathing techniques), which when performed correctly will cause *bandhas* to be automatically generated or formed around that particular joint or <u>joint complex</u>. The main instructions on how to safely perform the *asanas*, *mudras* and/or *pranayamas* required to create the *bandhas* are described and discussed in subsequent chapters. However, they are best learnt from an experienced teacher.

1.7.3.3 A Safe Approach to the use of *Bandhas* in *Yoga* Exercises:

sthira sukham asanam [Patanjali Yoga Sutra II.46; Iyengar, 1993]:
A prudent approach to *yoga asana* practice, with safety in mind, needs to be adopted when working with the *bandhas*. It is always important to practice *yoga* (or any similar exercise) keeping the face, neck and throat relaxed and shoulders generally moving away from the neck towards the hips. Before any major joint or <u>joint complex</u> is bent (flexed, extended etc) in any way, that joint needs to be protected by the stabilising grip of a *bandha*. In other words, do not bend more than just very gently unless you can have a firm muscular grip around the area you are about to bend. Only grip the *bandha* to the extent such that you can keep the face, neck and throat relaxed, and the internal physiology (such as <u>nervous system</u> and <u>blood pressure</u>) comfortable. If any <u>muscle activation</u>, including those related to the *bandhas,* is maintained too strongly or for too long it can lead to a significant increase in <u>blood pressure</u> or an over-stimulation of the nerves, which can be counter-productive and even dangerous.

This concept was clearly stated by the great yogic sage Patanjali [Patanjali Yoga Sutra II.46; Iyengar, 1993] in one of the few sutras mentioned regarding the asanas: *sthira sukham asanam*. Note the significance of the order of the words and their meanings. The sutra says first s*thira*, meaning be firm, or create a *bandha* around the region that is being bent. The sutra then says *sukham*, implying happy or comfortable, or relax the face, neck and throat and do not disturb the internal physiology. Finally, the sutra says *asanam*, or move into the next stage of the pose or exercise. In other words, one should not bend any further unless there is a firmness where it is being bent and yet an overall feeling of comfort. Alternatively, one should only bend a <u>joint complex</u> [Section 1.5.3] beyond one's everyday limits with the application of a *bandha* (<u>co-activation</u> of opposing muscles) around that joint.

1.7.3.4 *Bandha* States: *Ha bandhas* and *Tha bandhas*:

<u>Co-activations</u> of <u>antagonistic</u> (opposing) <u>muscle groups</u> around a <u>joint complex</u> (*bandhas*) are able to generate relatively high or relatively low pressures. Hence one can define two main *bandha* states, which may assist in the understanding of the principles that the *bandha* concept relates.

1.7.3.4.1 *Ha-bandhas* (hot or high pressure *bandhas*)
A *ha-bandha* or hot *bandha* state can be said to have been formed when the <u>co-activation</u> (simultaneous tensing) of <u>antagonistic</u> (opposing) <u>muscle groups</u> around a <u>joint complex</u> leads to the formation of uniform compressive forces (a relatively high pressure) around that <u>joint complex</u>.

Examples of stereotypical *ha-bandhas* include *mula bandha* as it is most typically practised

by tightening the region of the perineum and lower abdomen, and *jalandhara bandha* as it is usually practised with the neck flexors bringing the head into flexion and the neck extensors <u>co-activated</u> to simultaneously bring the neck into extension. *Ha-mula bandha* is able to push energy and matter in the form of blood and air away from the region of the lower trunk. Similarly, *ha-jalandhara bandha* is able to push energy and matter in the form of blood and air away from the region of the head and in so doing can prevent unnecessary pressure reaching the head during certain *kumbhakas* (breath retentions) of *yogic pranayama* (breath-control exercises) .

Two other main *ha-bandhas* involve <u>co-activations</u> of the <u>multi-joint muscles</u> crossing the feet and hands that produce a compressive effect from the fingers and toes:

- *Ha-mani bandha* involves the <u>co-activation</u> of the <u>multi-joint muscles</u> crossing the wrist and hand that activates <u>finger flexors</u> and <u>wrist extensors</u> [Section 3.9.1.2].

- *Ha-kulpha bandha* involves the <u>co-activation</u> of the <u>multi-joint muscles</u> crossing the ankle and foot that activates <u>toe flexors</u> and <u>ankle extensors (dorsi flexors)</u> [Section 6.7.1].

1.7.3.4.2 *Tha-bandhas* (cool or low pressure *bandhas*)

A *tha-bandha* or cool *bandha* state can be said to have been formed when the <u>co-activation</u> of <u>antagonistic</u> (opposing) <u>muscle groups</u> around a <u>joint complex</u> leads to the formation of uniform expansive forces (a relatively low pressure) around that <u>joint complex</u>. *Tha-bandhas* are usually formed when the <u>joint complex</u> involved is in a relatively neutral position or <u>anatomical position</u>.

An example of the stereotypical *tha-bandha* is *uddiyana bandha* as it is practised in its most usual form as an expansion of the chest that sucks the abdomen upwards usually after the breath is held out. *Tha-uddiyana bandha* is able to pull energy and matter in the form of blood and air towards the region of the chest and upper trunk.

Two other main *tha-bandhas* involve <u>co-activations</u> of the <u>multi-joint muscles</u> crossing the feet and hands that produce a stretching effect in fingers and toes:

- *Tha-mani bandha* involves the <u>co-activation</u> of the <u>multi-joint muscles</u> crossing the wrist and hand that activates <u>finger extensors</u> and <u>wrist flexors</u> [Section 3.9.1.2].

- *Tha-kulpha bandha* involves the <u>co-activation</u> of the <u>multi-joint muscles</u> crossing the ankle and foot that activates <u>toe extensors</u> and <u>ankle flexors (plantarflexors)</u> [Section 6.7.1].

1.7.3.5 *Bandha* inter-connectedness

Each *bandha* is in some way affected by the *bandhas* adjacent to it and even those more distant to it. Each *bandha* when formed can help stimulate the generation of *bandhas* adjacent to it, and subsequently onto more distant *bandhas*. Examples of *bandha* inter-connectedness are described below and in subsequent chapters.

Each *bandha* is generally enhanced if the *bandha* of the adjacent <u>joint complexes</u> are also <u>activated</u>. Due to the holistic nature of the body and, in particular, the connections between adjoining <u>muscle groups</u> by virtue of the <u>fascia</u> or <u>connective tissues</u> that cover the muscles and <u>tendons</u>, the <u>activation</u> of one muscle (say as part of one *bandha*) can cause a subtle pulling against an adjoining muscle, which may then be stimulated to undergo a <u>muscle activation</u> by virtue of the <u>myotatic (stretch) reflex</u>. Hence the <u>activation</u> of one *bandha* can enhance, stimulate and/or initiate the <u>activation</u> of an adjacent *bandha*.

1.7.3.6 Counter *bandhas*

When any of the *bandhas* are <u>activated</u>, the <u>tension</u> of the muscles involved needs to be isolated to the region of the *bandhas* only. There is a tendency for the untrained person to inadvertently and unnecessarily tense other muscles when they try and isolate *bandhas*. To counter this problem, one should consciously focus on the regions that inadvertently tense when a *bandha* is gripped and consciously relax those muscles. This conscious relaxation of regions during the process of creating a *bandha* may be termed a counter *bandha*. Counter *bandhas* and the regions they relate to will vary somewhat from person to person, but for most people the following regions tend to become tense when particular *bandhas* are <u>activated</u>.

- The counter-*bandha* for *mula bandha* generally relates to the need to relax the face, neck and throat.
- The counter-*bandha* for *uddiyana bandha* generally relates to the need to relax the shoulders and pull them closer to the hips. Therefore, the counter *bandha* for *uddiyana bandha* is the shoulder *bandha* (*amsa bandha*).

- The counter-*bandha* for *jalandhara bandha* generally relates to the need to relax the jaw as the chin moves down and in towards the throat.

1.7.3.7 Relationship between the *bandhas* and the respiratory system

The three central *bandhas* are intimately related with breathing.

Mula bandha (in its *ha*- form), the root lock that is essentially a compressive co-activation of lower abdominal muscles and lumbar multifidus muscles, is naturally formed with a complete exhalation that draws the navel in towards the spine.

Uddiyana bandha (in its *tha*- form), which is an expansion of the chest and rib cage via the intercostal muscles, is naturally formed during an inspiration, which causes an expansion of the chest. The expansion of the chest corresponding to *uddiyana bandha* is facilitated when an inhalation is begun with the abdominal muscles held in isometric muscle activation (i.e. while holding ha-mula bandha).

Jalandhara bandha (in its *ha*- form when the chin is brought down and into the throat) is important in *yogic* deep breathing to help stimulate the abdominal muscle activation (*mula bandha*) and also to help facilitate the thoracic expansion (*uddiyana bandha*) [Sections 8.2.8 & 8.4.2].

It is important to note that although formation of the three central *bandhas* is integral to the muscular sequence involved with breathing, they are not dependant on taking air into the lungs, i.e. *uddiyana bandha* and *mula bandha* can be made either while inhalation is taking place, after inhale retention or after exhale retention [Table A2], and even during the exhalation [Sections 8.2.8 & 8.4.2].

1.7.4 Increasing Strength, Flexibility and Relaxation with *Hatha Yoga*

Hatha yoga can be thought of as a balance between strength, flexibility and relaxation [Section 1.7.1]. When one has some understanding of nerve tensioning (stretching) and the principles of nerve reflex utilisation as practised in *nadi-hatha yoga* [Section 1.7.2], and when one understands how these concepts can be applied to create the co-activations of antagonistic (opposing) muscle groups used in *bandha-hatha yoga* [Section 1.7.3], then strength and flexibility can both be developed and increased while maintaining a controlled ability to relax.

In most conventional exercise, strength training and flexibility training are practised separately. In *hatha yoga,* however, strength and flexibility develop together in conjunction with joint stabilisation and general relaxation. By working holistically, *hatha yoga* exercises aim to improve performance of functional tasks, while decreasing the effort involved.

Synergistic muscle activations are used in *yoga* exercises to maximise the distance between proximal and distal attachments of the muscle to be stretched. Co-activations of muscles around a joint are engaged in order to help stabilise joints. Static *yoga* postures may utilise isometric muscle activations. Dynamic *yoga* exercises, with varied velocity of movements, help develop concentric and eccentric muscle activity.

Yoga includes many exercises that are weight-bearing or non-weight-bearing [Sections 1.6.5.9.3-4]. on any combination of upper and lower limbs. Hence, *yoga* incorporates both open-chain and closed-chain exercises [Sections 1.6.5.9.1-2]. *Yoga* exercises may require muscles to either generate tension or to relax completely in either a lengthened or shortened state [Section 1.6.6]. Hence, muscles are taught to function through a full joint range of motion (ROM).

Although strengthening, stretching and relaxation are usually inter-linked in *yoga* exercises, it is helpful to outline the main principles to consider for stretching, strengthening, and relaxation. These points will be discussed further in later chapters.

1.7.4.1 Principles of stretching in *yoga*

In order to safely and effectively stretch both muscles and tissues in *hatha yoga*, one must address four main areas. One must (1) establish correct positioning (*asana*), (2) understand nerves (as the physical manifestation of specialised *nadis*), (3) understand muscle co-activations (as the physical manifestation of *bandhas*), and (4) create the proper physiological environment through a combination of breath-control (*Pranayama*) and diet.

1. Establish correct positioning for maximum stretch or <u>tension</u>

- **Stretching muscles**: Establish correct local joint positioning in order to maximise the distance between <u>proximal</u> and <u>distal</u> attachments of individual muscles and <u>muscle groups</u>.
- **Tensioning (Stretching) nerves**: Establish correct whole body positioning (eg. curvature of the <u>spine</u>) in order to maximise <u>neural tensioning</u> (nerve stretching) [Section 1.7.2], especially of those nerves involved with the correct functioning of muscles that are being stretched, strengthened or relaxed [Figures 9.1-9.7].

2. Apply an understanding of <u>nerve reflexes</u>

- Inhibit the stretch or <u>myotatic reflex</u> in the muscles that are being stretched [Section 1.7.2.2.1.1].
- Take advantage of the <u>fascial connections</u> between muscles that can cause an <u>activation</u> of adjacent and distant <u>synergistic</u> muscles as a result of the <u>myotatic (stretch) reflex</u> [Section 1.3.2.1.3].
- Make use of <u>reflex reciprocal inhibition</u> [Section 1.7.2.2.1.2] by activating a muscle or <u>muscle group</u> that opposes the <u>action</u> of the muscle being stretched, in order to reciprocally relax the muscle being stretched (i.e. activate an <u>agonist</u> muscle in order to reciprocally relax the <u>antagonist</u>).
- Make use of <u>inverse myotatic reflex</u> [Section 1.7.2.2.1.3] by activating a muscle when it is already under <u>tension</u> to help stretch, strengthen and (later) relax it further.

3. Use joint *bandhas* to employ a stretch not squash principle

- Where possible create space rather than compression around joints, i.e. do not squash the side of the joint you are moving towards but instead stretch the side of the joint you are moving away from. This can be achieved with the coordinated use of the *bandhas*.
- For example, when raising the chin (i.e. <u>head extension</u>) maintain the length in the <u>cervical spine</u> and in the back of the neck by stretching the front of the neck and not by squashing the back of the neck.

This can be achieved with the *tha-jalandhara bandha* which involves lifting the chin using the <u>head extensors</u> while bringing the throat slightly forward (i.e. <u>neck flexion</u>) with the <u>neck flexors</u>.

4. Create an internal environment that facilitates greater fluidity in the <u>synovial-like fluids</u> around the joints and <u>cartilage</u>, between <u>fascia</u> and muscle, and within the sheaths of <u>tendons</u> and nerves:

- To increase the fluidity of <u>thixotropic</u> <u>synovial-like fluids</u>, use either heat from <u>muscle activations</u>, or use alkalinity generated either temporarily through <u>hyperventilation</u> (breathing more than the body actually needs) or more permanently through long-term change to a more <u>alkaline diet</u> [Section 10.3].
- Protect <u>cartilage</u> by creating heat and/or alkalinity around and within joint spaces in order to increase the fluidity of the <u>synovial fluid</u> and thus lubricate and increase the mobility of the joints [Section 1.3.2.2.3].

1.7.4.2 Principles of strengthening in *yoga*

In order to fully increase strength in the body, one must increase the strength of the bones and the muscles. **Strengthen bones** by applying <u>Wolffs Law</u> [Section 1.3.2.3.5], which states that increases in force through a bone will lead to increased deposition of bone in that area as a result of the force.

- Work towards <u>weight-bearing</u> on all parts of the body
- Generate muscle <u>tension</u> between bones
- Ensure correct alignment in the postures.

Strengthen muscles by applying the basic principles of a training schedule [Section 12.3] incorporated with many variations of basic *yoga asanas* (static postures) and *vinyasas* (dynamic exercises).

- Activate muscles (generate muscle <u>tension</u>) in three different ways
  - (i) Work against gravity using partial or full body weight as resistance
  - (ii) Work against other muscles or other body parts as resistance
  - (iii) Work <u>isometrically</u> against no external resistance (this involves an innate use of joint *bandhas*

eg to make a bulging biceps brachii against no resistance, one must generate a co-activation of triceps brachii with the biceps brachii that is part of *kurpara bandha*) [Section 3.9.1.1].

- Improve neural activation of muscles [Section 12.3.3.]. Often when a muscle is untrained in a particular task it does not fully become activated and cannot generate its maximum tension and strength. Improving neural activation of muscles is essentially training the brain and nervous system to get better at activating all the muscle fibres in the muscle in order to generate maximum tension and strength.
- Improve functional strength. Training is most effective if it is task specific [Carr & Shepherd, 1987], i.e. practice the muscle movement you wish to strengthen.
- Apply an optimal training load. *Asanas* (static postures) and *vinyasas* (dynamic exercises) can be modified where needed to be safer and more accessible or, conversely, more challenging for those who are ready for that.
- Use the appropriate number of repetitions for each *asana* or *vinyasa*, occasionally to the point of fatigue. Increases in muscle strength will not be provoked unless the muscle is exercised to a point where it cannot work as hard any more (fatigue) [Section 12.2.4].

- Utilise five types of muscle activations:
  - (i)   Isometric muscle activations in static postures
  - (ii) Isotonic muscle activations in dynamic exercises (concentric and eccentric)
  - (iii) Synergistic muscle activations
  - (iv) Co-activation of opposing muscles around joints (*bandhas*).
  - (v)   Postural muscle activations (including use of the muscular locks or *bandhas*).

1.7.4.3 Principles of relaxation in *yoga*

In order to fully relax one must address three (3) main areas. One must relax the muscles, the nerves and the brain.

Relax the muscles

- By bringing awareness to the muscles. One needs to feel and/or know where a muscle is before one can learn how to relax it. *Yoga* exercises bring an awareness or sensation to muscles through learning to activate or stretch these muscles in the different body parts.
- By first learning how to activate muscles it is then easier to relax them, i.e. you must be able to turn a muscle on before you are able to turn it off.
- By holding stretches for a reasonable length of time (at least 30 seconds) the myotatic (stretch) reflex can be overcome and the muscle is more able to relax.
- By applying a practical understanding of reflex reciprocal inhibition/relaxation, one is able to consciously relax a muscle, then relax even further by activation of the antagonist muscle.

Relax the nerves

- By knowing the paths of the main nerves and being aware of tensioning (stretching) them [Figures 9.1-9.7].
- By not over-tensioning (over-stretching) the nerves as this leads to their over-stimulation.

Relax the brain

- Relaxing muscles reduces stress. The basic concepts that *yoga* uses to help relax muscles translates to a reduction of stress in the brain.
- By maintaining an awareness of the breath in postures. This gives the brain something tangible to focus on.
- By keeping the face and neck relaxed throughout a *hatha yoga* practice. This can help to reduce the pressure and tension in the head.

- The supine *yoga* relaxation (*savasana*) for 5-15 minutes at the end of each *yoga* practice is important for many people. Recent studies [Bera *et al.*, 1998] have revealed that the effects of physical stress were reversed in significantly shorter time in *savasana*, compared to the resting posture in a chair and a supine posture. In *savasana* the muscles can be fully relaxed if they have been stimulated by either stretch or activation during the practice. However, if the <u>nervous system</u> was over-stimulated during the practice then relaxation will still be difficult. The <u>brain</u> can relax if it has been engaged throughout the practice in the process of either focusing on a particular type of breathing, or feeling the sensations of intelligently organised stretching and activation. If the <u>brain</u> was not engaged in the functioning of the body in the *yoga* exercises then it will be less able to relax and more likely to become either restless or sleepy.

1.8 *YOGA CIKITSA*: *HATHA YOGA* AS A FORM OF THERAPY [Sections 2.5, 3.9, 4.5, 5.6, 6.7, 7.5, 8.4, 9.7, 10.3, 11.4, 12.7]

A very experienced practitioner may be able to use *hatha yoga vidya* (*yogic* science) and *hatha yoga cikitsa* (*yoga* therapy) for specific diagnosis and treatment of musculoskeletal problems and medical conditions. However, this should not be attempted by most people and is beyond the scope of this book. Nevertheless, it is important to have a general idea of what you can do and what you should not do if you or someone you are teaching gets injured while practising yoga (perhaps in your class) or has a musculoskeletal problem or medical condition which is not as a result of yoga.

We have outlined some general principles below that may be applied when there are physical problems. This is an overview of what not to do in certain situations and what may help the healing process in other situations.

In dealing with any injury or illness, the most important thing is to not make things worse. If there is any uncertainty as to the nature of the problem, it is safest to rest the injured part, and if necessary, rest the entire body, then refer the person to a health professional. Never assume that, as the teacher of a class, you have to know how to cure someone.

First, it is important to learn the general principles of injury and healing. When there is some understanding of what is happening in a particular person's body, it becomes relatively safe to work with the holistic principle of improving the health of the body as a whole without really interfering with an injured part. As the overall health improves then the injured part often improves also. Therefore, improving overall level of strength, flexibility, musculoskeletal control and cardiovascular fitness is the first step in the process of more specific *yoga* therapy.

Generally, when dealing with someone who has a musculoskeletal injury or problem one needs consider the following factors:
*   Is the injury <u>acute</u> or <u>chronic</u>?
*   Is the injury <u>irritable</u> or <u>non-irritable</u>?

<u>Irritable conditions</u> are easily stirred up and must be treated very carefully or else they can become very sore after exercise or after a treatment.

<u>Non-irritable conditions</u>, on the other hand can be treated or exercised quite firmly. While they may have a sense of discomfort while exercising or while being treated, the discomfort settles down quickly after the treatment.

1.8.1 Treating Acute Injuries with *Hatha Yoga* [Table 1.6]

An acute problem usually shows the cardinal signs of inflammation [Sections 1.3.3 & 10.2.2.1], and is often quite recent.

The cardinal signs of <u>inflammation</u> usually seen in <u>acute</u> conditions are:

(i)   **Redness**
(ii)   **Pain**

(iii) **Heat**
(iv) **Swelling** and sometimes
(v) **Loss of function**

Acute conditions are usually treated in medical circles with the **R.I.C.E. principle** (**Rest**, **Ice**, **Compression** and **Elevation**).

If a musculoskeletal problem is acute in nature, it is usually best to rest the injured part, or if necessary, rest the entire body.

Hatha yoga can be still be practised in this situation if the problem area can be suitably bypassed and allowed to rest. Postures need to be suitably modified and a greater emphasis made towards a gentle more relaxed practice that does not generate too much excess heat.

Table 1.6 Treatment of acute injuries: Medical treatment versus *hatha yoga* therapy [Section 1.8.1]

MEDICAL TREATMENT OF ACUTE INJURIES (R.I.C.E.)	TREATMENT OF ACUTE INJURIES WITH *HATHA YOGA* [Section 1.8.1]
Rest	Rest injured part & keep working with the rest of the body (Or rest the whole body if necessary)
Ice	Do not generate excess heat with practice (Do a gentle *hatha yoga asana* & *vinyasa* practice)
Compression	Gentle isometric co-activations (*bandhas*) around a joint (Activate joint *bandhas* if possible and if appropriate)
Elevation	Inverted or semi inverted postures (*Viparita Karani*)

1.8.2 Treating Chronic Injuries with *Hatha Yoga* [Table 1.7]

Chronic injuries are usually long-standing injuries where the inflammation has subsided.

*   Chronic musculoskeletal injuries or conditions may be cautiously approached with the following general methodology [Table 1.7], when there are no signs of inflammation.
*   When there are no contraindications, one can use *hatha yoga* postures and exercises, breathing exercises, and relaxation to give general and specific improvements in circulation, strength, flexibility, and musculoskeletal alignment.

To improve circulation [Section 8.4.1] use:
*   **Breathing techniques** (*Pranayama*) to utilise the respiratory pump of circulation.
*   **Dynamic exercises** (*Vinyasa*), activating and relaxing muscles during movement to utilise the musculoskeletal pump [Section 1.0.4] of circulation and varying the speed of movements to utilise the centripetal pump of circulation [Section 1.0.4].
*   **Inverted and semi inverted postures** (*Viparita Karani*) to utilise the Gravitational pump of circulation [Section 1.0.4].
*   **Static postures** (*Asanas*), creating regions of relative high pressure (compression and/or isometric muscle activation) and relative low pressure (stretching and/or muscle relaxation) to utilise the postural pump of circulation [Section 1.0.4].
*   **Co-activation of opposing muscles around joints** (*Bandhas*) to utilise the muscle co-activation pump of circulation [Section 1.0.4].

To improve strength [Section 1.7.1.2] develop:
- **Muscle control**: develop the ability to fully relax or turn off a muscle and then smoothly activate or turn on a muscle to its maximum level of <u>muscle activation</u> in any of its states [Tables 1.4 & 1.5].
- **Muscle balance**: develop muscle symmetry and learn how to <u>co-activate</u> muscles for increased joint stability
    - **Symmetry**: restore and/or develop balance between:
        - Left side and right side of the body
        - <u>Agonist</u> and <u>antagonist</u> muscle groups
        - Anterior and <u>posterior</u>, <u>medial</u> and <u>lateral</u>, and <u>superior</u> and inferior musculature.
    - **Muscle <u>co-activation</u>**: develop the ability to <u>co-activate</u> (simultaneously tense) <u>agonist</u> and <u>antagonist</u> <u>muscle groups</u> for increased joint stability (*bandhas*) [Sections 1.7.3, 2.5.1, 3.9.1, 4.5.1, 5.6.1, 6.6.1, & 7.5].
- **Muscle specificity**: To develop functional task specificity:
    - Use <u>isometric</u>, <u>isotonic</u> and <u>isokinetic</u> exercises
    - Use varied velocities of joint movement
    - Move joints through their full <u>range of motion</u> (ROM)
    - Use <u>weight-bearing (WB) exercises</u> and <u>non-weight-bearing (NWB) exercises</u>
    - Use <u>open-chain (OC) exercises</u> and <u>closed-chain (CC) exercises</u>

To improve flexibility [Section 1.7.1.1, Chapters 1 – 7]
Develop:
- Joint mobility: ie develop ease of joint movement not just the ability to stretch further.
- Symmetry of flexibility: both inter-joint, ie between right and left sides of the body; and intra-joint (ie <u>superior</u> and <u>inferior</u>, <u>medial</u> and <u>lateral</u>, and <u>anterior</u> and <u>posterior</u>).

To improve musculoskeletal alignment [Chapters 1 – 7]
Work towards restoring and or developing normal:
- Joint structure
- Joint space
- Joint symmetry: both inter-joint, ie between right and left sides of the body; and intra-joint (ie <u>superior</u> and <u>inferior</u>, <u>medial</u> and <u>lateral</u>, and <u>anterior</u> and <u>posterior</u>).

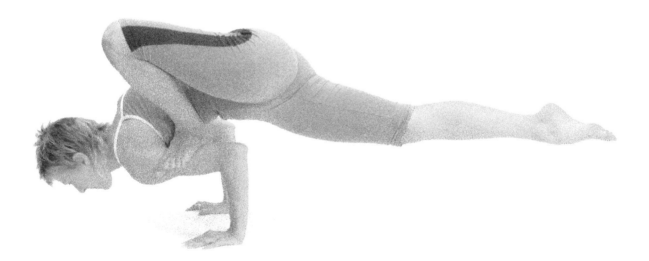

Bianca Machliss with spine flexed, left hip extended, right hip flexed, shoulders protracted, elbows flexed and wrists extended in *Urdhva Yoga Dandasana*. Photo courtesy of Alejandro Rolandi.

Table 1.7 Treatment of chronic injuries with *hatha yoga* [Section 1.8.2]

For Chronic Injuries	Method	
Improve Circulation	By using	
	1. *Pranayama*	= Breathing exercises [Section 1.0.4] **Respiratory pump**
	2. *Vinyasa*	= Dynamic exercises **Musculoskeletal pump & Centripetal pump** [Section 1.0.4]
	3. *Viparita karani*	= Inverted postures **Gravitational pump** [Section 1.0.4]
	4. *Asanas*	= Static postures **Postural pump** [Section 1.0.4]
	5. *Bandhas*	= co-activation of antagonistic (opposing) muscle groups around a joint complex **Muscle co-activation pump** [Section 1.0.4]
Improve Strength	By focusing on	
	1. **Control**	to be able to voluntarily activate or relax any muscle to a desired amount
	2. **Balance**	symmetry & co-activation
	3. **Specificity**	functional task specificity
Improve Flexibility	By focusing on	
	1. **Mobility**	of joints, muscles, nerves etc.
	2. **Symmetry**	equal flexibility on both sides of the body
Improve Alignment	By focusing on	
	1. **Structure**	of each joint
	2. **Space**	within each joint
	3. **Symmetry**	between both sides of a joint & both sides of the body

****

Chapter Breakdown

****

2.0 INTRODUCTION TO THE APPLIED ANATOMY OF THE SHOULDER JOINT COMPLEX IN *HATHA YOGA* POSTURES

In this chapter the bones, muscles, nerves and other tissues of the shoulder joint complex [Section 2.2.0] are examined. This information is then used to understand and apply the associated internal *yogic* lock, *amsa bandha* [Section 2.5.1], which is created by co-activation of opposing muscles crossing the shoulder joint complex.

The shoulder is a unique region of the body that has the versatility to manipulate objects in everyday life via the actions of the hand, but also has the strength to be weight-bearing in exercises such as *hatha yoga*. The shoulder has a tendency to become stiff, especially between the scapula or shoulder blade and the thorax or rib cage (the scapulothoracic joint); while often becoming loose and weak especially around the shallow ball and socket (glenohumeral) joint at the proximal ends of the humerus (upper arm bone). How the shoulder is best used in a *hatha yoga* practice in order to develop and maintain an appropriate balance between shoulder strength and flexibility is described and discussed. The balance between shoulder strength and flexibility can keep the shoulder functional both in a *yoga* practice and in daily life, and keep the shoulder safe from injury. The management of existing shoulder injuries and how to work towards healing them is discussed at the end of this chapter. How the shoulder can affect the functioning of other parts of the body is also described and discussed.

In *hatha yoga vidya* (the science of *hatha yoga*), the shoulder and upper limb are considered the organs of action for the upper back and the thoracic spine, the neck and the cervical spine, the heart and the lungs. Appropriate use of the muscles of the scapula (shoulder blade) and humerus (upper arm bone) in a *yoga* practice is the key to self-mobilisation (self-massage) of the upper back and the thoracic spine, as well as the neck and the cervical spine.

Correct use of the muscles of the shoulder joint complex is integral to learning how to move the ribs and thoracic vertebrae in order to expand the chest cavity. This helps create the important internal yogic

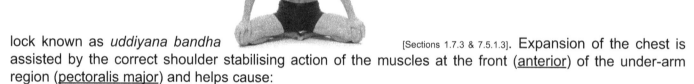

lock known as *uddiyana bandha* 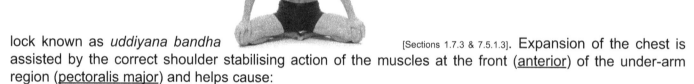 [Sections 1.7.3 & 7.5.1.3]. Expansion of the chest is assisted by the correct shoulder stabilising action of the muscles at the front (anterior) of the under-arm region (pectoralis major) and helps cause:

*   Reduction of pressure in the chest, which enhances the movement of blood into the heart, thereby promoting more efficient circulation
*   Movement of air into the uppermost and hardest to access regions of the lungs, thus further improving the oxygenation of all the bodys cells and the movement of *prana* (vital energy) throughout the body

Correct use of the muscles of the shoulder joint complex is integral in learning how to relax the neck muscles and the shoulder elevator muscles. This helps create the important internal yogic lock known as

jalandhara bandha 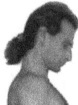 [Sections 1.7.3 & 7.5.1.2].

Correct use of the muscles of the <u>shoulder joint complex</u> is integral to learning how to firm the lower abdomen and help create the important internal yogic lock known as *mula bandha* [Sections 1.7.3 & 7.5.1.1]. Activation of the lower abdominal muscles is assisted by the correct shoulder stabilising action of the muscles at the rear (posterior) of the underarm region (<u>latissimus dorsi</u>) and helps cause:

- Stabilisation of the lower back (<u>lumbar spine</u>) which helps minimise the risk of injury and helps in the management and healing of people with lower back pain
- Increased abdominal strength and thus the ability to do a higher intensity of work in daily life and safely conduct a more intense *yoga* practice
- Improved exhalations, which allows greater elimination of wastes and stored toxins and improves the quality of inhalation
- Increased heat in the body that leads to a temporary increase in joint flexibility

Mastering control of the muscles at the rear (posterior) of the underarm region (<u>latissimus dorsi</u>) in all *yoga* postures is integral to learning how to connect the upper body to the lower body and create a tangible muscle union (*yoga*) between one's arms and one's legs. This is because <u>latissimus dorsi</u> is the only muscle that directly connects the upper and lower limbs.

Mastery of the use of the shoulders, in particular learning to control the movements of the <u>scapula</u> (shoulder blade) and <u>humerus</u> (upper arm bone) is the key to understanding how to gather energy rather than expend energy in one's *yoga* practice. This is partly due to two main reasons:

(i) Correct shoulder stabilisation work (*amsa bandha*) [Section 2.5] can assist in the activation of the 3 central *bandhas* as described above; and

(ii) The ability to control shoulder movements enables stimulation of the *nadis* (the subtle channels that carry the *prana* or vital energy) that we breathe in and absorb into our systems from the environment). This can be felt in a practical and tangible way when one tensions (stretches) the nerves of neck and upper arm (which encompasses related *nadis* and their *prana* in the form of electro-chemical energy) [Section 3.8, 3.9 & 9.7.3].

2.1 BONES OF THE SHOULDER JOINT COMPLEX [Figures 2.1 - 2.4]

The bones of the shoulder and upper limb are the <u>clavicle</u> (collar bone), <u>scapula</u> (shoulder blade) and <u>humerus</u> (upper arm bone) [Figures 2.1 - 2.4].

2.1.1 Clavicle
The <u>clavicle</u> (collar bone) connects the upper limb to the axial skeleton at the <u>sternum</u>. The <u>clavicle</u> has a crank shape, and it acts as a strut to hold the upper limb free from the trunk. The <u>clavicle</u> is the most commonly fractured bone in the body.

2.1.2 Scapula
The <u>scapula</u> connects the <u>clavicle</u> (collar bone) to the <u>humerus</u> (upper arm bone). It is the mobile base of the shoulder girdle. The <u>scapula</u> rests on the posterior upper thorax (back ribs).

The following features of the <u>clavicle</u> can be seen on a skeleton and identified with the help of Figures 2.1 - 2.4:
- Sternal end, <u>scapula</u> end, the crank shape
- **Posterior scapula:** <u>spine of scapula</u>, <u>acromion</u>, <u>supraspinous fossa</u>, <u>infraspinous fossa</u>, inferior and superior angles, medial border, lateral border
- **Anterior scapula:** <u>coracoid process</u>, <u>sub-scapula fossa</u>, inferior angle, medial border
- **Lateral:** <u>glenoid fossa</u> (the socket of the shoulders ball and socket joint)

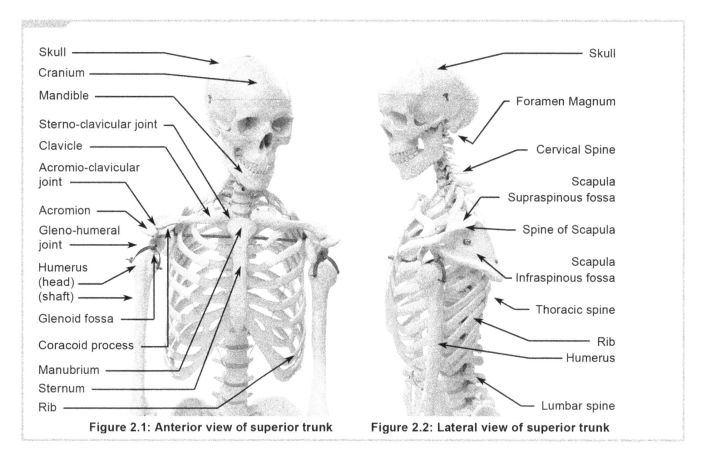

Skull

Cranium

Mandible

Sterno-clavicular joint

Clavicle

Acromio-clavicular joint

Acromion

Gleno-humeral joint

Humerus (head) (shaft)

Glenoid fossa

Coracoid process

Manubrium

Sternum

Rib

Skull

Foramen Magnum

Cervical Spine

Scapula Supraspinous fossa

Spine of Scapula

Scapula Infraspinous fossa

Thoracic spine

Rib

Humerus

Lumbar spine

Figure 2.1: Anterior view of superior trunk   **Figure 2.2: Lateral view of superior trunk**

2.1.3 Humerus

The humerus is the bone of the upper arm, which joins to the glenoid fossa (socket) of the scapula (shoulder blade). The humerus is the largest bone in the upper limb (UL).

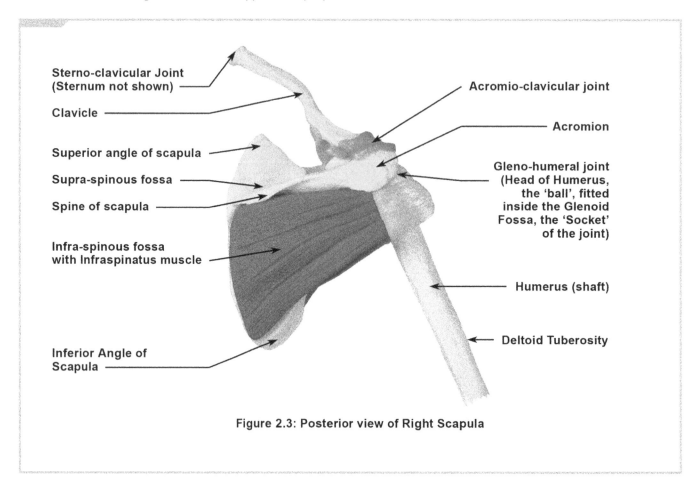

Sterno-clavicular Joint (Sternum not shown)

Clavicle

Superior angle of scapula

Supra-spinous fossa

Spine of scapula

Infra-spinous fossa with Infraspinatus muscle

Inferior Angle of Scapula

Acromio-clavicular joint

Acromion

Gleno-humeral joint (Head of Humerus, the 'ball', fitted inside the Glenoid Fossa, the 'Socket' of the joint)

Humerus (shaft)

Deltoid Tuberosity

Figure 2.3: Posterior view of Right Scapula

The following features of the humerus can be seen on a skeleton and identified with the help of Figures 2.1 - 2.4:
- **Proximal Humerus**: head, greater (lateral) and lesser (medial) tubercles, bicipital (inter tubercular) groove, anatomical and surgical necks, Deltoid tuberosity
- **Distal Humerus**: body/shaft, medial and lateral epicondyles

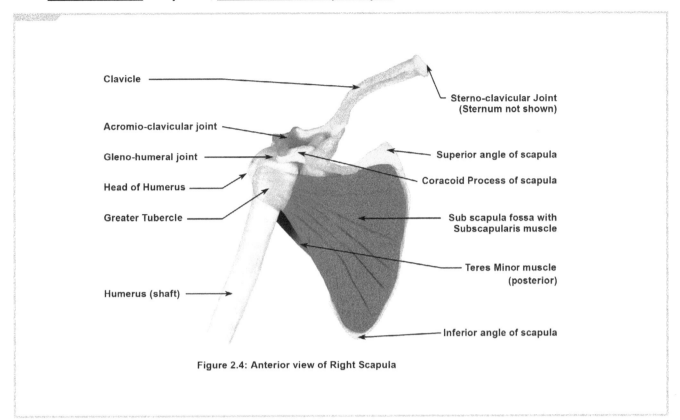

Figure 2.4: Anterior view of Right Scapula

2.2 JOINTS OF THE SHOULDER COMPLEX

The upper limb is the organ of manual activity. In the shoulder, stability is sacrificed to increase mobility.

2.2.0 The Shoulder Joint complex

There are four joints, which affect the shoulder, which we can define as the shoulder joint complex. These joints are:
- Sternoclavicular (SC) joint [Section 2.2.1]
- Acromioclavicular (AC) joint [Section 2.2.2]
- Scapulothoracic (ST) joint [Section 2.2.3]
- Glenohumeral (GH) joint [Section 2.2.4]

These four joints are considered to be a joint complex as they move and function together to achieve movements of the upper limb. In addition, many of the muscles of this region are multi-articular [Section 1.6.5.7], i.e. they act over several joints.

2.2.1 Sternoclavicular (SC) Joint

2.2.1.1 Classification of the sternoclavicular joint

The sternoclavicular (SC) joint [Figures 2.1 – 2.4] is classified as a synovial, sellar, bi-axial and complex joint. The sterno-clavicular (SC) joint:
- Is a very stable joint which joins the upper limb and pectoral (shoulder) girdle to the axial skeleton,
- Contains an articular disc.

2.2.1.2 Ligaments of the sternoclavicular joint
The main ligaments of the sternoclavicular joint are:
- **Sternoclavicular ligaments** (anterior and posterior), which join the sternum and clavicle,
- **Costoclavicular ligament**, which join the ribs and the clavicle.

2.2.2 Acromioclavicular (AC) Joint

2.2.2.1 Classification of the acromioclavicular (AC) joint

The acromioclavicular (AC) joint [Figures 2.1 – 2.4] is classified as a synovial, plane, multiaxial and complex joint. The acromioclavicular (AC) joint:

- Has a weak joint capsule,
- Has an articular disc,
- Is commonly dislocated in many sports.

2.2.2.2 Ligaments of the acromioclavicular (AC) joint

The main ligaments of the acromioclavicular joints are:

- Coracoclavicular ligament, which joins the coracoid process of the scapula with the clavicle
- Acromioclavicular ligament, which joins the acromion process of the scapula with the distal end of the clavicle
- Coracoacromial ligament, which joins the coracoid process of the scapula with the acromion process of the scapula.

2.2.3 Scapulothoracic (ST) joint

2.2.3.1 Classification of the scapulothoracic (ST) joint

The scapulothoracic joint [Figures 2.1 – 2.4] is not classified as a true joint; however, the gliding movements of the scapula (shoulder blade) over the rib cage (thorax) are very important as these movements involve the acromioclavicular (AC) and sternoclavicular (SC) joints.

2.2.3.2 Ligaments of the scapulothoracic (ST) joint

There are no ligaments between the scapula and the thorax.

2.2.3.3 Movements of the scapulothoracic (ST) joint [Table 2.2]

There are three pairs of primary movements of the scapulothoracic joint. Note that each pair has movements in opposite directions. These are:

- **Elevation** and **depression** (i.e. up and down respectively),
- **Protraction** (abduction) and **retraction** (adduction) (i.e. moving outwards away from the spine, and inwards towards the spine respectively),
- **External rotation** (lateral rotation) and **internal rotation** (medial rotation) (i.e. the inferior angle of the scapula turning outwards away from the spine, and inwards towards the spine respectively).

APPLICATION TO YOGA

No 2.1 **Keep scapula and thorax close in most weight-bearing arm-balancing postures for adequate force transfer between trunk and upper limb**

To allow complete range of motion (ROM) of the arm, and to allow adequate force transfer between the upper limb and the trunk, the scapula (shoulder blade) must be free to move in all three directions, while remaining firmly attached to the thorax (rib cage).

One of the best postures that trains the scapula to remain close to the thorax is the plank

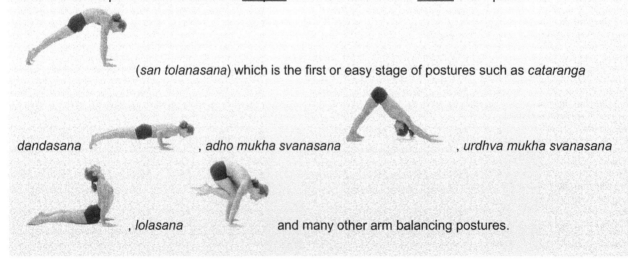

(*san tolanasana*) which is the first or easy stage of postures such as *cataranga*

dandasana , *adho mukha svanasana* , *urdhva mukha svanasana*

, *lolasana* and many other arm balancing postures.

2.2.4 Glenohumeral (GH) Joint

2.2.4.1 Classification of the glenohumeral (GH) joint

The glenohumeral (GH) joint [Figures 2.1 – 2.4] is classified as a synovial, ball and socket, multiaxial, and simple joint. The glenohumeral (GH) joint:

- Has articular surfaces covered in hyaline cartilage,
- Joins the glenoid fossa and head of humerus, and
- Has a joint capsule that is relatively thin and loose, and is weakest inferiorly.

2.2.4.2 Ligaments of the glenohumeral (GH) joint

The main ligaments of the glenohumeral joint are:

- The glenohumeral ligament, which joins the humerus to the glenoid fossa (the socket of the glenohumeral joint);
- The transverse humeral ligament, which traverses the bicipital groove at the head of the humerus in which the long head of the biceps brachii sits; and
- The coracohumeral ligament, which joins the coracoid process of the scapula to the humerus.

2.2.4.3 Bursae of the glenohumeral (GH) joint

The glenohumeral (GH) joint has two bursae (fluid filled sacs):

- The sub-acromial bursa separates the supraspinatus muscle from the acromion process of the scapula and the deltoid muscle; and
- The sub-scapula bursa

2.2.4.4 Movements of the glenohumeral joint

There are three pairs of primary movements of the glenohumeral joint [Table 2.3]. Note that each pair has movements in two opposite directions. These are:

- **Flexion** and **extension** (i.e. the humerus moving anteriorly away from the trunk towards the ears, and the humerus moving posteriorly away from the trunk respectively);
- **Abduction** and **adduction** (i.e. the humerus moving away from the trunk, and towards the trunk respectively); and
- **External rotation** (lateral rotation) and **internal rotation** (medial rotation) (i.e. from anatomical position the anterior humerus turning outwards away from the trunk, and the anterior humerus turning inwards towards the trunk respectively).

There are eight (= 2^3) possible **combined movements** of the glenohumeral (GH) component of the shoulder joint complex.

The articular surfaces of the glenohumeral (GH) joint can move in three ways, spin, slide and roll.

- **Spin** of the glenohumeral (GH) joint is where the head of the humerus turns around the longitudinal axis of the humerus to produce internal rotation or external rotation of the GH joint
- **Slide** of the glenohumeral (GH) joint is where the head of the humerus normally slides posteriorly in the glenoid fossa (socket) during GH flexion and slides anteriorly during GH extension.
- **Roll** of the glenohumeral (GH) joint is where the head of the humerus normally rolls anteriorly in the glenoid fossa (socket) during GH flexion and rolls posteriorly during GH extension.

Movement of the humerus is a combination of spin, slide and roll to prevent impingement of the humerus against the sides of the glenoid fossa or the inferior surface of the acromion process of the scapula.

Concave-convex rule

The concave-convex rule can be helpful if a joint is not functioning correctly and one needs to know how it should normally be moving.

For any synovial joint, if the moving surface is:

- **Convex** then the slide and roll are in **opposite** directions
- **Concave** then the slide and roll are in the **same** direction

2.2.4.5 Stability of the glenohumeral (GH) joint

- Due to large ROM there is decreased stability at the GH joint.
- The rotator cuff muscles hold the head of the humerus in place.
- The GH joint capsule is thin and loose and supported by the glenoid labrum.

- Inferior dislocation is common as there is no inferior support for the <u>humerus</u>.
- The position that is most likely to lead to GH dislocation involves both <u>abduction</u> and <u>external rotation</u>.

No 2.2 The eight possible combined movements of the glenohumeral (GH) component of the shoulder joint complex are all used in various *yoga asanas*

For example:

1. <u>Flexion</u>, <u>external rotation</u> (GH) and <u>adduction</u>: *urdhva namaskara mudra* (arms above head in prayer position) *adho mukha svanasana* (downward-facing dog pose);

2. <u>Flexion</u>, <u>external rotation</u> (GH) and <u>abduction</u>: *parsva virabhadrasana* (or standing with legs and arms wide), *trikonasana* (raised arm of triangle pose);

3. <u>Flexion</u>, <u>internal rotation</u> (GH) and <u>adduction</u>: *urdhva baddanguliyasana* (arms interlocked above head with palms facing up as in *parivatasana*), *urdhva hastasana* (arms above head facing away from each other);

4. <u>Flexion</u>, <u>internal rotation</u> (GH) and <u>abduction</u>: *Atanu puritat mudra* [Figure 9.1] (A radial nerve tensioning and a stretch of the large intestine meridian),

5. <u>Extension</u> and <u>external rotation</u> (GH) and <u>adduction</u>: *urdhva mukha svanasana* Appendix a];

6. Extension, external rotation (GH) and abduction: *ustrasana* 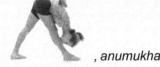 (with hands pointing backwards), *kloman mudra* [Figure 9.2] (a median nerve tensioning and a stretch of the lung meridian), *bukka puritat mudra* [Figure 9.3] (a median nerve tensioning and a stretch of the pericardium meridian), and *buddhizuddhi mudra* [Figure 9.4] (an ulnar nerve tensioning and a stretch of the heart meridian);

7. Extension and internal rotation (GH) and adduction: *namaskara parsvottanasana* 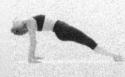, *anumukha puritat mudra* 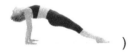 [Figure 9.5] (An ulnar nerve tensioning);

8. Extension and internal rotation (GH) and abduction: *purvottanasana* 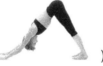 [Appendix A];

Many other possible movements exist which are intermediate between two extreme positions, for example in many standing positions eg *parsva virabhadrasana* [Appendix A] the arms are abducted but are neither flexed nor extended but somewhat neutral.

2.2.4.6 Combined movements of the shoulder joint complex

There is a large number of possible combined movements of the shoulder joint complex (i.e. combinations of glenohumeral (GH) joint movements and scapulothoracic (ST) joint movements). The following are some sets of combined movements and examples of postures which use these movements:

- Protraction (ST), depression (ST), flexion (GH), adduction (GH) and external rotation (GH)

  (eg *adho mukha svanasana*).
- Retraction (ST), depression (ST), extension (GH), internal rotation (GH) and adduction (GH)

  (eg *purvottanasana*)
- Protraction (ST), depression (ST), abduction (GH) and extension (GH) and external rotation (GH), as in *kloman mudra* (a median nerve tensioning and a stretch of the lung meridian), *bukka puritat mudra* (a median nerve tensioning and a stretch of the pericardium meridian), and *buddhizuddhi mudra* [Figures 9.3 & 9.4] (an ulnar nerve tensioning and a stretch of the heart meridian).

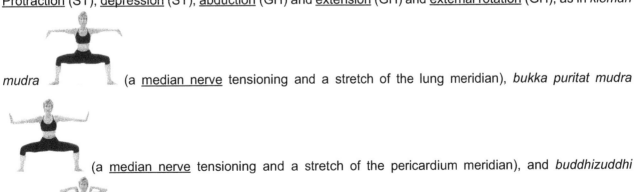

2.3 MUSCLES OF THE SHOULDER JOINT COMPLEX

The shoulder girdle includes the scapula (shoulder blade) and the clavicle (collar bone). Muscles of the shoulder girdle can be classified into three groups, as listed below [Sections 2.3.1, 2.3.2 & 2.3.3], and described in detail in Table form [Tables 2.1, 2.2, 2.3 & 2.4].

2.3.1 Muscles Connecting the Axial Skeleton and the Humerus

Muscles connecting the axial skeleton (ribcage and spine) to the humerus (upper arm bone) are:

• Pectoralis major (sternal head)	= Front under-arm muscle
• Latissimus dorsi	= Rear under-arm muscle

These two muscles are very important since they also affect the movements of the scapula and therefore affect shoulder stabilisation and the spine. In *yoga* classes, they are often referred to as the underarm muscles to describe them by their location to the layperson unfamiliar with anatomy.

2.3.2 Muscles Connecting the Axial Skeleton and the Shoulder Girdle

Muscles connecting axial skeleton (rib cage and spine) to shoulder girdle (scapula and clavicle) are:

• Trapezius	Located between the shoulder blades
• Rhomboid major	Located between the shoulder blades
• Rhomboid minor	Located between the shoulder blades
• Levator scapulae	Located between the sides of the neck and shoulder blades
• Pectoralis minor	A minor shoulder protractor
• Serratus anterior	The boxers muscle, a main protractor muscle
• Subclavius	

2.3.3 Muscles Connecting the Shoulder Girdle and the Humerus

Muscles connecting shoulder girdle (scapula and clavicle) to humerus (upper arm bone) are:

• Pectoralis major (clavicular head)	Important shoulder flexor at the front of shoulder
• Deltoid	Located at the top and side of the shoulder
• Coracobrachialis	
• Teres major	
• 4 Rotator cuff muscles [Section 2.3.6]	

2.3.4 Muscles of the Shoulder Joint complex: Scapulothoracic (ST) Component

The attachments and actions of muscles of the scapulothoracic (ST) component of the shoulder joint complex are shown in Figures 2.3 - 2.6 and in Table 2.1.

Table 2.1 Muscles of the shoulder joint complex (including the scapulothoracic (ST) joint component and the glenohumeral (GH) joint component) [Adapted from Moore, 1992]

MUSCLE	ORIGIN	INSERTION(S)	ACTIONS & *ROLES
Rhomboid major	• SPs T2-T5 vertebrae	• Medial border of scapula	• Retracts scapula at ST joint • Internally rotates scapula at ST joint
Rhomboid minor	• SPs C7-T1 vertebrae	• Medial border of scapula	
Trapezius	• SPs C7-T12 • Ligamentum nuchae • Occipital protuberance • Medial superior nuchal line	• Spine of scapula • Lateral clavicle • Acromion process of scapula	Superior fibres • Elevate scapula at ST joint • Externally rotate scapula at ST joint Middle fibres • Retract scapula at ST joint Inferior fibres • Depress scapula at ST joint • Externally rotate scapula at ST joint
Deltoid	• Lateral clavicle • Acromion process of scapula • Spine of scapula	• Deltoid tuberosity of humerus	Anterior fibres • Flex humerus at GH joint • Internally rotate humerus Middle fibres • Abduct humerus at GH joint Posterior fibres • Extend humerus at GH joint • Externally rotate humerus at GH joint
Serratus anterior	• Ribs 1-8, lateral ends	• Anterior surface of scapula - medial border	• Protract scapula at ST joint • Externally rotate scapula at ST joint
Pectoralis major (Sternal head)	• Anterior sternum • Ribs 2-6, costal cartilage	• Lateral lip of bicipital groove of humerus	• Adduct humerus at GH joint • Internally rotate humerus at GH joint • Extend humerus at GH joint (from a flexed position) • *Depress shoulder girdle
Pectoralis major (Clavicular head)	• Medial clavicle	• Lateral lip of bicipital groove of humerus	• Flex humerus at GH joint
Latissimus dorsi	• Iliac crest, • SPs T7-T12, • Inferior 3-4 ribs	• Floor of bicipital groove of humerus	• Adduct humerus at GH joint • Internally rotate humerus at GH joint • Extend humerus at GH joint (from a flexed position) • *Depress shoulder girdle
Levator scapulae	• TPs C1-C4 vertebrae	• Superior angle of scapula	• Elevate scapula at ST joint • Internally rotate scapula
Teres major	• Inferior angle of scapula	• Medial lip of bicipital groove of humerus	• Adduct humerus at GH joint • Internally rotate humerus at GH joint
Pectoralis minor	• Ribs 3, 4, 5	• Coracoid process of scapula	• Protract scapula at ST joint
Coracobrachialis	• Coracoid process of scapula	• Medial humerus	• Flex humerus at GH joint • Adduct humerus at GH joint

Abbreviations used in Table 2.1: SP = spinous process, TP = transverse process, T = thoracic vertebrae, C = cervical vertebrae, ST = scapulothoracic joint, GH = glenohumeral joint, *See Sections 1.6.4.2 1.6.5.6 for muscle roles and actions

The movements of the <u>scapula</u> and the <u>scapulothoracic (ST) joint</u> and the muscles that facilitate these movements are shown Table 2.2.

Table 2.2 Movements and muscle groups of the scapulothoracic (ST) joint of the shoulder joint complex *and amsa bandha*	
MOVEMENT PAIRS: Opposing (Antagonistic) Muscle Group Pairs	**MUSCLE GROUPS and individual muscles moving the scapula at the scapulothoracic (ST) joint of the shoulder joint complex**
	SHOULDER (ST) DEPRESSION 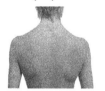 **Shoulder (ST) depressors**: trapezius (inferior), (latissimus dorsi and pectoralis major can also depress the scapula via their attachments on the humerus)	**SHOULDER (ST) ELEVATION** **Shoulder (ST) elevators**: trapezius (superior), levator scapulae
	SHOULDER (ST) PROTRACTION 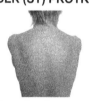 **Shoulder (ST) protractors**: serratus anterior, pectoralis minor, (pectoralis major can also protract the scapula via its effects on the humerus especially if the humerus is flexed at the glenohumeral joint)	**SHOULDER (ST) RETRACTION** 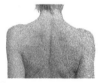 **Shoulder (ST) retractors**: trapezius (middle), rhomboids, (latissimus dorsi can also retract the scapula via its effects on the humerus especially if the humerus is extended at the glenohumeral joint)
	SHOULDER (ST) EXTERNAL ROTATION 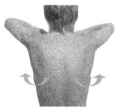 **Shoulder (ST) external rotators** : trapezius (superior and inferior), serratus anterior	**SHOULDER (ST) INTERNAL ROTATION** 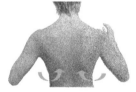 **Shoulder (ST) internal rotators**: rhomboids, levator scapulae, pectoralis minor

2.3.5 Muscles of the Shoulder Joint Complex: Glenohumeral (GH) Component

The attachments and actions of muscles that move the <u>glenohumeral</u> (GH) component of the <u>shoulder joint complex</u> are shown in Table 2.1. Many of these muscles can be seen in Figures 2.3 -2.6.

The movements of the shoulder and the muscles that facilitate these movements are shown Table 2.3.

Table 2.3 Movements and muscle groups of the glenohumeral (GH) joint of the shoulder joint complex and *amsa bandha*

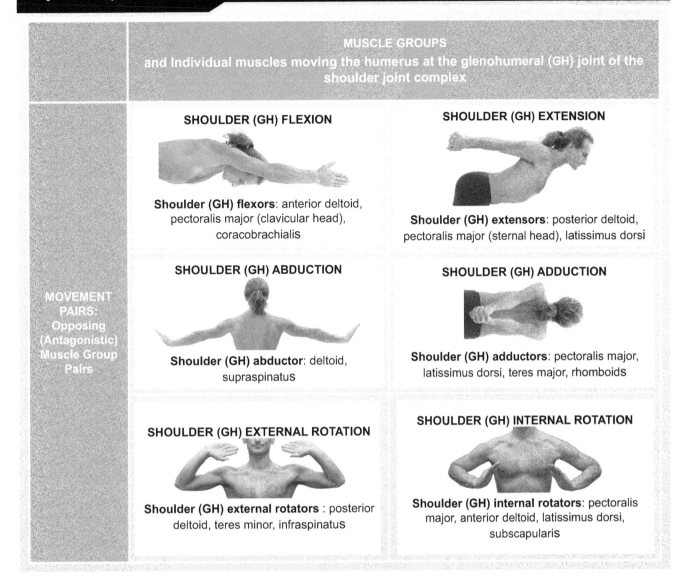

MUSCLE GROUPS
and Individual muscles moving the humerus at the glenohumeral (GH) joint of the shoulder joint complex

MOVEMENT PAIRS:
Opposing (Antagonistic) Muscle Group Pairs

SHOULDER (GH) FLEXION

Shoulder (GH) flexors: anterior deltoid, pectoralis major (clavicular head), coracobrachialis

SHOULDER (GH) EXTENSION

Shoulder (GH) extensors: posterior deltoid, pectoralis major (sternal head), latissimus dorsi

SHOULDER (GH) ABDUCTION

Shoulder (GH) abductor: deltoid, supraspinatus

SHOULDER (GH) ADDUCTION

Shoulder (GH) adductors: pectoralis major, latissimus dorsi, teres major, rhomboids

SHOULDER (GH) EXTERNAL ROTATION

Shoulder (GH) external rotators : posterior deltoid, teres minor, infraspinatus

SHOULDER (GH) INTERNAL ROTATION

Shoulder (GH) internal rotators: pectoralis major, anterior deltoid, latissimus dorsi, subscapularis

2.3.6 Rotator Cuff Muscles of the Glenohumeral (GH) joint

The four rotator cuff muscles [Figures 2.3 & 2.4] are teres minor, subscapularis, supraspinatus and infraspinatus. The main function of the rotator cuff muscles is the stabilisation of the ball and socket type glenohumeral joint. The rotator cuff muscles attach to the humeral head. The attachments and actions of the rotator cuff muscles of the glenohumeral (GH) Component of the shoulder joint complex are shown in Table 2.4.

Table 2.4 Rotator cuff muscles of the glenohumeral (GH) joint of the shoulder joint complex and *amsa bandha* [Adapted from Moore, 1992]

MUSCLE	ORIGIN	INSERTION	ACTIONS and *ROLES
Teres minor	• Lateral border of scapula.		• Externally rotate humerus at GH joint • *Stabiliser of GH joint
Supraspinatus	• Supraspinous fossa of scapula	• Greater tubercle of humerus	• Abduct humerus at GH joint • *Stabiliser of GH joint
Infraspinatus	• Infraspinous fossa of scapula		• Externally rotate humerus at GH joint • *Stabiliser of GH joint
Subscapularis	• Sub-scapula fossa of scapula	• Lesser tubercle of humerus	• Internally rotate humerus at GH joint • *Stabiliser of GH joint

*See Sections 1.6.4.2 1.6.5.6 for muscle roles and actions

The main function of the four <u>rotator cuff</u> muscles is to hold the head of the <u>humerus</u> in the glenoid cavity of the <u>scapula</u> (shoulder blade).

The <u>rotator cuff</u> may be damaged by injury or disease resulting in instability of the shoulder joint. Degenerative tendonitis of the rotator cuff muscles, a common disease especially in older people, is where calcium deposits in the muscle tendons resulting in stiffness and pain on shoulder movements.

Important muscles in the shoulder

The following muscles are important in the shoulder girdle. Their attachments and actions should be learnt. They are relatively easy to see and feel.

1. Rhomboids
2. Trapezius
3. Deltoid
4. Serratus anterior
5. Pectoralis major (sternal head)
6. Pectoralis major (clavicular head)
7. Latissimus dorsi.

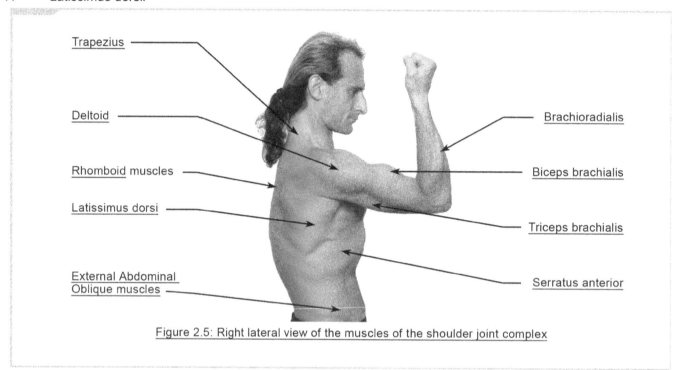

Figure 2.5: Right lateral view of the muscles of the shoulder joint complex

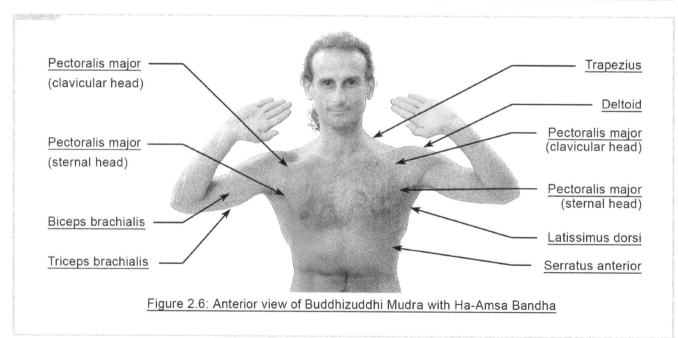

Figure 2.6: Anterior view of Buddhizuddhi Mudra with Ha-Amsa Bandha

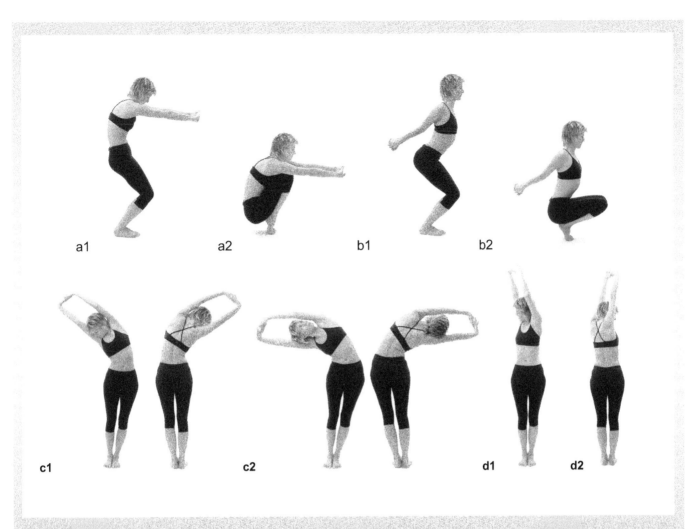

Figure 2.7 Shoulder movements and their effect on the spine

a) shoulder movements that include <u>scapulothoracic</u> (ST) <u>protraction</u> and <u>glenohumeral</u> (GH) <u>flexion</u> will facilitate <u>flexion</u> of the <u>thoracic spine</u> (T/Sp).

b) shoulder movements that include ST <u>retraction</u> and GH <u>extension</u> will facilitate <u>extension</u> of the T/Sp.

c) shoulder movements that include right ST <u>depression</u> and left ST <u>elevation</u> will facilitate right lateral <u>flexion</u> of the spine

d) shoulder movements that include right ST <u>retraction</u> and left ST <u>protraction</u> will facilitate right axial rotation of the spine

2.4 NERVES OF THE SHOULDER JOINT COMPLEX

2.4.1 The Brachial Plexus

The <u>brachial plexus</u> is the network of nerves that arises from the region of the neck and uppermost part of the back. The <u>brachial plexus</u>:

- Supplies (sends nerve information to, and receives information from) the shoulder and upper limb
- Is formed from the 5 <u>ventral rami</u> of **C5, C6, C7, C8 and T1**
- Has **three trunks** which are **derived from <u>C5+C6</u>, <u>C7</u>, and <u>C8 + T1</u>**, in the posterior of the neck.
  - o **Each trunk of the <u>brachial plexus</u>:**
    - – Forms **two divisions**, one goes anterior and the other posterior to the <u>clavicle</u>
    - – Has **three cords**: a **lateral cord (C5 +C6 +C7)**, a **posterior cord (C5 - T1)** and a **medial cord (C8 + T1)**
- <u>**Motor branches of the brachial plexus**</u> **supply** the **muscles of** the **upper back and upper limb**. The muscles they innervate and their root values are described in Table 2.5.

Table 2.5 Motor Branches of the brachial plexus and their root values
[Adapted from Moore, 1992]

Nerve (n.)	Nerve Roots	Muscle Supplied
Dorsal scapula n.	• C5 first branch	• Rhomboid major and minor
Long thoracic n.	• C5, 6, 7	• Serratus anterior
Supra scapula n.	• C5 + C6 junction/trunk	• Supraspinatus, infraspinatus,
Upper sub-scapula n.:	• Posterior cord (C5 - T1), first branch	• Subscapularis
Lateral pectoral n.	• Lateral cord (C5 +C6 +C7), first branch	• Pectoralis major
Medial pectoral n.	• Medial cord (C8 + T1), first branch	• Pectoralis major and minor
Thoraco-dorsal n.	• Posterior cord (C5 - T1), second branch	• latissimus dorsi
Lower sub-scapula n.	• Posterior cord (C5 - T1), third branch	• Subscapularis and teres major

• **Sensory branches of the brachial plexus** **receive information from the skin of the upper limb.** The regions they relate to and their root values are described in Table 2.6.

Table 2.6 Sensory Branches of the brachial plexus and their root values
[Adapted from Moore, 1992]

Nerve (n.)	Nerve Roots	Related Region of Skin
Medial cutaneous n. of arm	• C8 - T1 medial cord second branch	• Skin of medial arm (shoulder to elbow)
Medial cutaneous n. of forearm	• C8 - T1 medial cord third branch	• Skin of medial forearm (wrist to elbow, and posteriorly to the biceps)

No 2.3 Gentle nerve tensioning (stretching) in yoga postures may help relieve some problems, while over-stretching of the nerves may cause damage

Gentle tensioning (stretching) the nerves of the brachial plexus in *yoga* postures can help relieve some neck, shoulder, elbow and wrist problems, and can increase one's sense of well being. However, an over-stretch of the nerves of the brachial plexus can cause discomfort, pain and/or damage to these regions. Arm positions that tension (stretch) the nerves of the brachial plexus are shown in Figure 2.8.

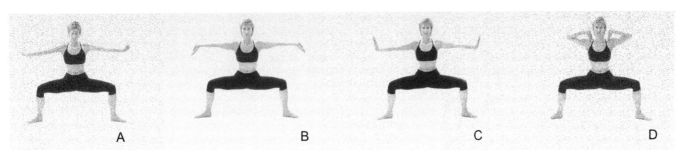

Figure 2.8 Shoulder movements and their effect on the nerves of the brachial plexus, and the effects on acupuncture meridians

Musculoskeletal or neurophysiological problems of the neck, shoulder, elbow or wrist and hand may be assisted by using four main nerve <u>tensionings</u> (stretches) of the <u>brachial plexus</u>, which are also called *yoga mudras* and are also stretches of <u>acupuncture meridians</u> [Figures 9.1- 9.7]

A. Atanu puritat mudra: <u>radial nerve</u> stretch and stretch of the <u>large intestine acupuncture meridian</u>: shoulder (ST) <u>depression</u> and <u>retraction</u>; shoulder (GH) <u>abduction</u>, <u>internal rotation</u> and slight <u>flexion</u>; elbow <u>extension</u> and pronation; wrist <u>flexion</u> and ulnar deviation.

B. Kloman mudra: <u>median nerve</u> stretch with <u>supination</u> and stretch of the <u>lung acupuncture meridian</u>: shoulder (ST) <u>depression</u> and <u>protraction</u>; shoulder (GH) <u>abduction</u>, <u>external rotation</u> and slight <u>extension</u>; elbow <u>extension</u> and supination; wrist <u>extension</u>.

C. Bukka puritat mudra: <u>median nerve</u> stretch with <u>pronation</u> and stretch of the <u>pericardium acupuncture meridian</u>: shoulder (ST) <u>depression</u> and <u>protraction</u>; shoulder (GH) <u>abduction</u>, <u>external rotation</u> and slight <u>extension</u>; elbow <u>extension</u> and pronation; wrist <u>extension</u>.

D. Buddhizuddhi mudra: <u>ulnar nerve</u> stretch and stretch of the <u>heart acupuncture meridian</u>: shoulder (ST) <u>depression</u> and <u>protraction</u>; shoulder (GH) <u>abduction</u>, <u>external rotation</u> and slight <u>extension</u>; elbow <u>flexion</u> and pronation; wrist <u>extension</u>.

2.5 APPLIED ANATOMY OF THE SHOULDER JOINT COMPLEX IN *HATHA YOGA* POSTURES

Correctly performed *hatha yoga* exercises can develop flexibility of the <u>shoulder joint complex</u> concurrently with muscle strength, joint stability and control of joint movement.

Strength and stability of the <u>shoulder joint complex</u> can be obtained by learning how to create <u>co-activation</u> (i.e. a simultaneous tensing) of muscles with opposing action (i.e. agonist and antagonist) in the shoulder. The concept of stabilising and strengthening the <u>shoulder joint complex</u> with <u>co-activations</u> is essentially the formation of a shoulder *bandha* analogous to the three central *bandhas* of the trunk (*jalandhara bandha, uddiyana bandha* and *mula bandha*) [Section 7.5.1], which are described in traditional *hatha yoga* texts such as the *Hatha Yoga Pradipika* [Devananda, 1987]. Ways of generating a shoulder *bandha* referred to as *amsa bandha* in *Sanskrit* are described below [Section 2.5.1].

2.5.1 Co-activation of Opposing Muscles of the Shoulder Joint Complex: *Amsa Bandha*

Amsa bandha is generated at the physical level when a series of opposing muscles or muscle groups crossing the <u>shoulder joint complex</u> are co-activated. In theory, a *bandha* can be generated whenever any two opposing muscles or muscle groups are activated together.

For example, *amsa bandha* may be formed by:
- <u>Co-activation</u> of <u>glenohumeral (GH) joint</u> <u>abductors</u> and <u>adductors</u>
- <u>Co-activation</u> of <u>glenohumeral (GH) joint</u> <u>internal rotators</u> and <u>external rotators</u>
- <u>Co-activation</u> of <u>glenohumeral (GH) joint</u> <u>flexors</u> and <u>extensors</u>
- <u>Co-activation</u> of <u>scapulothoracic (ST) joint</u> <u>protractors</u> and <u>retractors</u>

In practice, however it is very hard to will such seemingly opposing muscle activity for many people. Therefore, various tricks [Section 2.5.1.1] and special postures [Section 2.5.1.2, & 2.5.1.3] are available to assist in the generation of *bandhas*. These tricks take advantage of the fact that many of the key muscles in <u>joint complexes</u> are <u>multi-articular</u> [Section 1.6.5.7], and so may have multiple actions and roles at several joints in a <u>joint complex</u>.

To help achieve some of the valuable <u>co-activations</u> of *amsa bandha*, several <u>open-chain</u> and <u>closed-chain</u> exercises [Section 1.6.5.9.1] are available. Many people have relatively tight or stiff <u>shoulder elevators</u> and relatively weak <u>shoulder depressors</u>, therefore, simple <u>non weight-bearing</u> <u>open-chain</u> exercises may be attempted first [Section 2.5.1.1], which may then be progressed to <u>closed-chain</u> exercises.

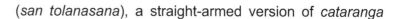

Two <u>closed-chain</u> exercises that may be practised to help achieve *amsa bandha* are *tolasana* [Appendix A] and the plank pose (*san tolanasana*), a straight-armed version of *cataranga dandasana* (push up position). The first exercise, *tolasana*, involves actively pulling the shoulders towards the hips while pressing the palms into the floor from a sitting position [Section 2.5.1.2]. The second exercise, the plank (*san tolanasana*) [Appendix A] involves learning to push the shoulders away from the upper back and spine into <u>protraction</u> whilst pressing down the palms onto the floor with the spine held parallel to the floor and pushing the upper back and spine away from the floor in the plank or cat positions [Section 2.5.1.3].

Formation of *amsa bandha* both during movement and in static postures while practising *hatha yoga* has the following benefits. *Amsa bandha*:
- Stabilises the <u>shoulder joint complex</u>
- Strengthens the muscles crossing the <u>shoulder joint complex</u>
- Allows safe and effective stretching of the shoulder muscles without putting undue strain on shoulder ligaments or joint capsule
- Improves coordinated control of the muscles crossing the <u>shoulder joint complex</u>
- Enables improved nerve tensioning of the nerves of the <u>brachial plexus</u> [Sections 2.5.1.5, 3.8.1 & 9.7.3]
- Generates body heat, making the synovial fluid less viscous (more runny) and hence makes the joints more flexible [Section 1.5.2.3]
- Improves the musculoskeletal pump effect in the body thereby increasing circulation [Sections 1.0.4 & 8.1.2.3.2]
- Helps stimulate the formation of all 3 central or spinal *bandhas*: *jalandhara bandha*, *uddiyana bandha* and *mula bandha* [Section 2.5.1.4]
- Helps stimulate the formation of other *bandhas* in the body, in particular the formation of *kurpara bandha* [Section 3.9.1.1] at the <u>elbow joint complex</u> [Section 3.2.0]

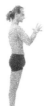

2.5.1.1 The use of *tadasana* : an open-chain exercise which allows co-activation of glenohumeral joint adductors and abductors, flexors and extensors, and internal and external rotators

Easy postures to begin to learn to create *amsa bandha* are those resembling *tadasana* (standing up). With time and regular practice, little mental or physical effort is required to form an *amsa bandha* in any posture and during movement. Initially however, the generation of *amsa bandha* utilises tricks that take advantage of the fact that many of the key muscles in the <u>shoulder joint complex </u>are multi-articular [Section 1.6.5.7], and have multiple actions and roles. To generate *amsa bandha* the most important muscles are probably pectoralis major and latissimus dorsi (the underarm muscles). These two muscles cross both the scapulothoracic (ST) joint and the glenohumeral (GH) joint, which are the main joints in the shoulder joint complex. Pectoralis major and latissimus dorsi have many different actions and roles in the shoulder joint complex [Table 2.1] but they are usually thought of as the primary GH joint adductors that oppose the action of the deltoid muscles, which are primary GH joint abductors. However, pectoralis major and latissimus dorsi are also very effective depressors of the scapula via their actions on the humerus. So, while it is relatively difficult for an untrained person to conceptualise how to try and raise one's arm (i.e. abduct the humerus) and simultaneously try to pull one's arm down (i.e. adduct the humerus), which would effectively form an abductor-adductor-type *amsa bandha*, it is practical and achievable for most people to stand and actively pull one's shoulders down (i.e. depress the scapula with the pectoralis major and latissimus dorsi) and simultaneous try and pull one's elbow up (i.e. abduct the humerus with the deltoid). Note, due to the multiple actions and roles these muscles have, this exercise also causes a co-activation of flexors and extensors (eg. pectoralis major and posterior deltoid) and also internal rotators and external rotators (latissimus dorsi and posterior deltoid).

Amsa bandha can also be generated in an anterior-posterior plane especially during postures that tension (stretch) the nerves of the arm [Figures 9.1 – 9.5]. Furthermore, the movements that generate *amsa bandha* also increase tension (stretch) on the nerves.

Amsa bandha can be generated in an anterior-posterior plane during *kloman mudra* (median nerve stretch) [Figure 9.2] by protracting the scapula at the ST joint while extending the humerus at the GH joint. Protraction of the scapula recruits serratus anterior and other protractors, while extension of the humerus recruits posterior deltoid. *Amsa bandha* is formed here because any deltoid activity causes shoulder (ST) retractors such as the rhomboids to tense in order to stabilise the scapula and prevent it from moving when the deltoid is activated [Norkin & Levangie, 1992]. Hence, protractors and retractors are co-activated in this case.

2.5.1.2 The use of *tolasana* : a closed-chain exercise which simultaneously stimulates shoulder depressor, abductor, adductor, and retractor activity

An easy way for most normal people to achieve a shoulder *bandha* is by performing an exercise resembling the *yoga* posture called *tolasana* [Appendix A]. *Tolasana* is classically performed in

padmasana (lotus posture) [Appendix A] but it may be done from any seated posture (eg cross-legged, kneeling or even from a chair). The palms are placed flat on the floor or chair lateral to the mid thigh region and an attempt is made to lift the body off the floor by pressing down with the palms. *Tolasana* is a closed-chain exercise of the upper limb that forces a co-activation of most of the major muscles of the shoulder joint complex. These muscles include:

* Pectoralis major and latissimus dorsi, the main muscles at the anterior and posterior of the armpits respectively, are active in *tolasana* and act as important depressors of the scapulothoracic (ST) joint, and adductors and internal rotators of the glenohumeral (GH) joint;
* the deltoid muscles, covering the superior, anterior, posterior, and lateral border of the shoulder are active in *tolasana* and act as abductors, flexors, extensors, and of the GH joint.
* The rhomboids and inferior trapezius are active in *tolasana*. They help stabilise the ST joint, and keep the scapula close to the rib cage so that the body may be lifted off the ground, rather than the proximal end of the scapula being lifted into the air and away from the rib cage by the abducting action of the deltoid [Norkin & Levangie, 1992].

Therefore, this simple exercise has formed a *bandha* (a muscle lock) around the shoulder joint complex by co-activating a significant number of opposing muscles groups. Thus, *amsa bandha* can help stabilise and strengthen the glenohumeral (GH) joint by generating compressive forces equally on the anterior and posterior regions, and the inferior and superior regions of this joint.

2.5.1.3 The plank pose and the benefits of protraction of the shoulder joint complex

When the classical *tolasana* [Appendix A] is performed accurately to its final stage, and the whole body is lifted into the air so that the upper thoracic spine becomes parallel to the floor, the scapulas will become protracted as well as depressed. Hence, the scapula stabilising and retracting roles of the rhomboids and trapezius are balanced by the muscles of protraction (in particular serratus anterior). In addition, the scapulothoracic (ST) joint becomes very stable, as the entire scapula remains firmly resting on the rib cage.

Initially most people do not have anywhere near the strength to achieve a full *tolasana*. Therefore, protraction

of the shoulder is best practised in the plank pose (*san tolanasana*) [Appendix A] (a version

of the push up position, *cataranga dandasana* [Appendix A], with the elbows extended and the shoulders placed directly above the palms, and with the knees resting on or off the floor). In the plank pose, pushing up between the shoulder blades encourages protraction of the scapula. If the *tolasana* movement of tightening the underarm muscles or pulling the shoulders towards the hips is well established and understood and it can be maintained in the plank pose, then a more complete *amsa bandha* will have been formed.

The following muscle groups, which help form *amsa* (shoulder) *bandha*, will be obliged to be active in the plank posture or the advanced *tolasana* due to the following reasons:

• **Shoulder (ST) protractor muscles** are actively tensing due to pushing up between the shoulder blades
• **Shoulder (ST) retractor muscles** are actively tensing to fix the proximal end of the scapula on to the rib cage in order to offset the abduction effect of the deltoid muscle
• **Shoulder (ST) depressor muscles** (the underarm muscles) are actively tensing as the body is lifted away from the floor in *tolasana* and as the shoulders are pulled towards the hips in the plank
• **Shoulder (GH) abductor muscles** (i.e. deltoid) are actively tensing in order to abduct the scapula and attempt to lift the body away from the floor in these closed-chain exercises
• **Shoulder (GH) adductor muscles group** (including the underarm muscles again) are actively tensing to try to adduct the humerus to the trunk, but since the humerus is attached to the scapula the underarm muscles, (pectoralis major and latissimus dorsi) serve also as shoulder (ST) depressors.

Note that this exercise does not cause tension in any of the shoulder elevator muscles such as the superior trapezius. On the contrary, activation of the shoulder (ST) depressors in the form of latissimus dorsi and pectoralis major tends to cause a reflex reciprocal relaxation of shoulder elevator muscles such as superior trapezius. Many muscles in a joint complex have multiple actions and roles. This is partly because most muscles are multi-articular [Section 1.6.5.7], i.e. they cross more than one joint. Multi-articular muscles in joint complexes facilitate the formation of a co-activation of antagonistic (opposing) muscle groups on several levels. For example, in the plank pose as described above there are three distinct levels of co-activation of opposing muscles which stabilise the shoulder joint complex or four types of *amsa bandha*. These antagonistic (opposing) muscle co-activations (*bandhas*) are described as follows:

• Pectoralis major and latissimus dorsi (the underarm muscles) can act as adductors of the humerus on the medial side of the glenohumeral (GH) joint; while the deltoid muscle group can oppose this action and act as abductor muscles on the lateral side of the glenohumeral (GH) joint
• Pectoralis major and latissimus dorsi (the underarm muscles) can also act as internal rotators of the

humerus at the <u>GH joint</u>, which is opposed by the action of the *posterior* <u>deltoid</u> muscle which can act as an external rotator of the <u>humerus</u> at the <u>glenohumeral</u> joint

•   <u>Pectoralis major</u> can also act as a <u>flexor</u> of the <u>humerus</u> at the <u>GH joint</u>, which is opposed by the action of the <u>posterior deltoid</u> muscle which can act as an <u>extensor</u> of the <u>humerus</u> at the <u>GH joint</u>

•   <u>Pectoralis major</u> can also act to protract the <u>scapula</u> (shoulder blade) on the anterior side of the <u>shoulder joint complex</u>, while <u>latissimus dorsi</u> can act to retract the <u>scapula</u> (shoulder blade) on the posterior side of the <u>shoulder joint complex</u>.

For the <u>ST joint</u> to remain stable throughout its range of movement, the <u>scapula</u> is best kept as close to the rib cage as possible while allowing movement to take place from extreme <u>protraction</u> to extreme <u>retraction</u>. In order to keep the anterior and posterior borders of the <u>scapula</u> on the rib cage, while moving from full <u>protraction</u> to full <u>retraction</u>, the <u>protractors</u> and <u>retractors</u> should ideally be kept simultaneously tensing in either a lengthened or a shortened condition. This <u>co-activation</u> of <u>shoulder (ST) protractors</u> and <u>shoulder (ST) retractors</u> (part of *amsa bandha*), whilst keeping the <u>scapula</u> evenly attached to the rib cage, is easiest for most people to master initially when the <u>scapula</u> is in its most protracted position. This <u>co-activation</u> (*amsa bandha)* can eventually be mastered in any position, either with the palms fixed and the trunk free to move (<u>closed-chain exercise</u>), or with the palms free to move and the trunk fixed in space (<u>open-chain exercise</u>). However, a beginner is more easily able to form *amsa bandha* in a <u>closed-chain exercise</u> since <u>closed-chain exercises</u> of the upper limb tend to promote a greater level of automatic <u>co-activation</u> of opposing shoulder muscle groups rather than <u>open-chain exercises</u>. This is due to the need for the <u>scapula retractors</u> to be active in holding the <u>scapula</u> to the rib cage to counter the effects of the <u>deltoid</u>, which acts as a <u>scapula abductor</u> and tries to lift the scapula away from the rib cage during <u>closed-chain exercises</u>.

2.5.1.4 *Bandha* inter-connectedness: *amsa* (shoulder) *bandha* assists in the formation and maintenance of the three central or spinal *bandhas*

An essential feature of the *amsa bandha* is the <u>depression</u> of the shoulder girdle by the under-arm muscles <u>latissimus dorsi</u> and <u>pectoralis major</u>.

Tendinous attachments of the <u>latissimus dorsi</u> join the <u>fascia</u> of the <u>lumbar spine</u>, which are contiguous with the <u>fascia</u> of the lower abdominal belt muscle, <u>transversus abdominis</u>, which is a key muscle in *mula bandha* (co-activation of lower trunk muscles). Therefore, activation of <u>latissimus dorsi</u> can stimulate a reflex activation of the <u>transverses abdominis</u>. Hence, *amsa bandha* can assist in the creation and generation of *mula bandha*.

Similarly, <u>pectoralis major</u> has attachments to the anterior chest wall and <u>sternum</u>, and acting as an accessory muscle of breathing, <u>pectoralis major</u> is able to be <u>activated</u> in such a way as to <u>adduct</u> the chest to the <u>humerus</u>. This is especially so when the upper limb is in a fixed position such as when the palm is

pressing onto the floor as in *urdhva mukha svanasana* (up-dog pose) or when the palm

is pressing onto the knees as in sitting poses such as *padmasana* (the lotus). Hence, *amsa bandha*

can assist in the creation and generation of *uddiyana bandha* (the expansion of the rib cage).

The combined action of both <u>latissimus dorsi</u> and <u>pectoralis major</u> is able to depress the shoulders and cause a lengthening in the neck and a <u>reciprocal reflex relaxation</u> of the <u>shoulder elevators</u>. Hence, *amsa* (shoulder) *bandha* can also assist in the creation and generation of *jalandhara bandha* (the maintenance of length in the back of the neck).

2.5.1.5 Use of *amsa bandha* for tensioning *nadis* and nerves of the brachial plexus

Amsa bandha may be easily achieved by using muscular effort to try to pull the scapulas toward the hips (scapula depression) while trying to abduct the arm at the glenohumeral joint. This generates a co-activation of opposing muscles around the shoulder joint complex because two important scapula depressors, latissimus dorsi and pectoralis major are also important adductors of the arm at the glenohumeral joint, opposing the deltoid, the main abductor of the arm.

Amsa bandha can be supplemented by making another co-activation of a similar nature that is useful for tensioning the nerves of the brachial plexus and lengthening all the *nadis* coming from the spine down the arm. Two possibilities exist:

2.5.1.5.1 *Amsa bandha* formed from scapulothoracic (ST) protraction opposing glenohumeral (GH) extension

Shoulder (ST) protraction can be opposed by shoulder (GH) extension. One can generate a co-activation of opposing muscles around the shoulder joint complex by trying to protract the shoulder (scapula) while simultaneously trying to extend the shoulder (GH joint). The reason for this is that some of the scapula protractors can either flex the arm or may trigger a myotatic reflex activation of some shoulder (GH) flexors, opposing the posterior deltoid, the main extensor of the arm. This supplement to the basic *amsa bandha* is a useful addition to the stretch of the median and ulnar nerves of the brachial plexus [Sections 1.7.2.2.1, 3.9.1.5, & 9.7.3].

2.5.1.5.2 *Amsa bandha* formed from scapulothoracic (ST) retraction opposing glenohumeral (GH) flexion

Shoulder (ST) retraction can be opposed by shoulder (GH) flexion. One can generate a co-activation of opposing muscles around the shoulder joint complex by trying to retract the shoulder (ST) while simultaneously trying to flex the shoulder (GH joint). The reason for this is that some of the scapula retractors can also either extend the arm or may trigger a myotatic reflex activation of some shoulder (GH) extensors, which oppose the action of the anterior deltoid (the main flexor of the arm). This supplement to the basic *amsa bandha* is a useful addition to the stretch of the *radial* nerve of the brachial plexus [Sections 1.7.2.2.1, 3.9.1.5, & 9.7.3].

2.5.1.6 Effects of *ha-amsa bandha* and *tha-amsa bandha* on the *cardiopulmonary system*

A powerful *ha-amsa bandha*, a compressive muscle lock [Section 1.7.3.4, Appendix c] of the shoulder, has scapulothoracic joint (ST) depression, (ST) retraction and (ST) internal rotation; and glenohumeral joint (GH) adduction, (GH) extension, and (GH) internal rotation. *Ha-amsa bandha* can restrict blood flow through the shoulder to the upper limb. This can be demonstrated by observing a reduction in radial pulse intensity of the pulse while making *ha-amsa bandha*.

A powerful *tha-amsa bandha*, an expansive muscle lock [Section 1.7.3.4, Appendix c] of the shoulder, has (ST) elevation, (ST) protraction and (ST) external rotation; and (GH) abduction, (GH) flexion, and (GH) external rotation. *Tha amsa bandha* does not limit the flow of blood through the shoulder to the upper limb. This can be demonstrated by observing an increase in radial pulse intensity when making *tha-amsa bandha*, which is especially noticeable subsequent to making *ha-amsa bandha*. This is best observed in a side lying posture, which negates the effects of gravity on blood flow through the shoulder joint complex.

2.5.2 Uses and effects of the shoulder muscles in *hatha yoga asanas*

2.5.2.1 Scapula depression assists in stabilising the shoulder in *hatha yoga* postures

Two major depressors to the shoulder complex, latissimus dorsi, and pectoralis major, may be isometrically activated at least briefly in almost all of the *yoga* postures. The activation of these muscles serves several functions:

- To strengthen the latissimus dorsi and pectoralis major muscles
- To assist the rotator cuff in stabilising the glenohumeral (GH) joint
- To assist in the reciprocal relaxation of the shoulder (ST) elevators which tend to be chronically overactive and tense in many people
- To depress the shoulder when the arm is engaged in an open-chain exercise, or to elevate the chest and thorax when the arms are engaged in certain closed-chain exercises.

2.5.2.2 Scapula elevation may assist in relaxing the neck in *hatha yoga* postures

It is unusual to tense the <u>shoulder elevator</u> muscles in classical *yoga* postures consciously, as it may bring more tension to an area where tension tends to build up. However, the <u>scapula</u> elevators can be used briefly to traction the neck while hunching the shoulders into the base of the skull especially in forward bending

postures such as *uttanasana* [Appendix A] and *pascimottanasana* [Appendix A].

Passive <u>shoulder (ST) elevation</u> can be achieved in seated postures such as *padmasana* [Appendix A] cross-legged or kneeling, where the hands can be placed onto the thighs and the elbow extensors used to force the elbow into <u>extension</u> and the shoulders into <u>elevation</u>. The neck can be tractioned (stretched or lengthened) in this manner.

<u>Shoulder (ST) elevators</u> can also be tensed in a lengthened state. This can be achieved while the shoulder is kept passively depressed by the action of the hands holding under the knees in seated postures such as

padmasana [Appendix A], cross-legged, or kneeling, while the <u>elbow flexors</u> try and passively <u>depress</u> the <u>scapula</u>. In this position, attempting to elevate the shoulders, thereby tensing them in a lengthened position, will lengthen or stretch them further, and this can trigger a subsequent relaxation response via the <u>inverse myotatic reflex</u> [Section 1.7.2.2.1.1].

In addition, <u>shoulder (ST) elevators</u> are used in making *tha-amsa bandha*, an expansive muscle lock, which has <u>scapulothoracic joint (ST) elevation</u>, (ST) <u>protraction</u> and (ST) <u>external rotation</u>; and <u>glenohumeral joint</u> (GH) <u>abduction</u>, (GH) <u>flexion</u>, and (GH) <u>external rotation</u>. However, in making *tha-amsa bandha* one must ensure that some (ST) <u>depressor</u> muscle activity is present even though these muscles will be in a lengthened state. Therefore one should gently tense (activate) (ST) depressors such as the underarm muscles (<u>latissimus dorsi</u>, and <u>pectoralis major</u>) even though the shoulder is being <u>elevated</u>.

2.5.2.3 Scapula protraction and retraction assists in mobilising the thoracic spine and opens the chest in *hatha yoga* postures

Many *yoga* poses require that the upper arm be kept flexed with the <u>scapula</u> protracted (eg. *urdhva hastasana*

utkatasana [Appendix A]). In this position, the <u>scapula</u> is able to exert a pressure against the *thoracic* cage, which can help mobilise the <u>thoracic spine</u>, especially if the upper limb is engaged in a <u>closed-</u>

<u>chain exercise</u> such as *adho mukha svanasana* [Appendix A].

Retraction of the shoulder blades, done with the upper limbs extended and adducted with the fingers interlocked, tends to lead to a stretching of the anterior chest wall, and a further mobilisation of the thoracic

spine. A similar effect is achieved in the *maricyasana* 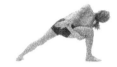 series of postures and in *baddha*

parsvakonasana 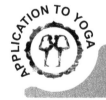 [Appendix A].

2.5.2.4 Effects of shoulder movements on the upper back and thoracic spine

The shoulder joint complex and the thoracic spine (T/Sp) are intimately related. Shoulder movements are able to affect the upper back and T/Sp:

- Unilateral shoulder flexion is accompanied by contralateral side flexion of the T/Sp.
- Bilateral shoulder flexion is accompanied by spinal extension.

Similarly, abnormalities of the T/Sp are able to affect the functioning of the upper limb and shoulder.

- Decreased T/Sp extensibility or increased T/Sp kyphosis often results in reduced shoulder range of motion (ROM).
- Increased T/Sp kyphosis (hunch back) often results in chronic protraction of scapula which may lead to:
  - o Increased resting length and hence decreased effectiveness of scapula retractors/stabilisers (eg. trapezius and rhomboids).
  - o Shoulder impingement problems.

2.5.2.5 Use of passive and active shoulder movements for mobilisation of the neck and cervical spine (C/Sp)

Chronic elevation of scapula or overuse of scapula elevators (upper trapezius and levator scapulae) can lead to immobility in the cervical spine (C/Sp). In order to mobilise the neck and C/Sp the following methods may be employed:

- Concentric activation of scapula elevators may help traction the C/Sp in some cases and help these muscles to fatigue and rest

No 2.4 Shoulder elevator muscles can traction the neck in forward bending postures

If one performs *uttanasana* and *padangusthasana* [Appendix A], and then intentionally hunches the shoulders and elevates the shoulder girdle and pulls them towards the base of the skull by using the shoulder elevator muscles, then the neck is given a type of self tractioning (stretching or lengthening).

- Stretch and relax <u>scapula elevators</u> by:
  o <u>Reflex reciprocal inhibition</u> due to activation of <u>scapula depressors</u> (especially <u>latissimus dorsi</u> and <u>pectoralis major</u> - the underarm muscles).

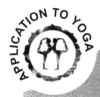

No 2.5 Arm balancing postures can be used to relieve neck tension

Tense, stiff or overused <u>shoulder elevators</u> may be relieved in postures such as *tolasana* (a pose in which hands are placed lateral to the thighs in a seated posture, and then muscles of the upper limb and trunk are used to lift the body off the floor). As the palms press down there is an activation of <u>scapula depressors</u> (especially <u>latissimus dorsi</u> and <u>pectoralis major</u>), which are acting to neutralise the actions of the <u>deltoid</u>, which is trying to <u>abduct</u> the <u>scapula</u> to the <u>humerus</u>. Activation of <u>scapula depressors</u> promotes the relaxation of the <u>scapula elevators</u> for two main reasons: (i) the <u>scapula elevators</u> are being stretched, which eventually relaxes them via <u>autogenic inhibition</u> (the <u>inverse myotatic reflex</u>); and (ii) there is <u>reciprocal inhibition</u> of the <u>scapula elevators</u> by the action of the <u>shoulder depressors</u>.

- PNF techniques [Section 1.7.2.2.4], with partner or intelligent use of posture by isometric activation of <u>scapula elevators</u> while <u>scapula</u> is kept <u>depressed</u> [Section 2.5.2.2].

2.5.2.6 Effects of shoulder movements and *amsa bandha* on the nervous system

Yoga practitioners in India are known for their ability to regulate the <u>autonomic nervous system (ANS)</u> [Section 9.5]. One of the ways control over the ANS can be achieved is by using shoulder movements and the various forms of *amsa bandha*.

A strong *ha-amsa bandha* can stop or reduce the flow of blood to the left arm [Section 2.5.1.6].

Due to the phenomenon known as <u>cerebral hemispheric contra laterality</u> [Section 9.7.5] reduction in blood flow to the left arm leads to inhibition of the <u>parasympathetic nervous system</u> [Section 9.5.2], which will stimulate nervous activity in general. Conversely, reduction of blood flow to the right arm leads to inhibition of the <u>sympathetic nervous system</u> [Section 9.5.1], which will reduce and calm nervous activity in general.

2.6 SHOULDER PATHOLOGY (SHOULDER PROBLEMS)

The <u>shoulder joint complex</u> is capable of a remarkably large range of motion. This is due to several important aspects of the shoulder structure, in particular:
- The shallow nature of the <u>glenohumeral cavity</u>, the socket of a very loose so-called ball and socket joint
- The non-fixed nature of the <u>scapulothoracic joint</u>.

The <u>shoulder joint complex</u> often becomes unstable, injured or irritable when:
- An excessive load is placed upon it
- It is moved through an excessive range of motion

Problems of the shoulder resulting from an excessive load or range of motion may be due to two main problems:
1. Weakness and/or lack of control of the muscles crossing the glenohumeral joint, and/or
2. Stiffness of the muscles and/or tissues crossing the <u>scapulothoracic joint</u>.

Before the second problem of shoulder muscle stiffness can be safely approached, the first problem of shoulder muscle weakness and /or lack of control must be first addressed. This necessitates the ability to co-activate the muscles crossing the shoulder joint and form *amsa bandha* [Section 2.5.1].

Most shoulder pathology relates in some way to impingement and/or instability.

2.6.1 Impingement of the Glenohumeral (GH) joint
The glenohumeral joint may become impinged because of:
- Encroachment from above (congenital abnormalities or osteophyte formation).
- Swelling of the rotator cuff tendons (tendonitis due to faulty biomechanics)
- Excessive elevation of the humeral head, perhaps due to an imbalance between muscular forces pulling the head of the humerus inferiorly (eg weak rotator cuff muscles, especially teres minor, infraspinatus, and subscapularis), and the muscular forces pulling the shaft of the humerus superiorly (deltoid and supraspinatus).

2.6.2 Chronic Anterior Instability of the Shoulder
Chronic anterior instability of the shoulder is a result of excessive joint laxity. It results in increased translation of the humeral head in an antero-superior direction, narrowing the subacromial space. Laxity of the anterior shoulder may develop over time, because of repeated stressing of the static stabiliser muscles at the extremes of motion.

The best *yoga* therapy for this problem usually revolves around training to master the co-activation of the shoulder muscles (*amsa bandha*) [Section 2.5.1], and learning how to maintain this co-activation through its range of joint movement. In addition, it may be necessary to address any lack of flexibility in the posterior aspect of the shoulder joint complex.

2.6.3 Frozen (or Very Stiff) Shoulder
A frozen shoulder is a problem which is directly opposite to the problem of instability. A *yoga* treatment should be directed at:
- Increasing shoulder flexion by stretching out the under-arm muscles in *yoga* postures such as the

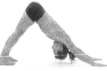

  adho mukha svanasana   [Appendix A].
- Increasing shoulder extension by stretching the front of the shoulder with postures which include

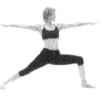

  interlocking the fingers behind the back as in *baddha prasarita padottanasana*   [Appendix A]
- Increasing shoulder abduction by learning how to take the arms out to the side and up to shoulder height while constantly pulling the shoulders downwards towards the hips. This can be practised

  alone or in many of the classical *yoga* postures such as *parsva virabhadrasana*
  [Appendix A]
- Increasing shoulder adduction with postures where one elbow is pulled to the opposite shoulder and then some gentle resistance from the shoulder being stretched is applied. This increases the stretch and strength of stiff abductors and and also of shoulder extensors which limits these movements eg

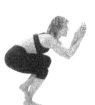 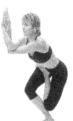 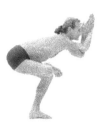

garudasana   , *vatayanasana*   and *utthita swastikasana*

- Increasing the range of <u>internal rotation</u> by stretching in postures resembling the *maricyasana*

series

- Increasing the range of <u>external rotation</u> by stretching <u>internal rotators</u> in postures resembling the first

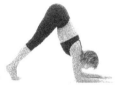

stage of *pinca mayurasana* 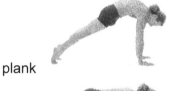 [Appendix A] i.e. similar to a dog pose with the elbows on the floor

- Mobilising the <u>scapula</u> and the <u>thoracic spine</u> (T/Sp) using <u>protraction</u> exercises such as the

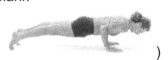

plank   (the first stage straight elbow version of *cataranga dandasana*

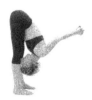

)

- Mobilising the <u>scapula</u> and the T/Sp using <u>retraction</u> postures which include interlocking the fingers

behind the back as in *baddha hasta uttanasana*
- Activation of the lower shoulder depressor muscles in particular <u>trapezius</u> to promote T/Sp <u>extension</u> and <u>scapula</u> control.

<u>Idiopathic adhesive capsulitis</u> is a commonly recognised but poorly understood cause of a painful and stiff shoulder. Recent studies have shown that a systematic four-way stretching programme for the shoulder similar to a generalised *yoga* approach given here gives relief in up to 90% of cases [Griggs *et al.*, 2000].

2.6.4 Problems Related to Faulty Scapulo-humeral Rhythm

Scapulo-humeral rhythm is the coordinated movements of the <u>humerus</u> and <u>scapula</u> resulting in full ROM during shoulder <u>elevation</u> (<u>abduction</u> + <u>flexion</u>). The normal person has:
- ***0 - 30°*** shoulder <u>elevation</u> involving mostly <u>humeral</u> movement
- ***30° - 180°*** shoulder <u>elevation</u> involving equal amount <u>scapula</u> and <u>humeral</u> movement
- Pain felt between 0 - 90° <u>abduction</u> may indicate GH or <u>scapula</u> problem
- Pain felt between 90 - 180° may indicate SC or AC joint problem
- Pain felt between 45 - 120° may indicate pinching of structures under AC joint (bursa, tendons)

Yoga therapy for correcting problems related to faulty scapulo-humeral rhythm is complex and depends on where the pain begins and ends during its range of movement (ROM). Therapy involves training to master the <u>co-activation</u> of the shoulder muscles known in *yoga* terms as *amsa bandha* [Section 2.5.1], and learning how to maintain this <u>co-activation</u> through its ROM.

2.6.5 Tears of the Shoulder Stabiliser Muscles: Rotator Cuff Injury

Rotator cuff tears can cause a lot of shoulder pain, both on rest and with movement. Although many people elect to take a surgical approach, a non-operative approach using gentle stretching and strengthening exercises has been shown to be affective in about 60% of cases [Goldberg et al., 2001]. A *yoga* exercise approach should work gently with postures that are directed at:

- Mobilising the thoracic spine (T/Sp)
- Mobilising the scapula
- Strengthening the shoulder depressor muscles (especially the under-arm muscles pectoralis major and latissimus dorsi) through a full range of joint motion
- Strengthening the elbow extensors, by tightening the triceps brachii while moving the arms even during open-chain exercises
- Gently tensioning (stretching) the nerves of the brachial plexus [Section 9.7.3].

****

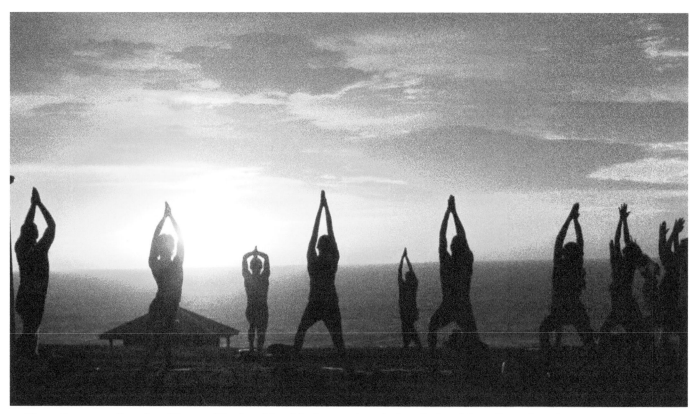

Yoga Synergy Sunrise Class with shoulder blades protracted and shoulders flexed and externally rotated in *Uttitha Virabhadrasana*. Photos courtesy of Melony Browell.

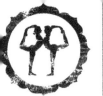
Chapter Breakdown

****

3.0 INTRODUCTION TO THE APPLIED ANATOMY OF THE FOREARM, WRIST & HAND IN *HATHA YOGA* POSTURES

In this chapter we examine the bones, muscles, nerves and other tissues of the elbow joint complex [Section 3.2.0], and the wrist joint complex [Section 3.5.0]. This information is then used to understand and apply the associated internal *yogic bandhas* (internal locks), *kurpara bandha* [Section 3.9.1.1] and *mani bandha* [Section 3.9.1.2], which are created by co-activation of antagonistic (opposing) muscle groups crossing the elbow joint complex and wrist joint complex respectively. These two *bandhas* are the key to improving the stability of the upper limb and are important in the control of circulation through the body.

In most anatomy courses, discussion on the upper limb is related to the arm being used primarily to take the hand into the appropriate position for manipulation of objects. The hand is also used for manipulation in *yoga* exercises, but the manipulation is usually of another part of the body, eg pulling the hand against the knee, or grabbing the big toe. However, in contrast to most other exercise forms, a great deal of the work done by the arms in *hatha yoga* is weight-bearing. Hence, many *yoga* exercises for the upper limb are closed-chain exercises [Section 1.6.5.9], ie the hand or forearm is fixed to the floor or wall and the movement or effect of the muscular effort affects the trunk and the spine. With intelligent and regular practise it becomes possible to use the arms to increase mobility of the spine.

3.1 BONES OF THE ELBOW JOINT COMPLEX

The main bones of the upper limb and the bones of the elbow joint complex are the:
- Humerus (upper arm bone)
- Radius (lower arm bone on thumb side of forearm)
- Ulna (lower arm bone on little finger side of forearm)

3.1.1 Humerus (distal end)
The following features of the humerus can be seen on a skeleton and identified with the help of Figures 3.1 – 3.5:
- **Posterior surface**: medial and lateral epicondyles, medial and lateral supracondylar ridges, olecranon fossa, and trochlea
- **Anterior surface**: medial and lateral epicondyles, medial and lateral supracondylar ridges, coronoid fossa, capitulum, and trochlea

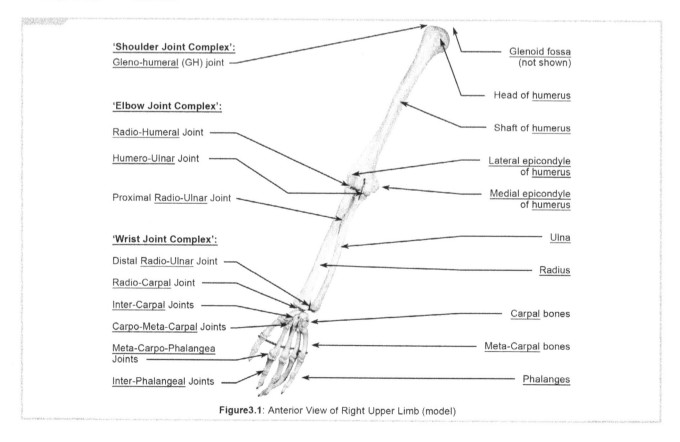

Figure3.1: Anterior View of Right Upper Limb (model)

3.1.2 Ulna

The following features of the <u>ulna</u> can be seen on a skeleton and identified with the help of Figures 3.1 – 3.5:
*   **Proximal end**: <u>olecranon process</u> (posterior), <u>coronoid process</u> (anterior).
*   **Distal end**: head of <u>humerus</u>, <u>styloid process</u>

3.1.3 Radius

The following features of the <u>radius</u> can be seen on a skeleton and identified with the help of Figures 3.1 – 3.5:
*   **Proximal end**: head of <u>radius</u>
*   **Distal end**: <u>styloid process</u>

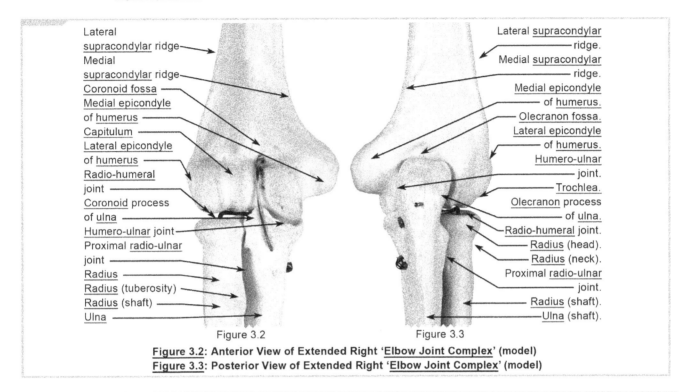

Figure 3.2

Figure 3.3

Figure 3.2: Anterior View of Extended Right 'Elbow Joint Complex' (model)
Figure 3.3: Posterior View of Extended Right 'Elbow Joint Complex' (model)

3.2 JOINTS OF THE ELBOW

3.2.0 The Elbow Joint complex

What is usually referred to as the elbow or elbow joint is actually a <u>joint complex</u>.

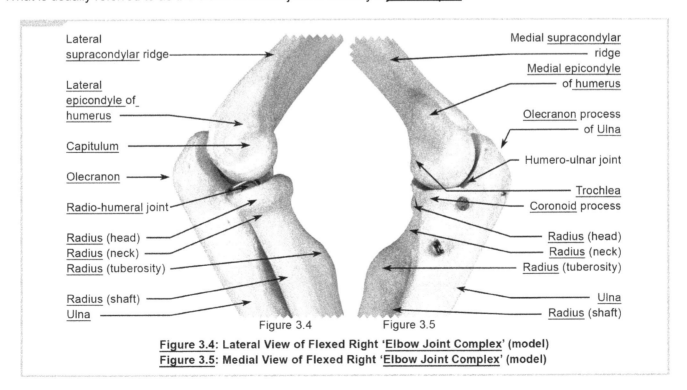

Figure 3.4

Figure 3.5

Figure 3.4: Lateral View of Flexed Right 'Elbow Joint Complex' (model)
Figure 3.5: Medial View of Flexed Right 'Elbow Joint Complex' (model)

The elbow joint complex consists of 4 articulations (joints):

-       Humeroulnar joint [Section 3.2.1]
-       Radiohumeral joint [Section 3.2.2]
-       Proximal radioulnar joint [Section 3.2.3]
-       Distal radioulnar joint [Section 3.3.4].

The 4th joint is actually closer to the wrist but since it moves in conjunction with the proximal radioulnar joint it is often thought of as a fourth joint of the elbow.

3.2.1 Humeroulnar (HU) Joint

Location   between trochlea of humerus and trochlea notch of ulna
Classification   synovial, hinge, uniaxial, simple joint
Movements   flexion and extension
Ligaments   Ulnar collateral ligaments

3.2.2 Radiohumeral (RH) Joint

Location   between capitulum of humerus and head of radius
Classification   synovial, hinge, uni-axial, simple joint
Movements   flexion and extension
Ligaments   radial collateral ligaments

3.2.3 Proximal Radioulnar (PRU) Joint

Location   between head of radius and radial notch of ulna
Classification   synovial, pivot, multi-axial, simple joint
Movements   pronation, supination
Ligaments   annular ligament

3.2.4 Distal Radioulnar (DRU) Joint

Location   between distal end of radius and ulna
Classification   synovial, pivot, multi-axial, complex joint
Capsule   weak transverse bands between radius and ulna across anterior and posterior borders
Articular disc   of distal radioulnar joint is the main uniting structure of the joint

3.2.5 Special Features of the Elbow Joint Complex

3.2.5.1 Articular capsule of the elbow joint complex

An articular capsule surrounds the elbow joint complex. This capsule surrounds the humeroulnar joint, the radio humeral joint and proximal radioulnar joint, but does not surround the distal radioulnar joint. The joint capsule is weak anteriorly and posteriorly, but is strengthened medially and laterally by collateral ligaments.

3.2.5.2 Bursae of the elbow joint complex

There are two bursae in the elbow joint complex. These are the:

- **Subcutaneous olecranon bursae** which sits subcutaneously over the olecranon and is exposed during falls on the elbow; and the
- **Subtendinous olecranon bursae** which sits between triceps tendon and olecranon, and is aggravated by repetitive flexion/extension of forearm resulting in pain on flexion due to pressure of triceps brachii.

3.2.5.3 Radioulnar interosseus membrane

The radioulnar interosseus membrane lies along the length of and between the radius and ulnar. It is classified as a fibrous syndesmosis (ie a non-synovial joint). Its functions are to:

- Bind the radius and ulna together, yet keeps them separate
- Provide attachment for forearm muscles
- Provide a tension that aids pronation and supination
- Allow the transmission of force from radius to ulna due to oblique downwards position, thus protects the radius

     [See Section 3.9.1.6 for the Application to Yoga].

3.2.5.4 Carrying angle of the arm

The <u>carrying angle of the arm</u> is the angle between the upper and lower arm when the body is in the <u>anatomical position</u>

(ie *savasana*). The carrying angle permits the forearm to clear the hip while carrying heavy loads with the least muscular effort. Females usually have a larger carrying angle.

3.3 MUSCLES OF THE ELBOW JOINT COMPLEX

The attachments and actions of the muscles of the <u>elbow joint complex</u> are shown in Table 3.1, and in Figures 2.5, 2.6, 3.7 and 3.8. The movements of the <u>elbow joint complex</u> are summarised in Table 3.2.

Table 3.1 Muscles that move the forearm [Adapted from Moore, 1992]

MUSCLE	ORIGINS	INSERTIONS	ACTIONS &/or ROLES
Triceps brachii	• **Long head**: infraglenoid tubercle of scapula • **Lateral head**: posterior surface of proximal humerus • **Medial head**: posterior surface of humerus	• Olecranon process of the ulna • Fascia of forearm	• Extends forearm • Long head steadies the abducted humerus
Biceps brachii	• **Short head**: coracoid process of scapula • **Long head**: supra-glenoid tubercle of scapula	• Tuberosity of radius • Fascia of forearm via bicipital aponeurosis	• Flexes forearm • Supinates forearm • Weak flexor of the arm at the shoulder joint
Brachialis	• Distal anterior humerus	• Coronoid process of ulna • Tuberosity of ulna	• Flexes forearm
Brachio-radialis	• Lateral supracondylar ridge of humerus	• Lateral surface of distal end of radius	• Flexes forearm
Pronator teres	• Medial epicondyle of humerus • Coronoid process of ulna	• Mid lateral surface of radius	• Pronates forearm • Flexes forearm • Binds radius and ulna
Anconeus	• Lateral epicondyle of humerus	• Lateral surface ulna, Olecranon process of ulna • Proximal part of posterior ulna	• Extends forearm • Stabilises elbow joint. • Abducts ulna during pronation
Supinator	• Lateral epicondyle of humerus • Posterior ulna	• Posterior, lateral & anterior surfaces of proximal radius	• Supinates forearm
Pronator quadratus	• Distal ¼ of ulna, anterior surface	• Distal ¼ of radius, anterior surface	• Pronates forearm at elbow joint • Binds radius & ulna

Table 3.2 Movements and muscle groups of the elbow joint complex and kurpara bandha

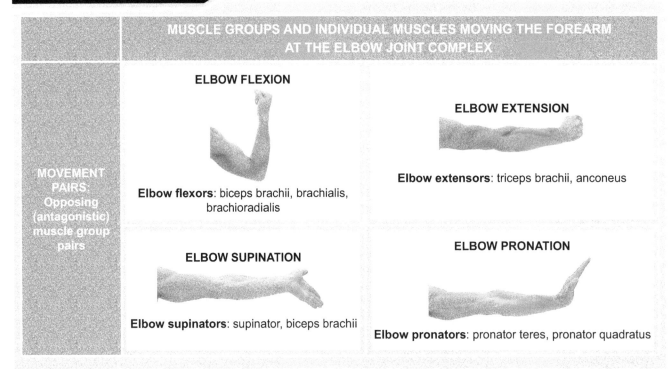

MOVEMENT PAIRS: Opposing (antagonistic) muscle group pairs	MUSCLE GROUPS AND INDIVIDUAL MUSCLES MOVING THE FOREARM AT THE ELBOW JOINT COMPLEX	
	ELBOW FLEXION **Elbow flexors**: biceps brachii, brachialis, brachioradialis	**ELBOW EXTENSION** **Elbow extensors**: triceps brachii, anconeus
	ELBOW SUPINATION **Elbow supinators**: supinator, biceps brachii	**ELBOW PRONATION** **Elbow pronators**: pronator teres, pronator quadratus

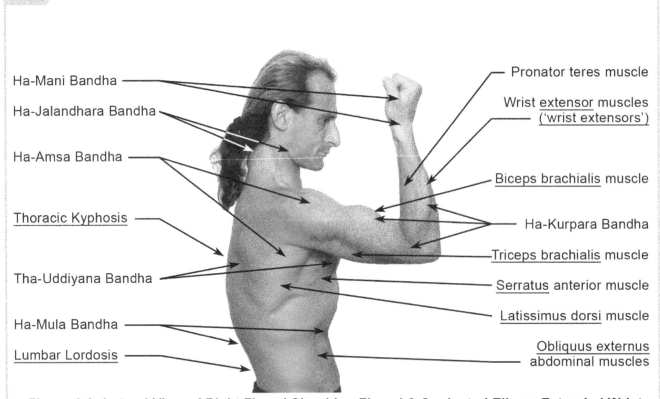

Ha-Mani Bandha — Pronator teres muscle

Ha-Jalandhara Bandha — Wrist <u>extensor</u> muscles ('wrist extensors')

Ha-Amsa Bandha — <u>Biceps brachialis</u> muscle

Thoracic Kyphosis — Ha-Kurpara Bandha

Tha-Uddiyana Bandha — <u>Triceps brachialis</u> muscle

Serratus anterior muscle

Latissimus dorsi muscle

Ha-Mula Bandha — <u>Obliquus externus</u> abdominal muscles

Lumbar Lordosis —

Figure 3.8: Lateral View of Right <u>Flexed</u> Shoulder, <u>Flexed</u> & <u>Supinated</u> Elbow, Extended Wrist & Flexed Hand showing the Bandhas of the Upper Body

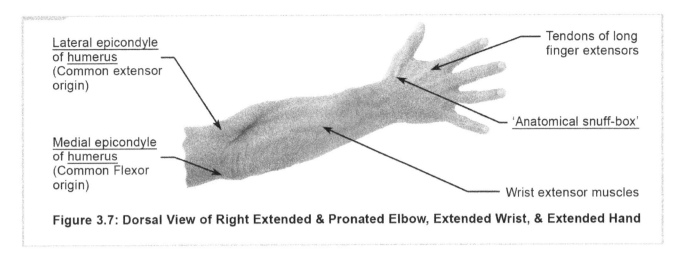

Lateral epicondyle of humerus (Common extensor origin)

Medial epicondyle of humerus (Common Flexor origin)

Tendons of long finger extensors

'Anatomical snuff-box'

Wrist extensor muscles

Figure 3.7: Dorsal View of Right Extended & Pronated Elbow, Extended Wrist, & Extended Hand

3.4 BONES OF THE WRIST & HAND

On a skeleton, and using Figures 3.1–3.5, identify the following features of the wrist and hand:

Carpal bones (8): start from left palm anterior <u>ulna</u> anti-clockwise:
- **Distal row:** <u>hamate</u>, <u>capitate</u>, <u>trapezoid</u>, <u>trapezium</u>
- **Proximal row:** <u>scaphoid</u>, <u>lunate</u>, <u>triquetrum</u>, <u>pisiform</u>.
- (Mnemonic: *How Can Tiny Tim Sing Looney Tunes Pissed*!!!)

Metacarpals (5): I (thumb), II (index), III (middle), IV (ring), V (little), all have a base shaft and head, forming the knuckles of the hand.

Phalanges (14): proximal, middle (not thumb) and distal, all have a base, shaft and head.

Sesamoid bones: usually two in thumb only, but sometimes there exist more in other digits, seen in radiographs only, these are thought to increase the mechanical advantage of the muscles that go over them.

Axis of the hand

The <u>axis of the hand</u> goes through the <u>capitate</u> and digit III. It is important for correct force transmission in positions where weight is taken on the hand

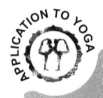

No 3.1 Correct hand positioning in weight-bearing postures of the upper limb maximises force transmission through the wrist

In postures such as down-dog pose *(adho mukha svanasana)* the middle finger (digit III) should point forward (parallel to a mat if it is being used) in order to maximise force transmission via correct positioning of the <u>axis of the hand</u>.

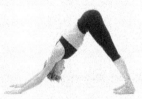

3.5 JOINTS OF THE WRIST & HAND

3.5.0 The Wrist Joint Complex

What is usually referred to as the wrist or wrist joint is actually a <u>joint complex</u> consisting of the <u>radiocarpal joint</u> [Section 3.5.1], the <u>midcarpal joint</u> [Section 3.5.2], and the <u>carpometacarpal joints</u> [Sections 3.5.3 & 3.5.4]. Many of the muscles that act across these three joints also act on the joints of the hand and fingers [Sections 3.5.5 & 3.5.6]. Therefore in this book, all the joints of the wrist, hand and fingers are referred to collectively as the <u>wrist joint complex</u>. The joints of the wrist and hand have articular surfaces which are not congruent and the <u>articular (joint) capsule</u> is partly lax. Hence, the wrist is not a very stable joint in its passive state and only becomes stable if there is <u>co-activation</u> (simutaneous tensing) of the muscles around the wrist joint complex. <u>Co-activation</u> of <u>antagonistic</u> (opposing) muscles of the <u>wrist joint complex</u> is referred to as *mani bandha* [Section 3.9.1.2].

3.5.1 Radiocarpal joint (Proximal Joint of the Wrist)

Location	between the distal end of the radius, triangular articular disc of distal radioulnar joint and the proximal row of carpal bones.
Classification	synovial, simple, bi-axial, ellipsoid/condyloid joint.
Articular (joint) capsule	fibrous and strengthened by ligaments.
Articular disc	triangular and located between the ulna and triquetrum bones.
Ligaments	Palmar radiocarpal ligament and dorsal radiocarpal ligament
	Radial and ulnar collateral ligaments limit abduction and adduction of the wrist.

Main movements at the wrist joint complex

The movements of the wrist joint complex are the movements of the radio-carpal, mid-carpal and inter-carpal joints together. These movements are flexion, extension, adduction (ulnar deviation), abduction (radial deviation) and circumduction (successive flexion, adduction, extension and abduction).

Close-packed position of the wrist joint complex

The close-packed position [Section 1.5.2.6] of a joint is the most stable but also the most susceptible to injury as the ligaments are fully taut. The close-packed position of the wrist joint is full extension and some radial deviation.

3.5.2 Midcarpal Joint

Location	between proximal and distal rows of carpal bones
Classification	synovial, compound, plane, multi axial joint
Movements	flexion, extension, abduction, and adduction
Ligaments	there are palmar, dorsal, and collateral ligaments.

3.5.3 Carpometacarpal (CMC) Joint of Thumb

Location	between trapezium and 1st metacarpal bone
Classification	synovial, simple, sellar, biaxial joint
Movements	flexion, extension, abduction, adduction, and opposition.
Ligaments	there are anterior, posterior and radial collateral ligaments.

3.5.4 Carpometacarpal Joints of Other Digits (2–4)

Classification	synovial, compound, plane, multiaxial joint

3.5.5 Metacarpophalangeal (MCP) Joints

Location	between metacarpal bones and proximal phalanx
Classification	synovial, simple, ellipsoid, biaxial joint
Movements	flexion, extension, abduction, and adduction
Sesamoid bones	These vary in number, but there are usually two sesamoid bones at the first MCP joint and one sesamoid bone at the second MCP joint. Their purpose is to increase the mechanical advantage of the muscles in which they sit.
Ligaments	There are collateral, deep transverse, and palmar ligaments, and a fibrous digital sheath that acts like a bracelet that prevents 'bow-stringing' (popping out) of long tendons when their muscles are activated.

3.5.6 Interphalangeal (IP) joints

Location	between head of proximal phalanx and base of distal phalanx.
Classification	synovial, simple, hinge, uniaxial joint
Movements	flexion and extension
Ligaments	there are collateral and palmar ligaments, the continuing fibrous digital sheath, which prevents 'bow-stringing' of long tendons; and an extensor aponeurosis.

3.6 MUSCLES OF THE WRIST & HAND

Hand muscles are either extrinsic or intrinsic. Extrinsic muscles of the hand have only their distal attachment (insertion) in the hand whereas intrinsic muscles of the hand have both attachments within the hand itself.

3.6.1 Extrinsic Muscles of the Wrist and Hand
The attachments and actions of the extrinsic muscles of the wrist and hand are shown in Tables 3.3 and 3.4.

Table 3.3 Flexors of the wrist & hand

MUSCLE	ORIGINS	INSERTIONS	ACTIONS
Flexor carpi Radialis	• Medial epicondyle, humerus	• Base of 2nd meta-carpal	• Flexes hand • Abducts hand
Palmaris longus	• Medial epicondyle, humerus	• Flexor retinaculum and palmar aponeurosis	• Flexes hand • Tighten palmar aponeurosis
Flexor carpi ulnaris	• Medial epicondyle of humerus • Olecranon process of ulna • Posterior ulna	• Pisiform bone • Hook of hamate • 5th meta-carpal	• Flexes hand • Adducts hand
Flexor digitorum superficialis	• Medial epicondyle of humerus • Anterior radius	• Medial four digits; bodies of middle phalanges	• Flexes middle phalanges • Flexes proximal phalanges of middle four digits
Flexor digitorum profundus	• Ulna medial surface • Ulna anterior surface	• Medial four digits • Base of distal phalanges	• Flexes distal phalanges of middle four digits
Flexor pollicis longus	• Anterior surface of radius	• Thumb • Base of distal phalanx	• Flexes phalanges of thumb

Table 3.4 Extensors of the wrist & hand

MUSCLE	ORIGINS	INSERTIONS	ACTIONS &/or ROLES
Extensor carpi radialis	• Lateral supracondylar ridge of humerus	• Base of 2nd meta-carpal	• Extends hand & • Abducts hand at wrist joint
Extensor digitorum	• Lateral epicondyle of humerus	• Extensor expansions of medial four digits	• Extends medial four digits at MCP joints • Extends hand at wrist joint
Extensor digiti minimi	• Lateral epicondyle of humerus	• Extensor expansion of 5th digit	• Extends digit 5 at MCP joint
Extensor carpi ulnaris	• Lateral epicondyle of humerus • Posterior ulna	• Base of 5th meta-carpal	• Extends hand & • Adducts hand at wrist joint
Abductor pollicis longus	• Posterior radius • Posterior ulna • Interosseus membrane	• Base of 1st meta-carpal	• Abducts and extends thumb at CMC joint
Extensor pollicis longus	• Posterior ulna • Interosseus membrane	• Base of distal phalanx of thumb	• Extends distal phalanx of thumb at MCP & IP joints
Extensor indices	• Posterior ulna • Interosseus membrane	• Extensor expansion of second digit	• Extends digit 2 • Helps extend hand

107

- Note that the common origin of the wrist flexor muscles (common flexor origin) is at the medial epicondyle of the humerus [Figure 3.1-3.5]
- Note, that similarly the common origin of the wrist extensor muscles (common extensor origin) is at the lateral epicondyle of the humerus [Figure 3.1-3.5].
- The movements of the wrist and hand are summarised in Table 3.5.

Table 3.5: Movements & muscle groups of the wrist joint complex and *mani bandha*

Movement pairs: Opposing (antagonistic) muscle group pairs	MUSCLE GROUPS AND INDIVIDUAL MUSCLES MOVING THE FOREARM AT THE WRIST JOINT COMPLEX	
	WRIST FLEXION **Wrist flexors**: flexor carpi radialis & ulnaris, palmaris longus, flexor digitorum profundus & superficialis, flexor pollicis longus, abductor pollicis longus	**WRIST EXTENSION** **Wrist extensors**: extensor carpi radialis longus & brevis, extensor carpi ulnaris, extensor digitorum, extensor pollicis longus, extensor indices, extensor digiti minimi
	WRIST RADIAL DEVIATION (ABDUCTION) **Wrist abductors**: flexor carpi radialis, extensor carpi radialis longus & brevis, abductor pollicis longus, extensor pollicis longus & brevis	**WRIST ULNAR DEVIATION (ADDUCTION)** **Wrist adductors**: flexor carpi ulnaris, extensor carpi ulnaris

3.6.2 Intrinsic Muscles of the Hand

Intrinsic muscles of the hand can be divided into three (3) groups:

(1) **THENAR EMINENCE** (thumb side muscle group)
- i) Flexor pollicis brevis (FPB)
- ii) Abductor pollicis brevis (APB)
- iii) Opponens pollicis (OP)

(2) **HYPOTHENAR EMINENCE** (little finger side muscle group)
- iv) Flexor digiti minimi (FDM)
- v) Abductor digiti minimi (ADM)
- vi) Opponens digiti minimi (ODM)

(3) **OTHER INTRINSICS**
- vii) Adductor pollicis (AP)
- viii) Lumbricals
- ix) Dorsal interossei
- x) Palmar interossei

Important muscles of the forearm, wrist and hand

The following muscles are important in the forearm, wrist and hand. Their attachments and actions are useful to learn. They are relatively easy to see and feel.

1. Triceps brachii
2. Biceps brachii
3. Brachialis
4. Brachioradialis
5. Pronator teres
6. Wrist flexor muscle group (wrist flexors) (learn as a group of muscles)
7. Wrist extensor muscle group (wrist extensors) (learn as a group of muscles)

3.7.1 Position of Function of the Hand

The position of function of the hand represents the position of the hand and wrist such that the bones have the best fit and muscle action is the most efficient. This includes:

*   Radial deviation and some extension at the wrist
*   Slight flexion of the fingers
*   Abduction of the thumb

3.7.2 Anatomical Snuff Box

The dorsal region (top) of the hand bordered by the tendons of extensor pollicis longus, extensor pollicis brevis and abductor pollicis longus is referred to as the anatomical snuff box.

Injury to the scaphoid bone (the most frequently fractured carpal bone) results in localised tenderness in the anatomical snuff box.

3.7.3 Retinacula

The flexor retinacula and extensor retinacula are strong thick fibrous bands that hold the long flexor and extensor tendons at the wrist and prevent a bow-stringing effect.

3.7.4 Digital Sweep: Role of the interossei and lumbricals

Four Lumbricals flex MCP joints and extend IP joints. **Eight Interossei**: 4 dorsal abduct (DAB) and 4 palmar adduct (PAD) the digits.

Together, via the extensor expansion, their role is to balance and moderate the effects of extensor digitorum (which extends the MCP joints) and flexor digitorum superficialis and profundus (which cause flexion at the IP joints).

3.7.5 Synovial Sheaths

Synovial sheaths are tubular sheaths surrounding the long flexor tendons and long extensor tendons across the wrist that act as a lubricating device (bursa) and permit smooth gliding of the tendons. The sheaths are filled with synovial fluid and, like articular (joint) capsules, are susceptible to inflammation.

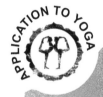

No 3.2 A heating *yoga* practice and an alkaline lifestyle help to keep tendon sheaths flexible

Synovial sheaths, which surround tendons, are filled with synovial fluid, which is thixotropic and therefore becomes less viscous with heat and alkalinity. Therefore, a *yoga* practice that develops body heat in conjunction with a diet that emphasises alkaline foods may assist in the smooth functioning of the tendons and minimise the risk of problems such carpal tunnel syndrome and other problems involving inflammation of the synovial sheaths.

3.7.6 The Carpal Tunnel

The carpal tunnel is formed by the flexor retinaculum and the anterior concavity of the carpus (carpal bones).

The digital flexor tendons and the median nerve pass through the carpal tunnel. The median nerve may become compressed after wrist trauma (eg fractures), from tenosynovitis of the flexor tendons (inflammation of the tender sheaths around the flexor tendons) or from metabolic/hormonal conditions (eg diabetes, menopause). Medial nerve compression in these circumstances is known as carpal tunnel syndrome.

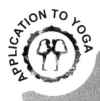

No 3.3 Yoga can help carpal tunnel syndrome

One research study [Garfinkel *et al.*, 1998] has shown that a *yoga*-based regimen was more effective than wrist splinting or no treatment in relieving some symptoms and signs of carpal tunnel syndrome.

3.7.7. Elbow Tendonitis: Tennis Elbow

Elbow tendonitis is a painful musculoskeletal condition that may result from forceful repetitive pronation supination of the forearm.

Elbow tendonitis is also known as lateral epicondylitis, or tennis elbow but is not confined to those who play tennis. It is characterised by pain or point tenderness at, or just distal to, the lateral epicondyle of the humerus. It appears to result from inflammation of the lateral epicondyle and premature degeneration of the common extensor tendon of the forearm. The pain is exacerbated by activities that put strain on the common extensor tendon.

3.8 NERVES OF THE FOREARM, WRIST & HAND

3.8.1 Peripheral Nerves of the Brachial Plexus:
Root Values, Courses, Sensory Distributions and Motor Distributions

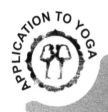

No 3.4 Nerve tensioning (stretching) can relieve many neck, shoulder, elbow and wrist problems

Understanding of the pathways of the peripheral nerves of the brachial plexus enables *yoga* to tension (stretch) these nerves and their associated *nadis*. This may help relieve some neck, shoulder, elbow and wrist problems and can increase one's sense of well being. However, an over-stretch of the nerves of the brachial plexus can cause discomfort, pain and/or damage.

POSTERIOR CORD of the brachial plexus
- **Axillary nerve** (= circumflex humeral nerve)
  - o **Spinal segments/nerve roots:** arise from nerves roots of C5 and C6
  - o **Muscular branches:** innervates deltoid and teres minor
- **Radial nerve:** the largest branch of the brachial plexus
  - o **Spinal segments/nerve roots:** arise from C5, 6, 7, 8, (T1)
  - o **Course:** passes between long and medial head of triceps brachii, passes obliquely across back of humerus then becomes posterior interosseus (deep terminal) branch of the radial nerve.
  - o **Cutaneous branches:** supply the skin on the dorsal surface of the arm as far as the olecranon process of the ulna, on the lateral part of the lower half of the arm, and along the dorsum of the forearm to the wrist.
  - o **Articular branches:** are distributed to the elbow joint.
  - o **Muscular branches:** supply triceps brachii, anconeus, extensor carpi radialis longus, and brachialis.
- **Posterior interosseus (deep terminal) branch of the radial nerve:**
  - o **Course:** reaches the back of the forearm round the lateral aspect of the radius
  - o **Articular branches:** supply carpal joints, distal radioulnar joints, some inter-carpal joints and inter-meta-carpal joints, MCP joints and PIP joints
  - o **Muscular branches:** supply extensor carpi radialis brevis, supinator, extensor digitorum, extensor digiti minimi, extensor carpi ulnaris, extensor pollicis longus, extensor indicis, abductor pollicis longus and extensor pollicis brevis.

LATERAL CORD of the Brachial Plexus:
- **Musculocutaneous nerve**
  - o **Spinal segments/nerve roots:** arise from C5, 6, 7
  - o **Course:** pierces coracobrachialis and descends laterally between the biceps brachii and the brachialis

to the lateral side of the arm.
  - o **Articular branches:** innervate the elbow joint
  - o **Muscular branches:** supply coracobrachialis, biceps brachii and brachialis.
- **Median nerve (lateral root)**
  - o **Spinal segments/nerve roots:** roots are dual: (lateral - C5, 6, 7 and medial – C8, T1)
  - o **Course:** runs on the lateral side of the brachial artery with no branches in the arm but passes to forearm as anterior interosseus branch of the median nerve.
  - o **Articular branches:** to the elbow joint.
  - o **Muscular branches** supply flexor muscles in forearm including flexor carpi radialis, palmaris longus, flexor digitorum superficialis, flexor pollicis longus, except lateral half of flexor digitorum profundus and all flexor carpi ulnaris; also supplies pronator teres and quadratus, and the thenar muscles and lumbricals.

MEDIAL CORD of the Brachial Plexus:
- **Median nerve** (medial root and anterior interosseus branch)
- **Ulnar nerve**
  - o **Spinal segments/nerve roots:** arise from C7, 8, and T1
  - o **Course:** passes anteriorly to the scapula (as do the others here) then passes distally, anteriorly to the triceps brachii, on the medial side of the brachial artery with no branches in the arm, then passes between the medial epicondyle of the humerus and the olecranon process of the ulna to enter the forearm, and passes between the heads of flexor carpi ulnaris, then descends deep to flexor digitorum profundus and accompanies the ulnar artery in the middle of the forearm.
  - o **Articular branches:** innervate the elbow joint.
  - o **Muscular branches:** supply flexor carpi ulnaris and the medial half of flexor digitorum profundus; also supply hypothenar muscles, adductor pollicis, palmar and dorsal interossei, palmaris brevis and lumbricals 4, 5.

3.8.2 Innervation of the Joints of the Upper Limb
A general rule for the **nerve supply to the joints** is **Hiltons Law**, which states that nerves that supply muscles acting on a joint usually send fibres to it.

The nerves that supply the joints of the shoulder, elbow and wrist are as follows:
- The shoulder joint complex is innervated by branches of the supra scapular, axillary and lateral pectoral nerves
- The elbow joint complex is innervated mainly by the musculocutaneous nerve and radial nerve but the ulnar nerve, median nerve and anterior interosseus nerve may also supply articular branches
- The wrist joint complex is innervated by the anterior interosseus branch of the median nerve, posterior interosseus branch of the radial nerve and deep branches of the radial nerve.

3.8.3 Functional Motor Loss and Deformity Resulting from Nerve Lesions
3.8.3.1 Radial nerve lesions
Lesion of the radial nerve in the axilla (armpit) leads to the syndrome known as wrist drop due to:
- Paralysis of triceps brachii, brachioradialis, supinator, and extensors of the wrist and digits
- Significant sensory loss in the skin of upper and lower arm
- The inability to extend wrist due to paralysis of the extensor muscles of the forearm (wrist drop)

3.8.3.2 Ulnar nerve lesions
Lesion of the ulnar nerve at the medial epicondyle of the humerus can lead to the syndrome known as claw hand due to:
- Extensive motor loss to the hand; paralysis of flexor carpi ulnaris, the hypothenar muscles, and the intrinsic hand muscles; when an attempt is made to flex the wrist the hand is drawn to the radial side by flexor carpi radialis; a fist cannot be made due to the inability to flex digits 4 and 5 at DIP joints because of paralysis of some lumbricals which moderate the effect of flexor digitorum and extensor digitorum via the extensor expansion (digital sweep) [Section 3.7.3]
- Extensive sensory loss to hand

3.8.3.3 Median nerve lesions
Lesion of the median nerve at the wrist frequently occurs just proximal to the flexor retinaculum [Section 3.7.3] due to wrist slashing. It can result in:

111

- The inability to oppose the thumb due to paralysis of the thenar muscles; loss of fine control of digits 3 and 4 due to loss of lumbricals.
- Cutaneous (skin) sensory loss in the lateral part of the hand.

3.9 APPLIED ANATOMY OF THE FOREARM, WRIST & HAND IN *HATHA YOGA* POSTURES

Many *yoga* postures such as the *cataranga dandasana* (push up) are weight-bearing on the upper limb (the arm). Upper limb weight-bearing postures have been shown to increase the strength of the elbow extensors and the forearm musculature, and to help improve bone density [Blimkie et al, 1996].

Similarly many *yoga* postures can utilise elbow flexors. Forward bending poses such as

supta pavanmuktasana and *pascimottanasana* that involve a pulling action of the upper limb against part of the lower limbs can be used to exercise the elbow flexors provided a sufficient bracing effect is given by a firmness from the trunk musculature (*mula bandha*) in order to protect structures in the spine.

To safely perform any of the *yoga* postures using the upper limbs, there needs to be a practical understanding of the muscles that cross the shoulder, elbow, wrist and hand. In addition, the ability to co-activate (simultaneously tense) antagonistic (opposing) muscles around the shoulder, elbow, and wrist is integral to the safe application of stretching and strengthening exercises for the upper limb.

3.9.1 *Bandhas* of the Elbow Joint complex and Wrist Joint complex

Co-activation of antagonistic muscles crossing the elbow joint complex can be termed an elbow *bandha* [Section 1.7.3.1]. Similarly co-activation of antagonistic (opposing) muscle groups crossing the wrist joint complex can also be termed a wrist *bandha*. Elbow and wrist *bandhas* are analogous to the three central *bandhas* described in the traditional *yoga* text, *Hatha Yoga Pradipika* [Devananda, 1987]. Application of these *bandhas* during movement and in static postures while practising *hatha yoga* has the following benefits:

- Increases stability of the elbow joint complex and wrist joint complex
- Increases strength of the muscles crossing the elbow joint complex and wrist joint complex
- Improves coordinated control of the muscles crossing the elbow joint complex and wrist joint complex
- Helps maintain bone density in the upper limb
- Enables improved nerve tensioning of the nerves of the brachial plexus [Sections 1.7.2.1, 3.8.1 & 9.7.3]
- Generates body heat, which makes the synovial fluid less viscous and joints more flexible
- Improves the effect of the musculoskeletal pump, increasing circulation
- Helps stimulate the formation of other *bandhas* in the body.

3.9.1.1 Co-activation of opposing muscles around the elbow joint: *kurpara bandha*

Co-activation of antagonistic (opposing) muscle groups crossing the elbow joint complex forms an elbow joint *bandha*, referred to as *kurpara bandha* in *Sanskrit* [Section 1.7.3.1]. *Kurpara bandha* is easiest for most people to

master in the open-chain exercise of making bulging biceps (i.e. tensing the biceps brachii) with a flexed elbow and supinated forearm. This exercise is familiar to most people. It is only possible to activate biceps brachii and make it bulge if there is a co-activation (simultaneous tensing) of the triceps brachii. Once this exercise has been mastered it can be progressed to slowly extending the elbow while maintaining the <u>co-activation</u> of <u>biceps brachii</u> and <u>triceps brachii</u>. This can be later progressed further by <u>pronating</u> the forearm and engaging the muscles of <u>pronation</u> (eg. <u>pronator teres</u>) along with muscles of <u>extension</u> and <u>flexion</u> (which includes <u>supination</u> from the <u>biceps brachii</u>).

Note that because the <u>biceps brachii</u> and <u>triceps brachii</u> both have elements which cross the <u>glenohumeral joint</u>, the formation of the *kurpara* (elbow) *bandha* assists in the stabilisation of the <u>glenohumeral joint</u> and hence in the formation of the of *amsa* (shoulder) *bandha*, which in turn assists the formation and maintenance of the three central *bandhas* (*mula, uddiyana,* and *jalandhara bandhas*) [Section 2.5.1.4].

3.9.1.2 Co-activation of opposing muscles around the wrist joint: *mani bandha*

<u>Co-activation</u> of antagonistic (opposing) muscle groups that cross the <u>wrist joint complex</u> can be referred to as a wrist *bandha*, or in *Sanskrit, mani bandha. Mani bandha* is formed when <u>wrist extensors</u> are co-activated with <u>wrist flexors</u>.

Mani bandha can be quite easily activated in both its *ha* (hot, compressive or pushing) form or in a *tha* (cool, expansive or pulling) form. The ability to form several types of *bandhas* at the one <u>joint complex</u> is because the <u>extensors</u> of the wrist joint also cross the joints of the hand and fingers. Therefore <u>wrist extensors</u> can also extend the fingers (<u>interphalangeal joints</u>) and palm (<u>carpal</u> and <u>meta carpal joints</u>). Similarly the <u>flexors</u> of the wrist also cross the joints of the hand and fingers. Therefore, <u>wrist flexors</u> can also flex the fingers (<u>interphalangeal joints</u>) and palm (<u>carpal</u> and <u>meta carpal joints</u>).

3.9.1.2.1 *Ha-mani bandha*: a compressive *bandha* of the wrist and hand [Appendix C]

Ha-mani bandha is a compressive <u>co-activation</u> of <u>antagonistic</u> wrist muscles. In effect it is a simultaneous tensing of <u>wrist extensors</u> and <u>finger flexors</u>.

The simplest *ha-mani bandha* can be generated when a clenched fist is made with the hand. To achieve the strongest clenched fist, and the most stable *ha-mani bandha*, the wrist should be held in slight <u>extension</u>, which requires some <u>wrist extensor</u> activity. At the same time <u>finger flexors</u>, (which can also act on the wrist and are in fact also <u>wrist flexors</u>), are actively <u>flexing</u> the fingers (<u>meta-carpal</u> and <u>interphalangeal joints</u>). Hence a <u>co-activation</u> of antagonistic (opposing) muscles of the wrist and hand (<u>wrist flexors</u> and <u>wrist extensors</u>) has been made. *Ha-mani bandha* (a compressive *bandha*) may be subjectively felt to push energy, especially in the form of blood, away from the hand and back towards the body when the elbow is extended. A noticeable increase in core body temperature can be immediately felt upon making a closed fist after first stretching the fingers.

3.9.1.2.2 *Tha-mani bandha:* an expansive *bandha* of the wrist and hand [Appendix C]

Tha-mani bandha is an expanive <u>co-activation</u> of <u>antagonistic</u> wrist muscles. In effect it is a simultaneous tensing of <u>wrist flexors</u> and <u>finger extensors</u>. The simplest *tha-mani bandha* can be generated when the palms are made to fully open and stretch out. If the muscles of the palm are left passive, the fingers will generally remain in <u>semi-flexed</u> position. Therefore, to fully extend the fingers requires the use of <u>finger extensors</u>, which include muscles that also cross the wrist and can extend the wrist (i.e. many <u>finger flexors</u> are also <u>wrist extensors</u>). To counter any unwanted <u>extension</u> at the wrist, the <u>wrist flexors</u> must become at least slightly active. Therefore, the simple act of stretching into the finger tips necessarily causes a <u>co-activation</u> (a *bandha*) of the <u>antagonistic</u> (opposing) <u>muscle groups</u> of the wrist and hand. This expansive or stretching *bandha* may be subjectively felt to pull or suck energy, especially in the form of blood and body heat, away from the body towards the hand.

The less these muscles can be tensed to achieve the feeling of straightening the fingers and palm or stretching into the finger tips, the more effective this *mani mudra* (wrist gesture) will be as a *tha-mani bandha* (i.e. a co-activation of antagonistic (opposing) muscle groups of the wrist joint complex which produces a suction effect towards the hand).

The feeling of the *ha-mani bandha* pushing energy or blood away from the hand to the body, while the *tha-mani bandha* pulls energy or blood from the body towards the hand may best be felt, when the two exercises (formation of *ha* or *tha-mani bandhas*) are performed with the arms abducted at the shoulder and extended at the elbows. In this position most people can feel a difference in central body heat and in sensation in which the stretched fingers and hand of *tha-mani bandha* acts as if it has a partial vacuum inside it, which pulls energy and blood towards the hand thus cooling the body, while the more compressed fist of the *ha-mani bandha* acts to push energy and blood away from the hand thus heating the body.

3.9.1.3 *Mudras* and *bandhas* of the wrist and hand

Many *yoga asanas* (postures) include *mudras* (controlled movements or gestures) of the wrist and hand, which can place a stretch on muscles and connective tissues. If the elbow joint complex and shoulder joint complex as well as the cervical spine are appropriately aligned, the *mudras* of the hands can also tension (stretch) nerves from the brachial plexus in the neck to the radial nerve, ulnar nerve and median nerve reaching the hand. In addition, acupuncture meridians and the more subtle *nadis* (energy channels) are also being stretched.

The radial nerve is tensioned in *atanu puritat mudra* [Figure 9.1], which also tensions

(stretches) the large intestine meridian. The median nerve is tensioned in *kloman mudra* [Figure 9.2], which also tensions the lung meridian. The median nerve is also tensioned in *bukka puritat mudra* [Figure 9.3], which also tensions the pericardium meridian. The ulnar nerve is tensioned in buddhizuddhi mudra [Figure 9.4], which also tensions the heart meridian. The ulnar nerve is also tensioned in *anumukha puritat mudra* [Figure 9.5], which also tensions the small intestine meridian.

It is important to note that it is not the position of a joint complex that makes it behave as a *ha-bandha* or *tha-bandha*, but rather the activities of the muscles crossing that joint complex. For example *ha-mani bandha* can also be formed with the wrist extension and the finger extension with the palm flat on the floor as in many

weight-bearing, closed-chain postures such as the *san tolasana* (plank position), *tolasana* (scales posture), the *urdhva mukha svanasana* (up-dog pose) and the *urdhva dhanurasana* (inverted bow position). These weight-bearing, extended wrist postures only remain stable in the wrist for prolonged periods if there is co-activation of antagonistic wrist muscles i.e. with *mani bandha*. In fact stability of the wrist may be jeopardised if finger flexors (or wrist flexors) are not active. This phenomenon represents a type of *ha-mani bandha* which is in wrist flexion and finger extension, but which for stability and strength of the wrist has active finger flexors (lengthened) and active wrist extensors (shortened). This type of *ha-mani bandha* is best performed as if you are trying to grab a section of the floor or by pressing the fingers into the floor while keeping the palm flat.

When this extended *ha-mani bandha* is performed with a firm muscular co-activation of finger flexors and wrist extensors its high pressure nature acts to push the body away from the ground. This is precisely what is needed in these postures to protect and strengthen the wrist joint complex. Also in postures such as the

adho mukha vrksasana (handstand), balance is far easier to achieve when there is this type of compressive co-activation of the antagonistic muscle groups (i.e. *ha-mani bandha*).

The position of the wrist joint complex in this type of *ha-mani bandha* resembles the nerve tensioning (stretching) exercises or *mudras* of the brachial plexus [Section 1.7.2.1]. When this type of weight-bearing or closed-chain *ha-mani bandha* is formed, depending on the position of the shoulders and elbows, the median nerve, the ulnar nerve and other elements of the brachial plexus may be tensioned (stretched) [Section 1.7.2.2.1 & 9.7.3]. If these *mudras* (gestures) are done as open-chain exercises (i.e. the hand is not fixed and is free to move) then *bandhas* are difficult to generate. However, if done as part of either a weight-bearing or closed-chain exercise then they can become very powerful bandhas and mudras at the same time and can significantly tension nerves as well as generating energy. This is especially the case for the floor hand in

utthita parsvakonasana 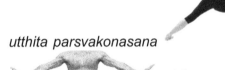 which can have a *ha-mani bandha* and *bukka puritat mudra* at the same time.

In postures such as the *adho mukha vrksasana* (handstand) both hands function best when they form a *ha-mani bandha* (a compressive pushing wrist *bandha*), which can push the body away from the floor.

In postures such as *utkatasana* both hands function best when they form a *tha-mani bandha* with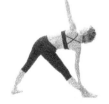

its effect of pulling blood and energy up against gravity. In postures such as *trikonasana*

and *parsvakonasana* 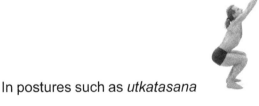 the lower hand, which may either squeeze the ankle or press onto the floor, acts as a *ha-mani bandha*, which can push heat, blood and the body away from the floor. At the same time the hand that is stretched up into the air acts as a *tha-mani bandha*, which acts to pull the body away from the floor. It is an interesting experiment to reverse the two *mani bandhas* in *trikonasana* and notice a dramatic change in circulatory flow and in how the posture feels.

3.9.1.4 *Bandha* inter-connectedness

When a *mani bandha* is generated and a <u>co-activation</u> of <u>wrist flexors</u> and <u>wrist extensors</u> is made, an effect is felt at the <u>elbow joint complex</u>. This is mainly due to two reasons:

*   Both the <u>flexor origins</u> and <u>extensor origins</u> are proximal to the elbow, and hence the <u>wrist flexors</u> and <u>wrist extensors</u> are also weak <u>elbow flexors</u> and <u>elbow extensors</u> respectively.
*   The <u>fascia</u> covering the <u>wrist flexors</u> and <u>wrist extensors</u> is contiguous with the <u>fascia</u> covering the <u>elbow flexors</u> and <u>elbow extensors</u>. Therefore, any activation of the <u>wrist flexors</u> or extensors will cause a minor stretching of the <u>elbow flexors</u> and <u>elbow extensors</u>, which may then be stimulated to activate or tense due to the effects of the stretch reflex [Section 1.7.2.2.1].

<u>Co-activation</u> of the muscles of the wrists (*mani bandha*) will assist in <u>co-activation</u> of the muscles of the elbow (*kurpara bandha*), which in turn assists in <u>co-activation</u> of the muscles of the shoulder (*amsa bandha*), which in turn assists in the formation of the three central *bandhas* (*jalandhara*, *uddiyana* and *mula bandhas*).

3.9.1.5 *Mani bandha* and *mula bandha* effects on the cardiopulmonary system

An English research group [Hughes et al., 1989] has studied the blood pressure of athletes when they perform <u>Valsalva manoeuvre</u> [Appendix E] and isometric handgrip. <u>Valsalva's manoeuvre</u> is to make an attempt at expiration with the glottis closed. Thus a <u>Valsalva manoeuvre</u> is essentially like performing a *ha-mula bandha* [Sections 1.7.3 & 7.5.1.1] and/or a *ha-uddiyana bandha* [Sections 7.5.1.3] while holding the breath in. An <u>isometric</u> handgrip is essentially like a *ha-mani bandha* [Section 3.9.1.2], like trying to make a closed fist. It was found [Hughes et al., 1989] that <u>stroke volume</u> (the amount of blood ejected from the heart in one beat) fell by almost 70% during <u>Valsalva's manoeuvre</u> alone, but fell only about 40% with simultaneous isometric handgrip. <u>Blood pressure</u> changes during isometric handgrip were also significantly modified by simultaneous <u>Valsalva's manoeuvre</u>. An isometric handgrip alone (*ha-mani bandha*) normally leads to a decrease in blood pressure until the grip is released (*tha-mani bandha*) when there is a brief increase in blood pressure, which triggers a <u>baroreceptor-mediated</u> fall in <u>heart rate</u>. However, during the simultaneous application of the <u>Valsalva's manoeuvre</u> there was much less change in blood pressure and <u>heart rate</u> throughout. Therefore <u>Valsalva's manoeuvres</u>, which resemble *ha-mula bandha* [Sections 1.7.3 & 7.5.1.1] and/or a *ha-uddiyana bandha* [Sections 7.5.1.3] invoked extreme falls in cardiac output and blood pressure in athletes. However, these falls were not as significant when there was a simultaneous isometric handgrip or *ha-mani bandha*. This suggests that a combined application of the *bandhas* regulates blood pressure and cardiac output in a complicated way.

3.9.2 Anatomical Principles of *Yoga* Therapy of the Forearm, Wrist and Hand

Yoga therapy for the forearm, wrist and hand should generally address the following issues:

*   Increase the strength of <u>elbow flexors</u>, <u>elbow extensors</u> and <u>elbow pronators</u>
*   Increase the flexibility of <u>elbow flexors</u>, <u>elbow extensors</u> and <u>elbow pronators</u>
*   Increase the strength of <u>wrist flexors</u> (and <u>finger flexors</u>) and <u>wrist extensors</u> (and <u>finger extensors</u>)
*   Increase the flexibility of <u>wrist flexors</u> (and <u>finger flexors</u>) and <u>wrist extensors</u> (and <u>finger extensors</u>)
*   Learn to <u>co-activate</u> <u>elbow flexors</u>, <u>elbow extensors</u> and <u>elbow pronators</u> (create *kurpara bandha*) in various joint positions of the upper limb [Sections 3.9.1 & 3.9.2]
*   Learn to <u>co-activate</u> <u>wrist flexors</u> and <u>wrist extensors</u> (create *mani bandha*) in various joint positions of the upper limb [Sections 3.9.1 & 3.9.2]
*   Learn to control and co-ordinate these muscle groups and both *mani* and *kurpara bandhas* when the arm is in different positions [Sections 3.9.1 & 3.9.2]
*   Learn to <u>tension</u> (stretch) the nerves of the <u>brachial plexus</u> [Sections 1.7.2.2.1 & 9.7.3]
*   Increase the mobility of the <u>thoracic spine</u> [Sections 2.5.3, & 7.5.2]
*   Increase the strength of the muscles of the <u>shoulder joint complex</u> [Section 2.5]
*   Increase the flexibility of the <u>shoulder joint complex</u> [Section 2.5].

3.9.2.1 Elbow flexor strength can be increased by resisting action of the arms with hip extensor activity

Many *yoga* postures are available for strengthening <u>elbow flexors</u>. For example, in standing or supine variations of the *pavanmuktasana* 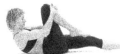 or *padangusthasana* 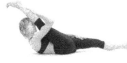 series of exercises, the arms can be used to pull one knee or leg toward the chest.

To increase <u>elbow flexor</u> activity the knee can be pushed away from the body, by activating <u>hip extensors</u>, in order to actively resist the efforts of the <u>elbow flexors</u>.

NB. For safety of the lower back, the lower abdominal muscles must also be activated during this exercise.

3.9.2.2 Elbow extensors and flexors can be used to stabilise the shoulder joint

The long heads of the main extensor (<u>triceps brachii</u>) and main flexor (<u>biceps brachii</u>) of the elbow cross over the shoulder joint and attach to the upper and lower rims of the socket (<u>glenoid fossa</u>) of the shoulder joint on the <u>scapula</u>. A <u>co-activation</u> of these two muscles around the <u>elbow joint complex</u> (*kurpara bandha*) [Sections 1.7.3.1 & 3.9] can help stabilise the <u>head of the humerus</u> in the <u>glenoid fossa</u> (the socket of the shoulder joint).

In this way, <u>triceps brachii</u> and <u>biceps brachii</u> can act as a <u>rotator cuff synergists</u>. When <u>rotator cuff muscles</u> are damaged or weak, <u>co-activation</u> of <u>elbow flexors</u> and <u>elbow extensors</u> can help to reduce and help manage this problem and the problems associated with it.

3.9.2.3 Elbow flexors can be used to rest the elbow extensors

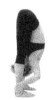

<u>Elbow flexors</u> such as the <u>biceps brachii</u> can be activated in postures such as *uttanasana* or

baddha hasta prasarita padottonasana . Postures such as these, which activate <u>elbow</u>

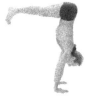

<u>flexors</u>, are good to perform before or after postures such as the *adho mukha vrksasana* (handstand) where <u>elbow extensors</u> such as <u>triceps brachii</u> have been generating tension.

<u>Biceps brachii</u> activation helps relax <u>triceps brachii</u> via <u>reciprocal reflex inhibition</u> [Sections 1.7.2.2.1.2 & 9.4.2.2], and thus allow the <u>triceps brachii</u> the chance to rest.

3.9.2.4 Forearm muscles can be used to stretch and release a stiff neck or upper back

An example of how *yoga* postures work holistically is seen with the use of the <u>forearm pronator muscles</u> in

a <u>closed-chain</u> exercise such as the *adho mukha svanasana* (down-dog pose). If the forearm is <u>pronated</u> while the palm is kept on the floor or wall in the downward-facing dog, it can result in a passive <u>external rotation</u> of the <u>shoulder (GH) joint</u>.

In other words, closed-chain pronation (the hand stays still and the forearm moves) in the downward-facing dog pose, can assist in keeping the shoulder blades spread without having to greatly activate, and thus harden, the muscles of the shoulders. This can in turn assist to stretch and relax a tight neck or stiff thoracic spine.

3.9.2.5 Forearm and wrist strength and stability can be increased with *mani bandha* in both contractile (weight-bearing) and tensile (pulling) exercises

Forearm and wrist muscles can be strengthened in both contractile (weight-bearing) postures and tensile (pulling) postures when a co-activation of the wrist flexors and wrist extensors (*mani bandha*) is made.

Wrist flexors and wrist extensors are usually automatically co-activated when the hand is used to grab or

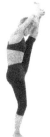

squeeze something. For example, in postures like *utthita padangusthasana*   your hand can pull and

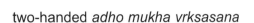

squeeze the foot, and in *parivrtta padmasana*   (or any simple twist) your hand can pull and squeeze the knee of the opposite lower limb to create a co-activation of the wrist flexors and wrist extensors (*mani bandha*). This can facilitate and increase in strength, stability and circulation.

By conscious co-activation of wrist flexors and wrist extensors (*mani bandha*) during weight-bearing postures, the wrist joint becomes strong and stable. This can be achieved by pressing down the fingers into the floor while attempting to lift the centre of the palm off the floor as if one is trying to grab the floor. Using this method it is relatively easy to balance on the hands in postures such as the traditional freestanding

two-handed *adho mukha vrksasana*   (handstand) and difficult one-handed balances

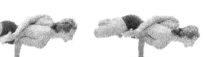

such as *eka hasta baddha padma mayurasana*   . Wrist stability is important for pain-free wrist movements, the ability to weight-bear on the hands, and the ability to free balance on the hands.

3.9.2.6 Co-activation of wrist flexors and extensors and forearm pronators assists in force transmission between the forearm and the hand

Co-activation of wrist flexors and wrist extensors (*mani bandha*) helps bind the bones of the forearm (radius and ulna) together because many of these muscles have attachments which cross over both these bones and thus pull these bones closer together when they are activated.

Binding radius and ulna is important for transmission of tensile (pulling) and contractile (pushing) forces down the arm since the radiocarpal joint is the main joint (transmitting 80% of force) between the forearm and hand, while the humeroulnar joint is the main joint between upper arm and forearm. In other words one should place most of the body weight on the radial side (thumb side) of the palm while co-activating the muscles around the forearm.

If the forearm is pronated in weight-bearing postures such as the *urdhva mukha svanasana*

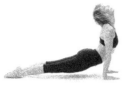

(up-dog pose) and *adho mukha svanasana* (down-dog pose) [Section 3.9.2.4] this further contributes to the binding of the radius and ulna while facilitating the external rotation at the glenohumeral joint and protraction at the scapulothoracic joint. Pronation is achieved by activation of the pronator teres in a closed-chain fashion by keeping the inner palm flat to the floor and turning the inner elbow towards the thumb and away from the floor. The resultant external rotation at the glenohumeral joint and protraction at the scapulothoracic joint causes an increase in the mobility of the thoracic spine.

3.9.2.7 Wrist flexibility, strength and stability can be increased by co-activating wrist flexors and extensors in both contractile (weight-bearing) and tensile (pulling) exercises

Wrist flexibility is best developed in conjunction with wrist strength. Wrist extension can be enhanced through weight-bearing postures where the wrist is placed in an extended position such as the *adho mukha vrksasana* (handstand). Tissue strength can be increased according to Wolffs law [Section 1.3.2.3.5] through weight-bearing postures of the wrist. When gravitational forces are placed on the joints and tissues this encourages or promotes increases in strength.

Strength can also be increased if muscles are voluntarily activated whilst being stretched [Sections 1.7.1, 1.7.2 & 9.4.2]. If the finger flexors (which are also wrist flexors) are activated in postures such as the handstand (*adho mukha vrksasana*) (by pressing the fingers into the floor) it can increase the strength of the wrist/finger flexors in a lengthened state and further stretch the wrist flexors by the inverse myotatic reflex [Sections 1.7.2.2.1.3 & 9.4.2.3] Similarly if the wrist extensors are activated in this posture by lifting the back of the hands away from the floor it can increase the strength of the wrist extensors in a shortened state and further stretch the wrist flexors by reciprocal reflex relaxation [Sections 1.7.2.2.1.2 & 9.4.2.2]. Co-activation of finger flexors in their lengthened state with wrist extensors in their shortened state (as in the handstand – *adho mukha vrksasana*) forms a type of *ha-mani bandha* [Section 3.9.1.2.1] which generates heat and pressure and can push blood and energy from the hand to the centre of the body and literally help lift the body into the air. This *ha-mani bandha* resembles *bukka puritat mudra* [Section 3.9.1.3; & Figure 9.3], which tensions (stretches) the median nerve and the pericardium acupuncture meridian.

Wrist flexion can be developed in postures such as *pada hastasana* where the feet are standing on the palms of the hands. If the finger flexors (which are also wrist flexors) are activated in postures such as *pada hastasana* (by pressing the fingers into the sole of the feet) it can increase the strength of the wrist/finger flexors in a shortened state and further stretch the wrist extensors by reciprocal reflex relaxation [Sections 1.7.2.2.1.2 & 9.4.2.2]. Similarly if the wrist extensors are activated in this posture by pressing the backs of the hands into the floor it can increase the strength of the wrist extensors in a lengthened state and further stretch the wrist extensors by the inverse myotatic reflex [Sections 1.7.2.2.1.3 & 9.4.2.3]. Co-activation of finger flexors in their shortened state with wrist extensors in their lengthened state (as in *pada hastasana*) forms a type of *ha-mani bandha* [Section 3.9.1.2.1] which generates heat and pressure and can push blood and energy from the hand to the

centre of body. This *ha-mani bandha* resembles *atanu puritat mudra* [Section 3.9.1.3; & Figure 9.1], which tensions (stretches) the radial nerve and the large intestine acupuncture meridian.

3.9.2.8 Elbows can be strengthened and stabilised in contractile (compressive and pushing) exercises by co-activating elbow extensors (which include triceps brachii) with supinators (which include biceps brachii)

Kurpara (elbow) bandha, which can be a co-activation of elbow extensors and elbow flexors, can strengthen and stabilise the elbow. If the arm is performing a non weight bearing posture, and is not pulling or pushing against resistance, co-activation can be achieved by making 'bulging biceps'. However, if the hand is pushing

into something like the floor in a pose such as *urdhva mukha svanasana* (upward facing dog pose) obligatory elbow extensor activity tends to disallow any co-activation with elbow flexors via the reciprocal relaxation relax. In this case biceps brachii (which is an elbow flexor and supinator) can be activated by squeezing the heel of the hand inwards as if trying to supinate the forearm.

3.9.2.9 Elbows can be strengthened and stabilised in tensile (pulling) exercises by co-activating elbow flexors (which include the supinator biceps brachii) with pronators

If the hand is pulling something like the big toe in a pose such as *utthita padangusthasana* obligatory elbow flexor activity tends to disallow any co-activation with elbow extensors via the reciprocal relaxation relax. In this case co-activation around the elbow joint can be created by simultaneously trying to pronate the forearm, which activates pronators, while actively flexing (bending) the elbow to activate biceps brachii, which is also a supinator.

****

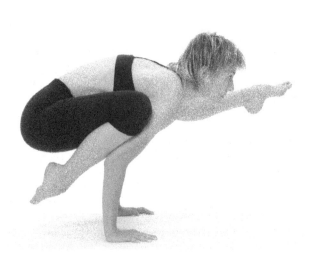

Bianca Machliss with wrists extended, elbows protracted and extended in *Eka Pada Bakasana*.
Photo courtesy of Alejandro Rolandi.

Chapter Breakdown

****

4.0 INTRODUCTION TO THE APPLIED ANATOMY OF THE PELVIS, HIP & LOWER LIMB IN *HATHA YOGA* POSTURES

In *hatha yoga vidya* (*yogic* science) the lower limbs are said to be the 'organs of action' for the lumbar spine, the digestive system and the reproductive system. It is therefore important for our overall health to understand the anatomy of the lower limb in order to most appropriately develop safe and effective *hatha yoga* sequences that can improve the strength, flexibility and general health of hips, knees and ankles.

In this chapter we examine the bones, muscles, nerves and other tissues of the pelvis and the associated hip joint complex [Section 4.2.0]. This information is then used to understand and apply the associated internal *yogic* lock, *kati bandha* [Section 4.5.1], which is created by co-activation (simultaneous tensing) of antagonistic (opposing) muscles crossing the hip joint complex.

The hip joint is generally a very strong and very stiff joint. Hip joint stiffness is a major contributing factor in lower back pain (LBP) and knee pain. Flexibility of the hip joint is very important in the *yoga* postures. Until a full range of movement is available in this joint, many *yoga* postures can only be attempted if they are modified or if they are done in conjunction with props.

4.1 BONES OF THE HIP JOINT COMPLEX

The pelvis is the inferior part of the trunk and creates the basin of the lower abdominal cavity. The pelvis consists of the paired hip-bones (the pelvic girdle), the fused sacrum, and the coccyx. The pelvis is shown in Figures 4.1 and 4.2.

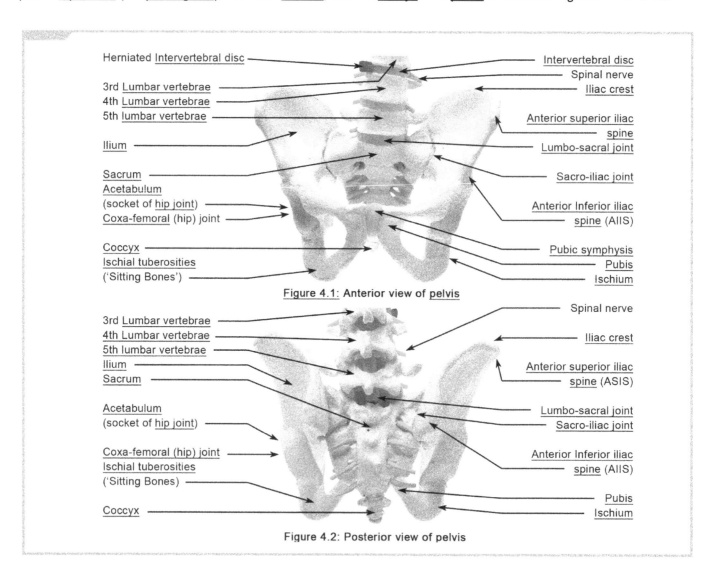

Figure 4.1: Anterior view of pelvis

Figure 4.2: Posterior view of pelvis

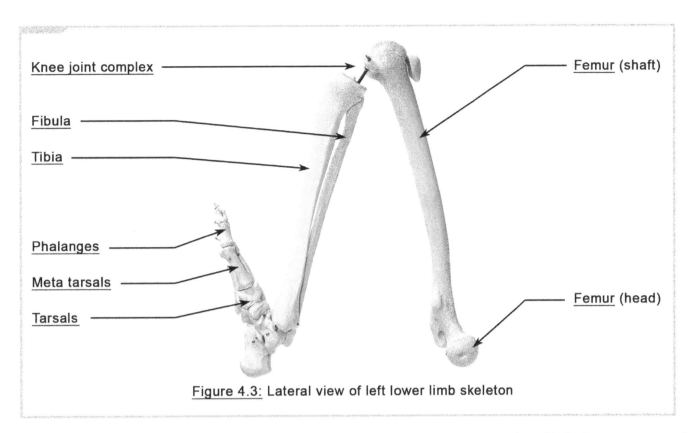

Knee joint complex

Fibula

Tibia

Phalanges

Meta tarsals

Tarsals

Femur (shaft)

Femur (head)

Figure 4.3: Lateral view of left lower limb skeleton

The bones of the lower limb are shown in Figure 4.3 but are discussed further in connection with the knee [Chapter 5] and in connection with the ankle [Chapter 6]. The bones of the lower limb include:
* Femur (thigh bone)
* Tibia and fibula (shin bones)
* Patella (knee cap)
* Tarsals (ankle and heel bones)
* Metatarsals (feet bones)
* Phalanges (toes)

4.1.1 Hip Bone (Coxal Bone)
Each adult hip or coxal bone consists of 3 fused bones called the ilium, the ischium, and the pubis.

The three bones forming the hip joint complex are initially separate bones that begin to fuse at the acetabulum between the ages of 15 and 17. The hip is completely fused by the age of 23. The acetabulum is the cup shaped cavity in the lateral surface of the hip-bone into which the femoral head fits.

The following features of the hip joint complex can be seen on a skeleton and identified with the help of Figures 4.1 and 4.2:
* **Ilium**: iliac crest, iliac fossa, iliac spine, anterior superior iliac spine (ASIS), anterior inferior iliac spine (AIIS), posterior superior iliac spine (PSIS), posterior inferior iliac spine (PIIS), greater sciatic notch.
* **Ischium**: ischial body, ramus, ischial tuberosity, lesser sciatic notch.
* **Pubis**: pubic body, superior ramii, inferior ramii, pectineal line, pubic tubercle, acetabulum, obturator foramen, inguinal ligament.

4.1.2 The Sacrum
The sacrum consists of the 5 fused sacral vertebrae between the 2 hip-bones
The following features of the hip joint complex can be seen on a skeleton and identified with the help of Figures 4.1 and 4.2:
* Sacral apex, sacral base, sacral foramina, median sacral crest, sacral promontory, 5 fused vertebrae.

4.1.3 The Coccyx
The coccyx or tail-bone is the most inferior or last part of the spine and it consists of 3-4 fused or semi-fused vertebrae. These can be seen on a skeleton and in Figures 4.1 and 4.2.

4.1.4 The Femur (proximal end)

The femur or thigh-bone joins the hip-bone at the acetabulum to form the hip joint.

The following features of the proximal end of the femur can be seen on a skeleton and identified with the help of the Figure 4.3:

- Femoral head, femoral neck, greater trochanter, lesser trochanter, gluteal tuberosity

4.2 JOINTS OF THE HIP & PELVIS [Figures 4.1 & 4.2]

The pelvis has 3 main joints or articulations:
- Hip joint (coxafemoral joint)
- Sacroiliac joint
- Pubic symphysis

4.2.0 The Hip Joint Complex

In order to assist in the understanding of how the hip and pelvic girdle functions it is helpful to consider all the joints of the hip and pelvic girdle as the hip joint complex. The hip joint complex therefore includes all the bones of the pelvis including the sacrum, and all the joints that move the pelvis including the hip or coxafemoral joints, the sacroiliac joints, the pubic symphysis and the joint between the first of the fused vertebrae of the sacrum and the lumbar spine (L5-S1).

Kati bandha [Section 4.5.1] is formed when the hip joint complex is supported and stabilised by a co-activation of antagonistic (opposing) muscle groups around this joint complex.

Note that the definitions of joint complexes may overlap each other. The sacroiliac joints can also be considered part of the lumbosacrococcygeal joint complex (referred to in these notes as the lumbar joint complex [Section 7.5.1]).

4.2.1 The Hip joint (Coxafemoral joint)

Location The hip joints (properly called the coxafemoral joints) are located between the two acetabula of the pelvis and the head of each femur.

Function The function of the hip joints and the pelvis is to support the weight of the head, arms, and trunk, both statically and during movement.

Classification The hip joint is classified as a synovial, ball and socket, multi-axial, simple joint.

Movements The movements of the hip joint are flexion and extension, abduction and adduction, and internal rotation and external rotation. The range of movement (ROM) of the hip joint is generally decreased relative to other joints, such as the shoulder (glenohumeral (GH)) joint, allowing greater stability and strength. *Hatha yoga* can in some poeple significantly increase hip joint flexibility with time and practice.

Ligaments

Anterior ligaments limit extension and abduction

- **Iliofemoral ligament**: inverted Y-shaped band from anterior inferior iliac spine (AIIS) to the inter-trochanteric line of the femur.
- **Pubofemoral ligament**: from superior pubic ramus to medial iliofemoral ligament.
- **Transverse acetabular ligament**: bridges the acetabular notch inferiorly forming a passage for vessels and nerves to enter the joint.
- **Ligament of the head of femur**: from fovea capitis on the head of femur to the transverse acetabular ligament and acetabulum. This ligament is weak but has an important function in carrying a branch of the obturator artery to the head of the femur. If this is severed necrosis (death) of the femoral head usually occurs.

Posterior ligament limits extension and medial rotation.

- **Ischiofemoral ligament**: from ischial portion of acetabular rim to neck of the femur at the base of the greater trochanter.

Special Features The fibrocartilaginous wedge-shaped rim called the acetabular labrum deepens the socket for the femoral head.

4.2.2 The Sacroiliac (SI) Joint

Location The two sacroiliac joints are located between the sacrum and the posterior hip bone.

Classification The sacroiliac joint is classified as a partly synovial, partly fibrous, plane, multi-axial, and simple joint.

Movements The movements of the sacroiliac joint are antero-posterior rotation and gliding. There is not a great amount of movement at these joints as stability is required for transmitting the weight of the body to the hip bones.

Ligaments of the sacroiliac joint

Anterior ligaments
- **Iliolumbar ligament**: joins the transverse process of L5 vertebra to iliac crest and sacrum, limits rotation and anterior glide of L5 on the sacrum.
- **Anterior sacroiliac ligament**: strong thin wide sheet of short transverse fibres from the iliac crest to tubercles of the first four sacral vertebrae.

Posterior ligaments
- **Interosseus sacroiliac ligament**: joins the iliac and sacral tuberosities; blends with the posterior sacroiliac ligament.
- **Posterior sacroiliac ligament**: unites the iliac crest and tubercles of the first four sacral vertebrae.
- **Sacrotuberous ligament**: joins the sacrum to the ischial tuberosity; prevents rotation of the sacrum and holds the distal sacrum down.
- **Sacrospinous ligament**: joins the sacrum and coccyx to the ischial spine; prevents rotation of the sacrum.

Function of the sacroiliac joint ligaments
The sacroiliac ligaments are for shock absorption and the transfer of weight to the limbs.

During pregnancy the sacroiliac ligaments, pubic symphysis and associated vertebropelvic ligaments become softened and more yielding due to the release of the hormone relaxin, thereby increasing the amount of movement at the sacroiliac joints and thus likelihood of injury at these joints. The combination of loosened posterior ligaments and an anterior weight shift caused by a heavy uterus may result in over-stretching of the sacroiliac joint capsules.

4.2.3 The Pubic Symphysis

Location The pubic symphysis is located between the superior pubic rami.

Classification secondary cartilaginous joint

- A thick fibrocartilage interpubic disc connects the pubic symphysis. This disc is usually thicker in women than in men; it also contains a small cavity that increases in size during pregnancy.

Ligaments
- **Superior pubic ligament** thickens the pubic rami superiorly
- **Arcuate pubic ligament** thickens the joint inferiorly
- **Tendinous fibres** of the rectus abdominis and obliquus externus abdominis muscles strengthen the joint anteriorly.

4.2.4 Movements of the Pelvis

The pelvis is able to move relative to the lower limb and the trunk. When the pelvis moves there is an accompanying hip joint motion and a compensatory lumbar spine motion. The movements of the pelvis and the associated movements of the hip joint and lumbar spine are shown Table 4.1. The movements of the hip joint and the muscles that facilitate these movements are shown Table 4.7.

Table 4.1 Relationship of pelvis, hip joint and lumbar spine during right leg weight-bearing and upright posture

PELVIC MOTION (weight bearing on the right leg)	Anterior pelvic tilt	Posterior pelvic tilt	Lateral pelvic elevation (hike) of Left pelvis	Lateral pelvic depression (drop) of Left pelvis	Anterior (Forward) rotation of Left pelvis	Posterior (Backward) rotation of Left pelvis
ACCOMPANYING HIP JOINT MOTION	Hip flexion	Hip extension	Right hip abduction	Right hip adduction	Right hip internal rotation	Right hip external rotation
COMPENSATORY LUMBAR SPINE MOTION	Lumbar spine extension	Lumbar spine flexion	Left spinal lateral flexion	Right spinal lateral flexion	Left spinal axial rotation	Right spinal axial rotation

4.2.4.1 Anterior pelvic tilt and posterior pelvic tilt

Anterior pelvic tilt and posterior pelvic tilt are movements in a sagittal plane about a coronal axis defined with respect to the anterior/posterior movements of the superior pelvis. In simple terms anterior pelvic tilt involves taking the top of the hip forward and posterior pelvic tilt involves taking the top of the hips backward. Posterior pelvic tilt has a similar effect to tucking the tailbone under.

In a standing position the naturally aligned pelvis has anterior superior iliac spines in a horizontal line with the posterior superior iliac spines, and on a vertical line with the pubic symphysis.

Anterior and posterior pelvic tilt can occur around both hip joints at the same time or it can occur on a single limb support around one hip joint. Anterior pelvic tilt is actively done by the hip flexors and may stretch the hip extensors as

in pascimottanasana 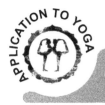 . Posterior pelvic tilt is actively done by hip extensors and may stretch the

hip flexors as in urdhva dhanurasana . In postures such as virabhadrasana the front leg undergoes a posterior pelvic tilt while the rear leg undergoes an anterior pelvic tilt.

No 4.1 Anterior and posterior pelvic tilt can improve twisting postures

When performing seated spinal twists to the left side, pelvic tilt alters the two hips. The left hip becomes posteriorly tilted (posterior pelvic tilt) and the right hip becomes anteriorly tilted (anterior pelvic tilt). This has the effect of reducing the spinal twist. Therefore, the right hip should be made to tilt posteriorly (posterior pelvic tilt) and the left hip should be made to tilt anteriorly (anterior pelvic tilt) for maximum twist of the spine.

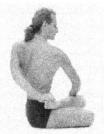

Parivrtta padmasana

4.2.4.2 Lateral pelvic tilt

These are movements in a <u>frontal plane</u> around an <u>anterior-posterior axis</u>. The normally aligned <u>pelvis</u> has a line between the <u>iliac crests</u> parallel to the floor while standing. One <u>hip joint</u> usually serves as the pivot point or axis and the opposite <u>iliac crest</u> <u>elevates</u> (<u>hip hiking</u>) or drops around that pivot point. A <u>hip tilt-hike</u> of the left leg will move the left <u>iliac crest</u> away from the floor while the right <u>pelvic crest</u> stays in the same place.

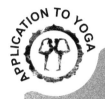

No 4.2 Lateral pelvic tilting can improve side-bending postures

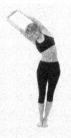

When performing side-bending postures to stretch the right side of the spine, <u>lateral pelvic tilting</u> alters the two hips. Therefore one can increase <u>spinal lateral flexion</u> by actively elevating the left <u>pelvis</u> which will increase the length of the right side of the spine by increasing <u>spinal lateral flexing</u> to the left.

parsva urdhva hastasana

4.2.4.3 Pelvic rotation

<u>Pelvic rotation</u> occurs in a transverse plane around a vertical axis. It can occur around a vertical axis through the middle of the <u>pelvis</u> but more commonly occurs when standing on one leg around the axis of the supporting hip. Anterior or forward rotation of an unsupported left hip occurs when the side of the <u>pelvis</u> of the unsupported <u>hip joint</u> moves anteriorly, and produces an accompanying <u>internal rotation</u> of the supported right <u>hip joint</u> and a compensatory spinal motion to the left.

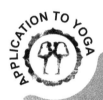

No 4.3 Pelvic rotation can improve twisting postures

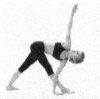

When performing spinal twisting postures (<u>spinal rotation</u>) such as the standing twist *parivrtta trikonasana* to the right side, the spine is turned to the right side and an inadvertent <u>anterior pelvic rotation</u> of the left hip usually also takes place, ie the left hip inadvertently moves closer to the floor thus reducing the <u>spinal rotation</u> to the right. <u>Posterior pelvic rotation</u> of the left hip, ie actively lifting the left hip away from the floor, increases in <u>spinal rotation</u> to the right.

parivrtta trikonasana

4.3 CLASSIFICATION OF THE PELVIS

Classification of the <u>pelvis</u> is based on two criteria:
1. **Measurements of <u>pelvic</u> diameters:**
   - <u>Pelvic</u> diameters are commonly measured either by <u>pelvic</u> examination, or by X-ray analysis, to provide information concerning the shape of the <u>pelvis</u> useful in predicting difficulty during childbirth,
   - Measurements are usually made of <u>transverse diameters</u> and/or <u>antero-posterior (AP) diameters</u>.
2. **Shape of the <u>pelvic</u> inlet**
   - **Gynecoid**: round, most spacious obstetrically, hence easiest for birth
   - **Android**: heart shaped, sacral promontory is prominent (not good for birth), wide transverse diameter
   - **Anthropoid**: long and narrow in the <u>antero-posterior</u> (AP) direction
   - **Platypelloid**: flat transversely; rare.

4.3.1 Differences between the Male Pelvis and Female Pelvis

The differences between the <u>male pelvis</u> and <u>female pelvis</u>, the most marked skeletal difference between men and women, are related to the heavier build and stronger muscles of men and the adaptation of the <u>pelvis</u> in women for childbearing. The main differences between the <u>male pelvis</u> and <u>female pelvis</u> are outlined in Table 4.2.

Table 4.2 Differences between the male pelvis and female pelvis

	FEMALE	MALE
GENERAL STRUCTURE	Thin and light	Thick and heavy
Muscle attachments	Poorly marked	Well marked
Shape of pelvic inlet	Gynacoid (~43%) Android (~32%) Anthropoid (~23%)	Android (most males) Anthropoid (some males)
Transverse diameters	Relatively large due to:	Relatively small due to:
• Pubic bones	• Wide	• Narrow
• Sacrum	• Wide	• Narrow
• Sub-pubic angle	• Large (~ 90 degrees)	• Small (~ 60 degrees)
• Ischial tuberosities	• Everted (ie pointing away from each other)	• Perpendicular/erect
AP diameters	Relatively large due to:	Relatively small due to:
• Sacral promontory	• Less prominent	• More prominent
• Sacral angle (L5-S1)	• Less than 180 degrees	• Close to 180 degrees
• Coccyx & sacrum	• Relatively straight	• Greater kyphosis
• Greater sciatic notch	• Wider	• Narrower
Pelvis major	Shallow	Deep
Pelvis minor	Wide and shallow	Narrow and deep
Superior pelvic aperture	Oval, rounded and relatively large	Heart shaped and relatively small
Inferior pelvic aperture	Relatively large	Relatively small
Obturator foramen	Oval	Round
Acetabulum	Narrow	Large

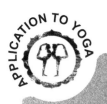

No 4.4 Hip flexibility differs between sexes

Due to the differences between the male pelvis and female pelvis [Table 4.2], women are often more flexible in the hip joint complex. Postures such as *baddha konasana* and most postures involving the hips including sitting in the cross-legged posture (*swastikasana*) tend to be easier for more women than men.

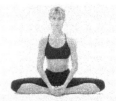

baddha konasana

4.4 MUSCLES OF THE HIP JOINT COMPLEX

4.4.1 Muscles Joining the Pelvis to the Torso
The main muscles joining the pelvis to the torso are quadratus lumborum, psoas minor, and the spinal extensors posteriorly; and the abdominal muscles anteriorly [Section 7.2.3, Table 7.4]. Strength and flexibility in these muscles is important to the health of the spine.

4.4.2 Muscles of the Gluteal Region
The attachments and actions of muscles of the gluteal (buttock) region are shown in Table 4.3. Strength and flexibility of the gluteal muscles is important to the health of the spine. Many of these muscles can be seen in Figures 1.2 -1.4 at the start of Chapter 1.

Table 4.3 Muscles of the gluteal region

MUSCLE	ORIGINS	INSERTIONS	ACTIONS & ROLES
Gluteus maximus	• Iliac crest • Sacrum • Coccyx	• Ilio-tibial tract (80%) • Gluteal tuberosity of the Femur (20%)	• Extends thigh at hip joint • Externally rotates thigh • Raises trunk from a flexed position • Tightens or compresses the sacroiliac joint
Gluteus medius	• External surface of ilium	• Greater trochanter of femur	• **Ab**ducts thigh at hip joint • Internally rotates thigh at hip joint • Stabilises the pelvis
Gluteus minimus	• External surface of ilium, deep to gluteus medius	• Greater trochanter of femur	
Piriformis	• Anterior surface of sacrum	• Greater trochanter of femur	• Externally rotates thigh • Abducts thigh from a flexed position • Steadies femoral head in acetabulum • Helps to stabilise the hip joint
Obturator internus	• Pelvic surface of obturator membrane		
Gemelli, superior & inferior	• Superior: ischial spine • Inferior: ischial tuberosity		
Quadratus femoris	• Ischial tuberosity	• Inter-trochanteric crest of femur	• Externally rotates thigh • Steadies femoral head in acetabulum

4.4.3 Muscles of the Posterior Thigh

Attachments and actions of posterior thigh (rear thigh) muscles are shown in Table 4.4. Strength and flexibility of posterior thigh muscles (mainly hamstrings) is important to the health of the spine. Many of these muscles can be seen in Figures 1.2 -1.4.

Table 4.4 Muscles of the posterior thigh

MUSCLE	ORIGINS	INSERTIONS	ACTIONS & ROLES
Semimembranosus	• Ischial tuberosity	• Posterior part of the medial tibial condyle • Medial meniscus	• Extends thigh at hip joint • Flexes leg at knee joint • Internally rotates leg • Extends trunk when thigh and leg are flexed
Semitendinosus	• Ischial tuberosity	• Posterior part of the superior tibia	
Biceps femoris	• Long head: ischial tuberosity and sacrotuberous ligament • Short head: posterior surface of femur	• Lateral side of the head of fibula • Lateral condyle of tibia	• Flexes leg at knee joint • Externally rotates leg at knee joint • Extends thigh (eg, when starting to walk)

Table 4.5 Muscles of the medial thigh

MUSCLE	ORIGINS	INSERTIONS	ACTIONS & ROLES
Adductor magnus	• Inferior pubic ramus • Ramus of ischium • Ischial tuberosity	Adductor part: • Medial femur Hamstring part: • Adductor tubercle of femur	Adductor part: • Adducts thigh at hip joint • Flexes thigh at hip joint Hamstring part: • Extends thigh at hip joint
Adductor longus	• Below pubic crest on the pubis body	• Middle third of linea aspera of femur	• Adducts thigh at hip joint • Internally rotates thigh at hip joint
Adductor brevis	• Body of pubis and inferior ramus of pubis	• Proximal part of linea aspera of femur	• Adducts thigh at hip joint • Flexes thigh at hip joint to some extent
Gracilis	• Body of pubis and inferior ramus of pubis	• Superior tibia, medial surface	• Adducts thigh at hip joint • Flexes thigh at hip joint • Internally rotates leg at knee joint
Pectineus	• Pectineal line of pubis	• Proximal femur	• Adducts thigh at hip joint • Flexes thigh at hip joint • Internally rotates thigh at hip joint
Obturator externus	• Margins of obturator foramen	• Trochanter fossa of femur	• Externally rotates thigh • Steadies femur head in acetabulum

4.4.3.1 Hamstrings

Semimembranosis, semitendinosis and biceps femoris have a common proximal attachment, the ischial tuberosity (sitting bone), and so are often grouped together as the hamstrings. One part of adductor magnus [Table 4.5], which also functions to extend the thigh at the hip joint, is sometimes included in the hamstring group.

4.4.4 Muscles of the Medial Thigh

All the medial thigh (inner thigh) muscles are adductors of the thigh at the hip joint (hip adductors), except for obturator externus which is an external rotator of the thigh at the hip joint (hip external rotator). The attachments and actions of these muscles are shown in Table 4.5. Strength and flexibility in the medial thigh muscles is important to the health of the spine and the knees. Many of these muscles can be seen in Figures 1.2 -1.4.

4.4.5 Muscles of the Anterior Thigh

The attachments and actions of muscles of the anterior thigh (front thigh) are shown in Table 4.6. Strength and flexibility in the anterior thigh muscles is important to the health of the spine and the knees. Many of these muscles can be seen in Figures 1.2 -1.4.

4.4.5.1 Quadriceps femoris

Rectus femoris, vastus lateralis, vastus medialis and vastus intermedius have a common distal attachment (insertion) and are therefore often grouped together under the name quadriceps femoris. In the quadriceps group only rectus femoris is bi-articular (ie a two-joint muscle) crossing both the hip joint complex and the knee joint complex and acting as a hip flexor and as a knee extensor. The rest of the quadriceps group only function as knee extensors and have a very important role in the healthy functioning of the knee joint complex [Section 5.3].

4.4.5.2 Iliopsoas

Iliopsoas is actually two muscles, iliacus and psoas major, with a common distal attachment to the lesser trochanter of femur (inner upper thigh bone). Both muscles are important hip flexors and hip external rotators . Psoas major is a multi-joint muscle that attaches proximally to the sides of the last thoracic and all five lumbar vertebrae. Therefore it is capable of producing spinal extension and spinal lateral flexion. If psoas major is stiff or lacking in flexibilty it can cause lower back pain and other problems by causing constant spinal extension (back arching). Maintaining flexibility of psoas major is one of the most important factors in relieving and preventing lower back pain. A good stretch for iliacus, psoas

Table 4.6 Muscles of the anterior thigh

MUSCLE	ORIGINS	INSERTIONS	ACTIONS & ROLES
Rectus femoris	• Anterior inferior iliac spine (AIIS)		• Extends leg at knee joint • Flexes thigh at hip joint • Stabilises hip joint
Vastus lateralis	• Greater trochanter • Linea aspera of femur • Lateral intermuscular septum		
Vastus intermedius	• Anterior and lateral surface of femur	• Base of patella and via patella ligament to tibial tuberosity	• Extends leg at knee joint • Stabilises knee joint
Vastus medialis longus	• Medial lip of linea aspera of femur		
Vastus medialis obliquus	• Tendon of adductor magnus • Fascia of adductor longus • Distal medial femur • Adductor tubercle		• Stabilises knee joint • Adducts patella
Sartorius	• Anterior superior iliac spine (ASIS)	• Medial surface of proximal tibia,	• Flexes leg at knee joint • Flexes thigh at hip joint • Abducts thigh at hip joint • Externally rotates thigh at hip joint
Tensor fasciae latae	• Anterior superior iliac spine (ASIS)	• , which attaches to lateral tibial condyle	• Flexes thigh at hip joint • Internally rotates thigh at hip joint • Stabilises pelvis
Psoas major	• T12 - L5 sides of vertebrae & intervertebral discs between them	• Lesser trochanter of femur	• Flexes thigh at hip joint • Externally rotates thigh at hip joint • Extends spine from T12 - L5 • Laterally flexes spine from T12 - L5 to the same side • Stabilise hip joint
Iliacus	• Iliac crest and fossa • Base of sacrum		• Flexes thigh at hip joint • Externally rotates thigh at hip joint • Stabilise hip joint

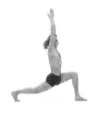

major, rectus femoris and other hip flexors is *utthita san calanasana* (the standing lunge).

4.4.6 External Rotators of the Thigh [Tables 4.3 & 4.5]

Six small external rotators (also known as lateral rotators) of the thigh are analogous to the rotator cuff muscles of the shoulder as they behave as effective joint compressor-stabilisers. These are obturator internus, obturator externus, superior and inferior gemelli, quadratus femoris, and piriformis. Obturator internus is a flat triangular muscle covering the lateral wall of the pelvis. Piriformis helps form the posterior pelvic wall. The sciatic nerve usually enters the gluteal region just posterior to piriformis; hence a tight piriformis may lead to sciatic nerve compression or impingement (sciatica). A

good stretch for piriformis and other hip external rotators is *adho mukha swastikasana* 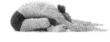 (the cross-legged forward bend).

Other external rotators of the thigh are <u>gluteus maximus</u> [Table 4.3] and <u>sartorius</u> [Table 4.6]. While these muscles are not specifically for <u>external rotation</u>, they are so large and strong that their effect is significant.

4.4.7 Hip Muscle Strengthening

The legs are responsible for bearing a great deal of weight and are subjected to intense vertical and lateral stresses. Consequently, the bones of the leg are often cracked or broken, and the hip, knee and ankle joint are particularly susceptible to fracture, strain, sprain and dislocation. Hence, it is considered beneficial to strengthen the bones and muscles of the legs. One method of strengthening the legs is through the use of the <u>unilateral stance</u> (one-legged standing) during exercise. There are many useful one-legged postures in *hatha yoga*.

4.4.7.1 Bilateral (2 leg) standing compared with unilateral (1 leg) standing

In erect <u>bilateral stance</u> (two-legged standing), each of the two hips carry a force equivalent to only one third of the total body weight. In erect <u>unilateral stance</u> one hip will carry a force approximately 2½ times the total body weight, and in the one-legged phases of walking and stair climbing the supported hip will carry up to 4 to 7 times the total body weight.

These massive increases in force while standing on one leg are due to the <u>abductors</u> of the supporting <u>hip joint</u>

Table 4.7 Movements and muscle groups at the hip joint

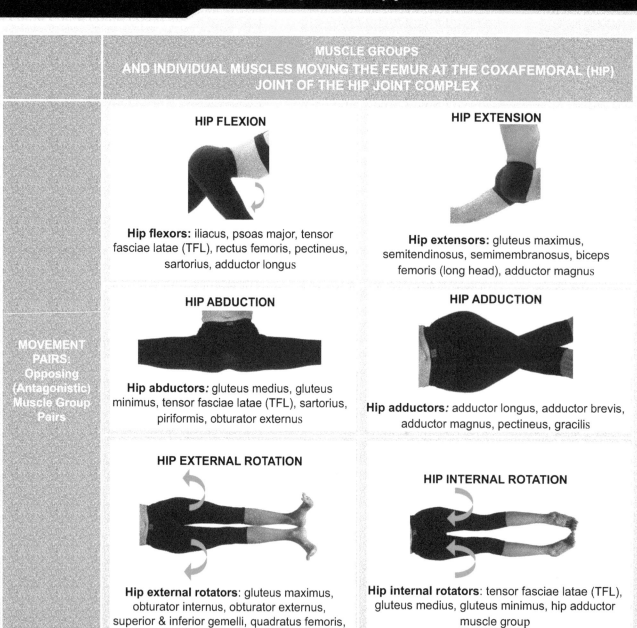

	MUSCLE GROUPS AND INDIVIDUAL MUSCLES MOVING THE FEMUR AT THE COXAFEMORAL (HIP) JOINT OF THE HIP JOINT COMPLEX	
MOVEMENT PAIRS: Opposing (Antagonistic) Muscle Group Pairs	**HIP FLEXION** **Hip flexors:** iliacus, psoas major, tensor fasciae latae (TFL), rectus femoris, pectineus, sartorius, adductor longus	**HIP EXTENSION** **Hip extensors:** gluteus maximus, semitendinosus, semimembranosus, biceps femoris (long head), adductor magnus
	HIP ABDUCTION **Hip abductors:** gluteus medius, gluteus minimus, tensor fasciae latae (TFL), sartorius, piriformis, obturator externus	**HIP ADDUCTION** **Hip adductors:** adductor longus, adductor brevis, adductor magnus, pectineus, gracilis
	HIP EXTERNAL ROTATION **Hip external rotators:** gluteus maximus, obturator internus, obturator externus, superior & inferior gemelli, quadratus femoris, piriformis, iliacus, psoas major, sartorius	**HIP INTERNAL ROTATION** **Hip internal rotators:** tensor fasciae latae (TFL), gluteus medius, gluteus minimus, hip adductor muscle group

having to create enough force to counteract the adduction of the unsupported hip joint by gravity. This abduction force further compresses the acetabulum into the head of the femur and has the same effect as if the person's weight had suddenly increased by a factor of 2½ to 7 times. In a unilateral stance gluteus medius acts as the main hip abductor but it also acts as a hip internal rotator.

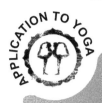

No 4.5 One-legged poses are a very effective in strengthening the standing leg and hip

One-legged postures usually oblige the hip abductors of the weight-bearing leg to generate powerful forces through the hip joint complex.

The adjacent diagram shows the easy and hard (*) versions of *pada mandala vinyasa*, a powerful one-legged sequence of postures that takes the non-weight-bearing (NWB) and the weight-bearing (WB) leg through movements involving hip flexion (fl), extension (ex), abduction (ab) adduction (ad), external rotation (er) and internal rotation (ir).

NWB Leg: 1.fl/ad/er; 2.fl/ab/er; 3. ex/ab/ir; 4.ex/ad/ir; 5.ex/ad/ir; 6.fl/ad/er

WB Leg: 1.ex/ad/ir; 2.ex/ad/er; 3. fl/ab/er; 4.fl/ad/er; 5. ex/ad/ir, 6.fl/ad/er

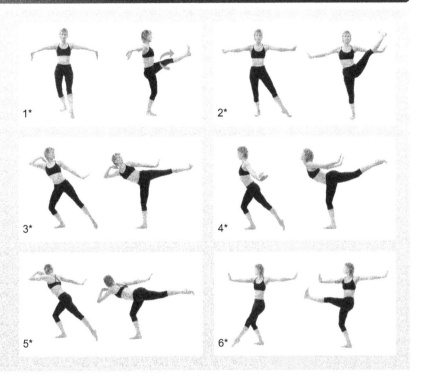

4.4.8 Muscles of the Pelvic Diaphragm (Pelvic Floor)

The pelvic diaphragm (pelvic floor) is the roof of the perineum [Section 4.4.9]. Muscles of the pelvis form the pelvic diaphragm (pelvic floor) and the pelvic wall. The pelvic wall is formed by sections of two hip : piriformis [Table 4.3] and obturator externus [Table 4.5].

4.4.8.1 Structure of the pelvic diaphragm (pelvic floor)

The pelvic diaphragm (pelvic floor) consists of 2 muscle groups, the levator ani and the coccygeus.

4.4.8.1.1 Levator ani muscles
The levator ani muscles consist of:
- **Iliococcygeus**
- **Pubococcygeus**
- **Puborectalis**
- **Levator vaginae/prostatae**

Levator ani help separate the pelvic cavity from the perineum [Section 4.4.9]. They arise anteriorly from the inner surface of the pubis and posteriorly from the obturator membrane and the pelvic surface of the ischial spine. They insert into the perineal body, sides of the anal canal and the anococcygeal ligament between the anal canal and the coccyx.

4.4.8.1.2 Coccygeus muscle
The coccygeus muscle arises from the ischial spine and attaches to the coccyx and the lower portion of the sacrum. The gluteal surface of coccygeus blends with the sacrospinous ligament.

4.4.8.2 Functions of the pelvic diaphragm (pelvic floor)

The muscles of the pelvic floor (levator ani and coccygeus) assist in micturition (urination), defecation, and parturition (childbirth). These muscles cover the pelvic outlet, providing support for the pelvic and abdominal organs.These muscles also assist in prevention of prolapsed uterus.

4.4.8.2.1 Functions of the levator ani muscles

Voluntary activation of the levator ani muscles help to constrict the openings of the pelvic floor (urethra and anus) and prevent unwanted micturition and defecation (stress incontinence). Activation of the levator ani (voluntary and involuntary) occurs when holding the breath, coughing, or whenever the intra-abdominal pressure (IAP) is increased.

In women, these muscles surround the vagina, thus helping support the uterus. During pregnancy these muscles can be stretched or traumatised and result in stress incontinence whenever IAP is increased. In men, damage to these muscles may occur following prostate surgery.

4.4.8.2.2 Functions of the coccygeus muscle

The coccygeus muscle assists the levator ani in supporting the pelvic viscera (organs) and maintaining the intra-abdominal pressure (IAP). Coccygeus exerts an anterior pull on the coccyx and may therefore contribute to posterior pelvic tilting [Section 4.2.4] of the pelvis or resistance to anterior pelvic tilting.

4.4.9 Muscles of the Perineum

The perineum is the region below the pelvic cavity, lying over the inferior pelvic aperture (pelvic outlet).
The roof of the perineum is the pelvic floor [Section 4.4.9]. The perineum is divided into uro-genital and anal triangles.

4.4.9.1 Urogenital triangle of the perineum

The urogenital triangle is the anterior triangle of the perineum and it contains:
- **External genitalia**
- **Urogenital diaphragm** composed of deep transverse perineal muscles
- **Superficial perineal space**, which contains the Ischiocavernosus and bulbospongiosus muscles, which aid in the erection of the clitoris/penis by ensheathing the roots of the erectile bodies of the clitoris/penis.

4.4.9.2 Anal triangle of the perineum

The anal triangle is the posterior triangle of the perineum. In the tendinous centre of the perineum is the fibrous perineal body, which is where several perineal muscles meet.

The posterior triangle functions to allow the anal canal to expand during defecation.

Important muscles of the pelvis and hip joint complex

The following muscles and muscle groups are important in the pelvis and hip joint complex. Their attachments and actions are useful to learnt. They are relatively easy to see and feel.
1. Iliopsoas (iliacus and psoas major)
2. Quadriceps
3. Tensor facia latae
4. Sartorius
5. Hamstrings
6. Hip adductors
7. Gluteus maximus
8. Gluteus medius
9. Muscles of the perineum and pelvic diaphragm (pelvic floor)

4.5 APPLIED ANATOMY OF THE HIP JOINT COMPLEX IN *HATHA YOGA* POSTURES

To enhance the functioning of the lower limb in *yoga* postures, there needs to be a practical understanding of the muscles which cross the hip joint complex (i.e. have attachments that are distal and proximal to the hip joint complex and which therefore affect the hip joint complex). In addition, the ability to tense at will any of the muscles around the hip joint complex and the ability to co-activate (simultaneously tense) antagonistic (opposing) muscle groups around the hip joint complex is integral to the safe and effective application of stretching and strengthening exercises for the lower limb and for the spine.

4.5.1 Co-activation of Opposing Muscles around the Hip Joint Complex: *Kati Bandha*

A hip *bandha*, referred to as *kati bandha* in *Sanskrit*, can be defined as [Section 1.7.3] the co-activation of antagonistic (opposing) muscle groups around the hip joint complex. Application of *kati bandha* during *asanas* (static postures) *vinyasas* (dynamic exercises) can help to increase the flexibility, strength and stability of the hip joint complex. Of particular importance is the increase in the stability of the sacroiliac joint and the flexibility of the hip (coxafemoral) joint.

Kati bandha can be created in many different ways. Different types of joint positions in various *yoga* postures require different manoeuvres to create co-activation of antagonistic muscle groups. Many of these co-activations rely on the fact that certain groups of the hip muscles have dual roles. In particular note that:
- **Hip adductors** may also act as **hip internal rotators, and**
- **Hip extensors** such as the large **gluteus maximus** also have a significant role as **hip external rotators.**

Due to the dual roles of these muscle groups, there are additional possibilities for muscle opposition in the hip joint compared to a hypothetical 'normal' ball and socket joint. In the hypothetical ball and socket joint, flexors only oppose extensors, abductors only oppose adductors, and internal rotators only oppose external rotators. In the hip joint, however, some hip adductors oppose not just hip abductors but also oppose hip external rotators and some hip extensors. Similarly, some hip extensors oppose not only hip flexors but also oppose some hip internal rotators and some hip adductors.

When creating *kati bandha* (hip joint *bandha*), there are many possible approaches and many types of partial and complete *bandhas*.

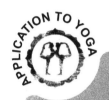

No 4.6 Many opposing muscle groups of the hip joint complex can be co-activated to form *kati bandha*

A hip joint *bandha* (*kati bandha*) can be made when opposing muscles of the hip joint are co-activated. The structure of the hip joint complex allows for more possibilities of muscle opposition than normal ball and socket joints because hip adductors can also act as hip internal rotators and large hip extensors, such as gluteus maximus, also have a significant external rotator effect. Therefore:

HIP FLEXORS	**ALL**	HIP EXTENSORS
HIP ADDUCTORS	OPPOSE	HIP ABDUCTORS
HIP INTERNAL ROTATORS	(are all antagonistic to)	HIP EXTERNAL ROTATORS

For example the non weight-bearing (NWB) limb in *niralamba padanghustasana*   is flexed but if it is also externally rotated (i.e. turned outward) then *kati bandha* is formed since hip flexors are opposed by hip external rotators .

Similarly, the non weight-bearing (NWB) limb in *niralamba virabhadrasana*   is extended but if it is also internally rotated (i.e. turned inwards) then *kati bandha* is formed since hip extensors are opposed by hip internal rotators.

Also, the rear (L) limb in *parsvottonasana*   can create *kati bandha* by pushing the (L) heel backwards as if trying to stretch the floor in order to activate hip extensors, and this action is opposed by squeezing the base of (L) big toe inwards in order to activate the hip adductors.

135

4.5.1.1 Creating *kati bandha* in non weight-bearing (NWB) lower limbs, in open-chain exercises

When the lower limb is engaged in a <u>non weight-bearing</u> (NWB) <u>open-chain exercise</u> (the body is fixed while the limb is free to move), several possibilities exist which can assist in creating a <u>co-activation</u> of <u>antagonistic</u> (opposing) <u>muscle groups</u>.

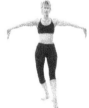

*1. **Kati bandha** can be formed in a <u>neutral</u> or <u>extended</u> position* eg. in *sirsasana* (headstand)

or *sarvangasana* 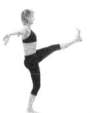 (shoulderstand), or *niralamba virabhadrasana* , by simultaneously trying to:

• <u>Internally rotate</u> the thigh inwards at the <u>hip joint</u>,
• Squeeze the buttock cheeks together (done mainly with <u>gluteus maximus</u>).

Kati bandha is made here as the <u>internal rotator</u> action of the inner thigh muscles opposes the <u>external rotator</u> action of the <u>gluteus maximus</u>.

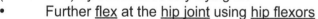

*2. **Kati bandha** can be formed in a <u>flexed</u> position* eg. as in *niralamba padangusthasana*

or the one-legged variations of *sirsasana* (headstand) by simultaneously trying to:

• Further <u>flex</u> at the <u>hip joint</u> using <u>hip flexors</u>
• <u>Externally rotate</u> at the <u>hip joint</u> using external rotators , which also have an <u>extensor</u> action, which can oppose the actions of the <u>hip flexors</u>.

*3. **Kati bandha** can be formed in an <u>abducted</u> position* (eg. as in the wide legs variations of headstand

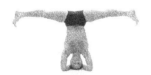

and shoulderstand) by simultaneously trying to:

• Turn the thighs inwards using the <u>internal rotators</u>, which also have a <u>hip adductor</u> action
• Actively <u>abduct</u> the thighs at the hips (push the thighs away from each other), which can oppose the actions of the <u>hip internal rotators/hip adductors</u>.

4.5.1.2 Creating *kati bandha* for weight-bearing (WB) lower limbs, in closed-chain exercises

Creation of *kati bandha* during a <u>weight-bearing</u> (WB) <u>closed-chain exercise</u> depends on the posture. There are many possibilities. Four of these are described below:

*1. **Kati bandha** can be formed around <u>WB flexed hips</u>* in all postures which have at least one WB leg

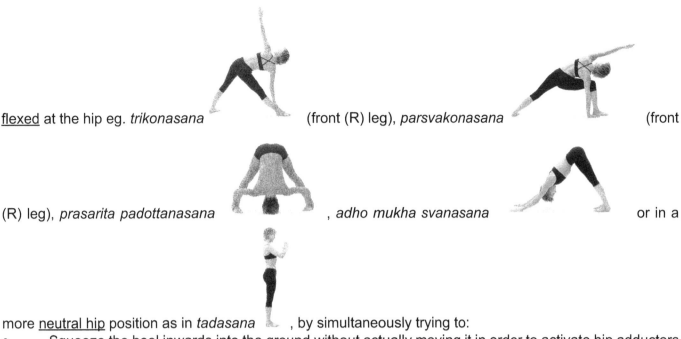

flexed at the hip eg. *trikonasana* (front (R) leg), *parsvakonasana* (front

(R) leg), *prasarita padottanasana* , *adho mukha svanasana* or in a

more <u>neutral hip</u> position as in *tadasana* , by simultaneously trying to:
- Squeeze the heel inwards into the ground without actually moving it in order to activate <u>hip adductors</u> <u>(hip internal rotators)</u>
- Push the front or ball of your foot outwards into the ground without actually moving it in order to activate <u>hip abductors</u> and <u>hip external rotators.</u>

2. Kati bandha can be formed around <u>WB extended hips</u> in all postures which have at least one WB leg in <u>hip</u>

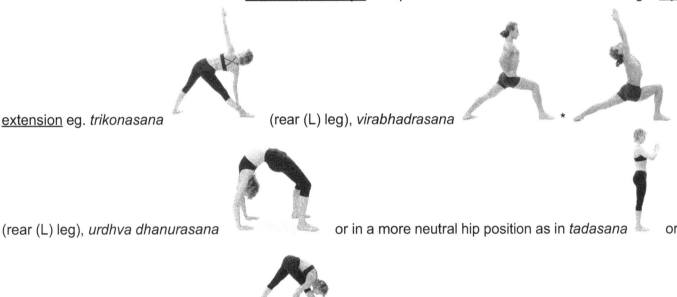

<u>extension</u> eg. *trikonasana* (rear (L) leg), *virabhadrasana* *

(rear (L) leg), *urdhva dhanurasana* or in a more neutral hip position as in *tadasana* or

trying to extend as in *parsvotonasana* (rear (L) leg)

- Squeeze the front or ball of each foot inwards into the ground without actually moving it in order to activate <u>hip adductors</u> and <u>hip internal rotators</u>
- Squeeze the heel of your foot outwards into the ground without actually moving it in order to activate <u>hip extensors</u> and <u>hip external rotators</u>

3. Kati bandha can be formed in *adho mukha swastikasana* (cross-legged forward bend) and similar postures, by simultaneously trying to:
- Press down with the feet to activate <u>hip extensors</u> and <u>hip external rotators</u>
- Lift the inner thighs to activate <u>hip flexors</u>, and <u>hip internal rotators</u>
- Squeeze the thighs towards each other to activate <u>hip adductors</u> and <u>hip internal rotators</u> **or** push the thighs away from each other to activate <u>hip abductors</u> and <u>hip external rotators.</u>

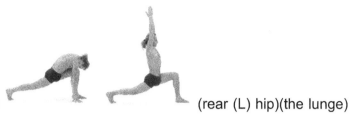

4. *Kati bandha* can be formed in *san calanasana* (rear (L) hip)(the lunge) and similar postures, by simultaneously trying to:

- Tense the buttocks muscles of the rear limb to activate the hip extensors, and hip external rotators
- Push the ball of the foot of the rear limb down into the ground and forward towards the front limb (as if trying to pull the two feet closer together) in order to activate the hip flexors.

4.5.2 Increasing Hip joint Flexibility with *Hatha Yoga*

The benefits of increasing the flexibility of the hip joint complex include minimising the risk of lower back pain [Section 4.5.2.1] and knee joint pain [Sections 4.5.2.3 & 5.6]. An understanding of the principles of hip muscle flexibility minimises the risk of hamstring tears and gives a methodology for helping recover from hamstring tears [Section 4.5.2.2].

4.5.2.1 Effect of hip flexibility on lower back pain

Lack of flexibility in the hip flexors and hip extensors is a major contributing factor in lower back pain. When these muscle groups are tight there is much more stress placed on the lumbar spine. Hip flexor flexibility

(stretching the front of the groin) is developed through postures such as *san calanasana* in which posterior pelvic tilt is taught while the thigh is kept in some hip internal rotation to increase the stretch on the the important hip flexor, iliopsoas [Section 4.4.5.2].

Hip extensor flexibility and in particular hamstring flexibility can be developed rapidly with correctly applied *yoga* stretches. During hamstring stretches the quadriceps should be kept active in order to keep the knee fully extended and in order to give reciprocal relaxation to the hamstrings. In order to increase the intensity of a hamstring stretch one should maximise the distance between the proximal and distal attachments of the hamstrings group by increasing anterior pelvic tilt rather than increasing spinal flexion. Hip flexor activations may be used in the forward bending (hip flexion and spinal flexion) postures as a means of increasing anterior pelvic tilt to decrease the spinal flexion and to increase the stretch on the hip extensors. However, the danger of this method is the risk of over stretching the hamstrings and reducing the stability of the lumbar spine.

4.5.2.2 Modifying hamstring stretches to prevent and recover from hamstring tears

In the case of a hamstring tear, over-stretching the hamstrings will discourage healing and almost always aggrevates the injury, making it take much longer to heal. Hence, it is prudent to decrease the intensity of hamstring stretches in forward bending postures (hip flexion and spinal flexion) such as *pascimottanasana*

. Clinical evidence suggests that it is only the most gentle of stretching, eliciting no hamstring pain, which may help to improve recovery and reduce inflamation, scar tissue and adhesions. In addition, recovery may be improved if the hamstrings are gently activated without eliciting pain in non-stretched

positions such as in the non-weight-bearing limb of *niralamba virabhadrasana* [Sections 4.5.1.1 & 4.5.3].

To reduce the stretch on the <u>hamstrings</u> to minimise risk of injury or to recover from injury three main methods may be employed:

(1)   Bend (<u>flex</u>) the knees in forward bends such as *pascimottanasana* 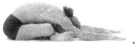 and/or

(2)   decrease the amount of <u>anterior pelvic tilt</u>, thereby decreasing <u>hip flexion</u> and increasing the amount of <u>spinal flexion</u> and/or

(3)   press or push the sitting bones (<u>ischial tuberosities</u>) towards the heels without actually moving the sitting bones (this activates <u>spinal flexors</u> thus contributing to anterior of *mula bandha*), and try and pull the lower back inwards without lifting the sitting bones (this activates <u>spinal extensors</u> thus contributing to posterior of *mula bandha*).

Note that for many people increasing <u>spinal flexion</u> with <u>knee extension</u> (as in (2) and (3) above) may cause an increased risk or an increase in pain to the <u>lumbar spine</u>. This may be protected against with a well-defined activation of the <u>lower abdominal muscles</u> and the <u>lumbar spine extensors</u> (*mula bandha*). For people with pronounced stiffness in the <u>hamstrings</u> or weakness in the spine or trunk muscles, bending the knees (alternative (1) above) is the safest option.

Many hamstring tears have also been shown to have a <u>sciatic nerve</u> component. Therefore, as a general rule in cases of apparent <u>hamstring tears</u> or <u>hamstring</u> pain, do not pull the foot towards you (<u>ankle dorsiflexion</u> [Table 6.3]) as this will increase the <u>tension</u> on the <u>sciatic nerve</u> [Figure 9.6]. Instead, push the base of the big toe away from you (ankle plantarflexion) to reduce the tension on the sciatic nerve and pull the heel towards you to help elicit *mula bandha* [Section 7.4.1.1].

If the aim is to stretch the <u>hamstrings</u> further, increasing the <u>anterior pelvic tilt</u> will achieve that, but to maintain safety and to enhance *mula bandha* the sitting bones (<u>ischial tuberosities</u>) should be pressed into the thighs towards the heels even though they may not actually move in that direction.

4.5.2.3 Effect of hip flexibility on knee pain

Lack of flexibility in the <u>hip external rotators</u> and <u>hip internal rotators</u> is a major contributing factor in knee pain during *yoga*. This is especially true for the many western *yoga* practitioners with stiff hips who force themselves

into poses such as the *padmasana* (lotus posture), which require large amounts of <u>hip external rotation</u>, and they overstress the knee joints in doing so. <u>Hip external rotation</u> can be enhanced by stretching

the <u>hip internal rotators</u> (and <u>hip adductors</u>) in postures such as *baddha konasana* and

samakonasana . Another common problem is the inability to safely perform postures

which require large amounts of <u>hip internal rotation</u> such as *supta virasana* (lying back between the legs). People with stiff hips can easily overstress their knees and lower back attempting such postures. <u>Hip internal rotation</u> can be enhanced by stretching the <u>hip external rotators</u> (and <u>hip extensors</u>) in

postures such as *adho mukha swastikasana* .

4.5.3 Increasing Hip Joint Strength with *Hatha Yoga*

Hatha yoga incorporates many one-legged postures. These poses are excellent strengthening exercises for the hip abductors of the standing leg and the hip joint in general [Norkin & Levangie, 1992][Section 4.4.7]. One-legged postures are also good to focus the mind. This is because a balance component is involved that requires attention on the present moment or balance will be lost.

In one-legged postures gluteus medius acts as the main hip abductor but it also acts as a hip internal rotator. Therefore if the buttock (gluteus maximus) of the standing leg is also activated (tensed) by squeezing the buttocks then an effective stabilising hip muscle co-activation (*kati bandha*) [Section 4.5.1] is generated because of the large hip external rotator component of gluteus maximus. In addition, because of the nature of multi-joint muscles and the interdependency between the *bandhas* [Section 1.7.3.5], one-legged postures are also excellent to help create the *bandhas* of the knee joint complex (*janu bandha*) [Section 5.6] and ankle joint complex (*kulpha bandha*) [Section 6.6] and bring strength and stability to these joints. According to kinetic chain theory [Section 1.6.5.9] co-activation of gluteus medius, vastus medialis obliquus and tibilis posterior [Section 6.3] is (or should be) hardwired into the descending tracts in the nervous system. Lack of this co-activation pattern has been shown to be a major factor in knee and hip and ankle joint pain.

A method for activating the hamstrings of the standing (WB) leg uses postures such as *utthita*

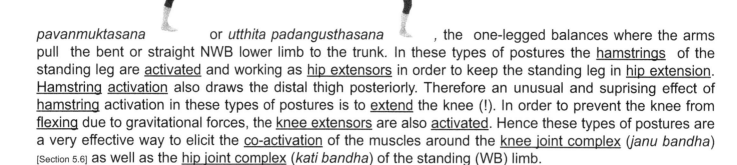

pavanmuktasana or *utthita padangusthasana* , the one-legged balances where the arms pull the bent or straight NWB lower limb to the trunk. In these types of postures the hamstrings of the standing leg are activated and working as hip extensors in order to keep the standing leg in hip extension. Hamstring activation also draws the distal thigh posteriorly. Therefore an unusual and suprising effect of hamstring activation in these types of postures is to extend the knee (!). In order to prevent the knee from flexing due to gravitational forces, the knee extensors are also activated. Hence these types of postures are a very effective way to elicit the co-activation of the muscles around the knee joint complex (*janu bandha*) [Section 5.6] as well as the hip joint complex (*kati bandha*) of the standing (WB) limb.

Studies have shown that the non weight-bearing (NWB) leg also gets a significant training effect in one-legged exercises [Kannus et al., 1992]. In many one-legged postures (*asanas*), the hamstrings of the NWB leg can be strengthened by using them to extend the thigh at the hip joint of the NWB leg. In order to maximise the use of the hamstrings as hip extensors, it is first necessary to reciprocally relax gluteus maximus (the main buttocks muscle) by internally rotating the thigh at the hip joint. One *asana* that works this way is *niralamba*

virabhadrasana . *Niralamba virabhadrasana* is a one-legged posture with the NWB knee extended and locked, the weight-bearing (WB) knee extended but unlocked, the WB hip flexed, and the NWB hip extended and internally rotated (N.B. arrow turning the left (rear) thigh inwards). When performed in the fashion described above *niralamba virabhadrasana* can have the following beneficial effects on the sacroiliac (SI) joint and the knee joint complex. These effects include the following:

- The inner thigh muscles become activated. Inner thigh muscles are generally thought of as hip adductors but they act here as hip internal rotators [Norkin & Levangie, 1992]. Hip adductor/internal rotator activity can help strengthen the lower back and often help relieve lower back pain. In addition, because one hip adductor (gracillis) has a distal attachment distal to (below) the knee, activation of the inner thigh muscles can also help to strengthen and stabilise the knee joint complex.
- Activation of the vastus medialis (a knee extensor) via its attachments to the hip adductor and adductor magnus [Table 4.6]. Adductor magnus activation causes a myotatic reflex activation of vastus medialis.

This can help strengthen and stabilise the knee and also relieve <u>patella mal-tracking</u> problems of the knee [Section 5.5.4].
- The <u>sacroiliac joint</u> is gently <u>tractioned</u> (stretched), due to active <u>internal rotation</u> of the thigh at the <u>hip joint.</u>
- <u>Reciprocal relaxation</u> of external rotators of the hip including <u>gluteus maximus</u>
- The <u>hamstrings</u> become <u>activated</u> as <u>hip extensors</u> becuse <u>gluteus maximus</u> activity has been inhibited. The <u>hamstrings</u> contribute to <u>co-activation</u> of the muscles around the <u>knee joint</u> (*janu bandha*) along with the <u>knee extensors</u> [Section 5.6] of the NWB limb.
- <u>Hip internal rotation</u> with <u>hip extension</u> causes <u>activation</u> of the inner thigh muscles (acting here as <u>hip internal rotators</u>) and the <u>hamstrings</u> (acting here as <u>hip extensors</u>) with a relaxed buttocks (<u>gluteus maximus</u>). However, for some people keeping the buttocks (<u>gluteus maximus</u>) relaxed may cause instability in the <u>sacroiliac joint</u> so once the <u>internal rotators</u> and the <u>hamstrings</u> have been activated it is then possible to <u>co-activate</u> (simultaneously tense) <u>gluteus maximus</u> by squeezing the buttocks muscle and thus effectively creating a *kati bandha* that can stabilise the <u>sacroiliac joint</u> as described in Section 4.5.1.1.

4.5.4 *Mula Bandha*: The Yogic Root Lock [Section 7.5.1.1]

The *yoga* postures are designed to give strength and flexibility to the spine. Strength in the spine is developed and maintained in *yoga* postures by a muscular contraction of the lower trunk, which is known in *yoga* as *mula bandha* or root lock. This *bandha* is essentially a gentle <u>tonic</u> (ongoing) <u>activation</u> of the following muscle groups:
- Muscles of the <u>perineum</u>
- Lower abdominal musculature, in particular <u>transversus abdominis</u>, and
- Lower back musculature, in particular the <u>lumbar multifidus</u>.

Initially obtaining an isolated contraction of the <u>perineum</u> without also tightening the <u>anal constrictor muscles</u> is difficult for most people. *Mula bandha* may be obtained by contracting the anus, but excessive use of this method often leads to constipation. Isolation of the <u>perineum</u> without the <u>anal constrictor muscles</u> can be approached in two main ways.
- By contracting the lower abdomen as part of controlled exhalations,
- By pressing (or trying to pull) the <u>coccyx</u> (tail-bone) inferiorly and anteriorly, and/or directing the base of the genitalia inferiorly and posteriorly, depending on the *yoga* posture and the practitioner's current level of flexibility.

4.5.5 Strengthening and Stretching Muscles and Healing Non-Acutely Injured Muscles with *Yoga* Postures: The hip flexors as an example

In general when trying to either strengthen a muscle or muscle group or when trying to heal a non-acutely injured muscle, one needs to consider the following types of postures:

- **Postures that cause an <u>obligatory active contraction</u> of a muscle group to a shortened position**
  [Appendix A].
  - o For example, the <u>hip flexors</u> (eg. <u>iliopsoas</u>, <u>sartorius</u>) must be active in *niralamba utthita*

  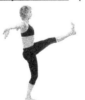

  padangusthasana (leg held up without the support of the hand).

- **Postures that are enhanced when a muscle group is voluntarily <u>activated</u> in a shortened position.**
  - o For example, <u>hip flexors</u> can be <u>activated</u> to enhance any of the forward bending postures such as

  pascimottanasana   in order to enhance <u>hip flexion</u> and <u>lumbar spine extension</u>.

This can be achieved by trying to lift the inner thighs from the floor without letting the knees lift off the floor.

- **Postures which cause an obligatory lengthening or stretching of a muscle group**
  - o   For example, the <u>hip flexors</u> must be stretched in a correctly applied lunge (*utthita san*

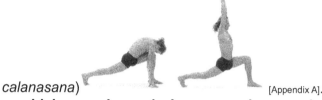

    calanasana)   [Appendix A].
- **Postures which are enhanced when a muscle group is lengthened or stretched**

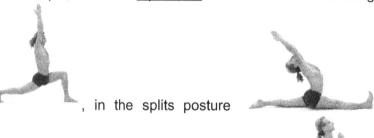

  - o   For example, when <u>hip flexors</u> are made to lengthen in the splits posture (*hanumanasana*) by increasing the <u>posterior pelvic tilt</u>, this brings the hips more into alignment and minimises the risk of injuring the lower back or the knees.
- **Postures which are enhanced when a muscle group is activated in a lengthened position**
  - o   For example, when the <u>hip flexors</u> are activated in a standing lunge (*utthita san calanasana*) , in the splits posture (*hanumanasana*), or in the advanced splits posture *kulpha hanumanasana* by trying to bring the thighs towards each other, this further increases the stretch of the <u>hip flexors</u> and assists in elevating the spine away from the floor.

Tables 4.8 – 4.11 at the end of this chapter describe how some of these principles can be used in various *yoga* asanas with respect to the movements and muscular actions of the <u>hip joint</u>. Study these tables and try and make tables of other postures of the <u>hip joint complex</u> and of the other major <u>joint complexes</u>.

****

Table 4.8 Postures which are enhanced by obligatory and non-obligatory hip muscle activation (Abbreviations: WB = Weight-bearing; NWB = Non-weight-bearing; R = Right; L = Left; LL = Lower Limb)

EXERCISE TYPE	HIP OPEN-CHAIN EXERCISES (Limb tries to move & body stays still)		HIP CLOSED-CHAIN EXERCISES (Limb stays still & body tries to move)	
MUSCLE LENGTH	**SHORTENED** muscle	**LENGTHENED** (stretched) muscle	**SHORTENED** muscle	**LENGTHENED** (stretched) muscle
MUSCLE GROUP (plus instructions on how to activate the muscle group)⇓				
HIP FLEXORS	*Niralamba padangusthasana* *Niralamba supta padangusthasana* (All of these postures have the shortened hip flexors of the NWB LL in obligatory activation)	*Padma janu dhanurasana* *Kulpha dhanurasana* *Natarajasana* (For all these postures push the NWB legs backwards, i.e. trying to flex the hips while keeping them in extension, or activate the hip flexors in a lengthened state)	*Utthita trikonasana* (Push R hip to R foot, try to stretch the mat with your feet to activate hip flexors in a shortened state) *Hamsa parsvottanasana* (Push R hip to R foot, try to stretch the mat with your feet to activate hip flexors in a shortened state) *Pascimottanasana* (Try to lift the thighs away from the floor to activate the shortened hip flexors)	*Utthita san calanasana* *Hamsa parivrtta san calanasana* (L leg) *Hanumanasana* (L leg) (For all these postures push rear LL to front LL, try to squash the mat with your feet in order to activte the lengthened hip flexors)

143

HIP EXTENSORS

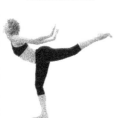

Salabhasana

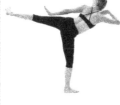

Niralamba virabhadrasana

(Both these postures have the shortened hip extensors of the NWB LL in obligatory activation)

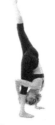

Urdhva prasarita eka padasana

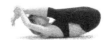

Urdhva mukha pascimottanasana

(For both these postures push the NWB legs upwards to activate the hip extensors in a lengthened state)

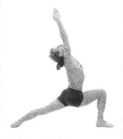

Utthita virabhadrasana (Push L hip to L foot, try to stretch the mat with your feet to activate hip extensors in a shortened state)

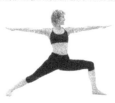

Niralamba setu bandhasana (Lift the hips higher by pushing down with the feet and/or tensing buttocks muscles to activate hip extensors in a shortened state)

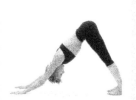

Adho mukha svanasana (Push the feet backwards into the floor to activate hip extensors in a lengthened state)

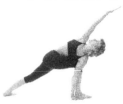

Uttana parsvakonasana (Push the R foot into the floor to activate hip extensors in a lengthened state)

HIP ABDUCTORS

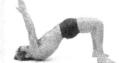

Niralamba ardha candrasana (The shortened hip abductors of the NWB LL are in obligatory activation)

Samakona adho mukha vrksasana (Activate the shortened hip abductors of the NWB LL by trying to push the legs wider apart)

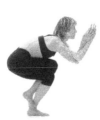

Garudasana (Try to push the thighs outwards and apart to activate the hip abductors in a lengthened state)

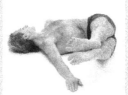

Jathara parivartanasana (The lengthened hip abductors of the NWB LL are in obligatory activation)

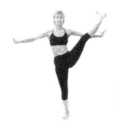

Parsva virabhadrasana (Push R hip to R foot, try to stretch the mat with your feet to activate hip abductors in a shortened state)

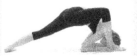

Niralamba parsva padangusthasana (The lengthened hip abductors of the WB LL are in obligatory activation)

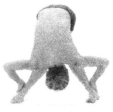

Parivrtta parsvakonasana (Push R hip to R side against L shoulder to activate hip abductors in a lengthened state)

Baddha kulpha meru danda vakrasasana (Try to squash the mat or the floor inwards with your feet to activate hip abductors in a lengthened state)

144

HIP ADDUCTORS

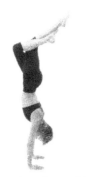

Garuda adho mukha vrksasana

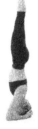

Sirsasana
(For both these postures activate the shortened hip adductors by pressing the thighs towards each other)

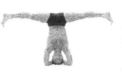

Upavistha kona sirsasana

Niralamba ardha candrasana

(For both these postures and all similar postures to activate hip adductors in a lengthened state try to turn the NWB thighs inwards as many hip internal rotators are also hip adductors)

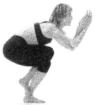

Garudasana

Adho mukha svanasana

(For these type of postures activate the shortened hip adductors by pressing the thighs towards each other)

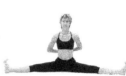

Hamsa samakonasana

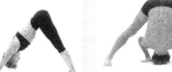

Prasarita padottanasana

(For these type of postures activate the lengthened hip adductors by pressing the thighs towards each other)

HIP EXTERNAL ROTATORS

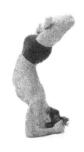

Padma sirsasana

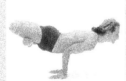

Padma mayurasana

(For these type of postures activate the shortened hip external rotators by trying to turn the NWB thigh more outwards)

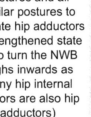

Pinda sirsasana

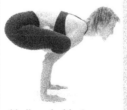

Urdhva kukkutasana

(For these type of postures activate the lengthened hip external rotators by tensing the buttocks muscles)

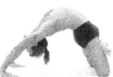

Padma urdhva dhanurasana
(Activate the shortened hip external rotators by tensing the buttocks muscles)

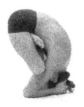

Utthita trikonasana
(In the front LL of asymmetrical standing postures activate the shortened hip external rotators by sqeezing the heel inwards and front of foot outwards)

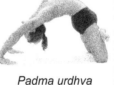

Yoga mudrasana

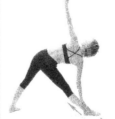

Adho mukha swastikasana

(For these type of postures activate the lengthened hip external rotators by pressing the feet down towards the floor)

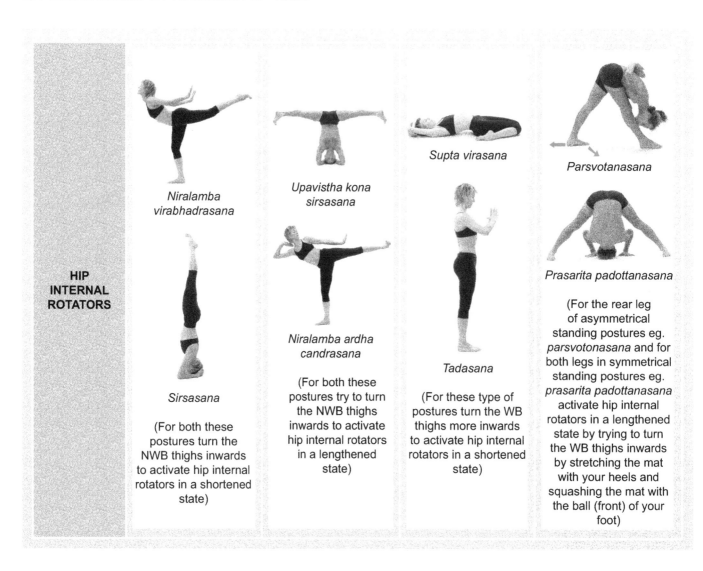

HIP INTERNAL ROTATORS

Niralamba virabhadrasana

Upavistha kona sirsasana

Supta virasana

Parsvotanasana

Sirsasana

(For both these postures turn the NWB thighs inwards to activate hip internal rotators in a shortened state)

Niralamba ardha candrasana

(For both these postures try to turn the NWB thighs inwards to activate hip internal rotators in a lengthened state)

Tadasana

(For these type of postures turn the WB thighs more inwards to activate hip internal rotators in a shortened state)

Prasarita padottanasana

(For the rear leg of asymmetrical standing postures eg. *parsvotonasana* and for both legs in symmetrical standing postures eg. *prasarita padottanasana* activate hip internal rotators in a lengthened state by trying to turn the WB thighs inwards by stretching the mat with your heels and squashing the mat with the ball (front) of your foot)

<u>Table 4.8</u>: Postures which are enhanced by non-obligatory hip muscle activation *(Continued)*

Table 4.9 An investigation into how various muscle groups can be used in a standing posture such as *trikonasana*

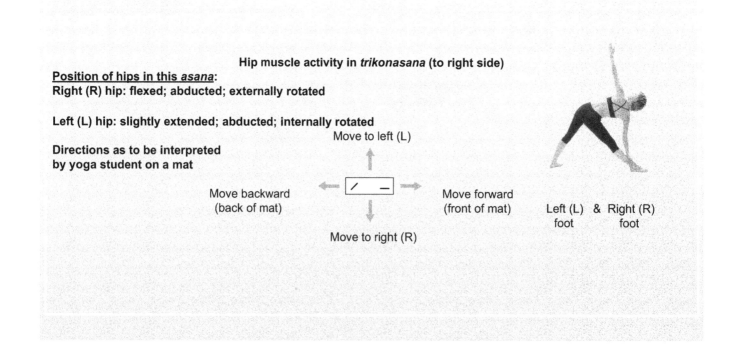

Hip muscle activity in *trikonasana* (to right side)

<u>Position of hips in this *asana*</u>:
Right (R) hip: flexed; abducted; externally rotated

Left (L) hip: slightly extended; abducted; internally rotated

Directions as to be interpreted by yoga student on a mat

Move to left (L)

Move backward (back of mat)

Move forward (front of mat)

Move to right (R)

Left (L) & Right (R) foot   foot

MUSCLE GROUP	POSSIBLE ROLE OF MUSCLE GROUP DURING THE POSTURE	INSTRUCTIONS TO ELICIT MUSCLE GROUP USE	PURPOSE OF MUSCLE ACTIVITY
R HIP FLEXORS	Closed-chain hip flexor activity	Push R hip into R foot towards the front of the mat	Increases hip flexion if L hip is allowed to internally rotate. Stabilisation of body; Enhances *mula bandha* by reflex activation of perineum and abdominal muscles
L HIP FLEXORS	Passive stretch which increases as R hip is brought to the left side of the mat	Move R sitting bone (ischial tuberosity) to L side of mat, and towards the L big toe	Lengthen the L hip flexors especially the psoas major which if tight can cause back problems
R HIP EXTENSORS	No muscle activity desired in gluteus maximus. Passive stretch of hamstrings which increases as R hip is brought into greater flexion i.e. hand comes closer to ankle	Slide R hand closer to foot; push R foot to R; pull up the knee cap; straighten the R knee more	Increased length of the hamstrings allows greater freedom of movement for the spine in this and other postures
L HIP EXTENSORS	No muscle activity desired in gluteus muscles especially due to internal rotation of L lhigh a L hip	Push L heel towards the back of the mat	Leads to an increased stretch in the L hip flexors
R HIP ABDUCTORS	Possibly working with hip flexors	Push R hip into R foot towards the front of the mat	As for R hip flexor group
L HIP ABDUCTORS	Closed-chain abductor activity	Push L hip into L foot towards the back of the mat	Strengthens L hip abductors; helps stabilise spine via myotatic reflex activation of abdominal muscles
R HIP ADDUCTORS	Passive stretch which increases as R hip is brought forward	Move R sitting bone (ischial tuberosity) to L side of mat, and towards the L big toe	Stretches the hip adductors; increases hip external rotation
L HIP ADDUCTORS	Passive stretch which increases if legs are brought further apart; Increased activity when L hip adductors are used as internal rotators of L hip	Press L ball (front) of foot inwards to R side of mat	Hip adductor activity and or stretching can help traction the spine due to location of the muscle attachments on the hip. Strengthens the knee joint complex
R HIP EXTERNAL ROTATORS	Increase activity of deep hip external rotators without activating gluteus maximus	Turn R thigh outwards; squeeze the R heel inwards and push the R ball (front) of foot outwards	To increase rotational ROM in the R hip; to facilitate the tractioning of the spine in this *asana*; increases stretch of the R hip internal rotators
L HIP EXTERNAL ROTATORS	Passive stretch of L hip external rotators which increases as L hip internal rotation increase	Turn L thigh inwards	To increase external rotational ROM in the L hip; to facilitate the tractioning of the spine in this *asana*
R HIP INTERNAL ROTATORS	Passive stretch of R hip internal rotators which increases as external rotation of R hip increases	Turn R thigh outwards	To increase external rotational ROM in the R hip; to facilitate the tractioning of the spine in this *asana*
L HIP INTERNAL ROTATORS	Increase activity of hip internal rotators including the hip adductor muscle group	Turn L thigh inwards; stretch the mat with your heel and squeeze the ball (front) of your L foot inwards	To increase internal rotational ROM in the L hip; to facilitate the tractioning of the spine and distraction of the sacroiliac joint in this *asana*

Chapter Breakdown

****

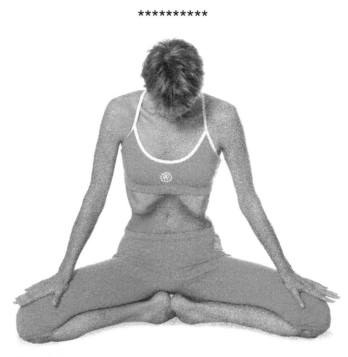

Bianca Machliss practicing *tha-uddiyana bandha* on exhalation retention in *Mulabandhasana*. This advanced pose requires extreme flexibility in hip abduction and internal rotation as well as extreme knee external rotation with a strong *ha-janu bandha* (compressive knee lock). Photo courtesy of Alejandro Rolandi.

5.0 INTRODUCTION TO THE APPLIED ANATOMY OF THE THIGH & KNEE IN HATHA YOGA POSTURES

The knee joint complex plays a major role in supporting the body during static and dynamic activities. The knee plays a supportive role in closed-chain activities and provides mobility for the foot in space during open-chain activities. The fact that the knee has to satisfy major stability and mobility requirements is reflected in its structure and function. The knee is not only one of the largest joints in the body but it is also the most complex [Norkin & Levangie, 1992].

Lack of mobility in the hip joint complex, weakness and lack of control in the muscles surrounding the knee joint complex and incorrect *yoga* practice are the main reasons why the knee is one of the most commonly injured parts of the body in *hatha yoga*. Safety of the knee joint complex should be as important an issue as protecting the lower back and the neck in both self-practise and teaching of *hatha yoga*.

5.1 BONES AROUND THE KNEE JOINT COMPLEX

The following features of the knee joint complex can be seen on a skeleton and identified with the help of Figures 5.1–5.6:

1. **Femur** (thigh bone)
2. **Tibia** (inner shin bone)
3. **Fibula** (outer shin bone)
4. **Patella** (knee cap).

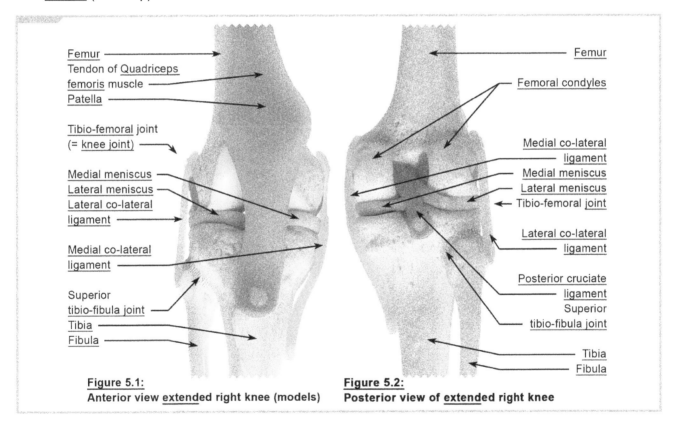

Figure 5.1:
Anterior view extended right knee (models)

Figure 5.2:
Posterior view of extended right knee

5.1.1 Femur (distal end)
The following features of the femur can be seen on a skeleton and identified with the help of Figures 5.1–5.6:
• Medial condyle, lateral condyle, epicondyles, adductor tubercle, patella surface and popliteal surface.

5.1.2 Tibia (proximal end)
The following features of the tibia can be seen on a skeleton and identified with the help of Figures 5.1–5.6:
• Tibial plateau, medial condyle and lateral condyle, intercondylar eminence, fibular articular facet, and tibial tuberosity.

5.1.3 Fibula (proximal end)

The following features of the fibula can be seen on a skeleton and identified with the help of Figures 5.1–5.6:
• Head, articular facet.

5.1.4 Patella

The patella is a sesamoid bone which functions to:
(i) protect the knee joint complex,
(ii) strengthen the quadriceps tendon and
(iii) increase the power of rectus femoris by increasing the leverage.

The following features of the patella can be seen on a skeleton and identified with the help of Figures 5.1–5.6:
• Anterior surface, articular surface, apex.

5.2 JOINTS OF THE KNEE

The knee has two main articulations (joints):
1. **Tibiofemoral joint**
2. **Patellofemoral joint**

The joints and ligaments of the knee are shown in Figures 5.1 – 5.6.

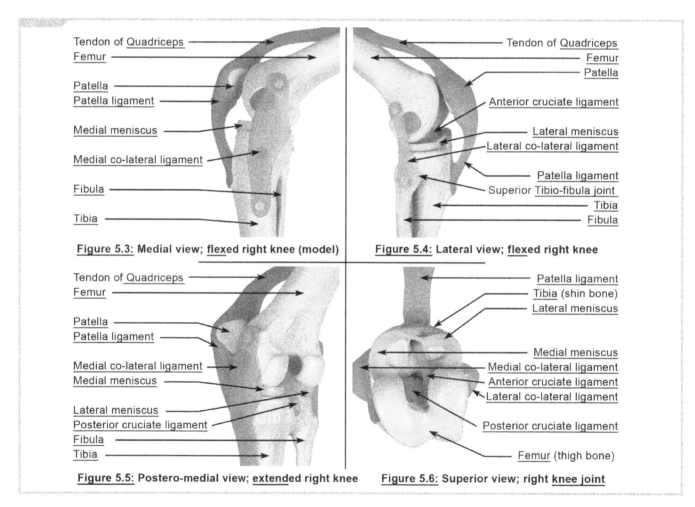

Figure 5.3: Medial view; flexed right knee (model)

Figure 5.4: Lateral view; flexed right knee

Figure 5.5: Postero-medial view; extended right knee

Figure 5.6: Superior view; right knee joint

5.2.1 Tibiofemoral joint

Location	between the two condyles of the femur and the two condyles of the tibia
Classification	synovial, condyloid, biaxial, complex
Movements	flexion, extension, internal rotation of the tibia on the femur, and external rotation of the tibia on the femur
Joint capsule	very strong with intrinsic ligament thickening and a complex synovial lining

Ligaments   Due to lack of bony restraint in virtually all of the knee motions, the <u>ligaments</u> play an important role in knee stability.

- The **patella retinacula ligament** joins the <u>patella</u> to the <u>tibial tuberosity</u>, and functions to stabilise the <u>patella</u>. It limits superior movement of the <u>patella</u> as the <u>quadriceps</u> are activated, and reinforces the capsule anteriorly.

- The **medial collateral ligament (MCL)** is a strong flat band (8–9 cm) extending from the <u>medial epicondyle</u> of the <u>femur</u> to the <u>medial condyle</u> and medial surface of the <u>tibia</u>. It attaches to the <u>medial meniscus</u> and is therefore <u>capsular</u>. It prevents <u>abduction</u> of the <u>tibia</u> and limits <u>extension</u> of the <u>knee joint</u>.

- The **lateral collateral ligament (LCL)** is a round cord about 5 cm long going from the <u>lateral epicondyle</u> of the <u>femur</u> to the lateral surface of the head of <u>fibula</u>. The tendon of the <u>popliteus</u> muscle separates it from the <u>lateral meniscus</u>, therefore it is <u>extracapsular</u>. The LCL prevents <u>adduction</u> and limits <u>extension</u> of the <u>tibia</u>.

- The **anterior cruciate ligament (ACL)** is an <u>intracapsular (extra-synovium) ligament</u> from the <u>anterior intercondylar</u> area of <u>tibia</u> to the posterior part of medial side of <u>lateral femoral condyle</u>. It prevents anterior glide of the <u>tibia</u> and limits <u>extension</u>. The ACL is usually weaker than the <u>posterior cruciate ligament</u> (PCL).

- The **posterior cruciate ligament (PCL)** is an <u>intracapsular (extra-synovium) ligament</u> from the posterior intercondylar area of the tibia to the anterior part of lateral surface of <u>medial femoral condyle</u>. It prevents posterior glide of the <u>tibia</u>, prevents <u>hyper-flexion</u> of the <u>knee joint</u>. It is the main stabiliser of the <u>femur</u> when going down stairs, and tightens during <u>flexion</u>.

- The **posterior meniscofemoral ligament** joins the <u>lateral meniscus</u> to the PCL, and moves the <u>lateral meniscus</u> out of the way during <u>knee flexion</u>, protecting the <u>lateral meniscus</u> from damage.
- The **oblique popliteal ligament** is a capsular broad band running supero-laterally from the <u>tibia</u> to the <u>femur</u> and serves to strengthen the capsule posteriorly.

- The **arcuate popliteal ligament** is a capsular Y-shaped band, running supero-medially from the <u>fibula</u> to the <u>femur</u> and <u>tibia</u>. It reinforces the capsule posteriorly.

- The **coronary ligament** has fibres running vertically holding the <u>menisci</u> to the <u>tibia</u>. It is stronger medially.

- The **transverse ligament** is an anterior connection between the <u>menisci</u>, which it holds together during <u>knee flexion</u>.

Articular discs (menisci)

There are two <u>articular discs</u> (<u>menisci</u>), one is the <u>medial meniscus</u> and the other is the <u>lateral meniscus</u>. They are crescent shaped plates of <u>non-contractile fibrocartilage</u> on the <u>tibial</u> surface. The discs are wedge shaped and thicker towards the periphery. As the knee moves, the <u>menisci</u> also move.

Functions of the menisci
The <u>menisci</u> function as shock absorbers. They increase stability of the knee, aid the mechanical fit of the knee, and help to spread <u>synovial fluid</u>.

- The **medial meniscus** is semicircular, broader posteriorly, attaches to the MCL, and is not very movable, which is one of the reasons why it is torn more frequently than the <u>lateral meniscus</u>.
- The **lateral meniscus** is nearly circular, smaller and more movable than the <u>medial meniscus</u>, and covers a larger articular surface. The <u>posterior meniscofemoral ligament</u> attaches the <u>lateral meniscus</u> to the PCL.

Infrapatella fat pad

Loose fatty tissue separating <u>patella ligament</u> from the <u>synovial membrane</u>

5.2.2 Patellofemoral Joint

Location between the patella and the femur.

Classification synovial, saddle (sellar), biaxial, simple.

Movements lateral and medial glide, cephalad and caudal glide.

Ligaments The quadriceps tendon and patellar tendon (also called patellar ligament) are components of the extensor mechanism of the knee. When the quadriceps is activated, force is transmitted through the quadriceps tendon, across the patella, through the patellar tendon, and the knee is extended.

Bursae The suprapatella bursa, subpopliteal bursa and gastrocnemius bursa are not usually separate entities, but are invaginations of the synovium, or communicate with the articular (joint) capsule through small openings.

- **Suprapatella bursa** – permits free movement of the quadriceps tendon over the distal femur during flexion and extension. Communicates with the knee joint.

- **Prepatella bursa** – sits subcutaneously on top of the patella. It can get friction bursitis from kneeling. This does not communicate with the knee joint.

Loading Loading of the patella and the patellofemoral joint will vary with activity. When walking, the pressure on the patella is 1/3 body weight, climbing stairs is three times the body weight and squatting in postures such

as *malasana* and *utkatasana* can be up to seven times body weight.

5.3 MUSCLES OF THE KNEE JOINT COMPLEX

The 16 muscles that cross the knee and therefore affect its functions are:

- **Quadriceps group**
  1. **Rectus femoris**
  2. **Vastus lateralis obliquus**
  3. **Vastus lateralis longus**
  4. **Vastus medialis obliquus**
  5. **Vastus medialis longus**
  6. **Vastus intermedius**

- **Hamstrings group**
  7. **Biceps femoris** (long head)
  8. **Biceps femoris** (short head)
  9. **Semitendinosus**
  10. **Semimembranosus**

  11. **Gracilis**
  12. **Sartorius**
  13. **Popliteus**
  14. **Gastrocnemius**
  15. **Plantaris** (which is absent in some people)
  16. **Iliotibial band (ITB)** (formed proximally from the fascia, attaching to the **tensor fasciae latae, gluteus maximus** and **gluteus medius**, and inserting distally into the lateral condyle of the tibia) [Section 5.4.2.].

Most of these muscles have already been described in Chapter 4 [Tables 4.2, 4.3, 4.4, 4.5]. The remaining muscles of the knee are described in Table 5.1. The movements and muscle groups around the knee joint complex are described in Table 5.2.

Table 5.1 Muscles of the posterior leg that cross the knee

MUSCLE	ORIGIN	INSERTION	ACTION
Gastrocnemius	• <u>Lateral head:</u> Lateral aspect of condyle of femur. • <u>Medial head:</u> Popliteal surface of femur superior to medial condyle.	• Posterior surface of calcaneus via tendocalcaneus (Achilles tendon).	• Plantarflexes foot • Raises heel during walking and • Flexes knee joint.
Popliteus	• Lateral condyle of femur. • Lateral meniscus.	• Posterior surface of proximal tibia.	• Weakly flexes the knee and unlocks it.
Plantaris (absent in some people)	• Lateral supracondylar line of femur. • Oblique popliteal ligament.	• Posterior surface of calcaneus via tendocalcaneus (Achilles tendon).	• Weakly assists gastrocnemius in plantarflexing foot and flexing knee joint.

Table 5.2 Movements & muscle groups at the knee joint

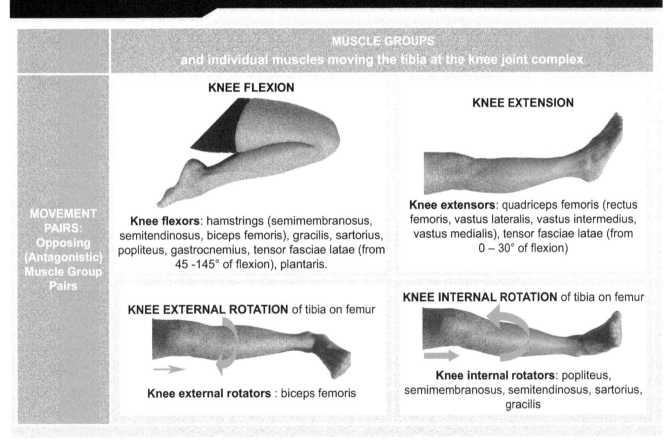

MUSCLE GROUPS
and individual muscles moving the tibia at the knee joint complex

MOVEMENT PAIRS: Opposing (Antagonistic) Muscle Group Pairs

KNEE FLEXION

Knee flexors: hamstrings (semimembranosus, semitendinosus, biceps femoris), gracilis, sartorius, popliteus, gastrocnemius, tensor fasciae latae (from 45 -145° of flexion), plantaris.

KNEE EXTENSION

Knee extensors: quadriceps femoris (rectus femoris, vastus lateralis, vastus intermedius, vastus medialis), tensor fasciae latae (from 0 – 30° of flexion)

KNEE EXTERNAL ROTATION of tibia on femur

Knee external rotators : biceps femoris

KNEE INTERNAL ROTATION of tibia on femur

Knee internal rotators: popliteus, semimembranosus, semitendinosus, sartorius, gracilis

Important muscles of the knee

The following muscles and muscle groups are important in the knee. Their attachments and actions are useful to learn. They are relatively easy to see and feel. Most of these muscles can be seen in Figures 5.7 and 5.8.

1. **Quadriceps femoris** group (rectus femoris, vastus lateralis longus, vastus lateralis obliquus, vastus intermedius, vastus medialis longus and vastus medialis obliquus)
2. **Hamstrings** group (biceps femoris, semimembranosus, semitendinosus)
3. **Gracilis** (and the other internal rotators and adductors of the hip, especially adductor magnus and adductor longus to which the origin of vastus medialis obliquus attaches)
4. **Sartorius**
5. **Gastrocnemius**

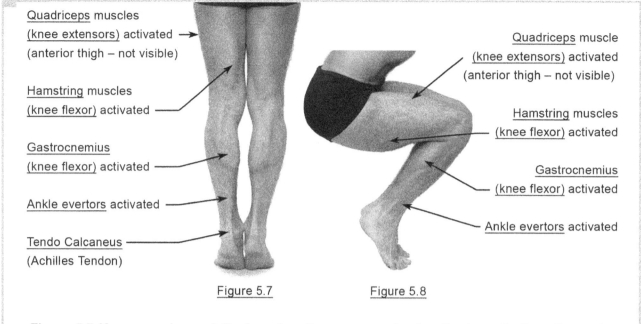

Quadriceps muscles
(knee extensors) activated →
(anterior thigh – not visible)

Hamstring muscles
(knee flexor) activated

Gastrocnemius
(knee flexor) activated

Ankle evertors activated

Tendo Calcaneus
(Achilles Tendon)

Quadriceps muscle
(knee extensors) activated
(anterior thigh – not visible)

Hamstring muscles
(knee flexor) activated

Gastrocnemius
(knee flexor) activated

Ankle evertors activated

Figure 5.7   Figure 5.8

Figure 5.7 Knee muscles and *tha-janu bandha*: an expansive *bandha* (co-activation of opposing (antagonistic) muscles) of the knee that enhances blood flowing through the knee joint complex.
Figure 5.8 Knee muscles and *ha-janu bandha*: a compressive *bandha* (co-activation of opposing (antagonistic) muscles) of the knee that prevents blood flowing through the knee joint complex.

5.4 SPECIAL FEATURES OF THE THIGH AND KNEE

5.4.1 Fascia Lata of the Thigh

The fascia lata of the thigh is a strong, dense, broad layer of fascia (as opposed to the tensor fasciae latae (TFL) which is a muscle) that arises from the body of the pelvis and invests several muscles of the thigh like an elastic stocking. It provides a dense tubular sheath for the thigh muscles, which prevents them from bulging excessively when they are activated and therefore improves their effectiveness.

5.4.2 Iliotibial Band (Tract) (ITB)

The iliotibial band (ITB) is part of the fascia lata. It is an extremely strong structure running laterally from the tubercle of the iliac crest to the lateral condyle of the tibia. It receives tendinous reinforcements from the tensor fasciae latae (TFL) and gluteus maximus muscles and is additionally supported by the lateral collateral ligament of the knee.

In biomechanical studies, the ITB and TFL have been shown to be instrumental in stabilisng the knee and preventing knee adduction, particularly in unexpected dodging and weaving exercises. The TFL has been shown to be deficient in patients with chronic knee arthritis and degeneration of the knee joint.

Tensor fasciae latae pulls on the ITB thereby steadying the trunk on the thigh and preventing posterior displacement of the ITB by gluteus maximus, three quarters of which insert into the ITB.

There exists much controversy about the role of the muscles attached to the ITB and fascia lata with respect to the movements of the knee. Some practitioners assert these muscles will have no effect on the knee but there is good clinical evidence to suggest that both tensor fasciae latae and gluteus maximus have an effect on knee flexion and extension via their attachments to the ITB.

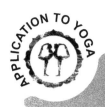

No 5.1 The outer thigh generally needs stretching not strengthening in order to assist in correct knee function

Many people have knee pain that is associated with a tightness of the structures of the outer thigh, in particular the iliotibial band (ITB). In such cases where hip adduction is limited, postures such as *meru danda vakrasana,* which can be a good hip abductor stretch, can reduce the incidence of knee problems. Once the ITB has been lengthened, the tensor fasciae latae and gluteus maximus, which both have attachments on the ITB, can perform their actions without the risk of adversely affecting knee function.

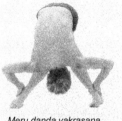

Meru danda vakrasana
(A hip abductor stretch)

5.4.3 Locking Mechanism of the Knee

The locking mechanism is an energy saving system. It is very stable and muscles do not need to be active when standing for a long time on two legs with knees extended. The locking mechanism of the knee allows the knee to remain in full extension with no muscular activity. This makes standing much more comfortable and energy efficient.

When the knee is being extended, incongruence of the femoral condyle and tibial condyle results in a rolling and gliding of the condylar surfaces on one another. On a fixed tibia, a rolling and gliding motion results in a medial rotation of the femur on the tibia during the last 5° of extension. Rotation within the knee joint, accompanying the end of knee extension, also brings the knee joint into the closed-packed or locked position [Section 1.5.2.6]. In the closed-packed (locked) position the tibial tubercles are lodged in the intercondylar notch, the menisci are tightly interposed between the tibial condyles and femoral condyles, and the ligaments are taut.

To initiate flexion, the knee must first be unlocked by the popliteus muscle, which initiates flexion. The popliteus unlocks the knee joint by medially rotating the tibia if the femur is fixed, or by laterally rotating the femur if the tibia is fixed, which would be the case in standing positions.

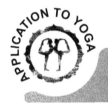

No 5.2 Disengage the locking mechanism of the knee in weight-bearing legs in order to stablise the knee joint complex with *janu bandha*

One-legged balancing poses are best initially practised with the standing (weight-bearing) leg kept slightly bent (flexed) at the knee, so the locking mechanism of the knee cannot operate. This forces at least some of the muscles which cross the knee joint complex to become active, which helps strengthen the knee, hip and ankle joints, and also facilities improvements in balance. When the muscles surrounding the knee joint complex can be voluntarily co-activated (*janu bandha*) then fully extending a weight-bearing knee can be safely practised.

5.5 ABNORMALITIES & INJURIES OF THE KNEE

5.5.1 Abnormal Angles between the Thigh and Leg
- **Genu varum** (bow-legged) is normal in children until 18-19 months of age, but it is abnormal in adults.
- **Genu valgum** (knock-kneed) is normal in children from about 18 months to three or four years of age. Children's limbs should be close to straight by age six, otherwise the situation is considered to be abnormal.
- **Genu recurvatum** (hyperextension of the knee) is generally thought to be an abnormal condition, which may result from lax posterior knee ligaments.

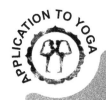

No 5.3 Always bend the knee slightly in weight-bearing postures when that knee is hyperextended

In cases of genu recurvatum (hyperextension of the knee), all weight-bearing postures of the lower limbs are best practised with the knee of a weight-bearing leg kept slightly bent (flexed), so the knee locking mechanism cannot operate and force the knees into hyperextension.

In straight legged postures such as *parsvottonasana* and *trikonasana* hyperextension of the most weight-bearing knee can be avoided by pressing onto the front of the foot of the leading leg in order to activate gastrocnemius (an ankle plantarflexor and a knee flexor) which increases knee stability and causes a slight knee flexion to alleviate the dangers of hyperextension.

5.5.2 Ruptured Knee Ligaments

The most commonly ruptured knee ligaments are the anterior cruciate ligament (ACL) and the medial collateral ligament (MCL). Rupture of the ACL and/or MCL leads to anteromedial instability of the knee joint complex.

The hamstring muscles act synergistically to the ACL (ie both the hamstrings and the ACL prevent the anterior movement of the tibia from the femur). Therefore, in cases of ACL tear or rupture, strength and control of the hamstrings is very important for aiding recovery and preventing further damage.

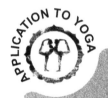

No 5.4 Activate the hamstrings to protect the knee in cases of ruptured or over-stretched anterior cruciate ligament (ACL)

In cases of ruptured or overstretched ACL, all poses that activate the hamstrings [Appendix A] either as knee flexors or as hip extensors are useful to support the loss of the ACL's main function, which is to prevent anterior translation (forward movement) of the tibia from the femur [Section 5.6.1.2]. All poses that assist in the generation of *janu bandha* [Section 5.6.1, Appendix C] will help stabilise the knee joint complex.

5.5.3 Meniscal Tears

Tears of the medial meniscus are often concurrent with tears of the anterior cruciate ligament (ACL) and medial collateral ligament (MCL). Medial meniscus damage and tears of the ACL and MCL are more common than lateral meniscus damage, which is often concurrent with tears of the posterior cruciate ligament (PCL) and lateral collateral ligament (LCL). If left untreated meniscal tears may lead to degenerative changes in later life. The menisci are well vascularised in children, but only vascularised on the periphery from age 10 to adult. 10-30% of the outside of the medial meniscus is vascularised, and 25% of the outside edge of lateral meniscus is vascularised. If torn, the periphery may heal. However, if the central portion is torn it is unlikely to heal. Only the outer 1/3 of each meniscus is innervated, whereas the inner portion is not, therefore any pain felt from a meniscal tear must be from a peripheral portion of that meniscus.

5.5.4 Patella Tracking Problems (Patella Mal-tracking)

When the patella (knee cap) does not track correctly (ie slide over its correct path of movement) over the femur this is refered to as patella mal-tracking. This painful problem can be due to imbalances in strength between vastus medialis obliquus (VMO) fibres, which are usually weak, and vastus lateralis fibres. The VMO originates on the adductor magnus tendon. This is the anatomic basis for recommending hip adductor strengthening in cases of patella mal-tracking. Hip abductor (gluteus medius) strengthening is also recommended as this helps to stabilise the pelvis by abductor-adductor co-activation (*kati bandha* [Section 4.6.1]). Recent studies [Witvrouw, 2000] have shown that, in the treatment of people with patellofemoral pain, a better response is achieved when closed-chain exercises [Section 1.6.5.9] are used over open-chain exercises.

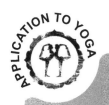

No 5.5 Activate the inner thigh and outer thigh muscles to protect and strengthen the knee in cases of patella mal-tracking

In cases of patella mal-tracking, all poses that activate the inner thigh muscles (hip adductors and hip internal rotators) [Sections 4.5.1 & 5.6.1] are useful to enhance the activation of vastus medialis obliquus (VMO). This is due to the fascial connections between adductor longus, adductor magnus and the VMO, and the myotatic (stretch) reflex activation of the VMO that can take place when the adductor longus or adductor magnus are activated as either hip adductors or hip internal rotators.

Co-activation of gluteus medius and vastus medialis is also very important in knee stability. Therefore a *kati bandha* (a hip *bandha*) [Section 4.5.1] in which there is co-activation of hip abductors (especially gluteus medius) and hip adductors (especially adductor magnus) is very important for the stabilisation of the knee joint.

5.6 APPLIED ANATOMY OF THE THIGH & KNEE IN *HATHA YOGA* POSTURES

Many people have damaged their knees doing *hatha yoga*. This is especially true of Western *yoga* practitioners who often start *yoga* late in life with very stiff hips. Hip stiffness is less common in non-Western cultures partly because of a lifestyle which includes squatting to go to the toilet and sitting cross-legged since childhood. Therefore, in any *yoga* practice and especially if teaching a mixed group of people the safety of the knee joint is an essential issue.

When considering the knees in *hatha yoga* strength, flexibility and alignmnent of the knee joint complex have to be addressed [Tables 5.3 & 5.4], but one must also address the strength and flexibility of the hips [Section 4.5] and ankles [Section 6.7]. To increase knee strength and stability, one needs to develop the ability to co-activate (simultaneously tense) antagonistic (opposing) muscle groups crossing the knee joint complex (*janu bandha*).

Correct alignment is an important issue for the correct flow of energy and also for the safety of the knee joint complex. The femur and the tibia must generally be kept in line without too much unprepared for knee internal rotation or knee external rotation of the tibia on the femur. For example, in postures such as *trikonasana*

it is important to ensure that in the lower limb on which you are bearing most weight, the leg (below knee) is not turning out alone while the thigh (above knee) is still turned in. Such a situation can not only damage the knee but can also compress that side of the lower back.

Vertical alignment is especially important for the beginner in *utthita san calanasana* and other lunge-like standing poses. The beginner should not let the knee bend more than 90° and not beyond the heel in order to minimise stress on the patellofemoral joint [Section 5.2.2].

In the straight-legged standing poses, hyperextension of the knee joint should be avoided by bending the knee very slightly untill it appears to a straight angle of only 180° (not more, which is hyperextension) by exerting greater pressure with the front of the foot on the floor. This activates gastrocnemius (a knee flexor), increasing knee stability and causing a slight flexion movement at the knee joint [Application to Yoga 5.3].

If knee extension or knee flexion is limited due to pain or immobilising injury then one should perform *yoga* postures only in the range of motion of the knee joint which is pain free and modify poses accordingly.

For example, postures such as *janu sirsasana*   should be practised with the flexed (bent) knee straightened as in *parivrrta upavistha konasana*. Note that it is best for symmetry of the hips and spine to practise both sides of a modified posture in the same way.

While knee flexibility and the ability to achieve full knee flexion and knee extension are important for most normal human activities, lack of knee flexibility is not usually the problem most people complain about with the knee during *hatha yoga*. Provided someone can either sit cross-legged, kneeling or hug the knees to the chest, then knee flexibility is not a problem for them. If this is not possible then there may be meniscal tear or some sort of joint problem and this should be addressed accordingly.

For most people with knee problems, the problems are either:
*   Instability of the knee due to over-stretched or torn knee ligaments [Section 5.5.2], usually combined with weakness or lack of control of the muscles around the knee. These types of problems are not always painful but can severely restrict what one can safely do in *yoga* and life in general.
*   Problems, such as patella mal-tracking [Section 5.5.4], resulting from an imbalance in the forces around the knee joint complex, including gravitational forces and forces generated by the muscles crossing the knee ankle and hip joint complexes. Strength and flexibility of hip abductors such as gluteus medius is important to prevent patella mal-tracking [Section 5.5.4].
*   Meniscal tears [Section 5.5.3] (knee cartilage tears) resulting in pain, instability or knee locking, which may have arisen from a combination of knee muscle weakness and/or an imbalance in the forces generated by the muscles crossing the knee joint complex.

Meniscal problems and ligament tears often manifest suddenly as a result of an accidental fall or sudden twist of the knee at a time when the muscles around the knee joint are either not sufficiently strong or not adequately controlled. Knee injuries are common in *yoga* practitioners who fail to realise the normal alignment of the knee joint and overstrain the knee joint capsule, knee ligaments and menisci by trying to stretch their knees into positions without having sufficient knee muscle strength or control for support. In addition, many new *yoga* enthusiasts with a keen desire to achieve postures that require large amounts of

flexibility in hip internal rotation, such as *supta virasana*   and postures that require

large amounts of flexibility in hip external rotation, such as *padmasana*   (lotus pose), can easily (and often do) overstrain and/or tear knee joint ligaments and damage their menisci if they approach their practice incorrectly.

5.6.1 Co-activation of Opposing Muscles of the Knee Joint Complex: *Janu Bandha*
Janu bandha is the co-activation (simultaneously tensing) of antagonistic (opposing) muscle groups that cross the knee joint complex. *Janu bandha* can stabilise and strengthen the knee joint complex as well help to generate and move energy through this region of the body.

The integrity of the knee joint complex is not derived from the bony fit of the femur (thigh bone) and tibia (shin bone). The main support for the knee joint comes from the ligaments, the joint capsule and the strength of the muscles that cross the knee joint. Since we have no direct control of the ligamentous structures around the knee, it is only the muscles that we can control and use to strengthen the knee joint.

There are 16 muscles that cross the knee [Section 5.3]. The most stabilising co-activation of the muscles around the knee joint complex (*janu bandha*) is when all 16 muscles are activated at the same time. Many of these muscles are multi-joint muscles [Section 1.6.5.7] and therefore also affect the hip and the ankle. In addition, there are several hip muscles (eg. the <u>abductor gluteus medius</u>) and ankle muscles (eg. the <u>ankle evertors</u>), which do not actually cross the knee but which are also important to activate for knee joint stability due to their <u>fascial connections</u> with the knee. In practical terms the best *janu bandha* is achieved if the following six <u>muscle groups</u> are activated at the same time:

1. **Knee extensors** (front of the thighs) [Section 5.6.1.1]
2. **Knee flexors** (back of the thighs) [Section 5.6.1.2]
3. **Hip adductors** (inner thighs) [Section 4.5 & 5.6.1.3]
4. **Hip abductors** (outer thighs) [Section 4.5 & 5.6.1.4]
5. **Ankle plantarflexors** (back of the leg) [Section 6.7 & 5.6.1.5]
6. **Ankle evertors** (outer leg) [Section 6.7 & 5.6.1.6]

Simple *yoga* exercises are described below that can help train each of these six <u>muscle groups</u> to become activated individually [Section 5.6.1.1- 5.6.1.6] and together to generate a complete *janu bandha* [Section 5.6.1.7].

5.6.1.1 Ways to activate knee extensors

Using <u>closed-chain</u> movements [Section 1.6.5.9], <u>knee extensors</u> (mainly the <u>quadriceps</u> group) can be easily

activated in <u>weight-bearing</u> (WB) <u>semi-flexed</u> knee postures such as *utkatasana* (half-squat pose). Once the <u>knee extensors</u> have been isolated and felt in this posture, which causes an obligatory <u>activation</u> of the <u>knee extensors</u> [Appendix A], the exercise can be progressed to the <u>extended knee</u> (straight leg) version of the position by trying to keep the muscles in the front of the thigh firm while slowly straightening the knees.

To activate the <u>knee extensors</u> on standing legs when the knees begin fully <u>extended</u> or locked (straight

knees) in postures such as *tadasana* is not as easy to elicit for a beginner. This is because when the <u>knee joint</u> is locked in this position, no <u>knee extensor</u> activity is required. In such situations, attempts should be made to use the <u>quadriceps</u> to try to move the <u>patella</u> <u>proximally</u>. Students inexperienced with anatomical jargon can be told to "pull up the kneecap", but perhaps somewhat surprisingly not everyone will respond to this instruction. The same instruction can also be applied in <u>non-weight-bearing</u> (NWB) postures where the anterior of the thigh is facing the floor and <u>knee extension</u> is assisted by gravity as in *niralamba*

virabhadrasana . Conversely, when the limb is in a NWB position with the anterior (front) of

the thigh facing away from the floor in postures like *niralamba padangusthasana*
then simply trying to straighten the NWB knee from a <u>flexed</u> position will elicit <u>knee extensor</u> <u>activation</u> since straightening the knee necessitates working against gravity. Note that the higher the leg is lifted from the floor, the more difficult it is to straighten the knee due to <u>passive insufficiency</u> of the <u>hamstrings</u> and <u>active insufficiency</u> [Section 1.6.5.8] of <u>rectus femoris</u> (the main quadriceps muscle).

5.6.1.2 Ways to activate knee flexors (especially hamstrings)

To elicit hamstring activation alone, the simplest way is to perform the hamstring curl exercise, as performed in

postures like *niralamba natarajasana* . This can be achieved by standing upright, taking one foot off the ground and then flexing the NWB knee as if trying to pull the heel to the backside. If some hip flexion (as opposed to hip extension) on the NWB hip is permitted (i.e. the NWB knee is brought closer to the chest), the exercise becomes easier as any active insufficiency [Section 1.6.5.8] of the hamstrings is reduced, as is any passive insufficiency [Section 1.6.5.8] of the quadriceps. The hamstring curl is a useful beginners' exercise and important for *yoga* practitioners to learn, as many *yoga* practitioners only ever think about stretching their hamstrings and never about strengthening them. The hamstring curl is only useful as a hamstring strengthening exercise for someone who has very weak hamstrings. For stronger people, the hamstring curl is often practised in gyms with weights attached to the ankles. A hamstring curl with weights is not recommended. It has been shown that unilateral muscle activations across a joint without antagonist co-activation, such as hamstring muscles activating without co-activation of quadriceps, may damage the joint. Learning how to co-activate hamstrings with quadriceps (*janu bandha*) [Section 5.6.1.7] is a far safer and more effective way of strengthening the hamstrings with the added benefit of conferring stability to the knee joint complex.

5.6.1.3 Ways to activate hip adductors (inner thigh muscles) [Section 4.5]

The hip adductors (inner thigh muscles) can be activated in a closed-chain fashion in postures such as

tadasana by simply squeezing the heels and thighs towards each other. The inner thigh muscles are also able to function as hip internal rotators. During an open-chain posture, such as having one leg in the air with no support for the NWB leg, as in *niralamba virabhadrasana* [Section 5.6.1.7] or *eka pada sarvangasana* [Figure 9.7C], it is better to take advantage of the internal rotator function of the inner thigh muscles. Turn the thigh inwards without moving the hip or pelvis. If done correctly, this should be able to elicit a controlled activation of the hip adductors as hip internal rotators, which should elicit a reciprocal reflex relaxation of the hip, mainly the gluteus maximus (the buttocks muscle). Once activation of the inner thigh muscles has been mastered in an open-chain exercise, such as in the NWB leg of *niralamba virabhadrasana*, the gluteus maximus can once again be co-activated to generate a type of *kati* (hip) *bandha* [Section 4.5.1.1].

5.6.1.4 Ways to activate hip abductors (outer buttocks muscles) [Section 4.5]

Strength and control of the hip abductors (outer buttocks muscles) is important for the stability of the knee. Hip abductor weakness is often a problem in cases of patella mal-tracking [Section 5.5.4]. Hip abductors, especially gluteus medius are best strengthened in the weight-bearing (WB) leg of most one-legged postures. Hip abductors can also be strengthened in all standing postures where the feet can be pressed apart into the floor as if the feet are trying to stretch the floor [Section 4.5.1.2]..

5.6.1.5 Ways to activate ankle plantarflexors (calf muscles) [Section 6.3; Tables 6.1, 6.2 & 6.3]

The only significant ankle plantarflexor that actually cross the knee is gastrocnemius. However, all the ankle plantarflexors [Tables 6.1, 6.2 & 6.3] can affect the function of the knee. This is due to fascial connections between gastrocnemius and the other main ankle plantarflexor soleus, which only crosses the ankle joint complex.

Ankle plantarflexors can be activated in several ways. The simplest way to activate these muscles is in a standing position. Standing in *tadasana* [Figures 1.3 & 1.4], bring the body weight onto the front of the feet and lean slightly forward as if you are about to raise the heels. Raising the heels is a further stage of this exercise [Figure 5.7 & 5.8]. The same effect can be achieved in any standing pose by pressing on the front of the foot.

5.6.1.6 Ways to activate ankle evertors (outer calf muscles) [Section 6.3; Tables 6.1, 6.2 & 6.3]

Although the ankle evertors do not actually cross the knee at all, they nevertheless affect the function of the knee joint complex by their actions on the ankle joint complex, and also because of fascial connections with the knee joint complex. Ankle eversion is also particularly useful for people who get inner knee pain presumably because it shortens the outer leg and thus lengthens the inner leg to the knee. Ankle evertor activity is perhaps most easily understood and experienced in the exercise described below [Section 5.6.1.5]. Stand with big toes touching and the heels slightly apart. Raise the heels with the ankle bones (medial malleoli) touching or pressing towards each other while the heels try and move apart as if one is lifting the outer feet . Ankle evertor activity is automatically elicited in postures such as *vasisthasana* [Appendix A] in order to pull the inner foot to the floor.

5.6.1.7 Ways to co-activate the muscles around the knee and create *janu bandha*

The hamstrings are the primary knee flexors, and are the antagonists of the quadriceps group. Hamstrings work synergistically with the anterior cruciate ligament (ACL). The ability to create a co-activation of the hamstrings with the quadriceps is crucial to the stability of the knee joint. Since the quadriceps work antagonistically to the ACL, it is important that one balances the extensor forces created at the anterior of the knee joint by the quadriceps with the flexor forces of the hamstrings. With practise, a co-activation of hamstrings and quadriceps (*janu bandha*) can be made with the same ease that most people can make a biceps bulge when they co-activate the biceps brachii with the triceps brachii in the upper arm [Section 3.3].

Janu bandha or co-activation of the muscles around the knee can be achieved using closed-chain exercises or open-chain exercises [Section 1.6.5.9]. A closed-chain method of knee muscle co-activation involves standing up straight in *tadasana* and bending the knees to *utkatasana* . First stand in *tadasana* and activate the quadriceps by trying to pull up the kneecap, then initiate knee flexion (i.e. try and bend the knees) to *utkatasana* without losing the tension of the quadriceps (i.e. keep trying to pull up the knee cap even as you bend the knee). This exercise forces a co-activation of the quadriceps and hamstrings, which one can learn to eventually control from just off full knee extension to greater than 90 degrees flexion.

Another closed chain-exercise that can generate *janu bandha* can be achieved from a unilateral stance in postures such as *utthita pavanmuktasana* (hugging the non-weight-bearing (NWB) flexed knee to the chest while standing) and *utthita padangusthasana* (pulling the NWB heel to the head, with extended NWB knee). These postures should be started with a slightly flexed WB knee so the knee joint is not locked and the quadriceps group (knee extensors) are active. Once the NWB leg and the trunk have been pulled as close together as possible, an attempt should be made to straighten the spine and the standing leg. This usually elicits an activation of the hamstring muscle group, which will act as hip extensors trying to extend the hip in a weight-bearing but closed-chain manner. This causes the femur to be drawn posteriorly resulting in an apparently paradoxical further <u>extension</u> of the <u>knee joint</u>. In other words, the <u>hamstrings</u>, which are normally considered important <u>knee flexors</u>, are in this case acting as <u>knee extensors</u>.

An <u>open-chain exercise</u> that helps elicit a <u>co-activation</u> around the <u>knee joint complex</u> is *niralamba*

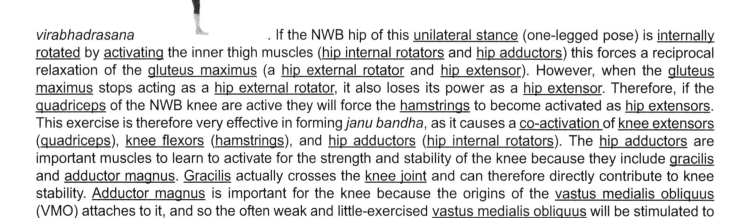

virabhadrasana   . If the NWB hip of this <u>unilateral stance</u> (one-legged pose) is <u>internally rotated</u> by <u>activating</u> the inner thigh muscles (<u>hip internal rotators</u> and <u>hip adductors</u>) this forces a reciprocal relaxation of the <u>gluteus maximus</u> (a <u>hip external rotator</u> and <u>hip extensor</u>). However, when the <u>gluteus maximus</u> stops acting as a <u>hip external rotator</u>, it also loses its power as a <u>hip extensor</u>. Therefore, if the <u>quadriceps</u> of the NWB knee are active they will force the <u>hamstrings</u> to become activated as <u>hip extensors</u>. This exercise is therefore very effective in forming *janu bandha*, as it causes a <u>co-activation</u> of <u>knee extensors</u> (<u>quadriceps</u>), <u>knee flexors</u> (<u>hamstrings</u>), and <u>hip adductors</u> (<u>hip internal rotators</u>). The <u>hip adductors</u> are important muscles to learn to activate for the strength and stability of the knee because they include <u>gracilis</u> and <u>adductor magnus</u>. <u>Gracilis</u> actually crosses the <u>knee joint</u> and can therefore directly contribute to knee stability. <u>Adductor magnus</u> is important for the knee because the origins of the <u>vastus medialis obliquus</u> (VMO) attaches to it, and so the often weak and little-exercised <u>vastus medialis obliquus</u> will be stimulated to become activated. <u>Vastus medialis obliquus</u> is a muscle important for correct <u>patella tracking</u> [Section 5.5.4].

The ability to create various types of *janu bandha* is also the means to generate energy and regulate its flow through the <u>knee joint complex</u>. <u>Co-activation</u> of opposing muscles around a fully flexed knee generates a compressive and heating *ha-janu bandha* [Figure 5.8 & Appendix C] which restricts the flow of blood and pushes energy (eg. heat) and matter (eg. blood and intracellular fluids) away from the knee. <u>Co-activation</u> of opposing muscles around a fully extended knee generates an expansive and cooling *tha-janu bandha* [Figure 5.7 & Appendix C] which enhances the flow of blood and pulls energy and matter towards the knee.

Learning how to create *janu bandha* in any position is also an important key to accessing advanced knee

postures such as *mulabandhasana*   and *kandasana*   (and others shown in Figures 11.1 and 12.5), which each require a balance between strength and flexibilty. *Mulabandhasana* requires extreme flexibility in <u>hip internal rotation</u> and <u>knee external rotation</u> with a strong *ha-janu bandha*. *Kandasana* requires extreme flexibility in <u>hip external rotation</u> and <u>knee internal rotation</u> with a strong *ha-janu bandha*.

5.6.2 *Hatha Yoga* for Acute and Chronic Knee Injuries
The main problems or injuries of the knee are:
- Pain
- Instability
- Loss of function.

- **To avoid or help fix knee problems/injuries:**
    - o   Consider whether the injury is <u>acute</u> or <u>chronic</u>, and treat accordingly [Section 1.8].

- **Avoid further aggravation by:**
    - o   Avoiding postures that irritate the injury, or modifying them till they do not irritate the injury
    - o   Avoiding <u>weight-bearing</u> postures in cases of swelling (do inversions if possible)

    - o   Using straight-legged versions of sitting postures like *janu sirsasana*   if the bent leg (<u>flexed knee</u>) postures cause pain
    - o   Using slightly <u>flexed knee</u> versions of straight-legged postures that cause pain in the knee (avoid knee hyperextension [Application to yoga 5.3]).

- **Reduce any swelling and improve circulation with:**
  - o   Inverted postures
  - o   <u>Co-activation</u> of muscles around the <u>knee joint</u> (*janu bandha*) [Section 5.6.1; Appendix C]
  - o   Gentle movement through full <u>range of joint motion</u> (<u>ROM</u>).
- **Then generally address:**
  1. Strength
  2. Flexibility
  3. Alignment
  4. Joint space

Tables 5.3 and 5.4 describe postures that may be used to increase strength and flexibility of the <u>knee joint</u>. The stability and safety of the knee can be enhanced, and the knee can improve its functional strength, if the following principles are applied in *yoga* postures:

1. Increased strength and control of all hip, knee and ankle muscles, but especially the six major muscle groups surrounding and affecting the function of the <u>knee joint complex</u> [Section 5.6.1].

In addition:
- **Learn to co-activate muscles surrounding the knee with:**
  - o   The knee in <u>extension</u> and <u>flexion</u>
  - o   <u>Weight-bearing</u> (WB) and <u>non-weight-bearing</u> (NWB) postures.
- **Balance strength of:**
  - o   Anterior and posterior knee muscles
  - o   Lateral and medial knee muscles.
- **Do <u>proprioceptive</u> training and muscle control exercises**
  - o   Dynamic balancing exercises.

2. Increase flexibility of all hip, knee and ankle muscles, but especially the following muscle groups:
- **Hip abductors** (lateral thigh)
- **Ankle invertors** (inner calf)
- **Ankle dorsiflexors** (front ankle)
- **Hip** (lateral and rear hip)
- **Hip internal rotators** (inner thigh)

In addition:
- **Improve symmetry of flexibility by balancing flexibility of:**
  - o   Anterior and posterior muscles and structures
  - o   Medial and lateral muscles and structures.

3. Correct structural alignment in *yoga* postures and daily life:
- Keep the <u>femur</u> correctly aligned with <u>tibia</u>
- Keep the same degree of rotation in <u>femur</u> and <u>tibia</u>
- Keep the <u>knee joint</u> directly over the heel in <u>weight-bearing</u> postures where possible.

4. Create and maintain adequate and uniform <u>joint space</u> using specific muscular activations and correct posture
- Lateral joint space = Medial joint space
- Anterior joint space = Posterior joint space (avoid knee hyperextension [Application to yoga 5.3]).

If a knee problem is persistant or serious it is important to refer to a knee specialist such as a physiotherapist or a doctor. Some knee problems will heal by themselves or with *yoga* therapy. Others, like ligament (eg. ACL) and mensical tears may be managed with *yoga* but are rarely, if ever, fully healed. In some cases surgery is a good option if all other avenues have been well explored.

****

Table 5.3 Postures that can or may use muscles of the knee joint complex

	KNEE FLEXORS (Hamstring muscle group and gastrocnemius)	KNEE EXTENSORS (Quadriceps group)
POSTURES THAT CAUSE AN **OBLIGATORY ACTIVATION** OF A MUSCLE GROUP IN A **SHORTENED POSITION**.	*Eka hasta bhujasana* (R leg)	*Tittibhasana* (both legs)
POSTURES THAT CAUSE AN **OBLIGATORY ACTIVATION** OF A MUSCLE GROUP TO A **LENGTHENED POSITION**.	*Urdhva prasarita eka padasana* (L leg (NWB) using hamstrings to extend the knee with an internally rotated NWB hip)	*Utkatasana, padangustha utkatasana* (both legs)
POSTURES THAT ARE **ENHANCED** WHEN A MUSCLE GROUP IS **ACTIVATED (TENSED)** IN A **SHORTENED POSITION**.	*Bakasana*	*Adho mukha svanasana*
POSTURES WHICH CAUSE AN **OBLIGATORY LENGTHENING OR STRETCHING** OF A MUSCLE GROUP	*Uttanasana*	*Supta virasana*

POSTURES WHICH ARE ENHANCED WHEN A MUSCLE GROUP IS **ACTIVELY LENGTHENED** (INTENTIONALLY STRETCHED)	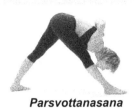 *Parsvottanasana*	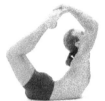 *Bhekasana*
POSTURES WHICH ARE ENHANCED WHEN A MUSCLE GROUP IS **ACTIVATED** (TENSED) **WHILE LENGTHENED** (STRETCHED)	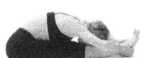 *Pascimottanasana* (press the heels downwards into the floor in order to activate the hamstrings)	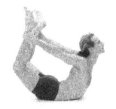 *Dhanurasana* (push the feet backwards towards the floor in order to activate the quadriceps)

Abbreviations used in Table 5.4:
X = Exercise; mm = Muscle; R = Right; L = Left; LL = Lower Limb, WB = Weight-bearing; NWB = Non weight-bearing

Table 5.4 Postures that may use knee muscles in a non-obligatory fashion

EXERCISE TYPE ⬜	KNEE **OPEN-CHAIN EXERCISES** (Limb tries to move and body stays still)		KNEE **CLOSED-CHAIN EXERCISES** (Limb stays still and body tries to move)	
MUSCLE LENGTH ⬜	**SHORTENED** muscle	**LENGTHENED** (stretched) muscle	**SHORTENED** muscle	**LENGTHENED** (stretched) muscle
MUSCLE GROUP ⇓				
KNEE FLEXORS (Hamstring muscle group and gastrocnemius)	***Niralamba natarajasana*** On L (NWB) limb trying to bring heel to backside	***Urdhva prasarita eka padasana***	***Urdhva dhanurasana*** Activate hamstrings (as hip extensors) by rolling thighs in (increase hip internal rotation), which relaxes buttocks, and trying to lift hips higher (increase hip extension)	***Adho mukha svanasana*** Pushing the feet down and backwards into the floor as if trying to stretch the floor
KNEE EXTENSORS (Quadriceps group)	***Niralamba padangusthasana***	***Urdhva prasarita eka padasana***	***Trikonasana*** pressing R hip towards R foot whilst pulling up the kneecap	***Uttana parsvakonasana*** pushing R heel into the ground as if trying to extend the R knee

165

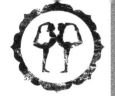

Chapter Breakdown

****

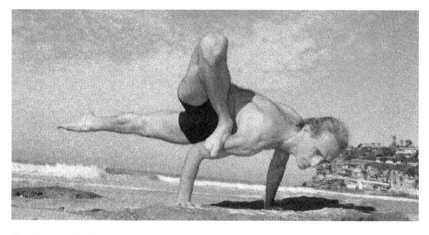

Simon Borg-Olivier in *Parivrtta Urdhva Yoga Dandasana*. This advanced pose requires extreme flexibility in hip flexion and spinal axial rotation. It also requires extreme flexibility with ankle inversion with lengthened ankle evertors. Photo courtesy of Ric Carter.

6.0 INTRODUCTION TO THE APPLIED ANATOMY OF THE ANKLE AND FOOT IN *HATHA YOGA* POSTURES

In *hatha yoga*, the feet and lower limbs are considered the 'organs of action' for the lower back and hips, and the digestive and reproductive organs. Strength, flexibility and appropriate use of the muscles of the feet and lower limbs are the key to self-mobilisation (self-massage) of the lower back and hips and integral to the healthy functioning of the digestive and reproductive organs.

6.1 BONES OF THE LOWER LEG, ANKLE AND FOOT

Each foot is made up of twenty eight bones that form the ankle, foot and toes. Foot bones are particularly specialised, allowing a wide range of flexibility, while being able to withstand the incredible amounts of stress placed upon them.

6.1.1 Functions of the foot
The foot allows upright stability and with no undue muscular effort, acts as a base of support. Flexibility of the foot allows shock absorption of body weight and accommodation of uneven ground. The foot acts as a rigid lever and thus helps with propulsion of the body through space. It is estimated that each stride of an adult places 60 kilograms per square centimetre on the bottom of the foot.

6.1.2 Bones of the Lower Leg, Ankle and Foot
The bones of the lower leg, ankle and foot are shown in Figures 6.1–6.4. They are the:
*   **Tibia** (inner ankle bone),
*   **Fibula** (outer ankle bone),
*   **Tarsals** (7),
*   **Metatarsals** (5),
*   **Phalanges** (14),
*   **Sesamoid bones** (2)

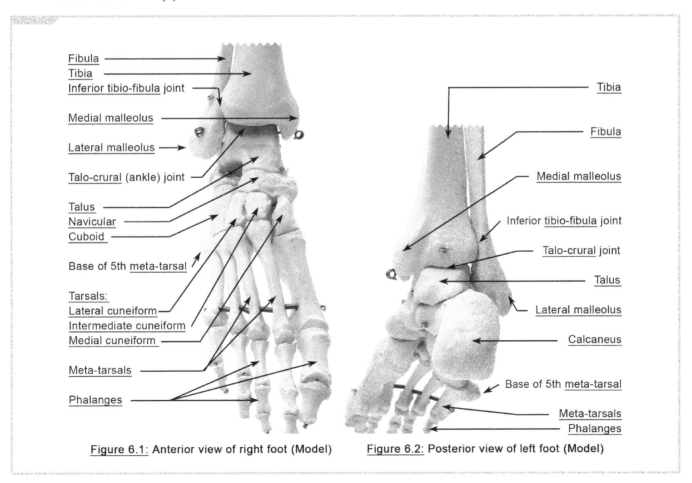

Figure 6.1: Anterior view of right foot (Model)   Figure 6.2: Posterior view of left foot (Model)

6.1.2.1 Tibia (shaft and distal end)

The following features of the tibia can be seen on a skeleton and identified with the help of Figures 6.1 – 6.4:
- Interosseus border, articular surface, popliteal surface, fibular notch, groove for tibialis posterior, medial malleolus

6.1.2.2 Fibula (shaft and distal end)

The following features of the fibula can be seen on a skeleton and identified with the help of Figures 6.1 – 6.4:
- Interosseus border, articular surface, groove for peroneal tendons, lateral malleolus

6.1.2.3 Tarsal Bones (7)

Starting from the dorsal, medial, anterior right foot moving clockwise:

Distal row: cuneiforms (3), cuboid
Proximal row: calcaneus (heel bone), talus (ankle bone), navicular
(Mnemonic: *3 Cunning Cubs Calculate Tall Novels!!!*)

The following features of the tarsal bones can be seen on a skeleton and identified with the help of Figures 6.1 – 6.4:
- **Calcaneus** (heel bone): sustenaculum tali, medial process, lateral process, groove for flexor hallucis longus, sulcus calcanei.
- **Talus** (ankle bone): head, body (trochlear), sulcus tali (which together with sulcus calcanei makes the sinus tarsi (= tarsal canal))
- **Navicular**: tuberosity
- **Cuboid**: tuberosity, groove for peroneus longus

6.1.2.4 Metatarsals (5)

I (base of big toe), II, III, IV, V (base of little toe). All have a base shaft and distal bulbous head; form the knuckles of the foot. Note the tuberosity on the fifth metatarsal head.

6.1.2.5 Phalanges (14)

Proximal, middle (not big toe) and distal, all have a proximal base, shaft and distal head.

6.1.2.6 Sesamoid bones

There are usually only 2 sesamoid bones and they are both in the big toe. The sesamoid bones are seen in radiographs only, they are found in the tendons of flexor hallucis brevis. Their functions include leverage and support, and we walk on these rather than our tendons.

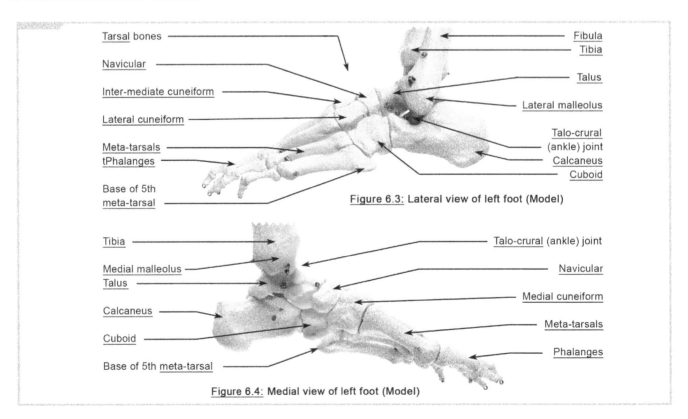

Figure 6.3: Lateral view of left foot (Model)

Figure 6.4: Medial view of left foot (Model)

6.1.3 The Axis of the Foot

The axis of the foot goes through <u>medial calcaneus</u>, <u>talus</u>, <u>navicular</u>, <u>intermediate cuneiform</u>, <u>metatarsals</u> and <u>phalanges</u> of <u>digit II</u>. The axis is important for correct force transmission when weight is taken directly on the foot.

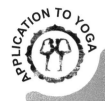

No 6.1 In standing postures keep the outer edge of the foot parallel to the line between the heels (or parallel to a mat – if one is used)

The axis of the foot is approximately parallel to the outer edge of the foot. Therefore, during *yoga* postures the outer foot is ideally placed in line with the direction the force of the body weight is being exerted. In this position, force transmission is most effective. Also, the muscles of the foot, in particular the <u>ankle evertors,</u> are able to function at their most effective length and thus confer greater stability to the ankle and hence more effective balance in standing postures especially.

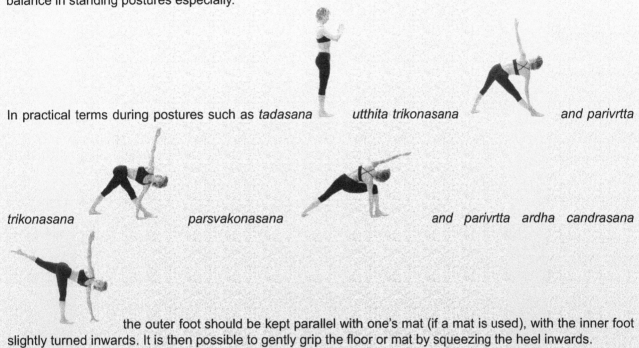

In practical terms during postures such as *tadasana*   *utthita trikonasana*   and *parivrtta*

trikonasana   *parsvakonasana*   and *parivrtta ardha candrasana*

the outer foot should be kept parallel with one's mat (if a mat is used), with the inner foot slightly turned inwards. It is then possible to gently grip the floor or mat by squeezing the heel inwards.

6.2 THE ANKLE JOINT COMPLEX

Each ankle and foot consists of 28 bones, which articulate at 35 joints in each leg. These joints are collectively referred to as the <u>ankle joint complex</u>.

The main movements of the <u>ankle joint complex</u> are:
- <u>Ankle extension</u> which is usually known as <u>ankle dorsiflexion</u>
- <u>Ankle flexion</u>, which is usually known as <u>ankle plantarflexion</u>
- <u>Ankle eversion</u>, which is sometimes called <u>ankle pronation</u>, and essentially involves turning the feet outwards
- <u>Ankle inversion</u>, which is sometimes called <u>ankle supination</u>, and essentially involves turning the feet inwards

For ease of study the joints of the <u>ankle joint complex</u> are divided into 3 Sections –

(A) HINDFOOT JOINTS: <u>tibiofibular</u>, <u>talocrural</u> and <u>subtalar</u> (<u>talocalcaneal</u>) joints; where most <u>flexion</u> (<u>dorsiflexion</u>) and <u>extension</u> (<u>plantarflexion</u>) of the ankle takes place.

(B) MIDFOOT (MIDTARSAL) JOINTS: <u>talocalcaneonavicular</u> (TCN) and <u>calcaneocuboid</u> (CC) <u>joints</u> (which together form the <u>compound transverse tarsal joint</u> where most <u>inversion</u> and <u>eversion</u> takes), <u>cuneonavicular</u>, <u>cuboideonavicular</u>, <u>intercuneiform</u>, and <u>cuneocuboid joints</u>.

(C) FOREFOOT JOINTS: <u>tarsometatarsal</u>, <u>intermetatarsal</u>, <u>metatarsophalangeal</u> and <u>interphalangeal joints</u>

For the purposes of studying the applied anatomy of *hatha yoga* the most important joints to understand are those of the hindfoot as that is where the main movements of the ankle joint take place.

(A) HINDFOOT JOINTS

6.2.1 Proximal tibiofibular (PTF) joint

Location	between head of fibula and lateral condyle of tibia
Classification	synovial, plane, multi-axial, simple joint
Articular (joint) capsule	fibrous with a synovial membrane

Ligaments　　　　The anterior and posterior ligaments strengthen the articular capsule. The tendon of the popliteus muscle is intimately related to the posterior – superior aspect of the PTF joint.

Bursa　　　　A pouch of synovial membrane which passes under the tendon of popliteus muscle, known as the popliteus bursa, sometimes communicates with the synovial membrane of the PTF joint, thus making the PTF joint and knee joint in direct communication.

6.2.2 Distal tibiofibular (DTF) joint

Location	between concave facet of tibia and convex facet of fibula
Classification	fibrous syndesmosis
Articular (joint) capsule	a small superior projection of the synovial capsule of the talocrural joint (ankle joint) that extends into the inferior part of the DTF joint

Ligaments:　　　　The ligaments of the DTF joint function to restrict the motion of both PTF joint and DTF joint and for maintaining a stable mortise [Section 6.2.2.1]. These include anterior and posterior tibiofibular ligaments, crural tibiofibular interosseus ligament and the interosseus membrane.

　　　　• 　　The crural tibiofibular interosseus ligament is the strongest of the ligaments at the DTF joint. Its short oblique fibres tightly bind the tibia and fibula and act as a fulcrum for fibula motion. As a result, small movements at the fibula malleolus result in large movements at the PTF joint.

　　　　• 　　The interosseus membrane is a fibrous membrane between tibia and fibula which directly supports both tibiofibular articulations.

6.2.2.1 Function of the tibiofibular joints

The tibiofibular joints serve to help create a mortise, or pincer grip (from the distal ends of the fibula and tibia) that holds the talus bone to create the talocrural joint [Section 6.2.3], which is the major joint in the ankle joint complex.

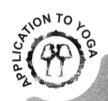

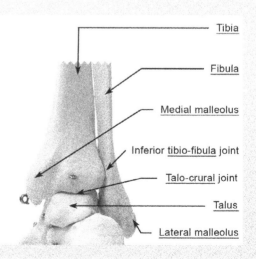

No 6.2: Tensing the muscles around the calf and ankle joint helps tighten the pincer-like grip of the talocrural joint by the tibiofibular mortise effect

The muscle tension that is created when one tenses the muscles of the calf and around the ankle joint helps to stabilise the ankle joint complex by squeezing the fibular and tibia against the talus. *Yoga* postures which require balance, especially one-legged standing postures, become more stable as the talocrural joint becomes more stable with an increased pincer grip effect from the pressure of the ankle muscles squeezing the fibular and tibia against the talus. The ankle muscles can become activated and this stabilising effect is enhanced in a number of different ways. For example when: (i) the arches of the feet are lifted, (ii) the toes are spread and slightly lifted, (iii) the toes are gripped into the floor, and often when the heel is gently squeezed inwards against the floor.

Tibia

Fibula

Medial malleolus

Inferior tibio-fibula joint

Talo-crural joint

Talus

Lateral malleolus

6.2.3 Talocrural (Ankle) Joint

Location   The <u>talocrural joint</u> is the articulation between <u>talus</u> and medial malleolus of the <u>tibia</u> (<u>tibiotalar</u> surface); and between the <u>talus</u> and the <u>lateral malleolus</u> of the <u>fibula</u> (<u>talofibular</u> surface).

Classification   The <u>talocrural joint</u> is a <u>synovial</u>, <u>modified hinge</u>, <u>uniaxial</u>, <u>simple</u> joint.

Movements   The movements of the <u>talocrural joint</u> are <u>plantarflexion</u> (<u>flexion</u>) and <u>dorsiflexion</u> (<u>extension</u>) are main movements, and there is also a small amount (7°) of rotation.

Ligaments   **Medial ligament** (deltoid ligament): This ligament has four (4) parts: tibionavicular, anterior – posterior tibiotalar and tibiocalcanean; functions to limit dorsiflexion and eversion, prevents abduction and lateral side of foot, helps to maintain the medial longitudinal arch

Lateral ligament: The lateral ligament actually consists of three (3 ligaments connecting the lateral malleolus of the fibula to the talus and the calcaneus; these are named according to their attachments
        (i) anterior talofibular ligament
        (ii) posterior talofibular ligament, and
        (iii) calcaneofibular ligament.

The <u>anterior talofibular ligament</u> is the ligament most likely to be damaged or torn in an ankle sprain; it functions to limit <u>dorsiflexion</u> and <u>inversion</u>, prevents <u>adduction</u> and medial slide of the foot, and helps to maintain the <u>lateral longitudinal arch</u> [Sections 6.6.5 & 11.4.3.1; Applications to Yoga 6.4]

Close packed position

The closed packed position of the <u>talocrural joint</u> is maximum <u>dorsiflexion</u>.

Stability   The <u>talocrural (ankle) joint</u> is very strong during <u>dorsiflexion</u> because:
- The ankle has powerful supporting ligaments.
- Several tendons that are tightly bound down by the thickenings of the <u>retinacula</u> cross the ankle.
- <u>Dorsiflexion</u> forces the anterior <u>trochlear</u> posteriorly, spreading the <u>tibia</u> and <u>fibula</u> slightly apart, this spreading is limited by the strong <u>interosseus ligament</u> that binds and unites the leg bones
- The <u>articular surfaces</u> between <u>tibia</u> and <u>talus</u> are main weight bearing surfaces, while those between the <u>articular facet</u> of the <u>fibula</u> and the <u>talus</u> are stabilising surfaces that prevent sideways movement.

Articular (joint) capsule fibrous capsule; thin anterior and posterior
- The capsule has strong collateral ligaments (medial <u>deltoid ligament</u> and <u>lateral ligament</u>)
- The capsule attaches to <u>tibia</u>, <u>fibula</u>, and <u>talus</u>.
- The <u>synovial cavity</u> of the <u>ankle joint</u> lies superficially on either side of the <u>tendocalcaneus</u> (Achilles tendon), hence, when the <u>ankle joint</u> is inflamed, the synovial fluid may increase, causing swelling in these locations.

Sections 6.2.4 – 6.2.12 are point-form-style notes on the details of the joints of the foot and the ankle. They are important as reference material. However, this information does not need to be memorised to understand the basic functioning of the foot as it is used in *hatha yoga*.

6.2.4 Subtalar (ST) joint (Talocalcanean joint)

Location between posterior inferior <u>talus</u> and posterior superior <u>calcaneus</u> bones
Classification synovial, simple, plane, multi-axial
Movements slight gliding and rotation that assists with <u>inversion</u> and <u>eversion</u> of the posterior part of foot
Closed packed position <u>inversion</u> (<u>supination</u>)
Ligaments weak lateral and medial <u>talocalcanean</u> ligaments, strong <u>interosseus talocalcanean ligament</u>; functions to form a pivot point for <u>inversion</u> and <u>eversion</u> to occur.

(B) MIDFOOT (MIDTARSAL) JOINTS

6.2.5 Talocalcaneonavicular Joint

Location where the head of <u>talus</u> articulates with the socket formed by the posterior surface of the <u>navicular</u>, the superior surface of the <u>plantar calcaneonavicular (spring) ligament</u>, <u>sustentacular tali</u>, and the articular surface of the <u>calcaneus</u>
Classification <u>synovial</u>, <u>simple</u>, <u>ball and socket</u>, <u>plane</u>, <u>multi-axial</u>
Movements gliding and rotation
Closed packed position <u>inversion</u> (<u>supination</u>)
Ligaments dorsal <u>talonavicular ligament</u>, <u>bifurcated ligament</u> and <u>plantar calcaneonavicular (spring) ligament</u>

6.2.6 Calcaneocuboid Joint

Location between <u>calcaneus</u> and <u>cuboid</u> bones
Classification <u>synovial</u>, <u>compound</u>, <u>sellar</u> (saddle), <u>biaxial</u>
Movements gliding with conjunct rotation
Closed packed position <u>supination</u>
Ligaments <u>bifurcated ligament</u>, <u>calcaneocuboid ligament</u> and the <u>long plantar ligaments</u>

6.2.7 Transverse tarsal joint

Classification <u>synovial</u>, <u>compound</u> joint formed by the union of the <u>talocalcaneonavicular joints</u> and the <u>calcaneocuboid joints</u>
Movements <u>inversion</u> and <u>eversion</u> of the foot

6.2.8 Other Midtarsal Joints (Cuneonavicular, Cuboideonavicular, Intercuneiform and Cuneocuboid)

Location between <u>tarsals</u>
Classification <u>synovial</u>, <u>simple</u>, <u>plane</u>, <u>multi-axial</u> (except for <u>cuboideonavicular</u>, a fibrous joint)
Movements: slight gliding and rotation
Closed packed position <u>inversion</u> (<u>supination</u>)
Ligaments <u>palmar ligament</u>, <u>dorsal ligament</u>, <u>collateral ligament</u>

(C) FOREFOOT JOINTS

6.2.9 Tarsometatarsal (TMT) Joints

Location between <u>tarsals</u> and <u>metatarsals</u>
Classification <u>synovial</u>, <u>simple</u>, <u>plane</u>, <u>multi-axial</u>
Movements gliding
Closed packed position <u>supination</u>

6.2.10 Intermetatarsal (IMT) Joints

Location between the <u>metatarsals</u>
Classification <u>synovial</u>, <u>simple</u>, <u>plane</u>, <u>multi-axial</u>
Movements gliding
Closed packed position <u>supination</u>

6.2.11 Metatarsophalangeal (MTP) Joints

Location between <u>tarsal</u> bones and proximal <u>phalanx</u>
Classification <u>synovial</u>, <u>simple</u>, <u>condyloid</u>, <u>biaxial</u>
Movements <u>flexion</u>, <u>extension</u>, <u>abduction</u>, <u>adduction</u> of toes
Closed packed position full <u>extension</u>
Sesamoid bones increases the <u>mechanical advantage</u> of muscles in which they sit in a way similar to <u>patella</u> (knee cap) assistance in <u>knee flexion</u> [Section 5.1.4].
Ligaments: <u>collateral ligament</u>, <u>palmar ligament</u>, <u>extensor aponeurosis</u>, <u>fibrous digital sheath</u> (prevents bow-stringing of long tendons)

6.2.12 Interphalangeal (IP) Joints

Location between head of proximal <u>phalanx</u> and base of distal <u>phalanx</u>
Classification <u>synovial</u>, <u>simple</u>, <u>hinge</u>, <u>uniaxial</u>.
Movements <u>toe flexion</u> and <u>toe extension</u>
Closed packed position full <u>extension</u>

6.3 MUSCLES THAT MOVE THE ANKLE AND FOOT

Extrinsic muscles of the foot [Tables 6.1 & 6.2] have only their distal attachment (insertion) in the foot whereas <u>intrinsic muscles</u> of the foot [Section 6.4] have both attachments within the foot itself. The attachments and actions of the extrinsic muscles of the ankle and foot are shown in Tables 6.1 and 6.2. Many of these muscles are visible in Figure 6.5.

The <u>bi-articular (two-joint) muscles</u> <u>gastrocnemius</u> and <u>plantaris</u>, which pass through both the <u>knee joint complex</u> and the <u>ankle joint complex</u>, are described in Chapter 5 [Table 5.1]. The movements of the ankle and foot, and the muscles that facilitate these movements are shown Table 6.3.

Table 6.1 Extrinsic muscles of the foot (anterior and lateral) [Adapted from Moore, 1992]

Muscle	Origin	Insertion	Actions & roles
Tibialis anterior	• Lateral superior condyle of tibia.	• Medial cuneiform bone • Base of first metatarsal.	• Dorsiflexes foot • Inverts foot.
Extensor hallucis longus	• Middle part of the anterior surface of fibula • Inter-osseous membrane.	• Dorsal aspect of base of distal phalanx of big toe (hallux).	• Extends big toe • Dorsiflexes foot.
Extensor digitorum	• Lateral condyle of tibia, • Anterior fibula • Inter-osseous membrane.	• Middle and distal phalanges of lateral four digits.	• Extends lateral four digits • Dorsiflexes foot.
Peroneus tertius	• Inferior, anterior surface of fibula • Inter-osseous membrane	• Dorsal surface of base of 5th metatarsal.	• Dorsiflexes foot • Aids in eversion of foot.
Peroneus longus	• Head of fibula • Lateral surface superior two thirds of fibular	• Inferior surface of the base of the 1st metatarsal and medial cuneiform bone.	• Everts foot • Weakly plantarflexes foot.
Peroneus brevis	• Inferior two thirds of lateral surface of fibula.	• Base of 5th metatarsal bone.	• Everts foot • Weakly plantarflexes foot.

Table 6.2 Extrinsic muscles of the foot (posterior) [Adapted from Moore, 1992]

MUSCLE	ORIGIN	INSERTION	ACTION & ROLES
Gastrocnemius	• Lateral head: Lateral aspect of condyle of femur • Medial head Popliteal surface of femur superior to medial condyle.	• Posterior surface of calcaneus via tendo-calcaneus (Achilles tendon)	• Plantarflexes foot • Flexes knee joint. • Raises heel during walking • Everts foot
Plantaris	• Lateral supracondylar line of femur • Oblique popliteal ligament	• Posterior surface of calcaneus via tendocalcaneus (Achilles tendon)	• Weakly assists Gastrocnemius in plantarflexing foot and flexing knee joint
Soleus	• Posterior head and surface of fibula, medial border of tibia.	• Posterior surface of calcaneus via tendo calcaneus (Achilles tendon).	• Plantarflexes foot & steadies leg on foot. • Everts foot
Flexor hallucis longus	• Posterior surface of fibula & inferior Inter-osseous membrane.	• Base of distal phalanx of big toe (hallux).	• Flex big toe • Plantarflexes foot • Supports longitudinal arch of foot.
Flexor digitorum longus	• Posterior surface of tibia.	• Bases of distal phalanges of lateral 4 digits.	• Flexes lateral four digits • Plantarflexes foot • Supports long arch of foot.
Tibialis posterior	• Interosseous membrane, posterior surface of tibia & fibula.	• Navicular, cuneiform and cuboid bones and bases of 2nd, 3rd and 4th meta-tarsal bones.	• Plantarflexes foot • Inverts foot.

Table 6.3 Movement pairs and muscles of the foot and ankle joint complex
[Adapted from Moore, 1992: & Norkin & Levangie, 1992]]

MUSCLE GROUPS
and individual muscles moving the foot at the ankle joint complex

MOVEMENT PAIRS: Opposing (Antagonistic) Muscle Group Pairs

ANKLE PLANTARFLEXION (EXTENSION)

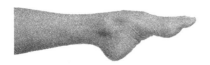

ANKLE PLANTARFLEXORS (PF):
Strong PF: gastrocnemius **(strong IN)**, soleus **(strongest IN)**,
Weak PF: plantaris, tibialis posterior **(strong IN)**, flexor hallucis longus **(strong big toe flexor) (weak IN)**, flexor digitorum longus **(strong toe flexor) (weak IN)**, peroneus longus **(strong EV)**, peroneus brevis **(strong EV)**,

ANKLE DORSIFLEXION (EXTENSION)

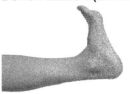

ANKLE DORSIFLEXORS (DF):
Strong DF: tibialis anterior **(strongest DF) (strong IN)**, extensor hallucis longus **(strong big toe extensor) (weak IN)**,
Weak DF: extensor digitorum longus **(strong toe extensor) (weak EV)**, peroneus tertius **(weak EV)**,

ANKLE EVERSION

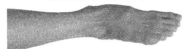

Ankle Evertors (EV):
Strong EV: peroneus longus **(weak PF)**, peroneus brevis **(weak PF)**,
Weak EV: peroneus tertius **(weak DF)**, extensor digitorum longus **(strong DF)**

ANKLE INVERSION

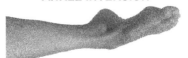

Ankle Invertors (IN):
Strong IN: tibialis anterior **(strongest DF)**, tibialis posterior **(strongest IN) (weak PF)**,
Weak IN: flexor digitorum longus **(weak PF)**, flexor hallucis longus **(weak PF)**, extensor hallucis longus **(weak DF)**

COMBINED MOVEMENTS

Muscle groups and individual muscles that can do combined movements of the foot (and their relative strengths) at the ankle joint complex

PLANTARFLEXION & EVERSION

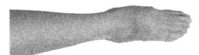

PF & EV: peroneus longus **(weak PF/ strongest EV)**, peroneus brevis **(weak PF/ strong EV)**,

PLANTARFLEXION & INVERSION

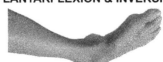

PF & IN: gastrocnemius **(strongest PF/ weak IN)**, soleus **(strong PF/ strongest IN)**, tibialis posterior **(weak PF/ strong IN)**, flexor hallucis longus **(weak PF/ weak IN)**, flexor digitorum longus **(weak PF/ weak IN)**,

DORSIFLEXION & EVERSION

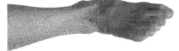

DF & EV: extensor digitorum longus **(weak DF/ weak EV)**, peroneus tertius **(weak DF/ weak EV)**

DORSIFLEXION & INVERSION

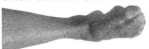

DF & IN: tibialis anterior **(strong DF/ strong IN)**, extensor hallucis longus **(strong DF/ weak IN)**

6.4 INTRINSIC MUSCLES OF THE FOOT

Intrinsic muscles of the foot have both attachments within the foot itself whereas extrinsic muscles [Tables 6.1 & 6.2] of the foot have only their distal attachment (insertion) in the foot.

Function of the intrinsic muscles of the foot can be better understood by comparing each foot muscle with its corresponding hand muscle. Although not as good at manipulation as the hand (in most people) the potential for similar function in the foot is limited only by the unopposable hallux (big toe) and the length of the digits.

The main roles of the muscles of the foot are as stabilisers of the toes and dynamic supporters of the transverse arch and longitudinal arches

The extensor mechanism of the toes is essentially the same as it is in the hand, as is the role of the Lumbricals, Palmar interossei and Dorsal interossei muscles in producing interphalangeal (IP) joint flexion.

Important muscles of the leg and foot:
The following muscles are important of the leg and foot. Their attachments and actions are useful to learn. They are relatively easy to see and feel. Most of these muscles can be seen in Figure 6.5.
1.   Gastrocnemius
2.   Soleus
3.   Tibialis anterior
4.   Tibialis posterior
5.   Extensor digitorum
6.   Flexor digitorum
7.   Extensor hallucis longus
8.   Peroneus longus
9.   Peroneus brevis
10.   Peroneus tertius

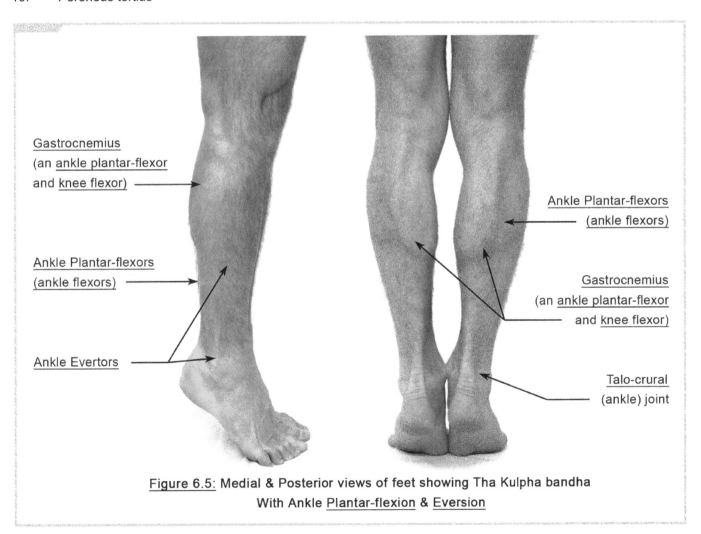

Figure 6.5: Medial & Posterior views of feet showing Tha Kulpha bandha
With Ankle Plantar-flexion & Eversion

6.5 SPECIAL FEATURES OF THE ANKLE AND FOOT

6.5.1 Arches of the Feet

There are three arches in the feet, the medial longitudinal arch , the lateral longitudinal arch and the transverse arch.

The medial longitudinal arch consists of the calcaneal tuberosity, talus, navicular, 3 cuneiforms, 1st, 2nd, 3rd metatarsals. The muscles tibialis anterior and tibialis posterior, flexor hallucis longus, abductor hallucis and flexor digitorum; the plantar fasciae and spring ligament maintain and support the medial longitudinal arch.

The lateral longitudinal arch consists of the calcaneus, cuboid, 4th and 5th metatarsals. The muscles peroneus longus, brevis and tertius, abductor digiti minimi, and flexor digitorum brevis; plantar fasciae and the long and short plantar ligaments maintain and support the lateral longitudinal arch.

The transverse arch consists of the navicular, cuneiforms, cuboid and metatarsal bones. The muscles tibialis posterior and tibialis anterior, peroneus longus and the plantar fasciae maintain and support the transverse arch.

6.5.2 Functions of the Arches of the Feet

Plantar arches of the foot have similar structure to palmar arches of the hand. The palmar arches are predominantly structured to facilitate grasping and manipulation while the arches of the foot are adapted exclusively for weight bearing functions. Functions of the foot include those of mobility and stability

Stability functions that can be performed by a foot with a fixed arch structure include:
  (i) Distribution of weight through the foot for proper weight bearing;
  (ii) Conversion of the foot to a rigid lever.

Mobility functions can only be performed by a non-rigid arch structure. These include:
  (i) Dampening of the shock of weight bearing
  (ii) Adaptation to changes in the supporting surface
  (iii) Dampening of superimposed rotations

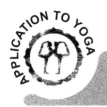

No 6.3: Lifting the three arches of the feet during *hatha yoga* practice helps stabilise the ankle joint complex

Lifting or emphasising the three arches of the weight-bearing feet during *hatha yoga* practice is important to strengthen and stabilise the ankle joint complex, improving balance in two-legged standing postures like *utthita*

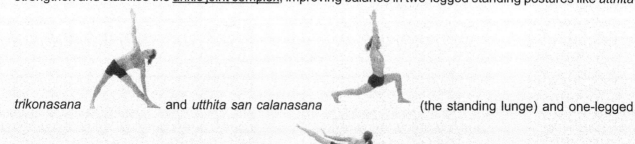

trikonasana and *utthita san calanasana* (the standing lunge) and one-legged

standing poses like *niralamba ardha candrasana* , and helps to activate *kulpha bandha* [Section 6.7.1] improving circulation of blood to the feet.

6.5.3 Plantar Aponeurosis (Fascia)

The plantar aponeurosis is a dense fascia that runs nearly the entire length of the foot beginning posteriorly on the calcaneus and going to the proximal phalanx of each toe. The main function of the plantar aponeurosis is to elevate the arches when the toes are extended. Toe extension can be done either by the toes actively extending or the heel lifting off the ground and thus causing the fascia to tighten.

6.6.1 Pes Planus (Flat Feet)

Pes planus may be congenital or due to muscle weakness, ligament laxity, pronated foot, trauma inducing paralysis, postural deformity such as hip medial rotation or medial tibial torsion, or genu varum (bow legs) of the knees. All infants have flat feet initially up to about two years old due to the fat pad in the longitudinal arch and the incomplete formation of the arches.

6.6.2 Pes Cavus (Hollow or Over-Arched Feet)

Pes cavus may be due to a congenital problem such as spina bifida, poliomyelitis, muscle imbalance, or a genetic factor. The foot has a shortened appearance, often associated with claw toes, high longitudinal arches and thickened and splayed forefoot. People with pes cavus may have difficulty tolerating prolonged activities such as ballet or long distance running.

6.6.3 Hallux Valgus

Hallux valgus is medial deviation of the 1st metatarsal in relation to the centre of the body. This syndrome may be due to a hereditary factor or some environmental factor, such as the fashion of wearing tight shoes.

6.6.4 Claw Toes

Claw toes are often associated with pes cavus [Section 6.6.2]. Because of defective action of the lumbricals and interosseus muscles there is hyperextension of the metatarsophalangeal joints and flexion of the proximal and distal interphalangeal joints.

6.6.5 Ankle Sprains [Sections 6.2.3 & 11.4.3.1; Applications to Yoga 6.4]

Ankle sprains are the most common sports injury in Australia. The anterior talofibular ligament is injured in 90% of cases. The anterior talofibular ligament is the major component of the lateral ligament group of the ankle joint complex. Due to its intracapsular attachment, ankle joint haemarthrosis (blood in the joint capsule) is common.

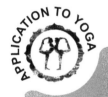

No 6.4: Yoga can help stabilise sprained ankles and allow them to recover

The most common ankle sprain is on the outside of the ankle. Exercises that encourage activation of the

muscles of the outer ankle (ankle evertors) such as the *padangustha* series of postures   and

the *vasistha* series of postures   , can help to stabilise the ankle joint and can allow over-stretched or torn lateral ligaments of the ankle to begin to heal.

6.6.6 Chronic Tendonitis

Chronic tendonitis of the Achilles tendon and the tendons of Tibialis posterior and the peroneal muscles are common.

Treatment of such injuries should aim to reduce inflammation, stretch the adhesions, restrengthen the weakened musculature, and control any abnormal biomechanics.

6.6.7 Shin splints

Shin splints is a poor term as it can be indicative of a number of causes such as tibial periostitis, tibial stress (fatigue) fractures and avulsion fractures, chronic compartment pressure syndrome and myofascial pain.

All of these conditions usually involve inflammation at the muscle – bone interface, which may produce oedema (swelling) with associated nerve compression complications.

6.7 APPLIED ANATOMY OF THE ANKLE AND FOOT IN *HATHA YOGA* POSTURES

The ability to balance in the one-legged and two-legged standing *yoga* postures depends to some extent on the ability to stabilise the ankle joint complex by strengthening the muscles around the ankle. As for the other major joint complexes it is important to learn how to co-activate (simultaneously tense) antagonistic (opposing) muscle groups crossing the ankle joint complex [Section 6.7.1].

Control over the joints and muscles of the ankle and feet in *hatha yoga* postures can help an experienced practitioner: improve balance, strengthen the ankle, stabilise the knees, create space in the medial knees, rotate the hips, stretch the groins, distract (separate) the sacroiliac joints, and lengthen the spine.

6.7.1 Co-activation of Opposing Muscles of the Ankle Joint Complex: *Kulpha bandha*

A co-activation (simultaneous tensing) of opposing (antagonistic) muscles crossing the ankle joint complex may be termed an ankle *bandha* [Section 1.7.3.1]. This *bandha*, which can be referred to by the *Sanskrit* name *kulpha bandha*, is crucial for the strength and stability of the ankle joint complex.

Kulpha bandha is formed when there is either:
- co-activation of ankle flexors (ankle plantarflexors) and ankle extensors (ankle dorsiflexors), or
- co-activation of ankle evertors and ankle invertors

Co-activation of antagonistic muscles is only possible for multi-joint (multi-articular) muscles [Section 1.6.5.7]. Studies have shown that co-activation of antagonistic pairs of one-joint (uni-articular) muscles is not possible, and only co-activation of antagonistic pairs of multi-joint muscles is possible [Herzog & Binding, 1993]. In the case of the ankle and the foot, the multi-joint nature of these muscles and their function in the foot and ankle is recorded in Tables 6.1, 6.2 and 6.3.

There are two main ways to create *kulpha bandha*. Both ways take advantage of the ability of multi-joint muscles to act independently at different joints, i.e. even though a particular muscle may cross two or more joints it may be seen to only have action at one joint.

The first way of making *kulpha bandha* takes advantage of the fact that some of the muscles that can extend (dorsiflex) the ankles (ankle dorsiflexors) can also extend (spread) the toes, while some of the muscles that can flex (plantarflex) the ankles (ankle plantarflexors) can also flex (grip with) the toes.

Therefore, the simplest way to create *kulpha bandha* is to either:

- actively extend (dorsiflex) the ankle joint while flexing (gripping with) the toes , or

- actively flex (plantarflex) the ankle joint while spreading the toes 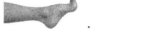.

The second way of making *kulpha bandha* takes advantage of the fact that some of the muscle groups in the ankle overlap in function. From Table 6.3 it can be seen that some ankle evertors such as Extensor digitorum longus can also act as ankle dorsiflexors. Therefore, it can be said that some ankle plantarflexors oppose ankle evertors in addition to ankle dorsiflexors. Therefore, active attempts to plantarflex and evert the ankle at the same time will cause the formation of *kulpha bandha*. By similar reasoning it can be seen that ankle dorsiflexor activity can be opposed by ankle invertor activity [Table 6.3] in addition to ankle plantarflexor activity.

Strength and stability of the ankle joint complex is important for three main reasons:
- To minimise the risk of ankle sprain in unstable conditions.
- To assist with balance in standing postures, especially balancing on one leg, by creating a stable base of support.
- To assist in the stabilising and strengthening of the knee by assisting in the creation of the *Janu bandha* (the co-activation of the opposing muscles of the knee joint complex) [Section 5.6].

Kulpha bandha can also make a significant contribution to the flow of energy, in the form of heat and blood, from and to the ankles and feet. This can be done, using the musculoskeletal pump [Sections 1.0.4, & 8.1.2.3] either through the alternations between ankle muscle activation and relaxation, or via alternations in the production of the *ha* (compressive) and *tha* (expansive) forms of *kulpha bandha* (below).

Like most *bandhas, kulpha bandha* has two main forms:
- *ha-kulpha bandha*, which is a compressive *bandha* that pushes energy and blood away from the ankle and foot, has ankle extensor and toe flexor activity eg. actively extending the ankles and flexing the toes 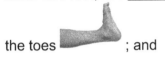 ; and

- *tha-kulpha bandha*, which is an expansive *bandha* that draws or pulls energy towards the ankle and foot, has ankle flexor and toe extensor activity eg. actively flexing the ankles and extending the toes.

Following is description of the main forms of *kulpha bandha* and their uses, but it should be noted that this analysis is a simplification and does not take into account the intrinsic muscles of the foot [Section 6.4].

Table 6.4 Muscle groups of the ankle joint complex that can co-activate (simultaneously tense) to oppose each other to form *kulpha bandha*	
PRIMARY ANKLE MUSCLE GROUP	OPPOSITION: Main muscle groups that can oppose each primary ankle muscle group to form a co-activation of opposing muscles around the ankle called *kulpha bandha*
Ankle plantarflexors (flexors)	Ankle dorsiflexors, Ankle evertors
Ankle dorsiflexors (extensors)	Ankle plantarflexors, Ankle invertors, Ankle evertors
Ankle evertors	Ankle invertors, Ankle plantarflexors
Ankle invertors	Ankle evertors, Ankle dorsiflexors

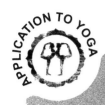

No 6.5 Many opposing pairs of ankle muscle groups can be co-activated to form *kulpha bandha*

An ankle *bandha* (*kulpha bandha*) can be made when opposing muscles of the ankle joint are co-activated. The structure of the ankle joint complex allows for more possibilities of muscle opposition than normal ball and socket joints because some ankle evertors also act as ankle dorsiflexors and many ankle plantarflexors also act as ankle invertors [Tables 6.1 -6.4]. Therefore:

ANKLE PLANTARFLEXORS	both OPPOSE	ANKLE DORSIFLEXORS
ANKLE INVERTORS	(both antagonistic to)	ANKLE EVERTORS

In addition

ANKLE DORSIFLEXORS	can also OPPOSE	ANKLE EVERTORS

Therefore, ankle plantarflexors can be opposed by ankle evertors to create stability in the ankle joint complex. For example better balance and ankle stability is achieved in postures such as *padangustha utkatasana*

when the heel is raised (using ankle plantarflexors) and the outer foot pulled towards the knee (using ankle evertors).

Similarly ankle dorsiflexors can be opposed by ankle invertors to create stability in the ankle joint complex.

For example, in *utthita swastikasana* (standing cross-legged forward bend), for most people, and especially for people with medial (inner) knee pain or instability, it is more effective to have the non weight-bearing top (L) leg dorsiflexed and inverted. This assists in creating *kulpha bandha* and also assists to stabilise the knee joint complex because it encourages the knee joint to internally rotate and bring firmness to the region around the medial (inner) knee.

However, ankle dorsiflexors can be opposed by ankle evertors to create stability in the ankle joint complex.

For example, in *utthita swastikasana* (standing cross-legged forward bend), for some people, mainly those with lateral (outer) knee pain or instability; it is more effective to have the non weight-bearing top (L) leg dorsiflexed and everted. This assists in creating *kulpha bandha* and also assists to stabilise the knee joint complex because it encourages the knee joint to externally rotate and bring firmness to the region around the lateral (outer) knee

6.7.1.1 *Ha-kulpha bandha*

Ha-kulpha bandha is a compressive *bandha* that pushes energy and blood away from the ankle and foot. *Ha-kulpha bandha* can be formed by co-activation of ankle flexors and ankle extensors, but because many of these muscles also extend or flex the toes, *ha-kulpha bandha* is simply created by co-activation of toe flexors (i.e. metatarsophalangeal flexors) and ankle extensors (i.e. ankle dorsiflexors). On a practical level, this can be achieved in several ways.

A weight-bearing (WB) closed-chain (CC) version of *ha-kulpha bandha* is most commonly used in the WB

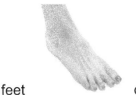

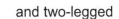

feet of both one-legged balances such as *utthita padangusthasana* and two-legged

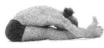

postures such as *parsvottonasana* . It can be created by pressing the toe tips into the floor, while attempting to lift the middle of the foot off the floor as if one is trying to grab the ground with the toes of the foot. This is particularly useful in maintaining balance on either one or both legs, as it stabilises the ankle joint while pushing energy and blood away from the floor.

Although many *yoga* teachers generally discourage this type of crunching the toes (pressing with the toe tips) during standing postures it is nevertheless a functional way to achieve balance especially in the more challenging standing positions. In addition the toe flexors are worked (activated) in their shorted position, and stale blood is pushed away from the toe tips allowing fresh blood to enter once the muscle is relaxed. *B.K.S. Iyengar* [1966] is seen to use this form of *ha-kulpha bandha* in many of the postures in *Light on Yoga*.

For example, *Sri Iyengar* is seen to be gripping with his toes in many of the difficult balancing postures such

as *eka pada urdhva dhanurasana* (one leg one arm back arch).t
A non weight-bearing (NWB) closed-chain (CC) version of *ha-kulpha bandha* can be created during the

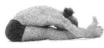

seated forward bending postures such as *ha-kulpha pascimottanasana* and *maha mudra*

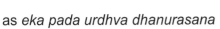

by actively extending the ankle joint (ankle extensor activity) while actively flexing the toes (toe flexor activity) as if one is trying to make a closed fist with the foot. This strengthens and stabilises the ankle joint complex and pushes energy away from the foot while increasing the tension (stretch) of the sciatic nerves and spinal cord, and the stretch of the gastrocnemius. A NWB CC version of *ha-kulpha bandha* can be created when the stretch is assisted by pressure from the hands, while actively pressing the toes against the hands (toe flexor activity) the stretch of muscles and nerves increases significantly. Body heat is significantly increased using this *bandha* during forward bending postures such as *ha-kulpha pascimottanasana*

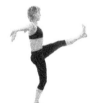 and it is not recommended for beginners or those with stiff <u>hamstrings</u>. It is also **not generally safe** for those with <u>intervertebral disc bulges</u> or <u>sciatic nerve impingement</u>. For beginners, and for those with stiff <u>hamstrings</u> or with <u>intervertebral disc bulges</u> or <u>sciatic nerve impingement,</u> it is <u>far safer</u> and easier to do a version of *tha-kulpha pascimottanasana* [Section 6.6.1.2] with the <u>ankle plantarflexion</u> and <u>toe</u>

extension 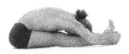 or even with <u>knee flexion.</u>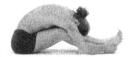

A special type of *ha-kulpha bandha* is formed when the heel is raised off the floor (ankle plantarflexion) and the outer arch of the foot raised (<u>ankle eversion</u>) in a WB CC exercise like the demi-point work in ballet. It is important to understand that a *bandha* forms with <u>co-activation</u> of <u>muscle activity</u>, and <u>muscle activity</u> is separate to <u>joint position</u>. For example in this type of *ha-kulpha bandha* the <u>toe joints</u> are in <u>toe extension</u>. However, the toes are still pressing into the floor, therefore in terms of muscles there is <u>toe flexor activity</u>. Some <u>toe flexors</u> are also <u>ankle flexors</u>, therefore there is some <u>ankle flexor</u> activity. Also lifting the outer feet activates some <u>ankle evertor activity</u> and therefore also some <u>ankle dorsiflexor activity</u> [Table 6.1 - 6.4]. This is a powerful *bandha* which is also a type of *mudra* as it <u>tensions</u> (stretches) nerves in the anterior leg. This *mudra* and *bandha* is used in many of the WB CC heel raised balances such as *padangustha*

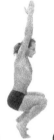

utkatasana (half squat on the ball of the foot).

6.7.1.2 *Tha-kulpha bandha*

Tha-kulpha bandha is an expansive *bandha* that draws or pulls energy towards the ankle and foot. *Tha-kulpha bandha* is formed by <u>co-activation</u> of <u>toe extensors</u> and <u>ankle flexors (plantarflexors)</u>. The *bandha* is supported and significantly strengthened with <u>active ankle eversion</u>. <u>Ankle evertors</u> (<u>peronius tertius</u> in particular) have some <u>ankle flexor (dorsiflexor) activity</u> which supports the work of the <u>toe extensors</u> (which also have some <u>ankle flexor (dorsiflexor) activity</u>). Therefore, together the toe extensors and ankle evertors can oppose the activity of ankle flexors to form *tha-kulpha bandha.*

Tha-kulpha bandha is most easily formed when the foot is engaged in <u>non weight-bearing</u> (NWB) <u>open-chain</u> (OC) movements or postures with <u>toe extensor activity</u> and <u>ankle flexor activity</u>. A NWB OC version of *tha-kulpha bandha* is most commonly used in the NWB foot of one-legged balances such as *niralamba utthita*

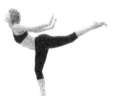

padangusthasana and *niralamba virabhadrasana* or in many variations of

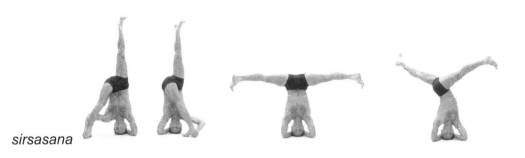

sirsasana

Tha-kulpha bandha in this same foot position can be adopted for nearly all two-legged postures in which the feet are on the floor where <u>ankle evertor activity</u> is possible. In this case blood and energy are pulled towards the feet which can feel quite grounding. Practically *tha-kulpha bandha* is practised on the floor by spreading the toes while lifting the arches of the feet [Sections 6.5.1 & 6.5.2].

6.7.1.3 Interrelationships between lower limb muscles; and between *kati bandha, janu bandha* and *kulpha bandha*

Bandhas are all inter-related. When one *bandha* is correctly applied it affects the adjacent *bandhas*

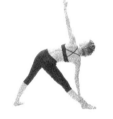

significantly. For example, during postures such as *utthita trikonasana*   *and parivrtta*

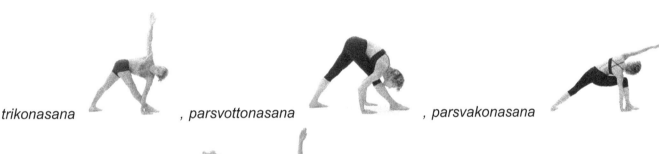

trikonasana   , *parsvottonasana*   , *parsvakonasana*

and parivrtta ardha candrasana   , the outer foot of the front (R) leg should be kept parallel with the edge of one's mat (if a mat is used), with the inner foot slightly turned inwards. It is then possible to gently grip the floor or mat by squeezing the heel inwards. In such postures:

- Exert pressure at the base of the big toe and the tips of the other toes to activate the <u>plantarflexors</u>. This contributes to creating *kulpha* (ankle) *bandha* [Section 6.6.1]) and *janu* (knee) *bandha* [Section 5.6.1].
- <u>Externally rotate</u> (try to turn out) the thighs at the <u>hip joints</u>. This lifts the inner arch of the foot, increases <u>traction</u> (stretch) of the spine, increases the length of the <u>hip extensors</u>, and contributes towards creating *kati* (hip) *bandha* [Section 4.5.1].
- Squeeze the heel gently inwards (<u>medially</u>). This activates the <u>hip adductors</u> and <u>hip internal rotators</u>, and contributes towards creating *kati* (hip) *bandha* [Section 4.5.1].
- Lift the outer edge of the foot off the floor to activate the <u>ankle evertors</u>. This assists to stabilise the <u>ankle joint complex</u> and contributes towards creating *kulpha* (ankle) *bandha* [Section 6.61] and *janu* (knee) *bandha* [Section 5.6.1].

6.7.2 Holistic (*Yoga*) Effects and Uses of Ankle joint Movements and Muscle Activations

In *yoga* the feet are said to be the organs of action for the lower trunk, the lower spine and the internal organs of digestion and reproduction. Following is a list of tangible things that the ankle and foot muscles and joints are able to assist in:

1. **To strengthen the ankle use:**
    *   <u>Isometric</u> and <u>isotonic</u> <u>activations</u> of ankle muscles
    *   <u>Co-activations</u> of opposing muscles crossing the ankle joints (i.e. learn to activate *kulpha bandha*) in static and dynamic exercises
    *   <u>Weight-bearing</u> (WB) and <u>non weight bearing</u> (NWB) postures.

2. **To improve balance use:**
    *   <u>Proprioceptive</u> (balance) training in one-legged balances such as *utthita padangusthasana*

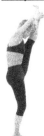

and two-legged poses such as *parsvottonasana.*

3. **To <u>traction</u> (lengthen) the spine use:**

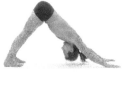

    *   <u>Closed-chain</u> (CC) <u>plantarflexion</u> in *adho mukha svanasana* (down-dog pose)

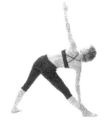

    *   <u>Closed-chain</u> (CC) <u>dorsiflexion</u> in *urdhva dhanurasana* (back arch).

4. **To <u>distract</u> (separate) the <u>sacroiliac</u> joints use:**

    *   <u>Inversion</u> of the ankle of the rear leg in standing postures such as *trikonasana*

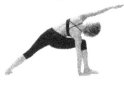

    (triangle pose) and *parsvakonasna* (sideways angle pose)

    *   <u>Closed-chain</u> <u>ankle dorsiflexion</u> of front leg in standing postures such as *parsva virabhadrasana*

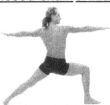

    (side-lunging warrior pose).

5. **To open or stretch the groin (<u>hip flexor</u> and <u>hip adductor</u> muscles) use:**
    *   <u>Ankle eversion</u> of front leg in conjunction with <u>hip external rotation</u> of front leg in postures such as

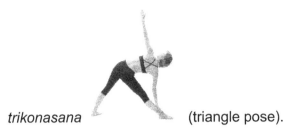

trikonasana (triangle pose).

6. **To stabilise the knee use:**
   - Closed-chain ankle plantarflexion in front leg of straight legged standing postures such as

     parsvottonasana in order to activate gastrocnemius muscle.

7. **To externally rotate the hip joints use:**
   - Ankle inversion of the rear leg in standing postures such as *parsvakonasana*

     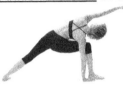

     (sideways angle pose).

   - Ankle dorsiflexion (extension) and knee extension of the rear lower limb in seated postures

     like *janu sirsasana* (NB. The ankle remains plantarflexed (flexed) but by attempting to dorsiflex (extend) the ankle there is activation of the ankle dorsiflexors in a lengthened state. The knee remains flexed but by attempting to extend the knee there is an activation of the knee extensors in a lengthened state).

8. **To make space in the knee use:**
   - Ankle eversion when knee is flexed and hip externally rotated in poses like *baddha*

     konasana 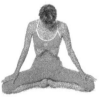 , *bhadrasana* 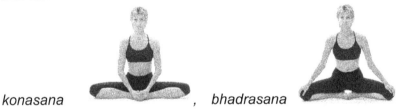 and *mulabandhasana*

     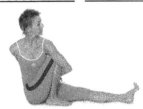

   - Closed-chain dorsiflexion in the standing leg of postures like *parivrrta maricyasana*.

9. **To increase hip flexion use:**
   - Closed-chain dorsiflexion in the standing leg of postures like *parivrtta padma*

maricyasana 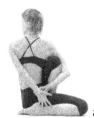 and *paripurna matsyendrasana*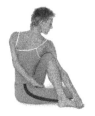

Appendix A describes postures in which ankle muscles are obliged to become active, and where muscles are obliged to at least be in a lengthened state if not stretched. Table 6.4 describes postures that use ankle muscles in a non-obligatory fashion to affect the body in various ways. Try and extend this table with your own postures and see how various adjustments in a posture can elicit different muscles to become active.

****

Table 6.5 Postures which use or may use the muscle groups of the ankle joint complex

MUSCLE GROUP	ANKLE PLANTARFLEXORS	ANKLE DORSIFLEXORS	ANKLE EVERTORS	ANKLE INVERTORS
Postures that cause an **obligatory activation** of an ankle muscle group to a **shortened position**	*Padangustha utkatasana* *Padangustha prasarita Padottonasana*	*Astavakrasana* *Bhujapidasana*	*Vasisthasana* R leg *Kasyapasana* R leg	*Parsva virabhadrasana* L Leg *Parsvakonasana* L leg
Postures that are **enhanced** when an ankle muscle group is **activated** (tensed) in a **shortened position**	*Niralamba padangusthasana* L leg *Parsvottanasana* R leg	*Urdhva dhanurasana* *Parsva virabhadrasana* R Leg	*Trikonasana* R leg *Baddha konasana*	*Parsva virabhadrasana* L Leg *Adho mukha baddha konasana*

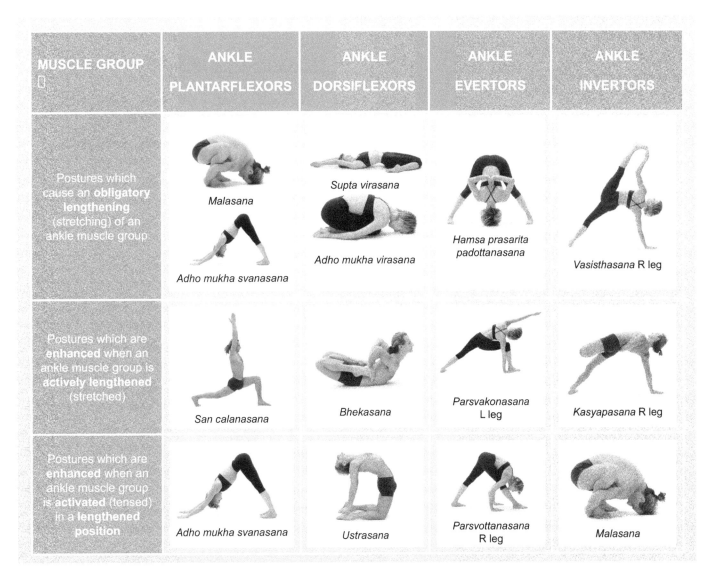

MUSCLE GROUP	ANKLE PLANTARFLEXORS	ANKLE DORSIFLEXORS	ANKLE EVERTORS	ANKLE INVERTORS
Postures which cause an **obligatory lengthening** (stretching) of an ankle muscle group	*Malasana* / *Adho mukha svanasana*	*Supta virasana* / *Adho mukha virasana*	*Hamsa prasarita padottanasana*	*Vasisthasana* R leg
Postures which are **enhanced** when an ankle muscle group is **actively lengthened** (stretched)	*San calanasana*	*Bhekasana*	*Parsvakonasana* L leg	*Kasyapasana* R leg
Postures which are **enhanced** when an ankle muscle group is **activated** (tensed) in a **lengthened position**	*Adho mukha svanasana*	*Ustrasana*	*Parsvottanasana* R leg	*Malasana*

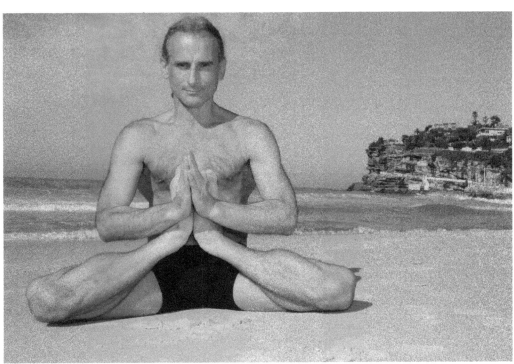

Simon Borg-Olivier in *Kandasana*. This advanced pose requires extreme flexibility in hip abduction and external rotation as well as extreme knee internal rotation with a strong *ha-janu bandha* (compressive knee lock). It also requires extreme flexibility with ankle inversion with lengthened ankle evertors. Photo courtesy of Ric Carter.

Chapter Breakdown

****

7.0 INTRODUCTION TO THE APPLIED ANATOMY OF THE SPINE & TRUNK IN *HATHA YOGA* POSTURES

When correctly performed, *hatha yoga* can improve the health of the <u>spine</u>. In many cases, however, *hatha yoga* is responsible for aggravating and even damaging the <u>spine</u>. Many practitioners either fail to achieve a balance between strength and flexibility, resulting in one part of the <u>spine</u> being compressed and perhaps damaged, and/or they do not adequately address pre-existing problems in the <u>spine</u>.

The movements of the <u>spine</u> are forward and backward bending (<u>flexion</u> and <u>extension</u>), side-bending (<u>lateral flexion</u> to left and right), and twisting (<u>axial rotation</u> to left and right). The most common mistake people make when trying to increase the flexibility of the <u>spine</u> is to assume that all these movements of the <u>spine</u> uniformly happen at all the various levels and joints of the <u>spine</u>. This is seldom the case. Most people bend more easily at some parts of their <u>spine</u> and are relatively immobile at others. *Hatha yoga* practised without caution and a real understanding (at least intuitive) of <u>spinal</u> anatomy will often make this situation worse. Those who practise *hatha yoga* with a lack of this awareness will only continue to bend the more flexible areas until they become over-lax, resulting in pain and/or injury.

At the same time, the less mobile regions of the <u>spine</u> become even stiffer with passing years due to the lack of movement. Practical use of the *bandhas* [Section 7.4.1] can help prevent this problem from occurring. However, unless the *bandhas* are applied from the correct starting position of the <u>spine</u> and the limbs, this problem can be made worse and the use of the *bandhas* may actually make the stiff parts of the <u>spine</u> stronger but stiffer and the flexible parts of the <u>spine</u> more flexible but weaker. The issue of how to correctly position the body and then direct your effort to safely increase <u>spinal</u> strength and flexibility is discussed later [Section 7.4.2].

7.1 BONES & JOINTS OF THE AXIAL SKELETON

<u>The axial skeleton</u> includes the <u>skull</u>, the <u>vertebral column</u>, the <u>bony thorax</u> and the <u>hyoid bone</u>. Figures 7.2–7.7 show the main features of the <u>axial skeleton</u>.

7.1.1 The Skull
7.1.1.1 Bones of the skull

The skull **[Figures 7.2 & 7.7]** has eight (8) <u>cranial bones</u>, which form a casing for the brain, and fourteen (14) <u>facial bones</u> including the <u>mandible</u> (jaw bone).

7.1.1.2 Joints of the skull

7.1.1.2.1 Temperomandibular joint (TMJ)

Location   the <u>temperomandibular joint</u> (TMJ) is the joint between the <u>mandible</u> (jaw) and the <u>skull</u>.

Classification <u>synovial</u>, condylar, hinge joint with an <u>articular disc</u>.

Excessive muscular tension in this joint can cause <u>TMJ syndrome</u>, which is characterised by pain around the ear and jaw, a clicking sound on opening and closing the mouth, headaches and teeth problems.

7.1.1.2.2 Sutures of the skull

The <u>sutures</u> of the <u>skull</u> are minimally movable joints with little connective tissue, nerves and blood vessels between <u>skull</u> bones. The sutures begin to <u>ossify</u> (close completely with bone) between 20 and 30 and may be completely <u>ossified</u> by the age of 60.

7.1.2 The Vertebral Column

The following features of the <u>vertebral column</u> can be seen on a skeleton and identified with the help of Figures 7.3–7.6:

* 7 <u>cervical vertebrae</u> (C1–C7), 12 <u>thoracic vertebrae</u> (T1–T12), 5 <u>lumbar vertebrae</u> (L1–L5), 5 fused <u>sacral vertebrae</u> (<u>sacrum</u>) (S1–S5), 3–5 fused <u>coccygeal vertebrae</u> (tailbone).

7.1.2.1 Curves of the vertebral column

The normal adult curvature of the spine is a <u>cervical lordosis</u> (anteriorly convex curvature), a <u>thoracic kyphosis</u> (anteriorly concave curvature), a <u>lumbar lordosis</u> and a <u>sacrococcygeal kyphosis</u>.

Up until the age of three months humans have a <u>single kyphosis</u>. As a baby learns to hold up its head, a <u>cervical lordosis</u> develops. As a baby learns to sit and stand, a <u>lumbar lordosis</u> develops. The <u>thoracic spine</u> and <u>sacrum</u> normally maintain a <u>kyphosis</u> throughout life.

7.1.2.2 Typical vertebrae

A normal <u>vertebra</u> comprises a weight-bearing anterior body, posterior <u>vertebral arch</u> with <u>vertebral foramen</u> for the <u>spinal cord</u> to pass through, 1 posterior <u>spinous process</u> (SP), 2 lateral <u>transverse processes</u> (TP) for muscle attachment and 4 processes with <u>articulating facets</u>.

7.1.2.3 Joints of the vertebral column

* **<u>Zygapophyseal (ZP) (facet) joints</u>**

Classification <u>synovial</u>, <u>plane</u>, <u>gliding</u> joints with thin loose capsules.

Location between the <u>inferior articulating facets</u> of superior <u>vertebrae</u> and the <u>superior articulating facets</u> of inferior <u>vertebrae</u>.

* **<u>Intervertebral joints</u>**
    o Articulating surfaces of adjacent <u>vertebral bodies</u> are covered with <u>hyaline cartilage</u>.
    o Adjacent <u>vertebral bodies</u> are bound most strongly by <u>fibrocartilaginous intervertebral discs</u> (IVDs) and are bound by strong <u>anterior</u> and <u>posterior longitudinal ligaments</u>.
    o <u>Intervertebral discs</u> (IVDs) have an external <u>annulus fibrosis</u> (AF), which has fibres running obliquely from one <u>vertebra</u> to the next, and an internal gelatinous <u>nucleus pulposis</u> (NP), which contacts the <u>hyaline cartilage</u> plates.
    o NP is normally very elastic and more cartilaginous than the fibrous AF
    o NP acts like a shock absorber for axial forces and like a semi-fluid ball-bearing during movements of the <u>vertebral column</u>.
    o NP is <u>avascular</u> (ie has no blood supply), receiving its nourishment by diffusion from the AF and adjacent surfaces of the <u>vertebral bodies</u>.
    o <u>Functions of the IVDs</u> are to:
        (i) bind <u>vertebrae</u> together
        (ii) allow motion
        (iii) absorb shock
        (iv) distribute load between segments
        (v) contribute to spinal curvature.

* **<u>Craniovertebral (CV) joints</u>**
    o The <u>craniovertebral (CV) joints</u> are the 2 <u>suboccipital joints</u>. The <u>atlanto-occipital joint</u> is between the <u>skull</u> and C1 (<u>atlas</u>). The <u>atlanto-axial</u> joint is between C1 and C2 (<u>axis</u>).
    o CV joints differ from other <u>vertebral joints</u> in that they are <u>synovial</u> but have no <u>zygapophyseal (ZP) (facet) joints</u>, and no IVDs.
    o <u>Atlanto-occipital joint</u> between the <u>axis</u> (C1) and the occipital condyles of the <u>skull</u> is a <u>synovial condyloid</u> type joint that permits <u>flexion</u> and <u>extension</u> movements such as nodding yes.
    o <u>Atlanto-axial joint</u> between C1 and C2 permits rotation as in the no movement.

7.1.2.4 Ligaments of the vertebral column

Figure 7.1 shows a diagrammatic representation (a cross section) of the ligaments of the vertebral column.

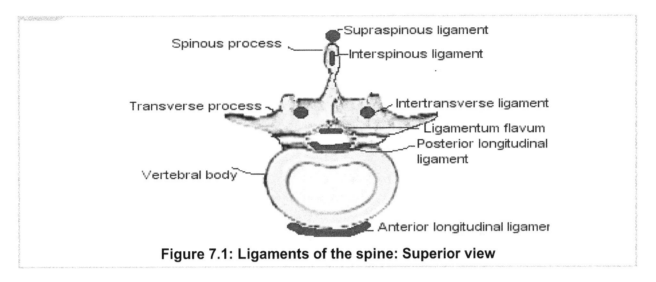

Figure 7.1: Ligaments of the spine: Superior view

Attachments and function of the main ligaments of the vertebral column are shown in Table 7.1

Table 7.1 Ligaments and ligamentous-like structures of the spine

LIGAMENT	LOCATION	FUNCTION
1. Anterior longitudinal ligament (continues as **Anterior atlantoaxial** from axis to atlas.)	• On anterior & lateral vertebral bodies from sacrum to axis • Well developed in lumbar & thoracic regions	• Limits extension of spine • Reinforces anterior portion of annulus fibrosis
2. Posterior longitudinal ligament (continues as the **Nectarial membrane** from axis to occipital bone.)	• Runs within the vertebral canal on posterior vertebral bodies from sacrum to axis	• Limits flexion of the spine • Reinforces posterior portion of annulus fibrosis
3. Ligamentum flavum ligament (continues as **Posterior atlanto-axial ligament** over atlas and axis.)	• On posterior surface of vertebral canal from sacrum to axis	• Limits flexion of spine, especially in lumbar area
4. Supraspinous ligament (continues as **Ligamentum nuchae** over cervical SPs.)	• Over thoracic & lumbar spinous processes (SPs)	• Limits flexion of spine
5. Interspinous	• From the base of one spinous process to another • Mainly in the lumbar region	• Limits flexion of spine
6. Intertransverse	• From one transverse process to another • Mainly lumbar region	• Limits lateral flexion of spine
7. Alar	• From the side of the dens of axis to lateral margins of foramen magnum of skull	• Limits rotation of skull to same side • Limits lateral rotation to opposite side
8. ZP joint capsules	• Over each ZP joint • Strongest in thoracolumbar & cervico-thoracic junctions	• Assists ligaments in providing stability • Limits the motion of spine

Abbreviations: SP = spinous process, TP = transverse process, ZP joint = zygapophyseal joint

191

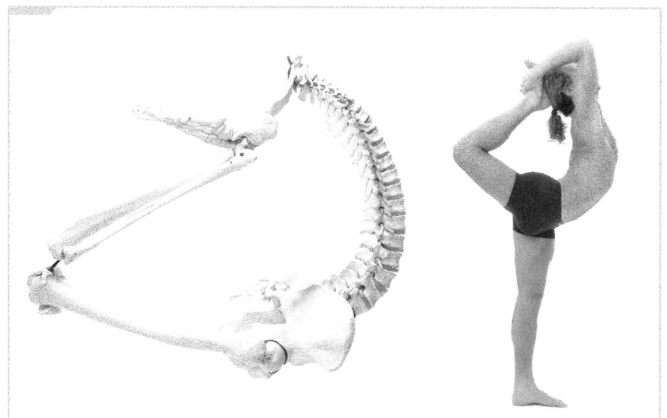

SPINAL FUN: Skeletal spine extended and right lower limb extended in *natarajasana* (backward bending posture) above right

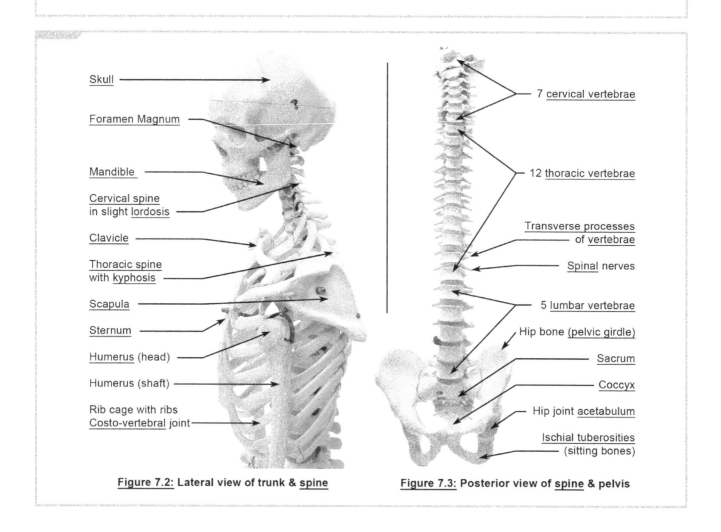

Skull

Foramen Magnum

Mandible

Cervical spine in slight lordosis

Clavicle

Thoracic spine with kyphosis

Scapula

Sternum

Humerus (head)

Humerus (shaft)

Rib cage with ribs
Costo-vertebral joint

7 cervical vertebrae

12 thoracic vertebrae

Transverse processes of vertebrae

Spinal nerves

5 lumbar vertebrae

Hip bone (pelvic girdle)

Sacrum

Coccyx

Hip joint acetabulum

Ischial tuberosities (sitting bones)

Figure 7.2: Lateral view of trunk & spine

Figure 7.3: Posterior view of spine & pelvis

192

7.1.2.5 Special features of lumbar vertebrae [Figure 7.4]

- Vertebral body is large with transverse diameters greater than anterior diameter.
- Spinous processes (SPs) are broad, thick, and extend horizontally.
- Transverse processes (TPs) are long slender, and extend horizontally.
- Superior facets are concave and face medially and posteriorly.
- Inferior facets are convex and face anteriorly and laterally.
- Both facets lie in a sagittal plane.
- Structure permits reasonable flexion and extension, some lateral flexion but little to no rotation.

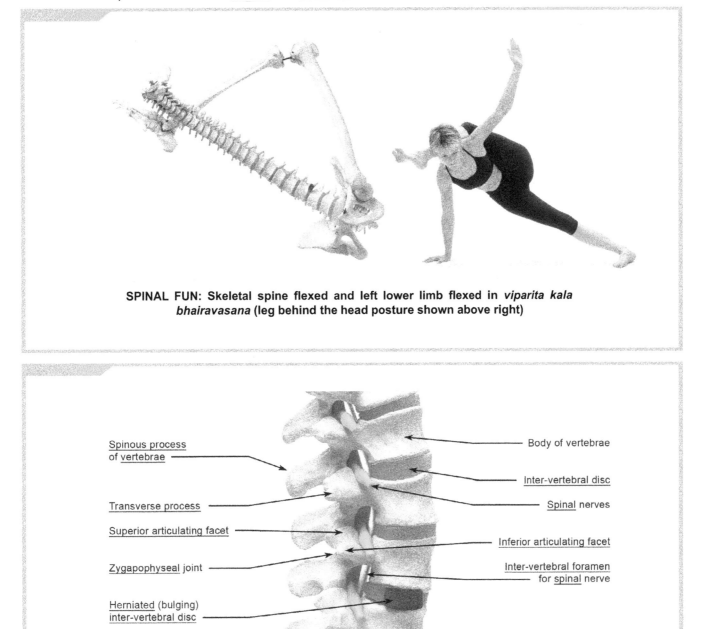

SPINAL FUN: Skeletal spine flexed and left lower limb flexed in *viparita kala bhairavasana* (leg behind the head posture shown above right)

Spinous process of vertebrae

Transverse process

Superior articulating facet

Zygapophyseal joint

Herniated (bulging) inter-vertebral disc

Body of vertebrae

Inter-vertebral disc

Spinal nerves

Inferior articulating facet

Inter-vertebral foramen for spinal nerve

Figure 7.4: Lateral view of lumbar spine

7.1.2.6 Special features of thoracic vertebrae [Figure 7.5]

- Vertebral body is slightly wedged anteriorly, and has equal transverse and anterior-posterior diameters, and has demifacets for articulations with ribs.
- Spinous processes (SPs) slope inferiorly and overlap the SP of the adjacent inferior vertebra.
- Transverse processes (TPs) have thickened ends for articulation with the costal tubercles.
- Superior facets face superiorly and laterally while inferior facets face anteriorly and medially.
- Structure permits limited flexion, extension, lateral flexion and axial rotation.

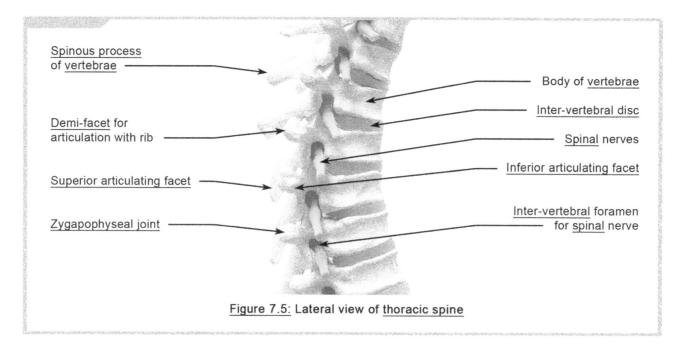

Spinous process
of vertebrae

Demi-facet for
articulation with rib

Superior articulating facet

Zygapophyseal joint

Body of vertebrae

Inter-vertebral disc

Spinal nerves

Inferior articulating facet

Inter-vertebral foramen
for spinal nerve

Figure 7.5: Lateral view of thoracic spine

7.1.2.7 Special features of cervical vertebrae [Figure 7.6]

- Except for C1 (atlas) and C2 (axis), which are atypical [Section 7.1.2.3 on craniovertebral joints], and C7 which is transitional between cervical and thoracic, the rest of the cervical vertebrae, C3–6 conform to the basic design for all vertebrae [Section 7.1.2.2] with the following regional variations:
    - o Cervical vertebral bodies are small with transverse diameters greater than anterior-posterior diameters and heights
    - o Spinous processes (SPs) are short, slender, horizontal, and bifid (split)
    - o Transverse processes (TPs) have a foramen for the vertebral artery
    - o Superior facets face superiorly and medially, while inferior facets face inferiorly and laterally
    - o The structure of cervical vertebrae permits large amounts of flexion, extension, lateral flexion and axial rotation
    - o Axial rotation and lateral flexion are coupled movements, ie when one movement takes place the other automatically happens at the same time. When the neck twists to the right side (right cervical spine axial rotation) there is associated side bending to the right side (right cervical spine lateral flexion). This has been shown to increase the size of the intervertebral foramina on the side that is being rotated away from and decrease the size of the intervertebral foramina on the side that is being turned towards.

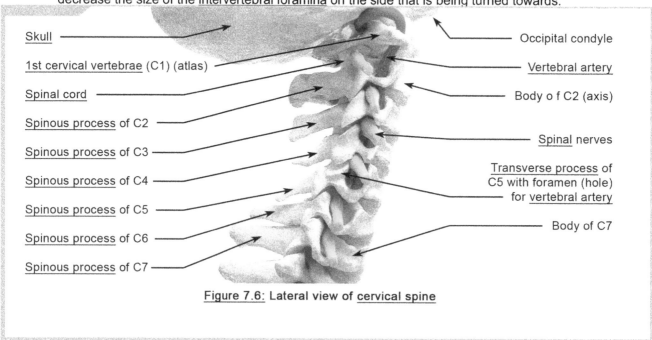

Skull

1st cervical vertebrae (C1) (atlas)

Spinal cord

Spinous process of C2

Spinous process of C3

Spinous process of C4

Spinous process of C5

Spinous process of C6

Spinous process of C7

Occipital condyle

Vertebral artery

Body o f C2 (axis)

Spinal nerves

Transverse process of
C5 with foramen (hole)
for vertebral artery

Body of C7

Figure 7.6: Lateral view of cervical spine

7.1.3 The Bony Thorax [Figure 7.7]

The bony thorax consists of a <u>sternum</u> (with superior <u>manubrium</u>, and inferior <u>xiphisternum</u>) and 12 ribs.

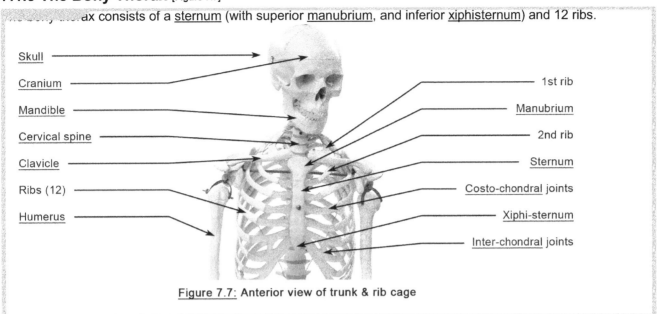

Skull
Cranium
Mandible
Cervical spine
Clavicle
Ribs (12)
Humerus

1st rib
Manubrium
2nd rib
Sternum
Costo-chondral joints
Xiphi-sternum
Inter-chondral joints

<u>Figure 7.7</u>: Anterior view of trunk & rib cage

Joints of the thorax
Manubrosternal (MS) and xiphisternal (XS) joints
- The <u>manubrosternal</u> (MS) and <u>xiphisternal</u> (XS) <u>joints</u> are <u>synchondroses</u>, which have a <u>fibrocartilaginous disc</u> between the joint
- The MS joint, which ossifies in 10% of adults, is sometimes called the <u>symphysis sterni</u> due to its similarity to the <u>symphysis pubis</u>
- The XS joint tends to ossify by the 5th decade.

Costovertebral (CT) joint
- The <u>costovertebral (CV) joint</u> is a plane <u>synovial joint</u>
- It lies between the head of a rib and the 2 <u>demi-facets</u> found on adjacent <u>thoracic vertebrae</u>
- The <u>costal</u> and <u>vertebral articular surfaces</u> are joined by thin <u>fibrous capsules</u> and supporting ligaments
- Motions of CV joints are rotation and gliding.

Costotransverse (CV) joint
- Plane <u>synovial joint</u>
- Joint between <u>costal tubercle</u> of a rib with the costal facet of the <u>transverse processes</u> of a <u>thoracic vertebrae</u>
- 3 major ligaments strengthen <u>joint capsule</u>.

Costochondral (CC) and chondrosternal (CS) joints
- Ribs 1–7 (true ribs) articulate with the <u>costal cartilages</u> at <u>costochondral (CC) joints</u> that articulate with <u>manubrium</u> at the <u>chondrosternal (CS) joints</u>
- CC joints are <u>synchondroses</u> with no ligamentous support
- The CS joints of ribs 2–7 are <u>synovial</u> but are often obliterated with age.

Interchondral (IC) joints
- <u>Costal cartilages</u> of ribs 8–10 articulate with the cartilages above them at the <u>interchondral (IC) joints</u>
- The IC joints are <u>synovial-like</u>, supported with capsule and ligaments but often get fibrous and fuse in old age.

7.1.4 The Hyoid Bone
The <u>hyoid</u> is a small U-shaped bone found at the level of the third <u>cervical vertebrae</u> (C3) between the <u>mandible</u> (lower jaw-bone) and the <u>larynx</u> (voice box). The <u>hyoid</u> bone functions to support and elevate the <u>larynx</u> (voice box) and trachea (wind-pipe). It also assists in the control of tongue movements, swallowing and speaking.

The <u>hyoid</u> bone is suspended by ligaments and does not articulate with any other bone. However, many important muscles are attached to the <u>hyoid</u> bone. These include muscles that also attach to the tongue, the <u>skull</u>, the <u>mandible</u> (jaw-bone), <u>scapula</u> (shoulder blade), <u>clavicle</u> (collar bone) and the <u>sternum</u> [Table 7.2]. Therefore, movements of the tongue can have a direct effect on the <u>skull</u>, <u>mandible</u>, clavicle, and <u>sternum</u> and, therefore, an indirect effect on the <u>spine</u>.

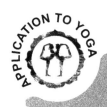

No 7.1 Movements of the tongue in *asana*, *pranayama*, *bandha* and *mudra* can indirectly affect the spine

Movements of the tongue can indirectly affect the spine through muscular connections between the tongue and the hyoid and between the hyoid and both the skull and the chest.

Pranayamas (breath-control exercises) that incorporate *mudras* (energy-control gestures) involving the tongue are therefore very powerful in their effects on the spine. *Mudras* such as *nabhi, kaki,* and *kecari* involve curling the tongue backwards towards the throat at different degrees; *simha mudra* involves stretching the tongue towards the chin, and *kakacandra mudra* involves rolling the tongue into a tube and is used to breathe through as in *sitali pranayama*. All these *mudras* should be applied with caution and only under the guidance of an experienced teacher.

7.1.5 Spinal Joint Complexes

In order to assist in the understanding of how the spine functions, it is helpful to sometimes refer to the spine as a linked series of three (3) spinal joint complexes relating mainly to the cervical region (the neck), the thoracic region (the upper back), and the lumbosacrococcygeal region (the lower back). These three regions or joint complexes are distinctly different and clearly delineated by the presence of the ribs in the thoracic regions.

The three (3) central or spinal *bandhas*, namely *jalandhara bandha, uddiyana bandha* and *mula bandha* are related to the cervical (neck), thoracic (upper back), and lumbosacrococcygeal (lower back) regions of the spine respectively [Sections 1.7.3.1 & 7.4.1].

7.1.5.1 Neck joint complex (cervical spine joint complex)

The neck joint complex is defined to include all the joints from the head to the start of the upper back including the atlanto-occipital joint between the skull and C1 (atlas) to the junction between the last cervical vertebrae and the first thoracic vertebrae (C7–T1).

Jalandhara bandha [Section 7.4.1.2] is formed when the neck joint complex (neck) is supported and stabilised by co-activation of antagonistic (opposing) muscle groups around these joints.

7.1.5.2 Upper back joint complex (thoracic spine joint complex)

The upper back joint complex is defined to include all the joints linked to spinal vertebrae which have ribs attached to them, from the joint at the start of the upper back (C7–T1) to the thoracolumbar junction, which is between the last thoracic vertebrae and the first lumbar vertebrae (T12–L1).

Uddiyana bandha [Section 7.4.1.3] is formed when the upper back joint complex (upper back) is supported and stabilised by co-activation of antagonistic (opposing) muscle groups around these joints

7.1.5.3 Lower back joint complex (lumbosacrococcygeal spinal joint complex)

What is defined in this text   as the lower back joint complex could more correctly be labelled the lumbosacrococcygeal spinal joint complex. This complex is defined to include all the joints linked to spinal vertebrae from the joint at the start of the lower back or lumbar spine (T12–L1) to the end of the coccyx (tail bone), including the sacrum and the sacroiliac joints.

Mula bandha [Section 7.4.1.1] is formed when the lower back joint complex (lower back) is supported and stabilised by a co-activation of antagonistic (opposing) muscle groups around the lumbar spine, sacrum and coccyx.

7.1.5.4 Joint complex overlap

Note that the spinal joint complexes slightly overlap each other. The distal end of the cervical spine complex is the start of the thoracic spine joint complex. The distal end of the thoracic spine complex is the start of the lumbosacrococcygeal spine joint complex. Also note that the sacroiliac joints can be also considered part of the hip joint complex [Section 4.2.0].

7.2 MUSCLES OF THE HEAD & TRUNK

The attachments and actions of muscles of the head and trunk are shown in Tables 7.2, 7.3 and 7.4.
The movements of the head and trunk and the muscles that facilitate these movements are shown in Tables 7.5, 7.6, 7.7 and 7.8.

Table 7.2 Muscles of the face, jaw, pharynx, larynx and hyoid bone

MUSCLE OR MUSCLE GROUP	ATTACHMENTS & DESCRIPTION	ACTIONS &/OR ROLES
Facial muscles (14 muscles)	• **From** fascia or bones of skull • **To** the skin	• Creates facial expression • Moves scalp, lips, and eyebrows • Closes eyes
Eyeball muscles (6 **extrinsic** muscles)	• **From** orbit of eye • **To** eyeball	• Rolls eyeball up and down • Rolls eyeball laterally and medially • Rotates eyeball
Lower jaw muscles (masseter, temporalis, & pterygoids)	• **From** cranium (mainly maxilla, parietal, and sphenoid bones) • **To** mandible	• Mastication • Biting • Chewing • Speech
Tongue muscles (4 **extrinsic** muscles) • **Genioglossus**	• **From** mandible • **To** hyoid bone, and underneath tongue	• Depresses tongue • Acting bilaterally – **protrudes** tongue • Acting unilaterally – moves tongue **laterally** (sideways)
• **Hyoglossus**	• **From** hyoid bone • **To** underneath tongue	• **Depresses** tongue • **Retracts** tongue • Turns sides of tongue downwards
• **Styloglossus**	• **From** styloid process of temporal bone of cranium and stylohyoid ligament • **To** side and under tongue	• **Retracts** tongue (pulls the tongue back and up) • **Elevates** tongue upward for swallowing
• **Palatoglossus**	• **From** soft palate • **To** side of tongue	• **Elevates** posterior tongue
Suprahyoid muscles (Muscles of pharynx or oral cavity; 2 of each) • **Mylohyoideus**	• **From** mandible (lower jaw bone) • **To** hyoid bone	• **Elevates** hyoid, floor of mouth, and tongue during swallowing and speaking
• **Geniohyoideus**	• **From** mandible • **To** hyoid bone	• **Protrudes** hyoid bone • **Elevates** hyoid bone • Helps open the jaw • Helps raise the tongue
• **Stylohyoideus**	• **From** styloid process of temporal bone of cranium • **To** hyoid bone	• **Elevates** hyoid bone for swallowing • **Retracts** hyoid bone
• **Digastricus**	• **From** mandible, and mastoid notch of temporal bone of cranium • **To** hyoid bone	• **Depresses** mandible • **Elevates** hyoid bone during swallowing and speaking
Infrahyoid muscles (Muscles below hyoid moving larynx; 2 of each) • **Sternohyoideus**	• **From** manubrium of sternum (first part of breast bone), and medial clavicle • **To** hyoid bone	• **Depresses** hyoid bone after it has been elevated during swallowing • Assists in flexion of head and neck • Opposes action of thyrohyoideus
• **Sternothyroideus**	• **From** sternum, and cartilage of rib 1 • **To** thyroid cartilage	• **Depresses** hyoid bone • **Depresses** thyroid cartilage and larynx
• **Thyrohyoideus**	• **From** thyroid cartilage • **To** hyoid bone	• **Depresses** hyoid bone • **Elevates** larynx • Opposes action of sternohyoideus
• **Omohyoideus**	• **From** superior border of scapula near supra-scapular notch • **To** hyoid bone	• **Depresses** hyoid bone • **Retracts** hyoid bone • Steadies hyoid bone • Moves hyoid sideways, assisting swallowing, speech, and chewing

197

7.2.1 Muscles of the Face, Jaw, Pharynx, Larynx and Hyoid Bone [Table 7.2]

The attachments and actions of muscles of the face, jaw, pharynx and larynx are shown in Table 7.2.

7.2.2 Muscles of the Neck and Back [Table 7.3]

The attachments and actions of muscles of the back and neck are shown in Table 7.3.

7.2.3 Muscles of the Thorax and Abdomen [Table 7.4]

The muscles of the thorax and abdomen are involved in breathing. These consist of obligatory muscles of breathing and accessory muscles of breathing.

Obligatory muscles of breathing are the diaphragm and intercostalis externus and intercostalis internus (external and internal intercostal muscles).

Accessory muscles of breathing are the scalenes (anterior, medial and lateral), sternocleidomastoid, pectoralis major, trapezius, abdominal muscles (obliquus externus abdominis, obliquus internus abdominis, transversus abdominis and rectus abdominis), quadratus lumborum. The attachments and actions of muscles of the thorax and abdomen are shown in Table 7.4.

APPLICATION TO YOGA

No 7.2 Spinal and trunk muscles are often more easily visible when spinal *bandhas* are applied during a breath retention

The abdominal muscles obliquus externus abdominis and rectus abdominis can be well defined using the central (spinal) *bandhas* during exhalation retention. The obliquus externus abdominis can be clearly seen

when *tha-uddiyana bandha* and *ha-mula bandha* are applied together 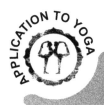. The rectus abdominis can be clearly seen when *tha-uddiyana bandha* and *ha-mula bandha* are applied together with resisted

spinal flexion in *nauli kriya* . These *bandhas* and muscle definitions can also be clearly seen in Figures 7.9b, 7.9c and 12.1.

7.2.4 Other Muscles Affecting the Head and Trunk

Many of the muscles that normally move the upper or lower limbs but have attachments to the axial skeleton (or even attachments to the hip joint complex since it is quite tightly bound to the sacrum) are also capable of moving the axial skeleton when the limbs are fixed. Such muscles include:

Upper limb/pectoral girdle muscles: trapezius, rhomboids, levator scapulae, latissimus dorsi, serratus anterior, and pectoralis major and minor.

Lower limb/pelvic girdle muscles: rectus femoris, psoas major, gluteus maximus, and the hamstring group in the lower limbs.

Hence, the arms and legs are known as the organs of action in *yoga* and correct use of the arms and legs during the *yoga asanas* (postures) allows functional mobilisation and manipulation of the spine.

Important muscles of the trunk (back spine, chest, and abdomen)

The following muscles of the trunk are important . Their attachments and actions are useful to learn. They are relatively easy to see and feel.

1. Scalenes (anterior, medius and posterior)
2. Sternocleidomastoid
3. Erector spinae
4. Rectus abdominis
5. Transversus abdominis
6. Obliquus externus abdominis and obliquus internal abdominis (external and internal abdominal obliques)
7. Intercostalis externus and intercostalis internus (external and internal intercostal muscles)
8. Diaphragm
9. Quadratus lumborum.

Table 7.3 Muscles of the neck and back

MUSCLE OR GROUP	ATTACHMENTS & DESCRIPTION	ACTIONS &/OR ROLES
Sternocleidomastoid (SCM)	• **From** sternum and clavicle • **To** mastoid process of temporal bone (below the base of the ear)	• Bilaterally **flex** cervical spine • Unilaterally **rotate** face to opposite side
Scalenes (anterior, middle and posterior)	• **From** TPs of C2-C7 • **To** ribs 1 & 2	• **Flex** head • **Axially rotate** head • Assists in inspiration
Splenius (capitis & cervicis)	• S. capitus – **from** ligamentum nuchae, SPs of T1-4 & C7 **to** occipital bone & mastoid process of temporal bone • S. cervicis – SPs of T3-6 **to** TPs C1-4	• Bilaterally they **extend** head and neck • Unilaterally laterally **flex, rotate** head to same side
Erector spinae (= sacrospinalis) 3 columns form large ridges on each side of the spine (a) Lateral column – Iliocostalis (lumborum. thoracic & cervicis) (b) Intermediate column – Longissimus (thoracis, cervicis & capitis) (c) Medial column – spinalis	• **From** one common origin (a broad tendon attaching inferiorly to the posterior iliac crest, posterior sacrum, sacroiliac ligaments, and the TPs of L1-S5) • **To (a)** all the posterior ribs and the posterior tubercles of C4-C6. • **To (b)** the TPs of C1-T12, the tubercles of the inferior 9 ribs, and the mastoid process of the temporal bone. • **To (c)** the SPs of T1-T6	• Bilaterally all three columns **extend** head and part or all of the spine • Unilaterally **laterally flex** the spine to same side • Acts concentrically to straighten the flexed spine • Acts eccentrically during spinal flexion • (Most commonly injured muscle during back strain)
Transversospinalis (Deep layer of intrinsic back muscles) (a) Semispinalis thoracis, cervicis & capitis (b) Multifidus (c) Rotatores	• Obliquely aligned fibres from inferior TPs to superior SPs • **(a)** TPs of T1-12 **to** SPs of T1-4 & C1-7, and occipital bone • **(b)** TPs to SPs of all vertebrae from S4-C2; fibres span 1-3 vertebrae • **(c)** TP of one vertebra **to** SP above	• **Extend** spine • **Rotate** spine to opposite side
Segmental muscles Interspinales & Intertransversarii	• SP **to** SP of consecutive vertebrae & • TP **to** TP of consecutive vertebrae	• Interspinales **extend** spine • Intertransversarii **laterally flex** spine

Abbreviations: C = cervical, L = lumbar, SP = spinous process, TP = transverse process, ZP joint = zygapophyseal joint

Table 7.4 Muscles of the thorax and abdomen

MUSCLE	ATTACHMENTS & DESCRIPTION	ACTIONS &/OR ROLES
Diaphragm	• **From** xiphoid process, cartilage of ribs 6-12, and L1-5 • **To** central tendon of diaphragm	• Forms floor of thoracic cavity • Inhale: Pulls central tendon of diaphragm down • Increases vertical length of thorax
Intercostalis externus	• **From** inferior border of rib above • **To** superior border of rib below	• May elevate ribs during inspiration • Increases width and depth of thorax
Intercostalis internus	• **From** superior border of rib below • **To** inferior border of rib above	• May pull ribs together in forced expiration • Decreases width and depth of thorax
Quadratus lumborum	• Iliac crest & iliolumbar ligament • **To** rib 12 and TPs of L1-4	• Lateral flexion of lumbar spine • Fixes rib 12 during respiration
Transversus abdominis	• Iliac crest, inguinal ligament, lumbar fascia and cartilage of ribs 6-12 (deepest abdominal muscle)	• Compresses abdomen • Important stabiliser of the lumbar spine • Normally activated before movement
Rectus abdominis	• **From** pubic crest and pubic symphysis • **To** cartilage of ribs 5-7 and xiphoid process	• Together compresses abdomen • Flexes lumbar spine • Aids defecation, urination, expiration, childbirth • Alone laterally flexes and rotates spine
Externus obliquus abdominis	• **From** ribs 5-12 • **To** iliac crest and anterior superior iliac spine	• Acting bilaterally flexes lumbar spine • Compresses and supports the abdominal viscera • Aids defecation, urination, expiration, childbirth • Acting alone laterally flexes and rotates the lumbar vertebral column to the contralateral side
Internus obliquus abdominis	• **From** ribs 5-12, inguinal ligament, iliac crest, and thoracolumbar fascia • **To** three or four ribs and their cartilages, being continuous with the intercostales interni and linea alba	• Acting bilaterally flexes lumbar spine • Compresses and supports the abdominal viscera • Aids defecation, urination, expiration, childbirth • Acting alone laterally flexes and rotates the lumbar vertebral column to the ipsilateral side

Abbreviations: C = cervical, L = lumbar, SP = spinous process, TP = transverse process, ZP joint = zygapophyseal joint

Table 7.5 Movements of the head and involved muscles

**MUSCLE GROUPS & INDIVIDUAL MUSCLES
MOVING THE HEAD AT THE ATLANTO-OCCIPITAL JOINT**

HEAD FLEXION

Head flexors: rectus capitus (anterior & lateralis), longus capitus, longus cervicis, hyoid muscles (suprahyoid and infrahyoid are synergists to head flexion), sternocleidomastoid (acting bilaterally)

HEAD EXTENSION

Head extensors: splenius capitus, longissimus capitus, semispinalis capitis, spinalis capitus, trapezius, rectus capitus posterior (major & minor), obliquus capitus (inferior & superior).

HEAD LATERAL FLEXION

Head lateral flexors (muscles on one side are activated): trapezius, splenius capitus, longissimus capitus, semispinalis capitis, obliquus capitus superior, sternocleidomastoid (acting unilaterally), rectus capitus lateralis, longus capitus.

HEAD AXIAL ROTATION

Head rotators (muscles on one side are activated): trapezius*, splenius capitus, longissimus capitus, semispinalis capitis, obliquus capitus inferior, sternocleidomastoid* (acting unilaterally)

* indicates movement to opposite side

Table 7.6 Movement pairs and muscles of the neck and cervical spine

**MUSCLE GROUPS & INDIVIDUAL MUSCLES
MOVING THE CERVICAL SPINE (NECK) AT THE NECK JOINT COMPLEX**

NECK FLEXION

Neck flexors: longus cervicis, scalenes (anterior, medius & posterior), sternocleidomastoid (acting bilaterally)

NECK EXTENSION

Neck extensors: splenius cervicis (c.), semispinalis c., longissimus c., levator scapulae, iliocostalis c., spinalis c., multifidus, interspinales c., trapezius, rectus capitus posterior major, rotatores (brevis & longi)

NECK LATERAL FLEXION

Neck lateral flexors (muscles on one side are activated): levator scapulae, splenius cervicis (c.), iliocostalis c., longissimus c., semispinalis c., multifidus, intertransversarii, scaleni, sternocleidomastoid (acting unilaterally), obliquus capitus inferior, rotatores (brevis & longi), longus coli

NECK AXIAL ROTATION

Neck rotators (muscles on one side are activated): levator scapulae, splenius cervicis (c.), iliocostalis c., longissimus c., semispinalis c., multifidus*, intertransversarii, scaleni*, sternocleidomastoid* (acting unilaterally), obliquus capitus inferior, rotatores (brevis & longi).

* indicates movement to opposite side

Table 7.7 Movement pairs and muscles of the upper back and thoracic spine

**MUSCLE GROUPS & INDIVIDUAL MUSCLES
MOVING THE CERVICAL SPINE (NECK) AT THE NECK JOINT COMPLEX**

THORACIC SPINE FLEXION

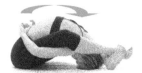

Thoracic spine flexors: rectus abdominis, obliquus externus abdominis, obliquus internus abdominis

THORACIC SPINE EXTENSION

Thoracic spine extensors: spinalis thoracis (t.), iliocostalis t., longissimus t., semispinalis t., multifidus, rotatores, interspinalis

THORACIC SPINE LATERAL FLEXION

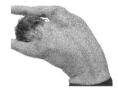

Thoracic spine lateral flexors: iliocostalis t., longissimus t., intertransverse, semispinalis t.*, multifidus*, rotatores*, obliquus externus abdominis, obliquus internus abdominis, transversus abdominis

* indicates movement to opposite side

THORACIC SPINE AXIAL ROTATION

Thoracic spine rotators: iliocostalis t., longissimus t., intertransverse, semispinalis t. *, multifidus*, rotatores*, obliquus externus abdominis, obliquus internus abdominis, transversus abdominis

* indicates movement to opposite side

Table 7.8 Movement pairs and muscles of the lower back and lumbar spine

**MUSCLE GROUPS & INDIVIDUAL MUSCLES
MOVING THE CERVICAL SPINE (NECK) AT THE NECK JOINT COMPLEX**

LUMBAR SPINE FLEXION

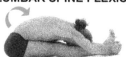

Lumbar spine flexors: rectus abdominis, obliquus externus abdominis, obliquus internus abdominis, transversus abdominis

LUMBAR SPINE EXTENSION

Lumbar spine extensors: latissimus dorsi, erector spinae, transversospinalis, interspinales, quadratus lumborum

LUMBAR SPINE LATERAL FLEXION

Lumbar spine lateral flexors: latissimus dorsi, erector spinae, transversospinalis, intertransversarii, quadratus lumborum, psoas major, obliquus externus abdominis

LUMBAR SPINE AXIAL ROTATION

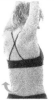

Lumbar spine rotators: transversospinalis (actually very little rotation occurs in the lumbar spine due to local muscle action)

7.3 ABNORMALITIES & INJURIES OF THE SPINE

7.3.1 Potential Causes of Back Injury

Potential causes of back injury include:

- Chronic stressful positions
- Repetitive loading
- Hard repetitive contact
- Heavy lifting, or incorrect lifting
- Sudden violent muscle activations.

7.3.2 Degeneration of an Intervertebral Disc (IVD)

Stresses on a normal intervertebral disc include (i) ageing, (ii) trauma, (iii) structural susceptibility, (iv) metabolic disorders, and (v) disease. Such stresses may result in structural changes and the transmission of asymmetric forces that may lead to disc degeneration. Smoking cigarettes has been shown to lead to dehydration and degeneration of intervertebral discs. Intervertebral disc degeneration can result in:

- Disc narrowing
- Disc protrusion (herniation)
- Facet joint syndrome (pain and synovitis)
- Spinal stenosis (encroachment of the spinal canal).

With increasing age, average fluid content of the intervertebral disc decreases and thus the discs narrow. This will lead to a loss in height leading to a lack of tension in the spinal ligaments and a reduction in stability of the spine.

Compressive loads on the intervertebral disc push the nucleus pulposis (NP) [Section 7.1.2.3] in a radial direction but the annulus fibrosis (AF) [Section 7.1.2.3] will restrain it. However, over a 24-hour period, discs are compressed due to gravity during the day, which means that we decrease in height up to a centimetre by the end of each waking day, and decompress (lengthen) when we sleep.

7.3.3 Age-Related Spinal Pathology

- **Young child** genetic disturbances of formation and growth, eg unsegmented vertebrae.
- **Adolescent** affected by growth spurt and increasing stress, eg scoliosis [Section 7.3.5.1], Scheuermanns kyphosis [Section 7.3.4.3], spondylolysis
- **Young adult** risk-taking activities, eg spinal fractures, muscle and ligament strains
- **Middle age** disc becomes vulnerable, eg disc protrusion
- **Elderly** degenerative changes and neoplasia, eg osteoarthrosis and secondary tumours.

7.3.4 Common Spinal Pathologies

7.3.4.1 Degenerative disc disease

Degenerative changes causing narrowing of the intervertebral discs commonly occur with age. These changes lead to increased stress on the facet joints, which may develop degenerative changes, synovitis, and osteophyte formation.

7.3.4.2 Ankylosing spondylitis (AS)

Ankylosing spondylitis (AS) is an inflammatory disorder of the synovial joints of the spine. People with AS complain of spinal stiffness, pain in the thoracolumbar area that is frequently proportional to activity; limited and decreased chest expansion.

7.3.4.3 Scheuermanns disease/kyphosis/osteochondritis

Scheuermanns disease is a relatively common condition active only in teenage years when inflammatory changes in the end plates of the vertebral bodies of the thoracic or lumbar spine allow herniation of the disc into the vertebral body.

Anterior wedging of vertebrae and discs leads to increased kyphosis in thoracic spine associated with compensatory increased lordosis of the lumbar spine, or increased kyphosis (decreased lordosis) of the lumbar spine with compensatory loss of thoracic kyphosis resulting in what appears to be a very flat back or straight spine.

Effects of anterior wedging appear not to change with time. Clinical evidence suggests that *hatha yoga* can be of great benefit to people suffering from the effects of Scheuermanns disease.

7.3.5 Musculoskeletal and Other Abnormalities of the Spine

7.3.5.1 Scoliosis

Scoliosis is a lateral flexion of the vertebral column, usually in the thoracic region, often accompanied by lateral rotation of the vertebrae. Compensatory curves may arise, helping to keep body mass over the base of support and eyes horizontal.

7.3.5.2 Torticollis

Torticollis (wry neck) is a lateral deformity of the cervical spine. It may be acute and resolve spontaneously or with treatment, or it may be congenital (from birth) caused by fibrosis of the sternocleidomastoid muscle.

7.3.5.3 Spina bifida

Spina bifida is a congenital defect of the vertebral column in which the laminae fail to unite at the midline. Protrusion of the membranes (meninges) or the spinal cord itself can result in paralysis, loss of urinary bladder control and absence of reflexes.

7.4 APPLIED ANATOMY OF THE SPINE AND TRUNK IN *HATHA YOGA* POSTURES

As for the other major joints, the health of the spine partly relates to maintaining adequate circulation, strength, flexibility and musculoskeletal alignment [Section 1.8.2].

7.4.1 Increasing Spinal Strength: The Central *Bandhas* of *Hatha Yoga*

The ancient *yoga* locking mechanisms known as *bandhas* [Section 1.7.3] are subtle internal locking techniques that are used to strengthen and protect crucial parts of the body, especially during the more strenuous *yoga* postures or exercises. *Bandhas* are also used to generate and move energy in the body through the differential pressures they create [Section 1.0.4].

As with the *nadis* [Section 1.7.2, 9.7], the *bandhas* deal with subtle energies and etheric principles in the body and, like *nadis*, which can be expressed physically as nerves, *bandhas* can also be expressed on a physical level, as the co-activation (simultaneous tensing) of antagonistic (opposing) muscle groups around a joint complex [Sections 1.7.3.1, & 7.1.5]. The *bandhas* that are most referred to in the ancient texts are those dealing with the strength and stability of the spine and the ability to generate and move energy through the spine. These central or spinal *bandhas* are *mula bandha* [Section 7.4.1.1], *uddiyana bandha* [Section 7.4.1.2] and *jalandhara bandha* [Section 7.4.1.3].

7.4.1.1 *Mula bandha* [Figure 7.10c & Appendix C] [Figure 7.10b & Appendix C]

Mula bandha, the *yogic* root lock, is a subtle internal locking technique that is used to strengthen and protect the lower trunk especially during the more strenuous *yoga* postures or exercises. *Mula bandha* is also used to generate and move energy through the body.

Mula bandha can be expressed in two distinct ways. *Ha-mula bandha* is a compressive (high pressure) co-activation of the circular (or circumferential) muscles of the lower trunk. This muscle group is essentially the muscles of forced abdominal exhalation (MFAE). *Tha-mula bandha* is an expansive (low pressure) co-activation of opposing muscles of the lower trunk. Both of these *bandhas* can increase spinal stability and trunk strength by increasing intra-abdominal pressure (IAP). This can be achieved in both cases by movement of the diaphragm toward the abdomen. The diaphragm can move towards the abdomen either due to diaphragmatic activation or via passive movement through voluntary compression of the chest (*ha-uddiyana bandha* [Section 7.4.1.3.2]) while retaining the breath inside (which is essentially a Valsalva manoeuvre [Section 7.4.1.3.2]).

7.4.1.1.1 *Ha-mula bandha*: a compressive *bandha* of the lower trunk [Figure 7.10c & Appendix C]

The *mula bandha* that is generally taught, practised and described in the texts is essentially a *ha-bandha* (a compressive *bandha*) [Section 1.7.3.4]. It is generally a heating *bandha*, ie it acts to generate heat by compression of the lower trunk, then dissipates this heat to the other parts of the body that are at relatively lower pressures [Section 1.0.4].

7.4.1.1.1.1 *Ha-mula bandha* via co-activation of opposing muscles [Appendix C]

The first type of *ha-mula bandha* can be generated via <u>co-activation</u> of opposing muscles around the <u>lower back joint complex</u> (<u>lumbosacrococcygeal spine</u>), which can give strength and stability to the lower trunk in *yoga* in the same way that the <u>co-activation</u> of <u>antagonistic</u> <u>flexor–extensor</u> pairs has been shown to have a stabilising effect on the <u>lumbar spine</u> [Richardson & Jull, 1995; Cholewicki *et al.*, 1997]. The muscles that are <u>co-activated</u> in *ha-mula bandha* are:

- <u>transverses abdominis</u>
- <u>lumbar multifidus</u>
- <u>obliquus externus abdominis</u> (<u>external oblique muscles</u>)
- <u>obliquus internus abdominis</u> (<u>internal oblique muscles</u>)
- <u>perineum muscles</u> [Section 4.4.8].

When *ha-mula bandha* is applied correctly the lower abdomen (inferior to the naval), the <u>lumbar spine</u>, and the perineum move inward towards each other and the waist narrows. This muscle group (engaged in *ha-mula bandha*) is essentially the muscles of forced abdominal exhalation (MFAE). It is important to note that this group (MFAE) opposes (is the <u>antagonist</u> of) the diaphragm, which is the single muscle of 'abdominal' inhalation. Therefore, if *ha-mula bandha* is engaged it is very difficult to activate the diaphragm (i.e. to breathe in a relaxed and natural way) because diaphragmatic activity is inhibited (via the reciprocal relaxation reflex [Section 12.7.2.2.2.1]) by the activity of the MFAE as they work to generate *ha-mula bandha*.

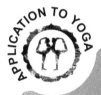

No 7.3 Breathe into the abdomen to help you relax your back muscles, relieve lower back pain increase trunk mobility

The diaphragm is the main muscle of breathing into the abdomen. Diaphragmatic activity (as in an abdominal inhalation) causes reciprocal relaxation or inhibition of the muscles of forced abdominal exhalation (MFAE) (which are also the muscles that can pull the navel to the spine). These muscles (MFAE) can be felt to be active all around the lower trunk. They tend to be overactive in many people with lower back pain and increase paraspinal muscle spasm. Breathing into the abdomen using your main muscle of inhalation (the diaphragm) can help relax (switch off) the muscles of forced abdominal exhalation (which include many muscles that tense the lower back), and allow the spine to be naturally tractioned (lengthened). This allows more uniform movements of each of the vertebrae in the spine and thus minimises any painful excessive movements in any one part of the spine.

During the mildest form of *ha-mula bandha,* the upper abdominal muscles, the <u>erector spinae</u>, the buttocks (<u>gluteal muscles</u>) and the <u>anal sphincter</u> muscles may be kept relaxed. However, if a particular *asana* requires additional <u>spinal</u> stability and/or support, then stronger <u>spinal extensor</u> muscles such as the <u>erector spinae</u>, and stronger <u>spinal flexor</u> muscles such as the <u>rectus abdominis</u>, may also be recruited and activated.

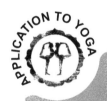

No 7.4 Avoid pulling the navel to the spine to enhance trunk stability, core strength and spinal mobility and to reduce stress

Pulling the navel to the spine and holding it there during inhalation can create a firm abdomen and give limited trunk stability and core strength but it tends to increase stress, inhibit natural (diaphragmatic) breathing, decrease trunk mobility and sometimes cause lower back pain to get worse. Pulling the navel to the spine is an important part of specific advanced breath-control exercises (pranayama) which are generally only of value if the practitioner has already mastered the posture, exercise or activity they are doing at the time. Otherwise natural (diaphragmatic) breathing (which does not include pulling the navel to the spine) is the best breathing in most instances for most people in yoga, exercise and in life.

7.4.1.1.1.2 *Ha-mula bandha* via increasing intra-abdominal pressure (IAP)

A second method that allows a *ha-mula bandha* to give stability and strength to the lower trunk in *yoga* is via the use of <u>intra-abdominal pressure</u> (IAP), which is primarily generated by the transverses abdominis

(Cholewicki et al., 1999) but also by obliquus externus abdominis and obliquus internus abdominis. The IAP effect is supplemented by the effects of other muscles and other *bandhas* – in particular by the compression of the chest that is used for a forced expiration as for *ha-uddiyana bandha* [Section 7.4.1.3]. This mechanism can increase spinal stability without the additional co-activation of specific spinal extensors and spinal flexors.

Voluntary generation of *ha-mula bandha* via the use of intra-abdominal pressure (IAP) can be achieved in two main ways:

- By making a forced expiration, which uses primarily the transversus abdominis, obliquus externus abdominis and obliquus internus abdominis to compress the abdomen.
- By making an attempt at a forced expiration while keeping the *glottis* closed. In other words making the same muscular tension one would generate to exhale, while holding the breath in and keeping the air passages closed. This is essentially the same as making what is referred to as a Valsalva manoeuvre [Astrand & Rodahl, 1986].

Increasing IAP while retaining the breath is practised in the more advanced forms of *pranayama* (eg *nadi avaroda pranayama* [Yogeshwarandaji, 1970]) and can also be incorporated into *asana* work. This method of generating a *ha-mula bandha* can be extremely effective in stabilising the spine. It is also able to manifest tremendous amounts of energy, which can be used to heat the body, and to generate the strength required to do many of the arm balancing postures and other exercises where much physical power is required.

However, if the body is not adequately prepared, and/or if this *pranayama* is not properly performed, **this *pranayama* can be extremely dangerous in its final form**. This method should not be attempted with fully inflated lungs unless instructed by an experienced teacher, and only after the body has been strengthened by years of regular *asana* and *pranayama* practice.

When IAP is increased while maintaining an internal breath retention (ie holding the breath in), the increase in pressure is able to move energy through the body with great force. *Hatha yoga* masters and others (such as the *Shaolin* monks) have used this method in many public demonstrations over the years to demonstrate great feats of strength, imperviousness to being pierced by sharp objects such as spears, and the ability to stop the heart. Many powerful acts can be achieved when this technique is mastered. However, it has to be contained in a safe way. Therefore, one must have a good practical understanding of all of the other *ha-* and *tha- bandhas* of the body. If the pressure generated inside the body is not adequately contained there is a grave risk of rupturing important blood vessels that can lead to paralysis, heart attack or stroke, depending on where the rupture takes place. The medical literature contains many citations of *yoga* practitioners being injured after practising breathing exercises or after doing related *bandha* style exercises [Corrigan, 1969; Hanus *et al.*, 1977; Fong et al., 1993].

A mild, gentle form of this method of increasing IAP with breath retention can be safely practised if one only inhales one quarter to one third of the full volume of the lungs and then makes only a gentle compression of the abdomen. This can be attempted by people with some experience of *asana* and *pranayama* but the effects should be constantly monitored and the practice temporarily or permanently discontinued if headache or other symptoms of high blood pressure are observed.

Although this type of *ha-mula bandha* appears to give some protective effect to the spine when it carries a load, research indicates this protective effect is most powerful when the spine is in its neutral position. When there is any axial rotation in the spine the ability to generate *mula bandha* using intra-abdominal pressure (IAP) is not as great as when the spine is in neutral. The ability to generate IAP and *mula bandha* is limited even further when the spine is flexed and axially rotated [Goldish et al., 1994]. Hence, the most dangerous sorts of postures are those that involve a combination of twisting (spinal axial rotation) and forward-bending (spinal forward flexion).

Therefore, there are two distinct mechanisms for generation of *mula bandha* and for the stability of the lower back joint complex (lumbosacrococcygeal spine) in general. One is the antagonistic (opposing) spinal muscle co-activation, and the second is abdominal muscle activation for the generation of intra-abdominal pressure (IAP) . Both mechanisms have been shown to be effective – both separately and in combination – for stabilising models of a lumbar spine (Cholewicki *et al.*, 1999). The critical load and the stability of spinal models increased with either increased antagonist co-activation forces or increased IAP along with increased abdominal spring force (Cholewicki et al., 1999). Both mechanisms are also effective in providing mechanical stability to the spinal models when activated simultaneously.

7.4.1.1.2 *Tha-mula bandha*: an expansive *bandha* of the lower trunk [Figure 7.10b & Appendix C]

Tha-mula bandha is an expansive bandha of the lower back joint complex that is able to draw energy towards the abdomen. *Tha-mula bandha* is rarely discussed in the texts but essentially involves an expansion of the same region that *ha-mula bandha* is generally compressing. The most commonly seen form of *tha-mula bandha* is the nauli kriya , which is the co-activation of the spinal flexor rectus abdominis and the spinal extensors done on an exhalation-retention with the chest expanded (*tha-uddiyana bandha*). The expansive nature of this *bandha* (*nauli*) was proven early in the twentieth century and published in the first Volume of the scientific journal Yoga Mimamsa in 1923. This expansion, or reduction in pressure, of the lower trunk can also be done in many postures such as *adho mukha svanasana* (downward dog pose) by simply pushing the hips towards the hands without the need to hold the breath out. However, the easiest way to generate a *tha-mula bandha* is to try to totally relax all the abdominal and lower back musculature, and then lengthen the spine. This is best achieved in the simplest version of the standing posture *utkatasana* with a straight spine perpendicular to the floor or in a sitting posture such as padmasana (lotus or cross-legged posture). A light downward pressure should be maintained on the sitting bones (ischial tuberosities) and the tail-bone (coccyx) while the spine is lengthened (tractioned) away from the floor. Lifting the shoulders as in *utkatasana* (shoulder elevation and flexion) can facilitate spinal tractioning. The muscles of the abdomen should be kept as relaxed as possible. When maximum height has been achieved, then the abdomen and lower back can be felt to have muscle tone reflecting a co-activation of the spinal flexors and spinal extensors. The lengthening of the lumbar spine using a co-activation of spinal flexors and spinal extensors to create t*ha-mula bandha* is analogous to the lengthening of the fingers using a co-activation of wrist flexors and wrist extensors to create *tha-mani bandha* [Section 3.9.1.2.2].

Co-activation of trunk flexor and extensor muscles is present around a neutral spine posture in healthy individuals. This co-activation is seen to increase as weight is added to the body, and is believed to be part of a neuromuscular system that provides mechanical stability to the lumbar spine (Cholewicki et al., 1997).

Voluntary generation of *tha-mula bandha* by co-activation of antagonistic (opposing) muscle groups can be achieved in three main ways. Each of these ways moves the spine one vertebra at a time without the help of gravity, momentum or another external force such as the assistance of your hands, in any of the three primary movement planes of the spine. i.e. flexion–extension, right–left axial rotation and right–left lateral flexion.

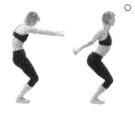

- o **Flexion–extension *tha-mula bandha*** can be generated in seated meditative postures (neutral or straight spine), forward bending postures (spinal flexion) or backward bending postures (spinal extension), by using anterior and posterior spinal muscles to move the spine one vertebra at a time in these directions. A good method is to try to move the whole spine from the base upwards. This method gives effective trunk muscle activation and power transfer. Also, it effectively moves blood out of the vertebral veins around the spine that are unique in the body because they do not have one-way back flow valves. It is important that when you bend forward the front does not get shorter but the back gets longer. Similarly when you bend backwards the front gets longer while the back does not shorten.

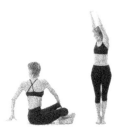

- o **Right–left axial rotation *tha-mula bandha*** can be generated in a right-sided twisting posture (spinal right axial rotation) by moving/turning each vertebra to the right side one at a time. You can further increase the twist by protracting the left shoulder and retracting the right shoulder. The effectiveness of the twist can be further increased by pushing the right sitting bone down and forward and the left sitting bone down and backwards. This creates *tha-mula bandha* because it effectively leads to co-activation of right internal abdominal oblique and left external abdominal oblique muscles that effectively firm the outer wall of the abdomen without hardening on the inside of the abdomen and/or inhibiting diaphragmatic activity and natural breathing.

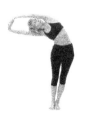

- o **Right–left lateral flexion *mula bandha*** can be generated in right-sided bending postures (spinal right lateral flexion) by using right and left lateral spinal muscles to move the spine one vertebra at a time laterally to the right side. Lateral spinal flexion can be enhanced by elevating the left shoulder and depressing the left pelvis [Section 4.2.4.2]. Lateral spinal flexion can also be enhanced by trying to pull the right sitting bone (ischial tuberosity) forwards and upwards towards the right side of chest to activate right spinal lateral flexors. Co-activation with left spinal lateral flexors (and hence a *tha-mula bandha*) can be achieved by laterally flexing the spine to the right in such a way that the left side of spine lengthens during right lateral flexion rather more than the right side of the spine shortens during right lateral flexion. While deep lateral spinal muscles are co-activated and maintain stability of the spine generally it is possible to make the trunk feel firm to the touch on the right side and feel relaxed at the front and left side. In this situation the increased activity in the right side causes reciprocal relaxation of the left side and assists in enhancing circulation.

Tha-mula bandha can be created in several other ways. The most effective of these ways involve using intelligent postures, and ways of getting into postures, to oblige co-activation of opposing muscles groups around the lower trunk (waist) joint complex. These types of *mula bandha*, which utilise co-activation of antagonists, can be significantly enhanced and strengthened by recruiting (activating) other muscles with fascial connections [Sections 1.3.2.1.3 & 1.7.2.2.1.1] to the muscles of *mula bandha* (transverse abdominis, lumbar multifidus, obliquus externus abdominis and obliquus internus abdominis). Activation muscles with fascial connections to *mula bandha* can make a reflex activation of *mula bandha*. Such muscles include:

- o muscles of the perineum [Section 4.4.9]
- o latissimus dorsi (eg generate *amsa bandha* [Section 2.5.1])
- o neck flexor and neck extensor muscles (ie generate *jalandhara bandha* [Section 7.4.1.2]).

Therefore, these methods often rely on stretch-reflex activation of trunk muscles via activation of upper and lower limb muscles. For example, by 'stretching the mat with your feet' in postures such as *parsvottonasana*

, this will activate hip flexors on the front lower limb and hip extensors on rear lower limb, which causes stretch-reflex activation of the spinal flexors and spinal extensors and hence a *tha-mula bandha*. In this instance the front and back of the trunk feel firm to touch while the sides can remain quite relaxed. Flexor-extensor co-activation (*bandhas*) such as this can effectively stabilise and protect the spine in all

postures that involve flexion or extension of the spine such as *pascimottasana* and *urdhva*

mukha svanasana . A similar effect can be achieved with stretch reflex activation of the side spine (lateral trunk) muscles when feet are used to stretch or squash the mat in a lateral plane using the hip abductors or hip adductors respectively to create a lateral flexion *tha-mula bandha*. In this instance the sides of the trunk feel firm to touch while the front and back are quite relaxed.

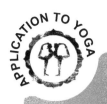

No 7.5 Use *tha-mula bandha* to enhance trunk stability, core strength and abdominal firmness whilst remaining relaxed

Trunk stability, core strength and abdominal firmness can be achieved without the need to pull the navel to the spine by:

- actively tractioning (lengthening) the spine using postural muscles and/or by moving the shoulders and hips away from each other
- actively rotating (twisting) the spine using postural muscles and/or by pushing one hip and the opposite shoulder forward
- actively side-bending (laterally flexing) the spine using postural muscles and/or one shoulder forward and up and the opposite hip forward and up
- activating hip abductors in a posture by 'trying' to push the thighs (or feet) away from each other
- activating hip adductors in a posture by 'trying' to squeeze the thighs (or feet) towards each other
- simultaneously activating hip flexors and extensors by, for example, stretching the mat with your feet in standing postures
- bringing the weight of the body towards the front of the foot as opposed to the heel when standing.

7.4.1.2 *Jalandhara bandha* [Appendix C, Figure 7.8]

A similar muscular locking device to that discussed for the <u>lumbar spine</u> and *mula bandha* [Section 7.4.1.1] exists for the stabilisation of the neck and head. This muscle locking system is known in *hatha yoga* as *jalandhara bandha* (the chin lock). *Jalandhara bandha* is essentially the same as the <u>co-activation</u> of <u>antagonistic</u> (opposing) <u>muscle groups</u> of the <u>neck joint complex</u>. Usually it is seen only as a <u>co-activation</u> of the <u>head/neck flexors</u> and the <u>head/neck extensors</u>, but similar effects can be also achieved for <u>right–left lateral flexion</u> and <u>right–left axial rotation</u> in a manner analogous to that described for *mula bandha* [Section 7.4.1.1.1]. *Jalandhara bandha* is maintained by fully lengthening from the <u>occiput</u> (base of the skull) to the <u>first thoracic vertebrae</u> (T1). In *jalandhara bandha* the jaw should be kept relaxed and the shoulders gently depressed and relaxed.

7.4.1.2.1 *Ha-jalandhara bandha*: a compressive *bandha* of the neck joint complex

Ha-jalandhara bandha [Appendix C, Figure 7.8a] is the more common form of *jalandhara bandha* that is usually seen in the texts. It is a compressive *bandha* of the <u>neck joint complex</u> that is able to push energy away from the neck, and restrict the flow of energy (including heat, pressure, blood etc) through the neck. Essentially it is an attempt at <u>head flexion</u> with <u>neck extension</u>. In an analogy with the hand, it would be like making the closed fist of *ha-mani bandha* [Section 3.9.1.2.1]. Practically, *ha-jalandhara bandha* is performed by gently <u>flexing</u> the head so that the chin descends, and then gently <u>retracting</u> (<u>extending</u>) the neck so that the chin moves towards the throat and towards the middle of the <u>cervical spine</u>. Application of *ha-jalandhara bandha* is essential in many *pranayamas* (breathing exercises) for preventing pressure changes to the head and brain. This is especially the case in *pranayamas* with *antara kumbhaka* (internal retention or holding the breath in) when the abdominal muscles are being engaged to increase <u>intra-abdominal pressure</u> (IAP) as described for *ha-mula bandha* [Section 7.4.1.1.1.2].

Figure 7.8 shows correct (safe) [Figure 7.8a] and incorrect (unsafe) [Figure 7.8b] versions of *ha-jalandhara bandha*. The correct form uses <u>head flexion</u> and <u>neck extension</u> (balanced <u>co-activation</u> of <u>antagonistic</u> (opposing) <u>muscle groups</u>) while the incorrect form uses <u>head flexion</u> and <u>neck flexion</u> (unbalanced overuse of <u>flexors</u> and underuse of <u>extensors</u> with possible risk of damage to the <u>spinal cord</u> or to the <u>vertebrae</u>)

7.4.1.2.2 *Tha-jalandhara bandha*: an expansive *bandha* of the neck joint complex

Tha-jalandhara bandha [Appendix C, Figure 7.8c] is an often used but rarely named form of *jalandhara bandha* that is sometimes called *urd-jalandhara bandha* by traditional *Indian yogis*. *Tha-jalandhara bandha* is used in postures such as *urdhva mukha svanasana* (up-dog pose) and many others [Appendix C]. It is an expansive *bandha* of the neck joint complex that is able to pull energy towards the neck and enhance the flow of energy (including heat, pressure, blood) through the neck. Essentially, it is an attempt at head extension with neck flexion. In an analogy with the hand it would be like stretching into the fingers like *tha-mani bandha* [Section 3.9.1.2.2]. Practically, *tha-jalandhara bandha* is performed by gently bringing the chin up and taking the throat slightly forward.

Figure 7.8 shows correct (safe) [Figure 7.8c] and incorrect (unsafe) [Figure 7.8d] versions of *tha-jalandhara bandha*. The correct form uses head extension and neck flexion (balanced co-activation of antagonistic (opposing) muscle groups) while the incorrect form uses head extension and neck extension (unbalanced overuse of extensors and underuse of flexors with possible risk of spinal nerve impingement or damage to the vertebrae).

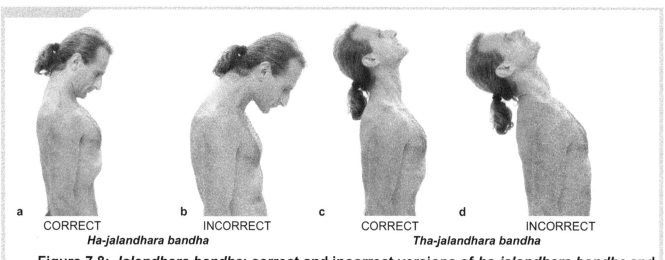

a CORRECT   b INCORRECT   c CORRECT   d INCORRECT

Ha-jalandhara bandha   *Tha-jalandhara bandha*

Figure 7.8: *Jalandhara bandha*: correct and incorrect versions of *ha-jalandhara bandha* and *tha-jalandhara bandha*

It is important to understand that the position of the neck joint complex is not as important as the activity of the muscle groups in the neck joint complex. For example, *tha-jalandhara bandha* should also be gently

applied in *sirsasana* (headstand) as head extensor activity with simultaneous and balanced neck flexor activity. Therefore, in a headstand the neck is made more stable by doing resisted head extension (trying to push, but not actually moving, the crown of the head gently into the floor in the direction of the back of the head) while doing resisted neck flexion (trying to move, but not actually moving, the throat very gently forward towards the chin).

7.4.1.3 *Uddiyana bandha* [Appendix C, Figure 7.9 & 7.10]

The third important *yogic* muscle lock is known as *uddiyana bandha* [Appendix C, Figure 7.9 & &.10]. *Uddiyana bandha* is essentially a co-activation of the intercostalis externus and intercostalis internus (external and internal intercostal muscles) with the small segmental flexors and extensors of the thoracic spine. This co-activation leads to a lift and expansion of the chest and slight rounding or kyphosing of the upper back. The throat should be kept relaxed with the shoulders gently depressed and relaxed. When *uddiyana bandha* is generated and held correctly, a reduction in the pressure of the chest cavity is created. This causes the upper abdomen to be passively drawn inwards towards the spine, pressure to be slightly reduced in the head and, if the nasal passages are open, air to be drawn into the lungs.

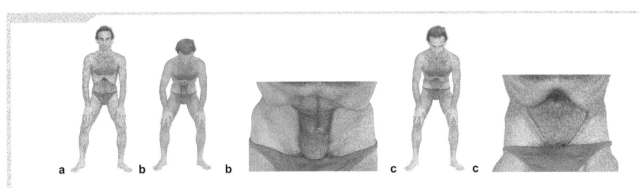

Figure 7.9 Three versions of *tha-uddiyana bandha* with *bahya kumbhaka* (exhalation retention)

(a) *Tha-uddiyana* with *tha-mula bandha* (ie trunk muscles used to lengthen <u>lumbar spine</u>);

(b) *Nauli* (= *tha-uddiyana* with *ha-mula bandha* defining the <u>rectus abdominis</u>);

(c) *Tha-uddiyana* with *ha-mula bandha* (defining the <u>obliquus externus abdominis</u>).

7.4.1.3.1 *Tha-uddiyana bandha*: an expansive *bandha* of the thoracic joint complex

Uddiyana bandha as described above and in most texts is essentially a *tha-bandha* (an expansive *bandha*), which generates a reduction in pressure in the <u>thoracic joint complex</u>. *Tha-uddiyana bandha,* therefore, has the ability to draw air into the chest exactly as in a <u>deep thoracic inhalation</u>, and it has the ability to draw the abdominal contents towards the chest when practised after the breath is held out (exhalation retention). *Tha-uddiyana bandha* alone can be done with a completely relaxed abdomen [Figure 7.9a]. This *bandha* can also be practised with *ha-mula bandha* in its <u>flexor-extensor antagonistic co-activation</u> form [Section 7.4.1.1.1.1] as in *nauli kriya* [Section 12.7.1.3.2, Figure 12.1] to clearly define the <u>rectus abdominis</u> [Figure 7.9b]. *Tha-uddiyana bandha* can also be practised with *ha-mula bandha* in its increasing <u>intra-abdominal pressure</u> (IAP) form [Section 7.4.1.1.1.2] to clearly define the <u>obliquus externus abdominis</u> [Figure 7.9c].

7.4.1.3.2 *Ha-uddiyana bandha*: a compressive *bandha* of the thoracic joint complex

Ha-uddiyana bandha is another type of <u>co-activation</u> of <u>intercostalis externus</u> and <u>intercostalis internus</u> (<u>external</u> and <u>internal intercostal muscles</u>) with the small segmental <u>flexors</u> and <u>extensors</u> of the <u>thoracic spine</u>. The same muscles that generate a <u>forced expiration</u> can form *ha-uddiyana bandha*. *Ha-uddiyana bandha* has the effect of compressing the chest as one would in a <u>forced expiration</u> or, if *ha-uddiyana bandha* is done with the breath held in (<u>inhalation retention</u>), it will increase the <u>intra-abdominal pressure</u> (IAP), as does *ha-mula bandha* [Section 7.4.1.1.1.2] in the same way the <u>Valsalva manoeuvre</u> works [Appendices C & E] .

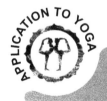

No 7.6 Use *ha-uddiyana bandha* and diaphragmatic breathing with *mula bandha* to enhance trunk stability, core strength and power (strength)

Trunk stability, core strength and power to lift into arm balances like handstand or *lolasana* can be enhanced by contracting the chest (as if you making a forced fast chest exhalation) to create *ha-uddiyana bandha* and by breathing into the abdomen using the <u>diaphragm</u>, while keeping the abdomen firm using a type of *mula bandha*. This increases the <u>intra-abdominal pressure</u> and brings the same type of strength to the arms and trunk that is seen using the <u>Valsalva maneouvre</u> without the associated potentially dangerous rapid increases in blood pressure.

In this case it is easier for most people to keep the abdominal wall firm by using *tha-mula bandha* as this does not inhibit the <u>diaphragm</u>, but an experienced practitioner can even use *ha-mula bandha* (which draws the navel closer to the spine) to keep the abdominal wall firm, because the chest compression of *ha-uddiyana bandha* inhibits chest inhalation (through chest expansion) and thus inhibits the <u>reciprocal relaxation</u> of the <u>diaphragm</u> by the *ha-mula bandha*.

7.4.1.4 *Maha bandha*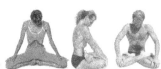

When all three central (spinal) *bandhas* are mastered and applied correctly and concurrently *maha bandha* is achieved [Figure 7.10]. To correctly practise *maha bandha,* whether sitting or standing, the following is required:

- The iliac crests (top of the hip) should be directly above the ischial tuberosities (sitting bones) ,
- The tip of the coccyx gently presses slightly anteriorly to the sacrum with the mid lumbar spine drawn inwards (*ha-mula bandha*)
- The waist narrows so that the lower abdomen and the lumbar spine move towards each other (*ha-mula bandha*),
- The chest and upper back expand and are positioned anteriorly and posteriorly an equal distance away from the central axis of the trunk (*tha-uddiyana bandha*)
- The back of the neck should maintain its maximum length whether the head is up (*tha-jalandhara bandha*) or down (*ha-jalandhara bandha*).

The positioning of the spine when the three *bandhas* are correctly applied in *maha bandha* while sitting re-creates the natural curvature of the spine from the coccyx to the base of the neck. This has the following effects:

- It generates a positive pressure at the base of the spine (*ha-mula bandha*) which helps push energy towards the head
- It generates a negative pressure in the chest and thorax (*tha-uddiyana bandha*) which pulls energy up the spine, and
- In *ha-jalandhara bandha,* when the head is down (head flexion) with the neck moving slightly backwards (neck extension), a protective downwards positive pressure is generated at the anterior of the neck. *Ha-jalandhara bandha* prevents unwanted increases of pressure to the brain as a result of increases in pressure from the abdomen (*ha-mula bandha)* and chest (*ha-uddiyana bandha*).

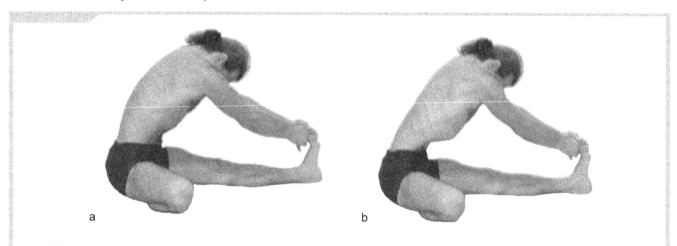

Figure 7.10 Two versions of *maha mudra* each with *maha bandha*

(*ha-jalandhara bandha, tha-uddiyana bandha* and *ha-mula bandha*)
(a) *Maha mudra* with *antara kumbhaka* (inhalation retention)
(b) *Maha mudra* with *bahya kumbhaka* (exhalation retention)

7.4.1.5 Interconnectedness of the *bandhas*

The three central *bandhas* actually help to generate and create each other:

- ***Ha-jalandhara bandha* helps generate *ha-mula bandha***: Bringing the chin towards the throat, or taking the head down (into flexion) and the neck back (into extension) (*ha-jalandhara bandha*) causes the lower abdomen to firm (*ha-mula bandha*). This effect is due to fascial connections and a nervous system connection down the spine and is especially noticeable in postures such as *uttanasana*

and *cataranga dandasasa* which is much more powerful and therefore easier to hold if the head and neck are kept in *ha-jalandhara bandha,* as opposed to *tha-jalandhara bandha* as demonstrated in B.K.S. Iyengar's *Light on Yoga* [1966].

- **Ha-jalandhara bandha** helps generate **tha-uddiyana bandha**: The lengthening of the back of the neck along with the flexing of the head in *ha-jalandhara bandha* also causes the upper back to lengthen and thus helps create *tha-uddiyana bandha*.

- **Tha-uddiyana bandha** helps generate **ha-mula bandha or tha-mula bandha**: *Tha-uddiyana bandha* creates an expansion in the chest and generates a negative pressure that draws the abdominal contents upwards allowing the lower abdomen to move inwards (*mula bandha*). This facilitates the creation of either the formation of a *ha-mula bandha* (if the transversus abdominis is also activated) or a *tha-mula bandha* (if transversus abdominis remains relaxed).

- **Tha-uddiyana bandha** helps generate **ha-jalandhara bandha**: As the chest expands in *tha-uddiyana bandha*, it also lifts and brings the sternum closer to the chin and helps to create *ha-jalandhara bandha*.

- **Ha-mula bandha** helps generate **tha-uddiyana bandha**: *Ha-mula bandha* can cause narrowing of the lower abdomen and lower half of the trunk due to the activation of the transverses abdominis muscle. This exerts a positive pressure on the diaphragm, which causes the chest walls to expand outward helping to generate *tha-uddiyana bandha*.

7.4.2 Increasing Spinal Flexibility

Spinal flexibility is achieved by the use of the various postures and breathing exercises which, when performed correctly, not only move the spine into flexion, extension, lateral flexion and axial rotation, but can also gently traction the spine.

A normal spine usually consists of flexible regions and stiff regions. In many of the *yoga* postures, *bandhas* [Section 7.4.1] are used to stabilise the more flexible and generally weaker areas of the spine (such as those commonly found in the lumbosacral region) so that less flexible areas of the spine, such as those that tend to occur near the region of the thoracolumbar junction, can be accessed.

7.4.2.1 Increasing flexion of the spine

Once the *bandhas* have been firmly applied, the spine may be flexed carefully. Care must be taken because if the flexion is excessive, that part of the spine has a risk of intervertebral disc herniation (rupture of the discs), or excessive neural tensioning (over-stretching of the nerves) (Section 9.7.3).

Spinal flexion is safest when the hips are not flexed and/or the knees are flexed. Unless one has a uniformly flexible spine and flexible hamstrings, or until one has a firm practical understanding of *mula bandha* and how to establish a grip of the lower abdominal and lower back muscles, spinal flexion should not be performed with the hips flexed and knees extended (straight).

Postures such as *uttanasana* (standing forward bend) and *pascimottanasana* (seated forward bend) are best performed with knees bent until the hamstring muscles have become flexible and the abdominal muscle grip has been established. If a person with stiff short <u>hamstrings</u> attempts a forward bend with <u>extended</u> (straight) knees, then the hips will be limited in the amount they can <u>flex</u> and so the <u>spine</u> will <u>flex</u> excessively. Since a person who is stiff in the <u>hamstrings</u> is also usually a beginner in *yoga,* they probably also do not understand the need to keep the <u>spinal</u> and abdominal muscles firm during this posture, nor do they have the ability to do so.

If, however, a practitioner with flexible hips and <u>hamstrings</u> attempts postures such as *uttanasana*

(standing forward bend) and *pascimottanasana* (seated forward bend), with the knees <u>extended</u> (straight), then the length in the <u>hamstrings</u> will allow the hips to <u>flex</u> sufficiently so that the <u>spine</u> is in only very minor <u>flexion</u>, hence negating the danger if these people have not tensed their abdominal muscles. If a flexible person wishes to <u>flex</u> their <u>spine</u> in a forward bend, they need to actually reduce their amount of <u>hip flexion</u> by increasing their <u>posterior pelvic tilt</u> (moving the top of their hips backwards).

7.4.2.2 The different approaches to spinal flexion and forward bending for beginners

Different teachers and different styles of *yoga* have approached this problem in various ways. Sri B.K.S. Iyengar (author of *Light on Yoga*) [1966] teaches people with stiff <u>hamstrings</u> to not <u>flex</u> the <u>spine</u> in forward bends. Instead, these people may be told to sit on a bolster or blanket to reduce <u>hip flexion</u>, and allow for the re-creation of the natural <u>lumbar lordosis</u>. These people may then be asked to hold their feet via the use of a belt or strap. For most stiff people, this will minimise the risk of danger to the <u>intervertebral discs</u> and also begin to stretch out the hamstrings. For very stiff people, however, the amount of support required to achieve this posture requires a great deal of prop support under the buttocks.

Sri T.V.K. Desikachar (author of *Heart of Yoga*) [1995] suggests that people with stiff <u>hamstrings</u> <u>flex</u> (bend) their knees in forward bends to increase hip <u>flexion</u> and allow less <u>lumbar spinal flexion</u>. This minimises the <u>tension</u> (stretch) on the <u>hamstrings</u> and the <u>sciatic nerves</u>) and allows the <u>spine</u> and the <u>spinal cord</u> to experience some lengthening.

Sri K. Patabhi Jois (author of *Yoga Mala*) [1999], who teaches *astanga vinyasa yoga,* minimises some of the risks of forward bends for beginners in three ways. First, he asks his students to keep the <u>neck extended</u> in order to minimise the <u>dural tension</u> (stretch on the <u>spinal</u> nerves). Second, he holds the postures only for a few moments so students are kept warm because of frequent movement. Third, he asks for breathing to be deep with firm abdominal muscle activation to instill the practice of *mula bandha*.

All three styles have their pros and cons in terms of their approach to <u>spinal flexion</u>. All three approaches are reasonably safe for most students if they follow the instructions of any of these three very experienced teachers exactly. Problems may arise, however, when people with limited understanding of anatomy and physiology attempt to mix these styles and the instructions of these teachings without an understanding of why the teaching was given.

7.4.3 *Hatha Yoga* for the Prevention and Relief of Lower Back Pain, Upper Back Pain and Neck Pain

Back pain may be caused by a number of things including:
* <u>Intervertebral facet joint</u> problems
* <u>Intervertebral disc joint</u> problems
* <u>Nerve root entrapment</u> or <u>spinal nerve entrapment</u>
* <u>Sacroiliac joint</u> problems (may cause <u>lower back pain</u>)
* <u>Spinal ligament</u> injury
* <u>Para-spinal muscle spasm</u>
* Internal organ dysfunction (may cause <u>referred pain</u> [Section 9.4.3.2] to the back).

A healthy back is associated with the following:
- Safe lifting practices
- Cardiovascular (aerobic) fitness
- Decreased weight (especially abdominal fat)
- Good posture.

7.4.3.1 Hatha yoga for lower back pain (LBP) and stiffness

Lower back pain (LBP) is one of the most common problems that a student may complain about in a *yoga* class. LBP may be the temporary result of working too hard in a *yoga* posture, or it may be an injury or condition unrelated to *yoga*.

The approach to effectively dealing with a person with LBP in *yoga* must be specific to the individual. When practising *hatha yoga* with a person with LBP, it is important to consider:
- The **person's age** (eg old versus young).
- The **person's sex** (eg females need to consider the effects of menstruation, pregnancy and menopause).
- Any **pathology** the person may have (eg rheumatoid arthritis or osteoporosis).
- The person's **level of aerobic fitness**, flexibility and strength (eg back pain in dancers and gymnasts, as opposed to back pain in a stiff untrained office worker).
- The **type of problem.**
- The **cause of the LBP**.

Refer to the notes following on the common causes of back pain and the type of approach one can take with exercise and *yoga*.

Intervertebral facet joint problem
In cases where LBP originates in the intervertebral facet joint, pain often increases during and/or after back bending (hip extension and spinal extension) postures and decreases following forward bending (hip flexion and spinal flexion) postures.

Intervertebral disc-related problem
In cases where the LBP is caused by an intervertebral disc-related problem, back bending usually relieves the problem (hip extension and spinal extension) while forward bending (hip flexion and spinal flexion) usually aggravates the problem.

Nerve root or spinal nerve entrapment
In cases of LBP caused by nerve root or spinal nerve entrapment, postures that traction the spine often give relief. *Rope sirsasana* (hanging upside down on a rope swing) and rope-supported *adho mukha svanasana* (down-dog pose with a rope pulling the hips back) are often useful postures in these situations. Forward bending postures done with a straight or neutral spine by an intelligent practitioner can also be of assistance. If these postures are not available then spinal twists (spinal axial rotation) with minimal spinal flexion (eg cross-legged twisting) may be useful. As a last resort, manually assisted traction (eg the teacher stretches the student) in *adho mukha virasana* or similar postures may be of assistance, but this can tend to make a student dependent on their teacher.

Sacroiliac joint (SIJ) problems
If the lower back pain (LBP) is originating from the sacroiliac joint, then pain may be relieved with hip internal rotation while the hips are in a neutral or extended position, and with hip external rotation while the hips are in a flexed position.

Ligamentous injuries

Ligamentous injuries of the spine should not be stretched but just rested for some time; otherwise healing of the ligament may be very slow.

Paraspinal muscle spasm

Paraspinal muscle spasms may be helped in various postures with a gentle combination of resting the muscles, then gently activating the muscles and gently relaxing and stretching the muscles.

Addressing lower back pain (LBP) and stiffness with *yoga*

Generally, the following things may be applied to a student with a LBP, with the provision that the simplest variation of a pose should be done first. Movements that aggravate the problem should be avoided or modified. There should be a gradual progression in the difficulty of the exercises as the condition starts to show improvement.

* Increase the **flexibility of the hip flexor** muscles (in particular, iliopsoas).
* Increase the **strength and control** of the **lower abdominal muscles** (in particular the transversus abdominis)
* Increase the **strength and control** of the **muscles of the perineum**
* Increase the **strength and flexibility** of the **paraspinal muscles** (in particular the multifidus and other spinal extensor muscles)
* Increase the **strength and flexibility** of the **hip extensor muscles** (in particular the hamstrings and gluteus maximus)
* Increase the **strength and flexibility** of the **hip adductor** (inner thigh) **muscles** (in particular the adductor magnus and adductor longus)
* Increase the **flexibility of the thoracic spine, neck, and shoulders** while stabilising the lower spine
* Gradually **increase aerobic capacity**, (increased aerobic capacity has been correlated with a reduced level of lower back pain).

A recipe of postures to relieve back pain does not exist. Certain postures may be of use if they are done appropriately to the condition. Any pose may either improve a condition or make it worse. Working cautiously initially is always advised. See what the effects of *yoga* exercises and postures are the next day before increasing the intensity or duration of the exercises or postures, or before changing the exercises.

Standing poses may be helpful in some cases of LBP, but often they help more if done with the support of a wall or chair. The following postures may be of assistance if performed appropriately (ie suitably simplified, modified and/or assisted):

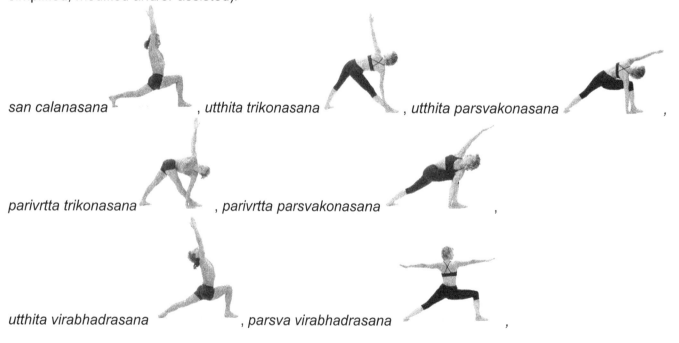

san calanasana , *utthita trikonasana* , *utthita parsvakonasana* ,

parivrtta trikonasana , *parivrtta parsvakonasana* ,

utthita virabhadrasana , *parsva virabhadrasana* ,

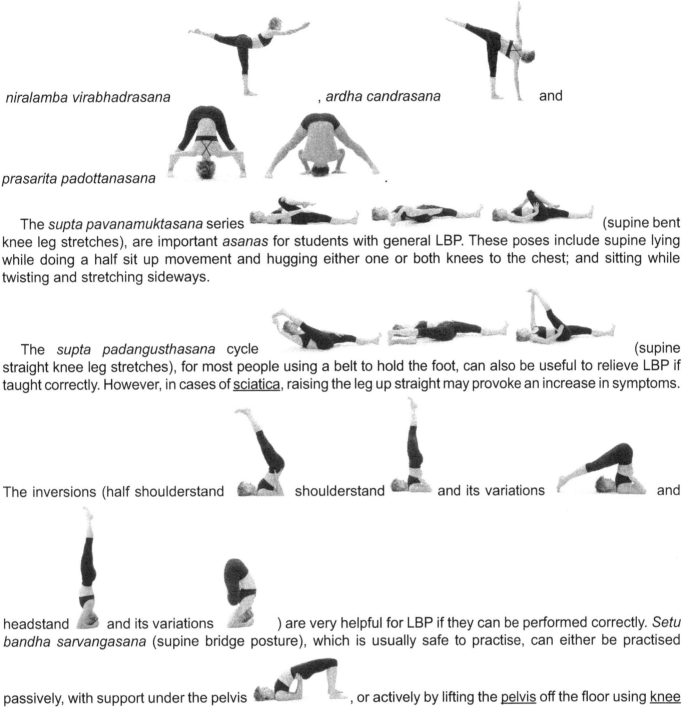

niralamba virabhadrasana   , *ardha candrasana*   and

prasarita padottanasana   .

The *supta pavanamuktasana* series   (supine bent knee leg stretches), are important *asanas* for students with general LBP. These poses include supine lying while doing a half sit up movement and hugging either one or both knees to the chest; and sitting while twisting and stretching sideways.

The *supta padangusthasana* cycle   (supine straight knee leg stretches), for most people using a belt to hold the foot, can also be useful to relieve LBP if taught correctly. However, in cases of <u>sciatica</u>, raising the leg up straight may provoke an increase in symptoms.

The inversions (half shoulderstand   shoulderstand   and its variations   and

headstand   and its variations   ) are very helpful for LBP if they can be performed correctly. *Setu bandha sarvangasana* (supine bridge posture), which is usually safe to practise, can either be practised

passively, with support under the pelvis   , or actively by lifting the <u>pelvis</u> off the floor using <u>knee</u>

<u>extensors</u> and <u>hip extensors</u> while contracting the lower abdominal muscles   .

7.4.3.2 *Hatha yoga* for upper back and thoracic spine (T/Sp) pain and stiffness

To self-mobilise the <u>thoracic spine</u> in *hatha yoga* the musculature of the area should be kept as relaxed as possible and the muscles of the arms and legs should be used in such a way as to lengthen the <u>spine</u>.

For example, in *adho mukha svanasana*   , <u>tractioning</u> (stretching) of the <u>spine</u> is due in part to gravitational effect of the semi-inverted position, but can also be encouraged by relaxing most of the <u>spine</u> and using the <u>plantarflexors</u> of the ankle as part of a <u>closed kinetic chain</u> to move the leg posteriorly.

To further address stiffness of the <u>thoracic spine</u> and other problems associated with such stiffness, focus on the following issues:

- Increase the mobility of the <u>scapulas</u> by moving and exercising the shoulder and arm joints
- Especially increase the ability to <u>protract</u> and <u>retract</u> the <u>scapulas</u> using both <u>open-chain exercises</u> (ie the upper limbs are free to move, while the trunk is kept still) and <u>closed-chain exercises</u> (ie the upper limbs are kept in a fixed position such as the floor, while the trunk is moved)
- Increase the strength and flexibility of the shoulder girdle
- Increase the mobility of the <u>thoracic spine</u>
- Increase the ability to <u>flex</u> the <u>thoracic spine</u>
- Increase the ability to <u>extend</u> the <u>thoracic spine</u>
- Increase the ability to <u>laterally flex</u> the <u>thoracic spine</u>
- Increase the ability to <u>axially rotate</u> the <u>thoracic spine</u>
- Avoid movements that aggravate the problem and rest the area in times of <u>acute pain</u> and <u>inflammation</u>.

7.4.3.3 *Hatha yoga* for neck and cervical spine (C/Sp) pain and stiffness

To address pain and/or stiffness of the neck and <u>cervical spine</u> and other problems associated with such stiffness, focus on the following issues:

- Increase the <u>mobility</u> of the <u>scapulas</u>. Especially increase the ability to <u>depress</u> and <u>elevate</u> the <u>scapulas</u> at will using both <u>open-chain exercises</u> (ie the upper limbs are free to move while the trunk is kept still) and <u>closed-chain exercises</u> (ie the upper limbs are kept in a fixed position such as on the floor, while the trunk is moved). Maintaining <u>amsa bandha</u> [Section 2.5.1] throughout a *yoga* practice is very important for the health of the cervical spine. In particular, it is very important to maintain activity of the underarm muscles <u>pectoralis major</u> and <u>latissimus dorsi</u> (<u>shoulder depressors</u>) [Section 2.5.1] as this helps to reciprocally relax the muscles on the side of the neck (<u>shoulder elevators</u>)
- Increase the strength and flexibility of the <u>shoulder girdle</u>. In terms of *yoga* therapy, the arms are the organs of action for the neck,
- Increase the mobility of the <u>thoracic spine</u> [Section 7.4.3.2]
- Increase the strength of the <u>cervical spine</u> musculature using the various types of *jalandhara bandha* [Section 7.4.1.2]
- Practise moving from *ha-jalandhara bandha* [Section 7.4.1.2.2] to *tha-jalandhara bandha* [Section 7.4.1.2.2] in various positions of the shoulder, upper arm and <u>thoracic spine</u>

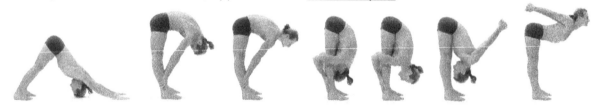

- For *ha-jalandhara bandha,* draw the chin gently towards the throat, and gently retract the middle of the posterior neck backwards. For *tha-jalandhara bandha,* raise the chin and move the throat slightly forward. Both these movements generate a <u>co-activation</u> of <u>neck flexors</u> and <u>neck extensors</u>, which act as <u>stabilisers</u> for the neck.
- When twisting the neck to the right side (<u>right cervical spine axial rotation</u>), lift the right ear away from the right shoulder (<u>left cervical spine lateral flexion</u>) and bring the chin slightly down and inwards (*ha-*

jalandhara bandha)   . This movement counters the non-vertical state of the <u>thoracic spine</u> as well as the non-linear relationship between the <u>thoracic spine</u> and the <u>cervical spine</u>. This also compensates for the natural <u>coupling</u> of <u>lateral rotation</u> with <u>axial rotation</u> in the <u>cervical spine</u> [Section 7.1.2.7]. During <u>axial rotation</u>, the <u>ipsilateral</u> (same) side becomes smaller indicating a lateral flexion towards that side, and the contralateral (opposite) side enlarges indicating a lateral flexion away from that side [Section 7.1.2.7].

- Avoid movements that aggravate the problem and rest the neck and the area around the neck in times of <u>acute pain</u> and <u>inflammation</u>.

7.4.4 Core stabilisation in Yoga

Core stabilisation is a physiotherapy term that has been used in many different ways to describe how the spine can be stabilised and protected by muscle activation. The general consensus is that the main muscles involved in core stabilisation are deep muscles such as the transverse abdominus, the lumbar multifidus and the muscles of the pelvic floor, as well as the diaphragm. Other muscles, closer to the surface, that help with core stabilisation include the other more superficial abdominal and back muscles, as well as muscles around the pelvis, hips and shoulders. Recent research using real-time ultrasound (RTU) imaging devices has shown that a major problem in low back pain is due to over-activity of the superficial core muscles and reduced activity of the deep core muscles. For some time this problem has been made worse because it was assumed that pulling the navel to the spine is the best way to activate deep core muscles such as transverse abominis. Informal surveys show that about two-thirds of people will pull their navel to the spine when asked to 'tighten their abdomen'. RTU has shown that pulling the navel to the spine, actually causes an over-tightening of more superficial and gross abdominal muscles such as the obliquus externus, which can be seen to push the pelvic floor downwards in a negative fashion as well as inhibit the natural function of the diaphragm. In traditional *hatha yoga* 'drawing the navel to the spine' is a type of compressive *ha-mula bandha* that is used to complete an exhalation in advanced *pranayama* (breath-control exercises) but it is not generally maintained throughout postures as it usually inhibits the diaphragm.

Although there is a relationship between breathing, *mula* and *uddiyana bandhas*, and core stabilisation, it is not as simple as one may imagine. As described in detail throughout this book a *bandha* is the co-activation (simultaneous tensing) of opposing muscles around a joint complex. From this definition there are always at least two opposing ways to create a *bandha*, one causing an increased local pressure (*ha bandha*) and one causing a decreased local pressure (*tha bandha*) in the body.

The existence of two types of *bandha* with opposing effects explains why in modern yoga texts *mula bandha* and *uddiyana bandha* are described in several ways that often seem in opposition. This is an ongoing source of confusion for many yoga practitioners and teachers especially if they are familiar with the concept of core stabilisation but not up to date with the latest research on the subject. For example, Sri B.K.S. Iyengar and Sri K. Pattabhi Jois, two of the most important *hatha* yoga teachers of the modern era, both use *mula bandha* and *uddiyana bandha* differently depending on whether the focus is on *pranayama* (breath-control exercises) or *asana* (physical exercise). In *asana*, it is the compressive *ha-uddiyana bandha* and the expansive *tha-mula bandha* that are mainly used to stabilise the spine and to generate internal power in a relaxed way.

This is typified by the posture *lolasana*   , which is the most common posture that is used in the *ashtanga vinyasa yoga* of Sri Pattabhi Jois and is also taught by Sri Iyengar. *Lolasana* obliges the average practitioner to compress the chest (*ha-uddiyana bandha*) and firm the abdomen without drawing the navel to the spine (*tha-mula bandha*). This action stabilises the spine, while allowing the diaphragm to be used to enhance both relaxation and strength especially during inhalation. In *pranayama*, the compressive *ha-uddiyana bandha* and the expansive *tha-mula bandha* are still used. However, there is more emphasis on the expansive *tha-uddiyana bandha*, which draws energy and information into the chest and upper spine

(and completes the inhalation) and the compressive *ha-mula bandha* , which pushes energy and information away from the abdomen and lower spine and completes the exhalation.

****

Chapter Breakdown

8.0 INTRODUCTION TO THE APPLIED ANATOMY & PHYSIOLOGY OF THE CARDIOPULMONARY SYSTEM IN *YOGA*

The coordinated actions of the cardiovascular system, which deals with the circulation of blood through the body, and the respiratory system, concerned with breathing and the exchange of gases, are together referred to as the cardiopulmonary system. One of the main aims of *hatha yoga* is to promote the circulation of *prana* (essentially the life force in the air we breathe) throughout the body. *Prana* is a subtle energy but in its gross manifestation is present in many forms [Goswami, 1980]. The flow of *prana* through the body, the circulation, is the flow of:

(i)   energy
(ii)   matter
(iii)   information

(i) The flow of *prana* as energy (as most people think of energy) is present in the body as heat mainly from muscle activations, but also from body chemistry (enzymatic reactions), electrochemical energy present in nerves and energy absorbed into the body from external sources such as the sun. (ii) The flow of *prana* as matter can be thought of as the latent or potential energy carried with the blood as energy-carrying molecules such as sugars and ATP (adenosine triphosphate) [Section 12.1.1.2]. (iii) The flow of *prana* as information is in the form of the acellular flow of nucleic acids (genetic material) such as DNA and RNA [Section 11.3.4], neurotransmitters, immunotransmitters, and hormones. Circulation can also be thought of as a flow of the more subtle yogic principle of *citta* (consciousness) throughout the body.

8.1 CARDIOVASCULAR SYSTEM

The **cardiovascular system** consists of blood, the heart, and the blood vessels.

8.1.1 Blood

8.1.1.1 Functions of Blood

- **Transportation** Transports oxygen (O_2) from lungs, nutrients from the gastrointestinal (GI) tract, and hormones from endocrine glands to tissues. Blood functions in the transport of heat, carbon dioxide (CO_2) and metabolic waste to lungs, kidneys and sweat glands for excretion.
- **Regulation** Helps regulate the body's pH and temperature.
- **Protection** Contains protective phagocytic white blood cells, and clotting factors which aid in the prevention of blood loss.

8.1.1.2 Characteristics of Blood

- Blood is heavier, and more viscous (thick and sticky) than water (H_2O).
- Blood is alkaline (pH 7.4); with a temperature of 38°C.
- Males have ~5-6 litres (L) of blood. Females have ~4-5 L of blood.
- Blood consists of 55% blood plasma, 45% cells and other formed elements.
- Blood plasma is a straw coloured, protein rich fluid. Most plasma proteins are synthesised by the liver and function to maintain the blood osmotic pressure.
- Blood cells are produced in red bone marrow of the humerus, femur, sternum, ribs, vertebrae, pelvis and cranium.

8.1.1.3 Types Of Blood Cells

8.1.1.3.1 Red Blood Cells (RBCs)

- Erythrocytes or red blood cells (RBCs) are flexible, biconcave discs that have a large surface area for diffusion of gases, but are small enough to squeeze through capillaries.
- Antigens (specific proteins) on the surface of RBCs determine blood groups.
- RBCs have no nucleus.
- There are 280 million haemoglobin (Hb) molecules per RBC.
- RBCs do not consume oxygen, they only transport it. They use anaerobically produced ATP as their energy source
- RBCs circulate for about 120 days and are then broken down by the liver and the spleen.
- After the destruction of a RBC, haeme molecules are broken down to iron. Iron goes back to the bone marrow to form new haemoglobin molecules and bilirubin. Bilirubin goes via the blood to the liver, and then to the bile duct where it is secreted in bile to the small intestine.

8.1.1.3.2 White Blood Cells (WBC)

- White blood cells (WBCs), also known as <u>leucocytes</u> have a nucleus, but do not have <u>haemoglobin</u>.
- WBCs are less numerous than RBCs, with a shorter life span.
- WBCs have important functions in the <u>immune system</u> [Section 10.2].

8.1.1.3.3 Platelets

- <u>Platelets</u> or <u>thrombocytes</u> are formed from <u>metamegakaryocytes</u> in <u>bone marrow</u> and are involved with blood clotting.

8.1.1.4 Haemostasis

- **Haemostasis** refers to the stoppage of bleeding.
- There are 3 basic mechanisms in prevention of blood loss:
    1. <u>Vascular spasm reflex</u> decreases blood flow
    2. <u>Platelet</u> plug formation sticks to the damaged area
    3. Blood <u>coagulation</u> (clotting) due to enzymes such as <u>fibrinogen</u>.

- **Blood clots** may occur in the <u>cardiovascular system</u> due to roughened <u>blood vessel</u> surfaces, slow blood flow, <u>atherosclerosis</u> [Section 8.1.2.1], trauma, or infection. These conditions induce <u>platelet adhesion</u>. A <u>clot</u> in a <u>vein</u> that is unbroken is called a <u>thrombus</u>. If dislodged, a <u>thrombus</u> can be carried with blood to the <u>lungs</u> or <u>arteries</u> of vital organs, where it may block the blood supply. If the <u>thrombus</u> lodges in the <u>brain</u> this can result in a <u>stroke</u>.

- **Haemophilia** refers to several different hereditary genetic deficiencies of <u>coagulation</u> in which spontaneous bleeding may occur, or bleeding after only a minor trauma. It is characterised by subcutaneous and intramuscular haemorrhaging, nosebleeds, blood in urine, joints etc. Treatment involves transfusions of fresh <u>plasma</u> or concentrates of the deficient <u>clotting factor</u>.

8.1.2 Blood vessels

8.1.2.1 Arteries

- <u>Arteries</u> take blood away from the <u>heart</u>.
- <u>Artery walls</u> have elastic and contractile tissue enabling them to pump the blood.
- Upon injury the <u>smooth muscle</u> in the <u>artery</u> wall goes into spasm to reduce blood loss.
    - o **Arteriosclerosis** is an imprecise term used for various disorders of arteries. It is generally thought of as thickening and hardening of <u>artery walls</u>, due to fibrosis or calcium deposition, resulting in a loss of elasticity and obstruction of blood flow. <u>Arteriosclerosis</u> is often used as a synonym for <u>atherosclerosis</u>.
    - o **Atherosclerosis** is a type of <u>arteriosclerosis</u> caused by a build-up of plaque in the inner lining of an artery.Plaque forms from the proliferation of <u>smooth muscle</u> cells and accumulation of fatty substances on the <u>artery walls</u>, especially <u>cholesterol</u> and <u>triglycerides</u>.

8.1.2.2 Capillaries

- <u>Capillaries</u> are microscopic vessels connecting <u>arterioles</u> (small <u>arteries</u>) and <u>venules</u> (small <u>veins</u>).
- <u>Capillaries</u> function in the exchange of nutrients, wastes, <u>oxygen</u> and <u>carbon dioxide</u>.
- Tissues with high metabolic activity require more <u>oxygen</u> and nutrients and therefore have large <u>capillary networks</u> eg liver and kidneys.
- Tendons and ligaments have smaller <u>capillary networks.</u>
- Linings of <u>visceral</u> organs and epidermis have no <u>capillary networks</u>.

8.1.2.3 Veins

<u>Veins</u> have thinner walls with less elastic tissue and larger <u>lumens</u> (central channels) than <u>arteries</u> and therefore a reduced ability to pump blood. <u>Valves</u> in the <u>veins</u> prevent backflow of blood. Blood is moved through <u>veins</u> via the <u>musculoskeletal pump</u> and the <u>respiratory pump</u>.

8.1.2.3.1 The musculoskeletal pump

The <u>musculoskeletal pump</u> works by skeletal muscles activating and pushing blood towards the <u>heart</u>. When muscles relax, <u>valves</u> prevent backflow.

8.1.2.3.2 The respiratory pump

The <u>respiratory pump</u> works during inhalation. The <u>diaphragm</u> descends resulting in a decrease in <u>intra-thoracic pressure</u> (ITP) and an increase in <u>intra-abdominal pressure</u> (IAP). Blood flows from high to low pressure, therefore from the <u>abdomen</u> to the <u>thorax</u>. During the exhalation the reverse would occur, however the <u>valves</u> prevent backflow.

8.1.3 The Heart

The heart is the size of a closed fist and weighs approximately 300g. Two thirds of the heart rests on the left side of the midline of the mediastinum. The heart is surrounded and protected by the pericardium.

8.1.3.1 Heart muscle

The myocardium is the striated muscle of the heart. Cardiac muscle fibres are involuntary, striated and branched. Each fibre physically contacts its neighbour by intercalated discs that allow muscle action potentials to spread from one fibre to another. The atrial unit contracts as one unit, and so do the ventricles. Intercalated discs prevent fibres from pulling apart during heart muscle activations. Like any muscle, the heart can hypertrophy (grow larger) when used extensively as in a fit person, and atrophy (become smaller) when left unused.

8.1.3.2 Heart chambers

The heart is the cardiovascular pump of blood in the body. Like any pump, it works by creating differential regions of relatively high and low pressures that assist in moving the blood through the heart. The pressure changes in the heart, resulting from cardiac muscle activation and relaxation, can be thought of as pushing the blood with high pressure, and pulling the blood with low pressure, through the heart.

The heart consists of four muscular chambers, two upper atria and two lower ventricles. When the cardiac muscle in a chamber is activated, the chamber is constricted which increases local pressure and squeezes, or pushes, the blood out of the chamber to the next chamber in the sequence. One-way heart valves [Section 8.1.3.3] prevent backward flow of the blood to the previous chamber and ensure blood is only pushed in a forward direction towards the aorta, which is the arterial exit from the heart. Conversely, every time the cardiac muscle of a chamber relaxes, this reduces the local pressure and acts to pull blood into it. Again because of one-way valves, blood can only be drawn in from the previous chamber

Atria have thin muscled walls and act mainly as collecting chambers. When the atria contract they push the blood they hold to the ventricles. When the right atrium relaxes, the local pressure reduces and this helps to pull the blood from the vena cava, the venous entrance to the heart. Note that the movement of blood into the heart is assisted by the actions of the other pumps in the body [Sections 1.04 & 8.4.1], in particular the musculoskeletal pump [Section 8.1.2.3.1] and the respiratory pump [Section 8.1.2.3.2]

Ventricles are thick-walled muscular pumps. The left ventricle is 2-4 times bigger than the right, as it pumps blood to the whole body while the right ventricle pumps blood to the lungs for oxygenation.

Pathway of blood in the body
The pathway of blood through the body is as follows:

Deoxygenated blood in superior and inferior vena cava ⇒right atrium ⇒ right ventricle ⇒ pulmonary artery ⇒ lungs ⇒ oxygenated blood ⇒ pulmonary vein ⇒ left atrium ⇒ left ventricle ⇒ aorta ⇒ arteries ⇒ capillaries ⇒ deoxygenated blood ⇒ veins ⇒ superior and inferior vena cava

8.1.3.3 Heart valves

Within the heart, the tricuspid valve (right) and bicuspid (mitral) valve (left) prevent backflow of blood between the atria and ventricles as the ventricles contract. The semilunar valves, between ventricles and arteries emerging from the heart, prevent backflow into the heart.

Rheumatic fever caused by Streptococcal bacteria inflames the heart and causes damage to the aortic valve, semilunar valve and bicuspid valve resulting in heart murmurs [Section 8.3.1]

8.1.3.4 Coronary arteries

Coronary arteries branch off the ascending aorta and supply the heart muscle with blood. Coronary veins drain into the coronary sinus on the posterior surface of the right atrium.

Coronary artery disease
Most heart problems are due to faulty coronary circulation caused by blood clots, fatty atherosclerotic plaques, or smooth muscle spasm in coronary artery walls, which can result in inadequate blood supply to the cardiac muscle, causing a heart attack.

8.1.3.5 Heart pacemaker

Specific cardiac muscle cells spontaneously fire impulses that trigger heart muscle activations. Normally the sinoatrial node in the right atrium is known as the pacemaker as it sets the rate of impulse conduction.

If a site other than the sinoatrial node develops abnormal self-excitability, there may be extra heartbeats or a different pace for a period of time known as arrhythmia. Caffeine, nicotine, alcohol, anxiety, drugs, hyperthyroidism, or potassium deficiencies may stimulate arrhythmias.

Parasympathetic nervous system decreases heart rate (HR) while the sympathetic nervous system increases HR [Section 9.5].

8.1.4 Blood Pressure

Blood pressure is the pressure exerted on the wall of the blood vessel by the blood. Clinically it refers to the pressure in the systemic arteries, which is generated by the ventricular muscles activation. Blood pressure is measured in millilitres of mercury (mmHg). A normal value is 120/80 and calculated as follows:

$$\frac{120\ mmHg}{80\ mmHg} = \frac{systole}{diastole} = \frac{pressure\ in\ arteries\ during\ contraction}{pressure\ in\ arteries\ during\ dilation} = normal$$

Blood pressure is **determined by** level of
- **Cardiac output (CO)** = heart rate (HR)   X   stroke volume (SV)
  (5.25 L/min   =   75 bpm   X   70 ml   is the normal value)
- **Systemic Vascular Resistance (SVR)**. This depends on blood viscosity, and blood vessel length and radius.

Increases in CO and/or SVR lead to an increase in blood pressure

8.1.4.1 Pulse

Pulse is a pressure wave through the arteries. The radial artery pulse is easily found at the wrist, common carotid artery pulse found in the neck.

8.1.4.2 Hypertension (high blood pressure)

Hypertension (high blood pressure) is a measure of the diastolic pressure (pressure in arteries during dilation). Mild hypertension is classed as diastolic 90 - 104 mmHg, moderate is 105 - 114mmHg, and high is > 115 mmHg. The heart uses more energy and requires more effort to pump against an increased after-load (amount of blood in the blood vessels after the heart), resulting in an increase in muscle thickness (enlarged heart) requiring more oxygen.

8.1.4.3 Hypotension (low blood pressure)

Hypotension (low blood pressure), medically defined as a diastolic pressure of less than 60mmHg, often makes people feel dizzy or faint when they stand up too fast due to insufficient blood flow to the brain [Applications to yoga 8.5].

8.1.5 Circulatory Routes
8.1.5.1 Systemic circulation

Systemic circulation includes the cardiac circulation, brain circulation and hepatic portal circulation. Oxygen and nutrients are carried to the tissues and wastes are removed from the tissues.

Hepatic portal circulation is between the gastrointestinal tract and the liver. Nutrient rich deoxygenated blood travels from the spleen, pancreas, stomach, intestines and gall bladder, via the hepatic portal vein to the liver, where glucose is stored as glycogen. The liver receives oxygenated blood via the hepatic artery; all blood leaves the liver via the hepatic veins to the inferior vena cava.

8.1.5.2 Pulmonary circulation

Pulmonary circulation transfers deoxygenated blood from the right ventricle via the pulmonary artery to the lungs where it is oxygenated and then sent back to the left atrium via the pulmonary veins. Pulmonary veins are the only veins carrying oxygenated blood.

8.1.5.3 Foetal circulation:

A foetus receives all blood and oxygen through the mother's blood via the placenta, because its lungs, kidneys and gastrointestinal tract are non-functional.

8.1.6 Cardiovascular Regulation

8.1.6.1 Baroreceptors [Section 9.4.3.4]

Baroreceptors are located in the walls of arteries, veins, and the right atrium. They are pressure sensitive receptors that monitor the stretch in the blood vessel wall. If pressure increases then parasympathetic NS output is stimulated to slow heart rate and thus reduce pressure and vice versa. In this manner, increasing blood pressure with *ha-bandhas* (compressive muscle co-activations) [Section 1.7.3.4] and some *kumbhakas* (breath retentions) in *hatha yoga* can be used to help calm the nervous system [Section 9.7.6.5].

8.1.6.2 Chemoreceptors [Section 9.4.3.3]

Chemoreceptors monitor the blood acidity, O_2 and CO_2 levels. They are located near the baroreceptors. For example, an increased ($\uparrow$) O_2, decreased ($\downarrow$) H^+ and a decreased ($\downarrow$) CO_2 results in vasoconstriction, which constricts blood vessels and therefore increases blood pressure.

8.2 THE RESPIRATORY SYSTEM

The respiratory system is involved with gas exchange, by oxygen uptake and carbon dioxide elimination, whereas the cardiovascular system is involved with gas transport in the blood between the lungs and cells. Pulmonary respiration is the exchange of gases between lungs and blood. Tissue respiration is the exchange of gases between blood and cells. The organs of the respiratory system (RS) include:

- **Upper respiratory system**: (i) nose, (ii) paranasal sinuses, (iii) pharynx (throat), (iv) larynx (voice box)
- **Lower respiratory system**: (v) trachea (windpipe), (vi) bronchi, (vii) lungs

8.2.1 The Nose

Blood capillaries in the nose warm the incoming air, hairs filter air, mucous membranes trap dust and moisten air. Conchae whirl air around. Olfactory stimuli (smells) are received in the nose. The nose also acts as a hollow resonating chamber for speech.

8.2.2 The Paranasal Sinuses

The skull contains a number of air-filled spaces called sinuses. They function to reduce the weight of the skull, provide insulation for the skull, and provide resonance for the voice.

Four pairs of sinuses, known as the para-nasal air sinuses, connect to the nasal passages (the two airways running through the nose). These sinuses are the frontal sinuses (behind the forehead), maxillary sinuses (behind the cheekbones), ethmoid sinuses (between the eyes) and sphenoid sinuses (behind the eyes).

The sinuses are lined with mucous membranes and can produce mucous which, if excessive, may lead to increases in local pressure and cause headaches.

8.2.3 The Pharynx [Table 7.2]

The pharynx is the portion of the airway at the back of the throat, connecting mouth, nasal cavity and larynx. The pharynx starts at the internal nares and ends just below the cricoid cartilage, inferior to the voice box. It is approximately 13 cm long.

The pharynx functions as a passageway for air and food, as a resonating chamber for speech and coordination of swallowing.

The divisions of the pharynx are as follows:
- Nasopharynx containing the adenoids (lymphoid tissue), moves mucus via cilia, exchanges air with the middle ear via the eustachian tubes and warms air.
- Oropharynx contains the palatine tonsils and lingual tonsils.
- Laryngopharynx connects with the oesophagus and contains a fossa (hole) where fish bones commonly get caught.

8.2.4 The Larynx

The larynx (voice box) is a valve-like structure between the trachea (windpipe) and the pharynx (the upper throat) which is the primary organ of voice production. The larynx is a cylindrical grouping of cartilage, muscles, and soft tissue which contains the vocal cords. The vocal cords are the upper opening into the trachea (windpipe), the passageway to the lungs.

The larynx is composed of 9 pieces of cartilage, connecting the pharynx to the trachea. Laryngeal cartilages include the epiglottis, which elevates during swallowing to close the glottis off and direct food to the oesophagus, the thyroid cartilage (Adams apple), and the cricoid cartilage which is inferior to the thyroid cartilage.

Skeletal muscles [Table 7.2] move the cartilage causing the vocal folds to contract or stretch, which changes the pitch of the voice. Males have thicker and longer vocal cords (due to hormones), resulting in slower vibration and lower pitch.

8.2.5 The Trachea

The trachea (windpipe) sits anterior to the oesophagus. It is a tube approximately 12 cm long and 2.5 cm diameter for the passage of air to the lungs. The walls of the trachea are lined with mucosa, ciliated epithelium and 16 - 20 C shaped hyaline cartilage rings that provide rigid support and prevent collapse of the airway. If the trachea is crushed or mucous membranes inflamed, then either a tracheostomy is performed by inserting a breathing tube inferior to the cricoid cartilage or intubation through the mouth or nose.

8.2.6 The Bronchi

The bronchi are the two main branches of the trachea (windpipe) that leads to the lungs. Primary bronchi (right and left) have incomplete cartilage rings. There are three secondary lobar bronchi going to the right lobes and 2 secondary lobar bronchi going to the left. Tertiary bronchi have plates of cartilage. These diverge into bronchioles, which have no cartilage, only smooth muscle. Bronchioles later become terminal bronchioles, alveolar ducts and then alveoli (air sacs).

Bronchial Tree: primary bronchi ➔ secondary bronchi ➔ tertiary bronchi ➔ bronchioles ➔ terminal bronchioles ➔ alveolar ducts ➔ alveoli (alveolar sacs)

Parasympathetic nervous system stimulation causes bronchoconstriction, a constriction of the vessels to the lungs, and smooth muscle spasm as in asthma and allergic reactions. Sympathetic nervous system stimulation causes bronchodilatation, an expansion of the vessels to the lungs. This is how adrenalin works, as do drugs to treat asthma.

8.2.7 The Lungs

The lungs are a pair of spongy organs contained within the chest that remove carbon dioxide from the blood and provide it with oxygen. The lungs extend from the diaphragm [Table 7.4] to just above the clavicle.

The left lung has a concavity called the cardiac notch where the heart sits. The hilus is where all the blood vessels and nerves enter and leave the lungs. The lungs are divided by oblique fissures in both lungs and the right lung is also divided by the horizontal fissure.

Two layers of the pleural membrane (parietal and visceral) enclose and protect the lungs. The space between the layers is known as the pleural cavity, which is filled with lubricating fluid to allow movement during breathing. The pleural cavity can fill with air, blood or pus.
- **Pneumothorax** is when the pleural cavity fills with air, due to surgery, gunshot, stabbing etc.
- **Haemothorax** is when the pleural cavity fills with blood due to malignancy or trauma.
- **Empyma** is when the pleural cavity fills with pus following bacterial infection eg pneumonia.

8.2.8 Mechanics of Respiration [Table 7.4]

Air moves into the lungs via a pressure gradient, from high to low pressures. To decrease the pressure inside the lungs, their volume must be increased via activation of the diaphragm and the intercostal muscles. Muscular activation (contraction) of the dome-shaped diaphragm causes it to shorten and flatten and thus increase the volume of the thoracic cavity [Table 7.4]. The dome of the diaphragm moves 1 cm during quiet breathing and 10 cm during heavy breathing. Activation of the intercostal muscles causes the thorax to expand and increase in volume. Obesity and pregnancy can prevent complete descent of the dome of the diaphragm resulting in shallow costal (thoracic) breathing.

Once the volume inside the thorax has increased due to the action of the diaphragm and intercostal muscles, the pressure of the thorax and the lungs decreases enough so that it is less than atmospheric pressure and air from the atmosphere is drawn into the lungs and fills them.

8.2.8.1 Mechanics of Inhalation

Inhalation (inspiration) occurs when the pressure in the lungs is less than that of the atmosphere and the air is free to enter the lungs via mouth or nose.

Normal inhalation from a standing position, involves the diaphragm moving down, and the ribs move up (pump handle effect) and out (bucket handle effect) by a combined action of internal intercostals and external intercostals.

On **forced inhalation,** accessory muscles of breathing may also be used [Section 7.2 & Tables 7.3 & 7.4].

8.2.8.2 Mechanics of Exhalation

Exhalation (expiration) occurs when the pressure in the lungs is greater than that of the atmosphere and the air is free to leave the lungs via mouth or nose.

Normal quiet exhalation is passive, muscles relax, diaphragm ascends and ribs move down. It depends on:
*   Recoil of elastic fibres in lungs and chest wall which were stretched on inhalation.
*   Inward pull of the surface tension due to alveolar fluid.

During **forced exhalation,** the abdominal muscles and intercostals are activated. On average, we breathe 12 - 16 tidal (normal and relaxed) breaths per minute, moving 5 - 6 litres of air in and out.

8.2.8.3 Abdominal and thoracic breathing

Abdominal breathing and thoracic breathing are terms sometimes used by people who teach breathing to indicate where on the body an expansion of the trunk should occur reflecting the primary activation of either the diaphragm (abdominal breathing) or the intercostal muscles (thoracic breathing). It is incorrect to think that air is actually coming into the abdomen during abdominal breathing. In both types of breathing, the air will only go into the lungs.

Abdominal breathing is seen as an outward movement of the abdomen on inhalation and an inward movement of the abdomen on exhalation. Abdominal breathing mainly uses the diaphragm muscle, which moves downwards (distally) as it generates tension. If the abdomen is relaxed, pressure from the diaphragm will move the abdominal contents downwards (distally) and also outwards (anteriorly).

Thoracic breathing is seen as an outward and upward movement of the rib cage on inhalation and an inward and downward movement of the rib cage and chest wall on exhalation. Thoracic breathing mainly uses the intercostal muscles.

Intercostal muscle expansion of the rib cage and chest wall in thoracic breathing is essentially the same as the muscular activation used in the *yogic* internal lock *uddiyana bandha* [Section 7.4.1.3].

8.2.9 Physiology of Respiration

Respiration is the exchange of gases from air to the blood and from the blood to the body cells. The main gases involved in respiration are oxygen and carbon dioxide.

8.2.9.1 Oxygen

Most (98.5%) of oxygen (O_2) is transported through the blood in combination with haemoglobin (Hb) in red blood cells, as oxyhaemoglobin. Some (1.5%) O_2 is dissolved in blood plasma.

Acid decreases the affinity of haemoglobin for O_2 (the Bohr effect) [Section 8.4.4] As the hydrogen ion (H^+) from the acid binds to the haemoglobin and alters its structure, causing it to release its O_2 into the tissues. Acid arises from lactic acid, an anaerobic metabolic by-product, and also from carbonic acid (dissolved carbon dioxide) [Section 9.2.9.2]. Carbon dioxide can also bind to haemoglobin and has a similar effect to the hydrogen ion. Also, as temperature rises oxygen releases from haemoglobin.

Hypoxia is low oxygen (O_2) availability caused by:
*   Low pressure of O_2 in arterial blood = Hypoxic hypoxia (eg from high altitudes, airway obstruction, or fluid in the lungs)
*   Failure of haemoglobin (Hb) to carry its normal O_2 complement = Anaemic hypoxia (eg from haemorrhaging, anaemia, or carbon monoxide poisoning).
*   Reduced delivery of blood and thus O_2 to tissues = Stagnant hypoxia (eg from heart failure, or circulatory shock).
*   Tissues unable to use O_2 brought to them = Histotoxic hypoxia (eg from cyanide poisoning).

8.2.9.2 Carbon dioxide (CO_2)

Carbon dioxide (CO_2) is carried in the blood in three forms:

- 70% in plasma as bicarbonate ions which is formed as follows:

$$CO_2 \quad + \quad H_2O \quad \Leftrightarrow \quad H_2CO_3 \quad \Leftrightarrow \quad H^+ \quad + \quad HCO_3^-$$
Carbon dioxide + water ⇔ carbonic acid ⇔ hydrogen ion + bicarbonate ion

- 20-30% of transported CO_2 as carried with haemoglobin as carboaminohaemoglobin ($HbCO_2$).
- 7% dissolved in plasma.

Decreases in arterial CO_2 can lead to vasoconstriction of arteries especially to the brain, hence less blood and oxygen gets to the brain, which may lead to dizziness. Decreases in arterial CO_2 can lead to bronchoconstriction and may lead to breathing difficulties and asthma in some people.

Increases in arterial CO_2 can lead to vasodilation of the arteries to the brain and the rest of the body and hence bring increased circulation to the tissues. Increases in arterial CO_2 can lead to bronchodilatation (expansion of the airways).

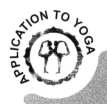

No 8.1 *Pranayama* which reduces minute ventilation can assist people with breathing difficulties

Pranayama, or breathing exercises, in which CO_2 is allowed to increase (such as breath retention exercises) can assist people with breathing difficulties and asthma if practised safely and taught by an experienced practitioner. To be effective at bronchodilatation (airway expansion), such pranayama would have to reduce the minute ventilation, ie involve breathing less air than normal [Section 8.2.9.4].

8.2.9.3 Carbon monoxide (CO)

Carbon monoxide (CO) is an odourless, colourless gas found in car exhaust, tobacco smoke and as a by-product of burning coal and wood. CO combines with the haeme molecule 200X stronger than O_2, thus a small concentration of CO will combine with lots of Hb molecules and can decrease the oxygen carrying capacity of blood by 50%.

8.2.9.4 Ventilation [Section 12.7.1.2.1]

Ventilation refers to how much air gets into the lungs. It is usually measured in terms of litres per minute of air that is inhaled and exhaled, or minute ventilation. Control of ventilation during *yogic* breathing is extensively discussed later [Section 12.7.1.2.1].

8.2.9.4.1 Hyperventilation
Hyperventilation is when one breathes more air than is actually required, ie increased minute ventilation. It will generally cause a decrease in the levels of carbon dioxide (CO_2) in the blood, which will lead to a decrease in carbonic acid in the blood, and therefore less blood to the brain and less air to the alveoli. Subsequent breath retentions are longer after hyperventilation. Hyperventilation makes the blood more alkaline [Sections 9.7.6.2, 10.3 & 12.7.1.2.1].

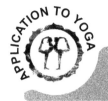

No 8.2 Hyperventilation during a yoga practice brings less oxygen to the brain [Section 12.7.1.2.1]

Hyperventilation (over-breathing) during a *yoga* practice causes CO_2 (carbon dioxide) to be expelled from the body. Reduced levels of CO_2 cause blood vessels going to the brain to contract and therefore less oxygen gets to the brain, and fainting or dizziness can be a consequence.

8.2.9.4.2 Hypoventilation
Hypoventilation is when one breathes less air than is actually required, ie decreased minute ventilation. It will generally cause an increase in the levels of carbon dioxide (CO_2) in the blood, which will lead to an increase in carbonic acid in the blood, and therefore more blood to the brain and more air to the alveoli. Hypoventilation makes the blood more acidic [Sections 9.7.6.3, 10.3 & 12.7.1.2.1].

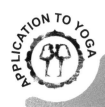

No 8.3 Mild hypoventilation during a yoga practice can bring more oxygen to the brain [Section 12.7.1.2.1]

Mild hypoventilation while practising *yoga* causes a build up of CO_2 (carbon dioxide) in the body. CO_2 acts as a chemical signal which causes the blood vessels going to the brain to dilate and therefore more blood and oxygen flows to the brain and thinking is clearer.

8.2.9.4.3 Stimuli that change the rate and depth of ventilation:

Stimuli that increase rate and depth of <u>ventilation</u> include the following:
- Increases in body temperature, <u>arterial</u> <u>blood acidity</u> or <u>arterial</u> CO_2
- Decreases in <u>blood pressure</u> or <u>arterial blood</u> O_2
- Prolonged pain
- Stretching of the <u>anal sphincter</u> (eg in defecation).

Stimuli that decrease rate and depth of <u>ventilation</u>:
- Decreases in body temperature, <u>arterial</u> <u>blood acidity</u> or <u>arterial</u> CO_2
- Increases in <u>blood pressure</u> or <u>arterial blood</u> O_2
- Absence of pain
- <u>Activation</u> of the <u>anal sphincter</u> and <u>anal constrictor muscles</u> (eg in *asvini mudra*, and through <u>fascial connections</u> also in *mula bandha* and *kati bandha*).

8.3 THE CARDIOPULMONARY SYSTEM

The coordinated actions of the <u>respiratory system</u> and the <u>cardiovascular system</u> are referred to as the <u>cardiopulmonary system</u>.

Ventilation refers to how much air is getting into a <u>lung</u> segment. **Perfusion** refers to how much blood flows past the <u>alveoli</u> in a segment. **Ventilation-perfusion mismatching** occurs in many disorders of the <u>cardiopulmonary system</u>. It is when well-<u>ventilated</u> <u>lung</u> units get little <u>perfusion</u>, or when well-<u>perfused</u> <u>lung</u> units have undergone <u>atelectasis</u> (alveolar collapse) and get little or no air.

8.3.1 Disorders of the Cardiopulmonary system
8.3.1.1 Valvular heart diseases
There are two basic types of <u>heart valve</u> defects:
(i) **Valvular stenosis** is the narrowing of one of the <u>valves</u> regulating blood flow to the <u>heart</u>.
- <u>Stenosis</u> may arise by scar formation or a <u>congenital defect</u>.
- All <u>stenosis</u> are serious because they place a severe burden on the <u>heart</u> by making it work harder to push blood through the abnormally narrow valve openings.

(ii) **Valvular insufficiency** (also known as <u>valvular incompetence</u>, or <u>valvular regurgitation</u>) refers to the backflow of blood through a valve (in the opposite direction to normal) because the valve leaflets do not fit closely together.

8.3.1.2 Right-sided heart failure
<u>Right-sided heart failure</u> (RHF) occurs when the <u>right ventricle</u> can no longer cope with the demands placed upon it, or if there is a major obstruction to the outflow from the <u>right atrium</u>, as in <u>tricuspid valve stenosis</u>. RHF may also result following <u>myocardial infarction</u> (heart attack) of the <u>right ventricle</u>, <u>pulmonary disease</u> (especially <u>bronchitis</u> and <u>emphysema</u>), <u>pulmonary valve disease</u> and <u>tricuspid insufficiency</u>.

Signs and Symptoms of RHF include increased systemic venous pressure, enlarged spleen and liver (which may become cirrhotic if the enlargement is <u>chronic</u>), <u>ascites</u> (fluid in the <u>peritoneal cavity</u>), and <u>oedemous</u> (swollen) ankles and other dependent areas.

8.3.1.3 Left-sided heart failure
Left sided <u>heart</u> failure (LHF) occurs when the <u>left ventricle</u> can no longer cope with the demands placed upon it or if there is an obstruction to the outflow from the <u>left atrium</u> as in <u>mitral stenosis</u>. LHF may result following <u>myocardial infarction</u> of the <u>left ventricle</u>, <u>aortic valve disease</u> and <u>mitral valve insufficiency</u>, and <u>hypertension</u>.

Signs and Symptoms of LHF are generally the result of <u>pulmonary congestion</u>. Symptoms include <u>dyspnoea</u> (shortness of breath on exertion), <u>orthopnea</u> (shortness of breath while lying down), and <u>acute pulmonary oedema</u> (excess fluid in the <u>lungs</u>). Signs and symptoms of LHF may sometimes be difficult to differentiate from respiratory symptoms, but a correct differential diagnosis is essential as the treatment is quite different for the two conditions.

8.3.1.4 Asthma, Bronchitis & Pneumonia

<u>Asthma</u> involves the <u>chronic inflammation</u> or <u>smooth muscle</u> spasm of the <u>bronchiole</u> wall resulting in narrowing of the airways. Triggers of <u>asthma</u> include pollen, dust mites, sulphites in wine and emotions such as laughing or stress. Symptoms of <u>asthma</u> include wheezing, difficulty exhaling (as air is trapped in the <u>alveoli</u>) and by excessive mucous secretion.

<u>Asthma</u> is often provoked with an increase in the amount of air taken into the <u>lungs</u> per minute (<u>hyperventilation</u>). With an increase in the amount of air leaked in every minute there is also an increase in the amount of <u>carbon dioxide</u> removed each minute. Since <u>carbon dioxide</u> (in the dissolved form of <u>carbonic acid</u> in the blood) is a trigger for <u>bronchodilatation</u>, its absence tends to encourage <u>bronchoconstriction</u>.

8.3.1.5 Bronchitis

<u>Bronchitis</u> involves <u>inflammation</u> of the <u>bronchi</u> resulting in an increase in size of the mucous secreting glands in the airway. A typical symptom is a cough with thick greenish-yellow sputum.

8.3.1.6 Pneumonia

Pneumonia refers to an <u>acute inflammation</u> or infection of the <u>alveoli</u>. <u>Alveolar sacs</u> fill up with fluids reducing air space in the <u>lungs</u> and thus reducing the ability for <u>oxygen</u> to diffuse into blood.

8.4 APPLIED ANATOMY & PHYSIOLOGY OF THE CARDIOPULMONARY SYSTEM IN HATHA *YOGA*

8.4.0 The Reasons for Breathing

The ultimate state of *pranayama* (yogic breath-control) and meditation is a state where breathing is reduced as much as possible without force. However this is a process that can for most people take a life time. In order to work towards the mastery of yoga it is sometimes useful to breathe more than normal (<u>hyperventilation</u>) but eventually the aim to be able to comfortabley live and practice while breathing less than normal (<u>hypoventilation</u>).

In yoga and life breathing may guided or controlled for six main reasons. These are:

1.　　Physical
2.　　Neurological
3.　　Mental
4.　　Emotional
5.　　Cardiovascular
6.　　Physiological

Pranayama (yogic breath-control) is the art of learning how to breathe less than normal (<u>hypoventilation</u>). Although sometimes fast, deep and/or complete breaths have benefits, the less you breathe overall the better your mental capacity is and the greater is the blood flow to nourish the brain and the heart. The <u>haemoglobin</u> also transfers oxygen more efficiently to all the cells of the body (the Bohr effect). Many studies on meditation have shown that focus and concentration are better when you breathe less! Additionally, the nervous system is much calmer when you breathe less and this is reflected in a reduced desire to eat. Breath-control is also useful on a mental level. Any type of focus on your breathing can help you concentrate, but the nervous system works best if you breathe less than normal.

Breath-control works on the <u>cardiovascular</u> and <u>circulatory system</u>. You can enhance the movement of energy and information through your subtle channels and enhance the movement of blood and heat through your blood vessels by breathing differentially from your <u>abdomen</u> (<u>diaphragmatic breathing</u>) or from your chest (<u>thoracic breathing</u>). You can also bring more blood and oxygen to the brain and heart and less blood and oxygen to the arms and legs by breathing less than normal (<u>hypoventilation</u>). Conversely, you can bring less blood and oxygen to brain and heart and more blood and oxygen to the arms and legs by breathing more than normal (<u>hyperventilation</u>).

A brief summary of the the different possible effects of breathing is outlined below:

1. Physical
- Mobilising the spine
- Deep inhalation tends to cause spinal flexion (bends your spine more forward) while deep exhalation tends to cause spinal extension (bends your spine more backwards)
- Stabilising the spine
- The muscles of breathing out (especially from the chest) can make your spine more stable
- Strengthening the spine and body
- The diaphragm (the main muscle of inhalation) can be used as powerful strength muscle

2. Neurological
- Control of the autonomic (automatic) nervous system via the diaphragm which can be controlled either by the conscious mind (somatic) or unconscious mind (autonomic)
- Reciprocal relaxation of the muscles of abdominal exhalation (which include many of the muscles that can tend to over-tense and contribute to lower back pain) by the main muscle of inhalation (the diaphragm)

3. Mental
- Focus on any type of breathing can help with concentration
- Reduced breathing (hypoventilation) leaves the body slightly more acidic (with carbonic acid), which gives the physiological effect of calming the nervous system and the mind in general

4. Emotional
- Slow abdominal (diaphragmatic) breathing tends to enhance parasympathetic control of relaxation response with *ahimsa* (non-violence) and/or love and peace and happiness as dominant emotions
- Faster chest (thoracic) breathing tends to enhance sympathetic control of 'flight or fight' response with *tapas* (passion to do your best) and/or fear anger and aggression as dominant emotions

5. Cardiovascular
- Deep breathing with the abdomen relaxed (which can be diaphragmatic and/or thoracic provided the abdomen is relaxed) causes an increase in blood flow. With this type of breathing heart rate and blood pressure increases on inhalation and decreases on exhalation
- Deep breathing with the abdomen relaxed causes increased pressure into the abdomen on inhalation and decreased pressure on exhalation that increases blood flow and nervous system stimulation to the abdominal organs

6. Physiological
- Reduced breathing (hypoventilation) for:
  - Calmer nerves
  - Increased oxygenation and blood flow to brain and heart
  - Reduced hunger
- Increased breathing (hyperventilation) for:
  - Stimulation of nerves
  - Decreased oxygenation and blood flow to brain and heart
  - Increased hunger

8.4.1 The Effect of *Hatha Yoga* on Circulation

Beneficial side-effects of practising *hatha yoga* include claimed increases in strength, flexibility, and the ability to relax. However, one of the main physiological purposes of *hatha yoga* is to improve the circulation in the body. In fact, stimulating the circulation is one of the main ways *hatha yoga* actually works.

The word *hatha* means force in *Sanskrit*, and can represent pressure (Pressure = Force per unit Area). The sound *ha* is *Sanskrit* for the sun, which represents heat or high pressure. The sound *tha* (pronounced ta) is *Sanskrit* for the moon, which represents coolness or low pressure [Borg-Olivier & Machliss, 1997] [Section 1.04; Figure 1.5].

Hatha yoga sets up regions of relative high pressure and low pressure within the body, which help stimulate circulation in a manner similar to the way that the heart works [Section 8.1.2.3.1].

Through *hatha yoga* one can make the heart (the cardiovascular pump) beat faster and stronger by making the cardiac muscle contract more often. However, *hatha yoga* aims to increase and improve circulation not by pumping the heart harder, but instead by enhancing the effects of the other six pumps of circulation described. This is achieved with the various *yogic asanas*, *pranayamas*, and techniques.

The six pumps of circulation are:

- **Musculoskeletal pump** [Section 8.1.2.3.1]

  Dynamic exercises (*vinyasas*), which activate and relax muscles during movement, can be utilised to enhance the musculoskeletal pump of circulation.

- **Respiratory pump** [Section 8.1.2.3.2]

  Breathing techniques (*pranayamas*) can be utilised to enhance the respiratory pump of circulation.

- **Gravitational pump**

  Inverted and semi inverted postures (*viparita karani*) can be utilised to enhance the gravitational pump of circulation.

- **Postural pump**

  Static postures (*asanas*), creating regions of relative high pressure (physical compression of a body region during a pose) and relative low pressure (stretching of a body region during pose) can be utilised to enhance the postural pump of circulation.

- **Muscle co-activation pump**

  Co-activation (simultaneous tensing) of antagonistic (opposing) muscles (*bandhas*) [Section 1.7.3,], in *asanas* and *vinyasas* to create regions of relative high pressure (*ha-bandhas*) and relative low pressure (*tha-bandhas*) can be utilised to enhance the muscle co-activation pump of circulation.

- **Centripetal pump**

  Changes in movement (*vinyasa*) during a *yoga* practice create centripetal centrifugal and inertial forces in the body which can enhance the centripetal pump of circulation.

8.4.1.1 The balance between muscle activation and relaxation: How much should one tense the muscles in *yoga*?

One of the greatest difficulties in a *yoga* practice is to know how much one should leave the main effects of a posture to be dependant on the relaxed version of a pose alone, and how much one should supplement this with conscious tension or activation of various muscles. The answer is not simple and depends on many factors. The intensity of any posture can be greatly enhanced when any of the muscles are activated isometrically.

The effects of a posture can change significantly when an exercise goes from having the muscles relaxed to having them active. Body heat and blood pressure can increase significantly when muscular tension is added to a practice. The nervous system becomes more profoundly affected [Section 9.7] due to activation of spinal reflexes, stimulation of the sympathetic nervous system and perhaps an increase in tensioning (stretching) of nerves.

If there is complete muscle relaxation in a pose, minimal effort is required; the body remains cool but tends to remain quite stiff. Also if one moves too far or too fast into an *asana* (static posture) or *vinyasa* (dynamic exercise) while completely relaxed in the muscles, there can be a danger of over-stretching the weaker, more flexible parts of one's body without stretching the more stiff regions, and injury may result. Also some people who stay completely relaxed in a pose will remain calm in the mind while others will find their minds distracted and not engaged by their *yoga* practice.

Some conscious tension or muscle activation in the body during *asanas* and *vinyasas* can stabilise joints, increase body heat and therefore flexibility, generate energy, promote circulation, and engage the mind. Excess tension or muscle activation can overheat the body, prevent movement, stop circulation, increase blood pressure [Section 8.4.1.3], stress the nervous system and the mind, and drain the body of energy.

In order to attempt the deeper or more difficult variations of postures, appropriate muscular tension in the form of *bandhas* [Section 1.7.3], co-activation of antagonistic (opposing) muscle groups, must be present or the poses can actually be damaging for the body. A general rule is that the more any part of the body is bent, the stronger the *bandha* around that part should be made, until such a time that alternate means of protecting the joints are available, eg. controlled miminisation of stretching the weak parts.

A good guide is to only tense the various parts of the body and only move into a posture as much as you can while remaining relaxed in the face, neck and throat. Also, only bend any part of your body more than you would in everyday life with the proviso that you have a little tension around the region you are bending in a way that will stabilise and protect your joints.

8.4.1.2 *Hatha yoga* for people with vertebral artery insufficiency (VAB)

The vertebral arteries are two important arteries that pass through the vertebral foramen to supply the brainstem. On some people one vertebral artery may be compromised. If this is the case then certain neck postures such as neck extension, neck lateral flexion and neck axial rotation can compromise the other vertebral artery leading to brainstem symptoms such as spots before the eyes, dizziness, fainting, and double vision.

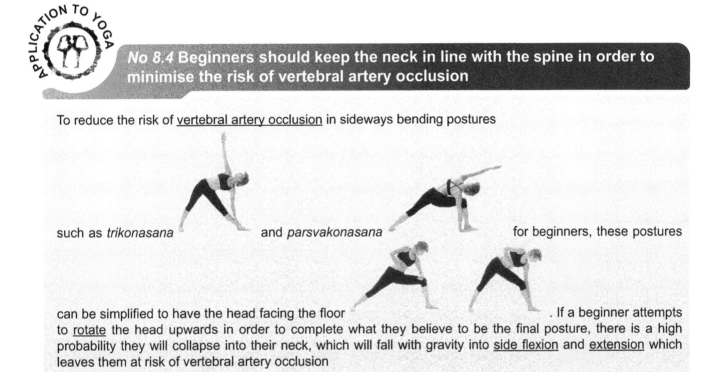

No 8.4 Beginners should keep the neck in line with the spine in order to minimise the risk of vertebral artery occlusion

To reduce the risk of vertebral artery occlusion in sideways bending postures

such as *trikonasana* and *parsvakonasana* for beginners, these postures

can be simplified to have the head facing the floor . If a beginner attempts to rotate the head upwards in order to complete what they believe to be the final posture, there is a high probability they will collapse into their neck, which will fall with gravity into side flexion and extension which leaves them at risk of vertebral artery occlusion

8.4.1.3 *Hatha yoga* for people with high blood pressure (hypertension) and headache

Hypertension (high blood pressure) is a serious concern as it is the underlying problem that may lead to heart attack, stroke and kidney failure. Hypertension may be present for many reasons, including stress, diet, lifestyle, lack of sleep etc. At the most physical level, blood pressure tends to become elevated with increased heart rate, increased cardiac output, increased fluid retention, increased viscosity (thickness) of blood (perhaps due to dehydration), increased blood vessel length (perhaps due to obesity), and decreased blood vessel radius (perhaps due to particular food matter lining blood vessel walls).

Headache may be caused by hypertension, but even if it is not, it will almost certainly be made worse if there is a further increase in blood pressure. Therefore, a *hatha yoga* practice at times of hypertension or headache should be done in such a way as to not further increase blood pressure. Do not aggravate the situation by making the heartbeat increase. In extremely bad cases, all active postures should be avoided and only passive poses performed. No standing poses should be done if blood pressure is very high, as they can be very strenuous and lead to a further increase in blood pressure. Postures that cause the abdominal muscles to become activated should not be performed when blood pressure is very high. Arm balancing postures and postures with the arms raised up should also be avoided as these postures place a lot of stress on the heart.

Initially it is sufficient to give such students very simple passive forward bends such as *pascimottanasana* , with the backside elevated and the head resting on a bench, supported *ardha halasana* if possible, *setu bandha sarvangasana* and s*avasana* (supine relaxation in the anatomical position).

As a patient's condition improves, and for people who only have a mild <u>hypertension</u>, the following *asanas* and *pranayama* may be slowly incorporated into the practice; *uttanasana* (with head support initially) *adho mukha svanasana* (with head support initially), *ardha salamba sarvangasana* ,

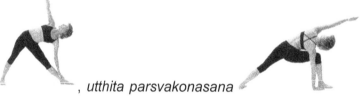

salamba sarvangasana , *ujjayi pranayama* and *nadi sodhana pranayama* [Figure 8.1]. Gradually simple variations of the less stressful standing poses may be added. These include *utthita trikonasana* , *utthita parsvakonasana* and *prasarita padottanasana* (with head support initially). When the standing poses are added the student should initially be asked to look down, not to look up, and to rest the hands on the hips rather than taking the hands into the air. It is also important that students with <u>hypertension</u> maintain a relaxed <u>abdomen</u> so that the <u>diaphragm</u> is free to function correctly.

<u>Blood pressure</u> is elevated when the <u>sympathetic nervous system</u> is overactive. Therefore postures and practice that calm the <u>nervous system</u>, in particular the forward bending postures, are useful to help reduce <u>hypertension</u>.

In situations where <u>hypertension</u> may be an issue, all *ha-bandhas* [Section 1.7.3] should be held only very gently, or not held at all. <u>Isometric</u> <u>muscle activations</u>, such as those in *bandhas*, are able to constrict the flow of blood if the <u>activation</u> is greater than 25% of the maximum possible <u>isometric</u> <u>activation</u>. However, the less each *bandha* is applied, the less one should try to bend that region as the <u>joint complex</u> in that region may be less stable. When professional weight-lifters perform their sometimes extreme exercises they have been shown to generate <u>isometric</u> <u>muscle activations</u> similar to those applied in strong *bandhas*. In some cases the <u>blood pressure</u> in some Olympic level weight lifters has been shown to increase to an astonishing 380/260 (normal is about 120/80).

Finally, the lifestyle conditions that lead to <u>hypertension</u> should also be addressed. For example, address diet, work conditions, sleeping patterns and attitudes to life.

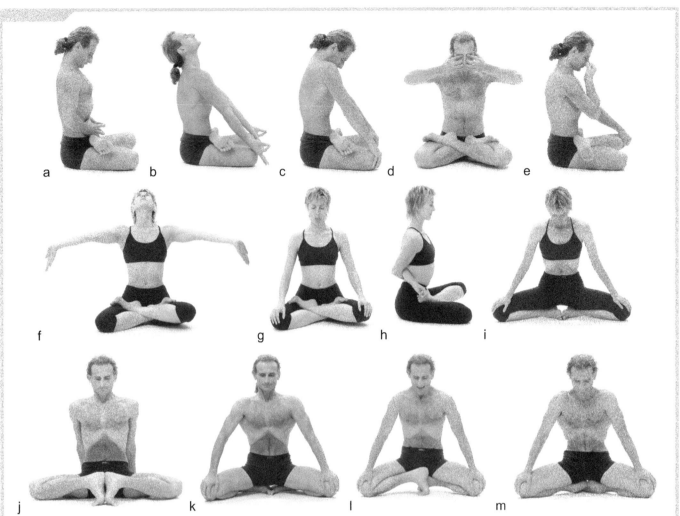

Figure 8.1: Seated *pranayama* (*in padmasana unless otherwise stated*)**:**
(A) *ujjayi pranayama* in *antara kumbhaka* (inhalation retention) with *ha-jalandhara bandha, ha-uddiyana bandha, ha-mula bandha, dharana mudra* (b) *puraka* (inhalation) in *sitkali pranayama* with *tha-jalandhara bandha*; (c) *ujjayi* with *antara kumbhaka, ha-jalandhara bandha, tha-uddiyana bandha, ha-mula bandha*; (d) *ujjayi pranayama* with *san mukhi mudra*; (e) *nadi sodhana pranayama*; (f) *kloman mudra* with *tha-jalandhara bandha*; (g) *sitali pranayama* with *kaki mudra*; (h) *kevala kumbhaka* (minimal breathing) in *baddha padmasana*; (i) *bahya kumbhaka* (exhalation retention) with *ha-jalandhara bandha, tha-uddiyana bandha, ha-mula bandha* in *bhadrasana*; (j) *bahya kumbhaka* with *ha-jalandhara bandha, tha-uddiyana bandha, tha-mula bandha* in *bhagasana*; (k) *bahya kumbhaka* with *ha-jalandhara bandha, tha-uddiyana bandha, tha-mula bandha* in *bhadrasana*; (l) *bahya kumbhaka* with *ha-jalandhara bandha, tha-uddiyana bandha, ha-mula bandha* (<u>obliquus externus abdominis</u> isolation), and *simha mudra* in *yoni dandasana*; (m) *bahya kumbhaka* with *ha-jalandhara bandha, tha-uddiyana bandha* and *tha-mula bandha* in the form of *nauli* (<u>rectus abdominis</u> isolation) in *mulabandhasana*.

8.4.1.4 *Hatha yoga* for people with low blood pressure (hypotension) and dizziness

<u>Hypotension</u> (<u>low blood pressure</u>) can be dangerous as the blood flow to the <u>brain</u> can be reduced and this can lead to fainting and falling to the floor. Also there can be dizziness and <u>nausea</u>. Care should be taken when sitting up or standing up from the floor, especially after inverted positions as the blood tends to rush suddenly away from the head and fainting can occur. Deep fast breathing or any sort of <u>hyperventilation</u> [Section 8.2.9.4.1] should be avoided as this will reduce blood flow to the <u>brain</u> due to the reduction in <u>carbon dioxide</u>. Passive supine postures

(with or *without support as needed) such as *supta baddha konasana* 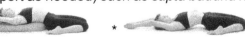 *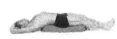

, *supta virasana* 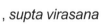 * , *setu bandha sarvangasana*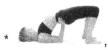

* 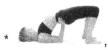 , are recommended, as is *ardha sarvangasana* (half shoulderstand) [Iyengar, 2001].

235

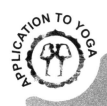

No 8.5 Exhale before standing up from a semi-inverted posture to minimise the loss of blood from the head and reduce the risk of fainting

After inversions or semi-inverted postures such as *uttanasana* it is important to note that blood pressure in the head tends to decrease when standing up. To minimise the risk of fainting it is important to stand up slowly. This allows some time for the body to compensate for the change in gravitational forces.

Another useful tool for preventing the loss of pressure to the head is to exhale fully before standing up, then stand on an empty breath. Once you have stood up, take only a little breath in without expanding the chest (*tha-uddiyana bandha*) as this would draw blood away from the head. Then, hold the breath in and gently contract the abdomen (*ha-mula bandha*) and the chest (*ha-uddiyana bandha*).

Exhaling before standing up and holding the breath out helps to increase carbon dioxide in the blood, which tends to increase blood flow to the head. If, once you have stood up, the intra-abdominal and intra-thoracic pressure is increased by contracting the abdomen and chest while holding the breath in, this can also increase blood flow to the head.

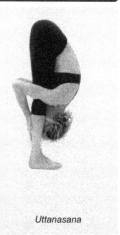

Uttanasana

If, on the other hand, you inhale while standing up, then the decreased pressure caused by the expansion of the chest (*tha-uddiyana bandha*) during the inhalation would result in a drop in pressure in the head and increase the likelihood of fainting.

8.4.2 Cardiopulmonary Considerations in *Hatha Yoga* Exercises

There are many reports in the literature of yogis who can control autonomic functions by controlling their breathing. Experienced *hatha yoga* practitioners are able to perform a variety of advanced breathing techniques, such as very slow deep breathing. However, these advanced breathing techniques are not suitable for beginner *yoga* practitioners, as they are potentially dangerous. New *yoga* students are best advised to breathe in a normal, relaxed fashion. Students should be taught how to keep their faces and necks relaxed while breathing and avoid the use of their accessory muscles of breathing [Section 7.2.3].

In the initial stages students are also warned against breathing too deeply, as this may lead to hyperventilation (over-breathing), unless the increase in their tidal volume is associated with a decrease in the number of breaths per minute. Students should be warned against activating their abdominal muscles towards the end of inhalation (i.e. performing a Valsalva manoeuvre) as this has been shown to increase blood pressure during and after isometric exercise [OConnor, Sforzo & Frye, 1989] and can also lead to an increase in inter-cranial pressure (ICP).

8.4.2.1 *Hatha yoga* for asthmatics and people with breathing difficulties

The scientific validity of *yoga* and *yoga* therapy for asthma is quite well established [Singh *et al.*, 1990; Nagendra & Nagarathna, 1986; Nagarathna & Nagendra, 1985: Goyesche *et al.*, 1980, 1982]. Studies have shown that *yoga* therapy is beneficial for bronchial asthma [Jain & Talukdar, 1993] and *yoga* training results in increased lung function and exercise capacity in young asthmatics [Jain *et al.*, 1991].

People with breathing difficulties, such as asthmatics, tend to develop poor physical posture. *Hatha yoga* postures can be used to help strengthen, stretch and relax the following muscles and stretch the regions associated with them:

* Accessory muscles of breathing such as the muscles of the shoulders and chest, which are often tight in asthmatics;
* Spinal musculature, which is often tight in asthmatics and often manifests as abnormal spinal curvature;
* Abdominal muscles and other abdominal tissue (commonly tight in asthmatics), which can prevent the diaphragm from being able to function correctly by preventing its descent due to its activation (here a contraction).

Asthmatics often do little physical activity for fear of provoking an asthma attack. Many asthmatics fall into a vicious cycle of inactivity that makes them progressively weaker and sicker, and makes it harder for them to participate in any physical activity. *Yoga asanas* (static postures) and *vinyasas* (dynamic exercises) can slowly strengthen the muscles of the arms, legs, and trunk. In addition, because *yoga* exercises are often weight-bearing on the arms, legs or trunk, they can help increase bone mineral density (BMD) and help strengthen bones in younger asthmatics. With increased bone and muscle strength, it is easier for asthmatics to participate in other physical life activities.

Yoga is essentially the art of learning how to regulate and be comfortable with one's breath in all situations. Initially *yoga* for people with breathing difficulties should focus on becoming aware of normal breathing in simple postures such as lying, sitting, or standing. Then, once relaxed natural breathing is comfortable in the simple postures, a slower breathing may be introduced. Slower breathing prevents drying of airways (a known trigger of asthma), allows less resistance in the airways and is less likely to reduce the normal levels of carbon dioxide, which acts as a natural bronchodilator. Carbon dioxide acts to open the bronchial tubes thus allowing more air to get to the lungs and eventually every cell in the body.

Supine postures are useful postures for allowing the asthmatic to learn to breathe normally. Supine passive *yoga*

postures such as *savasana*   or supported *setu bandhasana*   , allow the chest and abdomen to be passively stretched. Other passive poses that may be useful include leaning forward over a chair to stretch the spine and posterior trunk while resting the diaphragm. Once able to regulate the breathing in passive postures, relaxed breathing in more strenuous postures can be practised.

Progression can later be made to first natural then regulated breathing in standing postures such as

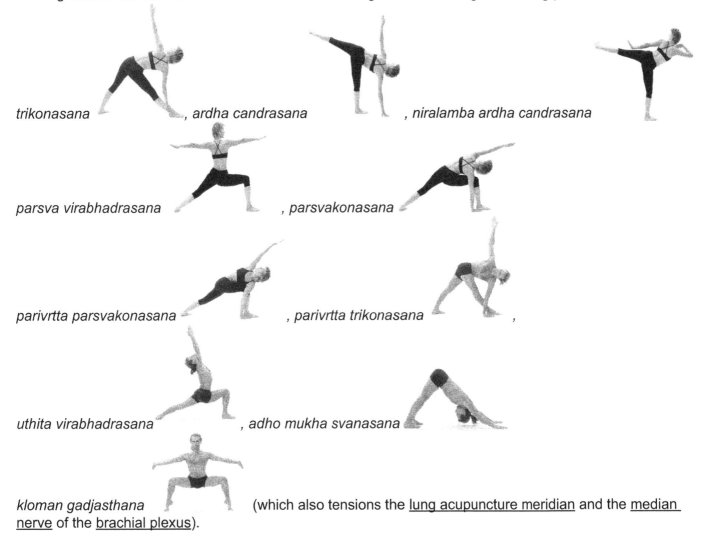

trikonasana   , *ardha candrasana*   , *niralamba ardha candrasana*

parsva virabhadrasana   , *parsvakonasana*

parivrtta parsvakonasana   , *parivrtta trikonasana*   ,

uthita virabhadrasana   , *adho mukha svanasana*

kloman gadjasthana   (which also tensions the lung acupuncture meridian and the median nerve of the brachial plexus).

Learning how to remain as relaxed as possible while performing both passive and active postures helps people with breathing difficulties learn to remain relaxed in their everyday life activities. With regular *yoga* practice asthmatics often find it easier to remain relaxed during an acute asthma attack, and not make breathing more difficult by panicking.

8.4.3 The Effects of Breathing Rate on Various Body Systems

Some types of *pranayama* (*yogic* breathing exercises) require slow breathing that fills and empties the entire lungs. This is sometimes referred to by other authors as complete breathing. Complete breathing requires full use of the diaphragm, the thoracic intercostal muscles and the abdominal muscles:

- The **diaphragm** [Table 7.4] is the main muscle used in what is referred to as abdominal breathing [Section 8.2.8]. On inhalation the abdomen gets larger as the diaphragm is activated (tenses and shortens), and on exhalation the abdomen gets smaller as the diaphragm relaxes (lengthens) and returns to its original position.

- The **thoracic intercostal muscles** (intercostals) [Table 7.4] are used in what is referred to as thoracic breathing [Section 8.2.8]. On inhalation the thorax (chest and upper back) gets larger as the intercostals are activated (tensing and shortening), and on exhalation the thorax gets smaller as the intercostals relax (lengthen) and return to their original position.

- The **abdominal muscles** [Table 7.4] are used to make a forced exhalation or a complete exhalation. By maintaining the grip (tension and shortness) of the abdominal muscles after the exhalation it makes it easier to expand the chest on a subsequent inhalation.

Many people have difficulty breathing with both the diaphragm and the intercostal muscles and are unable to expand their thorax unless they breathe quite forcefully with relatively fast and deep breathing [Table 8.1]. Fast, deep breathing forces the abdominal muscles to become activated (tense) to get the air out quickly and fully and, since the abdominal muscles have no time to relax after the exhalation, the subsequent inhalation is done with the abdomen firm, thus forcing the thorax (chest and upper back) to expand.

Similarly, there are many people who can not easily relax their abdomen. Their abdominal muscles hold so much tension that these people are unable to breathe into their abdomen, and are hardly able to use their diaphragm at all, unless they spend time focusing on relaxation and slower breathing [Table 8.1]. These people tend to be doing mainly thoracic breathing while doing any physical activity.

In terms of the *bandhas*, the complete inhalation, i.e. the maximum possible inhalation, can be done with a *tha-uddiyana bandha* (chest expansion) followed and supplemented by a *tha-mula bandha* (abdominal expansion), while the maximum possible exhalation can be done with a *ha-mula bandha* (abdominal contraction) followed and supplemented by a *ha-uddiyana bandha* (chest contraction).

Table 8.1 compares the effects of two extreme types of breathing (fast deep breathing compared to slow shallow or tidal breathing) on the various body systems. These are only two of the many breathing possibilities that exist and each have varying effects. There is no such thing as right or wrong breathing but one must use the type of breathing that is appropriate for the situation.

Both the thoracic breathing and abdominal breathing confer possible benefits and disadvantages. Ideal yogic breathing is a combination of the most advantageous aspects of both fast, deep breathing and slow, shallow breathing [Table 8.1]. In ideal yogic breathing, the three central *bandhas* (*jalandhara*, *uddiyana*, and *mula*) [Section 7.4.1] are held throughout the breath cycle. To initially learn to maintain a grip on the three *bandhas*, the thorax should be kept expanded (*tha-uddiyana bandha*) throughout the breath cycle as it would be during thoracic breathing inhalation; the lower abdomen should be kept firm and drawn inwards (*ha-mula bandha*), as in a forced exhalation; while the back of the neck is kept long and the chin kept slightly down and inwards (*ha-jalandhara bandha*) [Section 7.4.1].

In optimal *yogic* breathing, slow relaxed diaphragmatic breathing is used to respire only a small amount of air per minute, but with the chest and abdomen held in such a way that only a small volume of air is needed to fill and then empty the lung. In the most advanced stages of *pranayama* the key emphasis should be not on increasing lung volume from breath to breath but rather on increasing the pressure in the chest with each inhale without increasing the volume.

Table 8.1 The effects of two extreme types of breathing on the musculoskeletal anatomy and neurophysiology of the body: Fast deep breathing compared to slow shallow (tidal) breathing

EFFECT ON...	FAST DEEP (FORCED) BREATHING RESULTING IN HYPERVENTILATION	SLOW SHALLOW (RELAXED TIDAL) BREATHING RESULTING IN HYPOVENTILATION
Minute ventilation (ml air/min)	**Increased (↑)** amount of air inspired (breathed) / minute (☐ hyperventilation)	**Decreased (↓)** Amount of air inspired (breathed) / minute (☐ hypoventilation)
Breathing Type	↑ Thoracic (intercostal) breathing	↑ Abdominal (diaphragmatic) breathing
CO_2 Levels	↓ CO_2 levels → Bronchoconstriction & Vasoconstriction	↑ CO_2 levels → Bronchodilation & Vasodilation
pH of blood and in intracellular fluids	↑ **pH,** ie more alkaline blood and intracellular fluids	↓ **pH,** i.e. more acidic blood and intracellular fluids
Overall Muscular Effort	↑ Muscular Effort	↓ Muscular Effort
Abdominal Muscle Strength	↑ Abdominal muscle strength with practice	No change in abdominal muscle strength with practice
Intercostal Muscle Strength	↑ Intercostal muscle strength with practice	Little increase in intercostal muscle strength with practice
Nervous System	Stimulates Sympathetic nervous system (☐ ↑ Tension)	Stimulates Parasympathetic nervous system (☐ ↑ Relaxation)
Time (Subjective)	Time appears to pass slowly	Time appears to pass quickly

There exist several reasons (some esoteric) for working towards this system of *yogic* breathing which maintains the *bandhas* throughout. Correct application of the *bandhas* allows for:

(i) the spine and its musculature to be held in its most biomechanically advantageous position for strength and mobility.

(ii) the circulatory channels of the body (*nadis*) including blood vessels, nerves and acupuncture meridians to be able to flow without impediment.

(iii) the body to become like a capacitor, able to draw energy from the air (*prana*) and use it where needed in the body.

(iv) the mind to become focused or still, which enables it to more readily to enter a state of deep meditation.

(v) the esoteric energy centres (*cakras*) along the spine to become activated and, as the upper parts of the lung become activated, stimulates the esoteric glands of the brain such as the pineal gland.

Complete *yogic* breathing in which the *bandhas* are held throughout the breath, and which does not cause the symptoms of hyperventilation, takes years to master and should not be practised by beginners. This type of breathing is most easily available to those who adopt the classical *hatha yoga* diet (a low protein vegetarian diet with an emphasis on fresh fruit, salads, sprouted grains, and steamed vegetables) that leaves alkaline ash in the blood so the blood can tolerate the larger amounts of carbonic acid generated by the large amounts of carbon dioxide (CO_2) that this type of breathing generates [Section 10.3.4]. To work towards the optimum yogic breathing, the beginner should simply practise expanding the chest on the inhalation (*tha-uddiyana bandha*), and then contracting the waist by activating <u>abdominal muscles</u> on the exhalation (*ha-mula bandha*). With time and practice, the expansion of the chest can be maintained on the exhalation and the firmness of the lower <u>abdomen</u> can be maintained on the inhalation. Once this has been mastered the most useful effects of both fast, deep breathing and slow, shallow breathing [Table 8.1] can be obtained.

Pranayama (*prana* = breath, life force, energy; *ayama* = extension, cessation , control) means the <u>extension</u> of the breath. The aim of *pranayama* is to reduce <u>minute ventilation</u> (the amount of air breathed per minute). This requires the ability to tolerate larger amounts of CO_2 in system. The ancient texts state that "**the *yogi* measures his life not by the number of years he lives but by the number of breaths he takes.**" The main message of these ancient yogi stories is the less air you use the better. This implies that an excess of air actually may shorten life.

8.4.4 Breath-control and Regulation: *Pranayama*

The *yogic* science of breathing is termed *pranayama*. *Prana* has been described as the life-force in the air that we breathe. *Prana* is not actually the breath, but it has something to do with the way we breathe and what happens to the air that we take in. *Ayama* means to control, to regulate, to cease or to extend [Iyengar, 1966]. Therefore, the art and science of *pranayama* is ultimately not about breathing more air, but actually learning to breathe less air over a longer space of time. Like a car that is considered to be more efficient when it runs just as far on less fuel, the human body eventually works better on less fuel (air). Hence, *pranayama* is the art of learning how to make the most effective use of every bit of air that we breathe in and the *prana* we absorb. This involves learning how to make the air reach parts of the <u>lungs</u> and parts of the body that are often not reached in everyday life.

By retaining less air for a longer period of time, <u>carbon dioxide</u> concentrations in the blood are increased. <u>Carbon dioxide</u> acts as a chemical signal that causes <u>vasodilation</u> (i.e. causes the <u>blood vessels</u> going to the <u>brain</u> to expand and therefore take more blood to the <u>brain</u>). An increase in <u>carbon dioxide</u> in the blood causes an increase in the amount of blood and *prana* (life force or energy) flowing to the <u>brain</u>. Similarly, <u>carbon dioxide</u> is a known <u>bronchodilator</u> (i.e. causes expansion of the small tubules which transport gases to and from the <u>lungs</u>). An increase in the blood concentration of <u>carbon dioxide</u> will also cause an increase in the amount of air and *prana* going to the <u>lungs</u> and therefore also to the cells of the rest of the body. Studies in India have demonstrated that, when most people begin a *yoga* practice, initially over the first few years there is a tendency to breathe a greater volume of air per minute than when at their resting state, i.e. beginner *pranayama* practitioners often tend to <u>hyperventilate</u>. These studies have also shown that most experienced *yoga* practitioners (after many years of regular practice) tend to take in less air per minute on average than they do in their normal resting state, and less air generally than the beginner or non *yoga* practitioner, i.e. experienced *pranayama* practitioners tend to <u>hypoventilate</u>. The normal person takes about 12 –16 breaths per minute in the resting state when not doing a *yoga* practice. These resting state breaths are generally <u>tidal breaths</u> of about 500 ml (0.5 litres). Therefore the average breath rate is about 6 – 8 litres per minute. The average <u>lung</u> capacity is about five litres. A beginner who chooses to breathe deeply (i.e. complete inhalations and exhalations) throughout their *yoga* practice, and yet maintains a normal breath rate of up to 12 – 16 breaths per minute, will therefore be breathing up to 60 litres per minutes (ten times as much air as normal). Such excess levels of fuel in a car engine would almost certainly 'flood the engine' or, at best, render it less efficient than it should otherwise be, and the body responds in a similar way to excess breathing. Such high levels of breathing do not allow a build-up of <u>carbon dioxide</u> (CO_2) in the blood. With such high levels of breathing, the <u>carbon dioxide</u> gets 'blown off' before it can reach levels that enable it to act as a chemical signal to <u>vasodilate</u> (expand) the <u>blood vessels</u> going to the <u>brain</u> and <u>bronchodilate</u> (expand) the tubules going to the <u>lungs</u>. Also, because of the <u>Bohr effect</u> [Section 8.2.9.1], there is an inhibition of transfer of <u>oxygen</u> (O_2) from <u>haemoglobin</u> to <u>tissue cells</u>. The <u>Bohr effect</u> states that an increase in <u>alkalinity</u> (a decrease in CO_2) increases the affinity of <u>haemoglobin</u> to oxygen. So the paradox of *pranayama* and breath-control is that one actually gets more <u>oxygen</u> and *prana* to the <u>brain</u>, <u>lungs</u> and into <u>tissue cells</u> by taking in less, rather than more, air. However, when the effort required to maintain difficult postures dramatically increases, more fuel (greater amounts of air) obviously needs to be taken in.

The purpose of deep breathing then is not to take in **more** air, but rather to aerate those parts of the <u>lungs</u> that are not aerated in everyday breathing. For the beginner, a complete (full and deep) inhalation is the only way they can aerate the uppermost parts of the chest. A complete breath that does actually fully expand the chest, automatically creates *uddiyana bandha*. Once *uddiyana bandha* is learnt however it can be practised even with little or no air in the lungs. When the intercostal and/or the accessory muscles of breathing are used during inhalation to expand the chest, as in *tha-uddiyana bandha*, then even the smallest amounts of air and *prana* are drawn to the upper lungs, where, for a normal person, only the complete breath will have the chance of reaching. In order to complete a full exhalation, *ha-mula bandha*, which includes an activation of the lower abdominal muscles, needs to be established. Once *ha-mula bandha* can be maintained during the inhalation and *tha-uddiyana bandha* can be maintained during the exhalation, and both *bandhas* held in place over many inhalations and exhalations, then the maximum amount of air that can be taken in can only be about as small in volume as the tidal breath of the normal person at rest (about 50 - 500ml). However, even though the complete or full breath one can take while retaining *ha-mula* and *tha-uddiyana bandhas* is only small, the very nature of the *bandhas* will direct the air to parts of the lung where it hardly ever goes in everyday life and where it is needed the most.

Kevala kumbhaka

The *yoga* texts speak often of the highest form of *kumbhaka* (breath retention) called *kevala kumbhaka*. It is written that in this *pranayama* the breath is suddenly stopped without *puraka* (inhalation) and *rechaka* (exhalation). The student can retain his breath as long as he likes through this *kumbhaka*. He attains the state of *raja yoga*. Through *kevala kumbhaka*, the knowledge of *kundalini* (energy inside the spine) arises. To enable this to take place physically the practitioner's skin must breathe easily and the practitioner must have sufficient alkaline reserves to tolerate increased amounts of CO_2. The phenomenon may be able to be explained in terms of the anatomical dead space. The anatomical dead space is that region in the trachea and in the beginning of the bronchial tubes which must be filled with air first before any air gets to the alveoli and the functional parts of the lungs. The anatomical dead space occupies a volume of about 150 ml. This means that if one takes a deep breath (say 3000 ml), the greater proportion of the air will get to the lungs (2850 ml or 95% of the breath) and the less proportion (150 ml or 5% of the breath) will occupy the anatomical dead space. If, on the other hand, one takes a shallow breath (say 300 ml) then only half the breath (150 ml or 50% of the breath) goes to the functional part of the lungs while the other half of the breath (150 ml or the remaining 50% of the breath) will fill the anatomical dead space and not actually reach the functional parts of the lungs at all. If you can have a tidal breath of less than 150 ml (the volume of the anatomical dead space) then it is essentially like not breathing and may be precisely what the yogic texts describe as *kevala kumbhaka*.

8.4.5 Research on *Pranayama* (Breath-Control), *Kumbhaka* (Breath Holding) and the *Bandhas*

There is quite a lot of published scientific research available based on experiments that have been done on breath-holding. Much of this research considers the effect of the Valsalva manoeuvre (an expiratory effort with a closed glottis) on the cardiopulmonary system. The Valsalva manoeuvre is similar to making an *antara kumbhaka* (inhalation retention) with *ha-mula bandha* and *ha-uddiyana bandha*.

Athletes had their blood pressure monitored while cycling while simultaneously performing the Valsalva manoeuvre resulting in a significant inclrease in blood pressure [Nobrega et al., 1994]. A similar magnitude blood pressure increase was observed during Valsalva alone.

The Valsalva manoeuvre is also a widely used test for autonomic nervous system function as it consists of a physiologic effort, which can be performed in everyday life [Bazak, 1990]. However, Bazak [1990] has warned that extreme effort in making a Valsalva manoeuvre, in effect making an *antara kumbhaka* (inhalation retention) with *ha-mula bandha* and *ha-uddiyana bandha* may cause faintness or fainting, even in normal persons. Bazak [1990] also points out the similarity of the effect of Valsalva manoeuvre to that of hyperventilation (over-breathing) on the cerebral circulation, i.e. the Valsalva manoeuvre and hence *antara kumbhaka* (inhalation retention) with *ha-mula bandha* and *ha-uddiyana bandha* can cause a reduction in the supply of blood to the brain.

In another study on athletes [Hughes et al., 1994] maximum Valsalva manoeuvres caused extreme falls in cardiac output (the amount of blood leaving the heart) and blood pressure. The advanced *yoga* practitioner can feel the radial pulse weaken and actually disappear when performing an *antara kumbhaka* (inhalation retention) with *ha-mula bandha* and *ha-uddiyana bandha*. It was further found [Hughes et al., 1994] that the reduction in cardiac output seen in the athletes was attenuated (lessened) by simultaneous isometric handgrip. The *yoga* practitioner can also substantiate this by monitoring the radial pulse then performing an *antara kumbhaka* with *ha-mula bandha* and *ha-uddiyana bandha* (Valsalva manoeuvre) then adding a *ha-mani bandha* (simultaneous handgrip) [Section 3.9.1.2].

Effect of Hyperventilation and Hypoventilation On ↓	HYPERVENTILATION	HYPOVENTILATION
Minute ventilation (ml air/min)	**Increased (↑)** amount of air inspired (breathed) litres / minute (☐ hyperventilation)	**Decreased (↓)** Amount of air inspired (breathed) litres / minute (☐ hypoventilation)
Types of breathing (approximate values based on an average lung size of 5 litres and resting breath of 10 breaths per minute x 0.5 litres per minute)	At rest: any breathing which has more than 5 litres per minute for the average person eg. More than one full breath per minute, or more than 2 half breaths per minute	At rest: any breathing which has less than 5 litres per minute for the average person eg. Less than one full breath per minute, or less than 2 half breaths per minute
Carbon dioxide (CO_2) Levels	↓ CO_2 levels → Bronchoconstriction and Vasoconstriction	↑ CO_2 levels → Bronchodilatation and Vasodilation
Effect of CO_2 Levels on Colonic Tone	↓ CO_2 levels → ↑ Colonic tone; may cause constipation, may relieive diarrhoea	↑ CO_2 levels → ↓ Colonic tone; may promote bowel movements, may cause diarrhoea
Carbonic acid levels of blood and in intracellular fluids	↓ carbonic acid levels in blood and intracellular fluids	↑ carbonic acid levels in blood and intracellular fluids
pH of blood and in intracellular fluids	↑ pH, i.e. more alkaline blood and intracellular fluids	↓ pH, i.e. more acidic blood and intracellular fluids
pH effect on Blood Vessel Diameter	↓ blood vessel diameter i.e. Vasoconstriction	↑ blood vessel diameter i.e. Vasodilation
pH effect on Bronchial Tube Diameter	↓ bronchial tube diameter i.e. Bronchoconstriction (which can lead to asthma)	↑ bronchial tube diameter i.e. Bronchodilation (which can relieve asthma)
Cellular ventilation	↓ Blood flow to cells (due to Bohr effect)	↑ Blood flow to cells (due to Bohr effect)
Alveolar ventilation	↓ Air flow to lungs	↑ Air flow to lungs
Nervous System	Stimulates sympathetic nervous system (☐ ↑ Tension, ↑ Pain)	Stimulates parasympathetic nervous system (☐ ↑ Relaxation, ↓ Pain)
pH Effects on Nervous System	↑ pH ☐ ↑ over-excitability of nervous system, ↑ hypersensitivity of nerves	↓ pH ☐ depression of nervous system ↓ sensitivity of nervous system
pH effect on synovial fluid in joints and surrounding nerves and muscles	↑ pH ☐ ↑ flexibility (temporary) of joints and also greater mobility of muscles and nerves over the connective tissue sheaths that surround them (temporary)	↓ pH ☐ ↓ flexibility (temporary) of joints and also reduced mobility of muscles and nerves over the connective tissue sheaths that surround them (temporary)
pH effect on food habits	↑ pH ☐ ↑ levels of hunger; ↑ desire more acid producing foods, such as high protein foods, complex carbohydrates, fats and processed foods ↓ tolerance and desire for alkaline producing foods (eg.t fruits, salads and vegetables)	↓ pH ☐ ↑ suppresion of appetite; ↓ desire for acid producing foods (eg. high protein foods, complex carbohydrates, fats and processed foods); ↑ tolerance and desire for alkaline producing foods (eg. fruits, salads and vegetables)

Table 8.2 The effects of hyperventilation (increased ventilation) versus hypoventilation (decreased ventilation) on the musculoskeletal anatomy and neurophysiology of the body.

Cardiac patients with <u>tachycardia</u> (faster than normal <u>heart</u> beat) could have their <u>tachycardia</u> permanently and reproducibly terminated with a <u>Valsalva manoeuvre</u> [Waxman *et al.*, 1994]. The speed with which the <u>Valsalva manoeuvre</u> terminated the <u>tachycardia</u> increased in direct proportion to the strength of the <u>Valsalva manoeuvre</u>. This evidence helps explain the scientific basis of what happens, and part of the mechanism involved, when the advanced *yoga* practitioner is able to briefly stop their <u>heart</u>.

Another study [Bartlett, 1977] showed that seated subjects were able to hold their breath at the functional residual capacity (about half the <u>lungs</u> full) for longer times when they applied either a <u>Valsalva manoeuvre</u> (sustained effort at exhalation without actually breathing) or a <u>Mueller manoeuvre</u> (sustained effort at inhalation using the <u>diaphragm</u>, without actually breathing). These manoeuvres both resemble *ha-* and *tha-* versions of *mula* and *uddiyana bandhas*. Interestingly, the subjects were also asked to see the effect of squeezing rubber bulbs with their hands as a control for the experiment. Squeezing a ball, essentially like *ha-mani bandha* (a closed fist or handgrip), [Section 3.9.1.2] was shown to be equally effective in prolonging breath-holding time. The *bandhas* are intimately related, therefore this result is not a surprise for a *yoga* practitioner but the experimenter has suggested that since the <u>Valsalva manoeuvre</u>, the <u>Mueller manoeuvre</u> and the handgrip all prolonged breath-holding time, the effect is due to the influence of psychological factors. Furthermore, conclusive research from a *yogic* perspective would be relatively easy to conduct by repeating these experiments but using the handgrip as part of the experiment and getting a suitable non-muscular control to test for presence of psychological factors.

8.4.6 Progressive *Pranayama* (Yogic Breathing Exercise) Sequence for the Development of Breathing with Use of the *Bandhas* (Yogic Muscular Locks)

The following exercises can systematically develop the central *bandhas*. The easiest exercises are done in a supine lying position, while the more difficult exercises are done in a sitting position such as *padmasana* (lotus) [Figure8.1] or any comfortable sitting posture.

WARNING: Progress with the following progressive series of *pranayama* (breath-control) exercises with caution. NEVER FORCE THE BREATH. Do not continue these exercises beyond step #8 without the guidance of an experienced teacher. For safety master one step before proceeding to the next.

1. **Supine relaxed <u>abdominal (diaphragmatic) breathing</u>:** Breathe naturally with a relaxed <u>abdomen</u> (natural small breaths into the <u>abdomen</u> with natural pauses). Inhale and exhale are both completely passive and incomplete. This is generally invisible and inaudible breath.

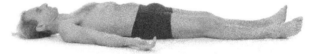

2. **Supine deep <u>abdominal breathing</u>:** slow inhale relax and expand the <u>abdomen</u> by contracting the <u>diaphragm</u> away from the chest. Chest must remain totally still and relaxed throughout. First exhale passively, when no more air comes out passively, actively bring the navel towards the spine (*ha-mula bandha)* to exhale fully. Relax the <u>abdomen</u> completely before the next breath begins.

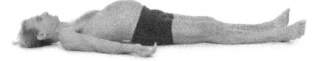

3. **Seated deep abdominal breathing:** as for # 2 but in any comfortable seated posture (sitting).

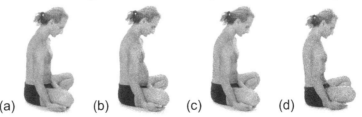

(a) Relaxed; (b) <u>diaphragmatic (abdominal)</u> inhale; (c) passive <u>abdominal</u> exhale; (d) active <u>abdominal</u> exhale

4. **Supine <u>thoracic breathing</u> (if possible have a bolster or rolled blanket under the chest):** Keep the <u>abdomen</u> and your shoulders completely relaxed. Inhale by expanding the chest (*tha-uddiyana bandha*). Do not let the <u>abdomen</u> expand during inhalation. Exhale passively by relaxing the chest, then, if possible, gently exhale actively contracting the chest further (*ha-uddiyana bandha*) using the <u>intercostal muscles</u>.

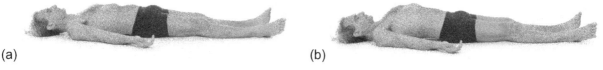

(a)   (b)

(a) relaxed breathing; (b) <u>thoracic</u> inhale

---

5. **Seated <u>thoracic</u> breathing:** As for # 4 but in sitting

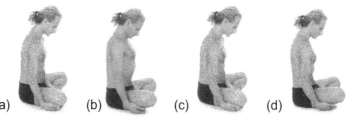

a)   (b)   (c)   (d)

(a) relaxed breathing; (b) <u>thoracic</u> (chest) inhale; (c) passive <u>thoracic</u> exhale; (e) active <u>abdominal</u> exhale

---

6. **Supine complete breathing (<u>abdominal breathing</u> then <u>thoracic breathing</u>):** First inhale using the <u>diaphragm</u> and relax and expand the <u>abdomen</u>. Then expand the chest (*tha-uddiyana bandha*) without letting the <u>abdomen</u> become tense or collapse closer to the floor (i.e. keep the <u>diaphragm</u> actively descended and contracted). Inhale for as long as possible in this way (even up to one minute to strengthen the muscles on inhalation). Then first exhale passively from the chest, then passively from the <u>abdomen</u> by letting the chest then <u>abdomen</u> relax and drop down. Then actively exhale the rest of the way by gripping the <u>perineum</u> and then drawing the first the lower <u>abdomen</u> and then the upper <u>abdomen</u> closer to the spine.

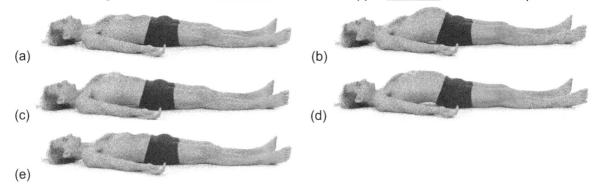

(a)   (b)

(c)   (d)

(e)

(a) passive; (b) <u>diaphragmatic</u> inhale; (c) <u>thoracic</u> inhale (complete inhale); (d) passive <u>thoracic</u> exhale;
(e) passive <u>abdominal</u> exhale

---

7. **Seated complete breathing:** As for # 6 but in a seated posture with the option that after the air has been actively exhaled from the <u>abdomen</u> more air may be exhaled by compressing the chest with the chest exhalation muscles (*ha-uddiyana bandha*) (not shown).

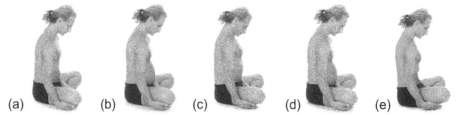

(a)   (b)   (c)   (d)   (e)

(a) relaxed breathing; (b) <u>diaphragmatic</u> inhale; (c) <u>thoracic</u> inhale (complete inhale); (d) passive <u>thoracic</u> exhale;
(e) active <u>abdominal</u> exhale

---

8. **Exhalation retention (bahya kumbhaka):** Initially when holding the breath (in or out) simply focus on being erect in the spine and being as relaxed as possible. Initially practice all breath retentions with *ha-jalandhara bandha*. First learn exhalation retention in a seated position by exhaling passively (an incomplete exhalation)

and learn to get comfortable with this for up to at least 30 seconds before proceeding with further breath retention. Once this is mastered then attempt full exhalation retention (having drawn the navel to the spine with <u>abdominal</u> exhalation muscles then again relaxed the <u>abdomen</u>). Finally, attempt <u>thoracic</u> inspiratory effort (*tha-uddiyana bandha*) (this is like trying to breathe into the chest without actually breathing) Hold out for as long as you comfortably can and allow enough time to relax (collapse) the chest before inhaling calmly. Attempt this exercise first in standing then in a seated posture.

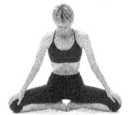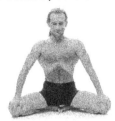

9. **Inhalation retention (*antara kumbhaka*):** First learn inhalation retention in a seated position by inhaling passively (an incomplete <u>abdominal</u> inhalation) and learn to get comfortable with this for up to at least 60 seconds before proceeding further with breath retention. Once this is mastered then attempt full inhalation retention (using the complete breath as described previously). Finally, once you can comfortably hold the breath in for at least 2 minutes attempt <u>abdominal</u> expiratory effort (*ha-mula bandha*) and <u>thoracic</u> expiratory effort (*ha-uddiyana bandha*) (this is like trying to actively breathe out from <u>abdomen</u> and from the chest without actually breathing). Attempt this exercise in a seated posture.

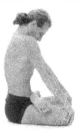

10. **_Ujjayi pranayama_ in sitting with _ha-jalandhara bandha_ (head down and neck back) and _antara kumbhaka_ (inhalation retention):** Exhale completely, contract the <u>abdomen</u> (*ha-mula bandha*) then contract the chest (*ha-uddiyana bandha*); then inhale expanding the chest (*tha-uddiyana bandha*) keeping the <u>abdomen</u> firm (*ha-mula bandha*); hold the breath in (*antara kumbhaka*), relax the face, neck and throat, enhance *ha-jalandhara bandha, tha-uddiyana bandha,* and *ha-mula bandha*; relax the face, neck and throat again; begin exhalation (first tense the perineum then lower <u>abdomen</u> to begin exhale) from the <u>abdomen</u> (*ha-mula bandha*) then relax (drop down) chest, then gently contract chest (*ha-uddiyana bandha*) by activating <u>intercostal muscles.</u>

11. **_Ujjayi pranayama_ in sitting with _ha-jalandhara bandha_ (head down and neck back) and _bahya kumbhaka_ (exhalation retention):** Exhale completely, contract the <u>abdomen</u> (*ha-mula bandha*) then contract the chest (*ha-uddiyana bandha*); then begin first round of the exercise; inhale and expand the chest (*tha-uddiyana bandha*) keeping the <u>abdomen</u> firm (*ha-mula bandha*); hold the breath in (*antara kumbhaka*), relax the face, neck and throat. Enhance *ha-jalandhara bandha, tha-uddiyana bandha,* and *ha-mula bandha*, then relax the face, neck and throat again; begin the exhalation (first tense the perineum then the lower <u>abdomen</u> to begin exhalation) from the <u>abdomen</u> (*ha-mula bandha*) then relax (drop down) chest then, if possible, gently contract chest (*ha-uddiyana bandha*) by activating the <u>intercostal muscles</u>. At end of exhale hold the breath out (*bahya kumbhaka*), then relax upper <u>abdomen</u> (so lower ribs are free to move), then expand the chest and upper back (*tha-uddiyana bandha*), then contract <u>abdomen</u> (*ha-mula bandha*) then relax (drop down) chest then, if possible, gently contract chest (*ha-uddiyana bandha*) by activating <u>intercostal muscles</u>. Then begin next round of exercise, or rest with normal breathing.

12. **_Ujjayi pranayama_ in sitting with _antara kumbhaka_ (inhalation retention) and _bahya kumbhaka_ (exhalation retention):** Combine #13 and #14.

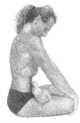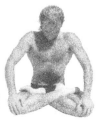

A common problem during most people's yoga practice and in everyday exercise is the over-tensing of the trunk musculature (<u>abdominal</u> muscles and <u>paraspinal</u> muscles). This is made worse by the over-activity of the <u>muscles of forced abdominal exhalation</u> (MFAE), which is usually due to habitual drawing the navel to the spine either because it looks better (e.g. one's trunk looks slimmer) than letting the <u>abdomen</u> relax, or because it is believed to help reduce risk of back pain.

The first and most important breathing type to learn during exercise is natural relaxed <u>diaphragmatic</u> breathing where only a relatively small number of relatively small breaths are taken each minute - the inhalation is purely <u>diaphragmatic</u> (i.e. no chest expansion) and the exhalation is purely passive (i.e. no muscles are used to exhale in natural breathing).

Many (perhaps most) normal people (as opposed to natural people) do not have very much control over their muscles of breathing. Five of the most common limitations or inabilities with learning breath-control (pranayama) techniques are as follows:

- Different people respond in at least two different ways to the instruction to 'firm', 'tense' or 'tighten' the <u>abdomen</u> (e.g. some people firm the <u>abdomen</u> by drawing or pulling the navel closer to the spine by using the <u>muscles of forced abdominal exhalation</u> (MFAE), while other people simply firm the <u>abdomen</u> using postural muscles, without drawing or pulling the navel towards the spine and without using the MFAE).

- Many people do not realise that to exhale fully in many postures they generally need to compress or contract the <u>abdomen</u> by pulling the navel towards the spine, or they are simply not able to do this action (until they are suitably trained to do so).

- Many people can compress or contract the <u>abdomen</u> by pulling the navel towards the spine on exhalation but they generally don't release it in every day life and it brings them a lot of tension, and prevents them from using their <u>diaphragm</u> to breathe into their <u>abdomen</u>.

- Many people can only draw the navel to the spine to make a complete exhalation by making the <u>abdomen</u> firm while it is in fact possible to exhale fully without hardening the <u>abdomen</u> yet still using the MFAE.

- Many people can not breathe into their chest unless they are holding their <u>abdomen</u> firm by compressing or contracting the <u>abdomen</u> by pulling the navel towards the spine.

- Many yoga practitioners don't realise that many postures, especially those using active movements, do not need the use of the MFAE to exhale fully because some postures physically compress the relaxed <u>abdomen</u> to cause deeper than normal exhalation, while other postures achieved through the activation of postural trunk muscles that allow the passive exhalation of natural breathing to be almost complete exhalation without the need for any additional thought or muscle activity (this is also true for daily activities such as natural brisk walking).

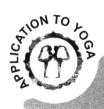

APPLICATION TO YOGA

No 8.6 Abdominal, chest and complete inhalation can be achieved with combinations of mula bandha and uddiyana bandha

Abdominal (diaphragmatic) inhalation can be achieved (in increasing order of difficulty) with:

- abdomen relaxed and chest relaxed (this is easiest type of abdominal breath for most people to achieve)
- abdomen relaxed and chest expanded with *tha-uddiyana bandha*
- abdomen relaxed and chest compressed with *ha-uddiyana bandha*
- abdomen firm with *tha-mula bandha* and chest relaxed
- abdomen firm with *tha-mula bandha* and chest expanded with *tha-uddiyana bandha*
- abdomen firm with *tha-mula bandha* and chest compressed with *ha-uddiyana bandha*
- abdomen firm with *ha-mula bandha* and chest expanded with *tha-uddiyana bandha*
- abdomen firm with *ha-mula bandha* and chest compressed with *ha-uddiyana bandha* (this is the hardest type of abdominal breath for most people to achieve)

Chest (thoracic) inhalation (tha-uddiyana bandha) can be achieved with (in increasing order of difficulty):

- abdomen firm with *ha-mula bandha* and under-armpit muscles (the shoulder depressors latissimus dorsi and pectoralis major) active (this is the easiest type of chest inhalation for most people to achieve)
- abdomen firm with *ha-mula bandha* and under-armpit muscles relaxed
- abdomen firm with *tha-mula bandha* and under-armpit muscles active
- abdomen firm with *tha-mula bandha* and under-armpit muscles relaxed
- abdomen relaxed and under-armpit muscles active
- abdomen relaxed and under-armpit muscles relaxed (this is the hardest type of chest inhalation for most people to achieve)

Complete (diaphragmatic then thoracic) inhalation (the complete yogic breath) is when the diaphragm is active first to breathe 'into the abdomen' then keeping the diaphragm active (i.e. keeping a sense of 'breath in the abdomen') the thorax becomes active to 'breathe into the chest'. A complete breath is easiest for most people to achieve:

- once it is possible to breathe into the abdomen alone and chest alone
- once the strength of the diaphragm and chest muscles are sufficient to allow them to remain active at the same time (i.e. to be able to activate and shorten the diaphragm and move it away from the chest, while a chest expansion (*tha-uddiyana bandha*) is exerting a negative (upwards) pressure on the chest during inhalation).

****

Chapter Breakdown

****

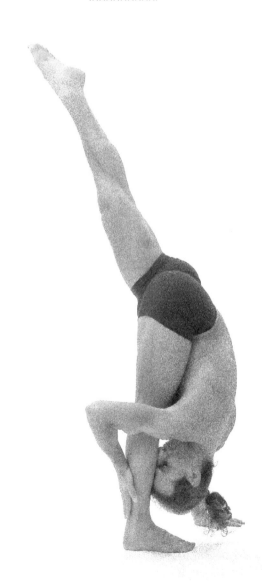

Simon Borg-Olivier tensioning (stretching) the spinal cord, femoral nerve and sciatic nerve in *Urdhva Prasarita Eka Padasana*. Photo courtesy of Alejandro Rolandi

Hatha yoga effects the nervous system (NS) in several ways, and for several reasons:

(i) The *asanas* (postures) and *mudras* (gestures) can facilitate nerve tensioning (stretching of specific nerves) [Section 1.7.2, 9.7.3, Figures 9.1 – 9.7], which can improve their ability to function and correctly conduct electrochemical signals, especially if they have been slightly impinged.

(ii) Specific stretching of muscles and tissues causes a number of nerve reflexes [Sections 1.7.2 & 9.4.2] to take place. In addition, by applying a practical understanding of nerve reflexes, such as the myotatic reflex (stretch reflex), reciprocal relaxation reflex and the inverse myotatic reflex, the *yoga* practitioner is able to simultaneously train for strength, flexibility and relaxation.

(iii) Specific breathing patterns have a number of different effects on the nervous system by virtue of their effect on the pH (acid-alkali levels) of the blood [Section 10.3.4], the effect on the heart [Section 8.1.3], the effect of pressure on the baroreceptors [Section 8.1.6.1], and the effect of oxygen and carbon dioxide levels on the chemoreceptors [Section 8.1.6.2].

If during a *hatha yoga* practice, *asanas*, *pranayama*, *bandhas* (muscle co-activation) [Section 1.7.3] or *mudras* are overworked or if their combined effect is excessive, then the sympathetic nervous system (SPNS) may become over stimulated, and the autonomic nervous system (ANS) may be left out of balance. This may lead to random firing of the nerves and a certain amount of shakiness. Care should be taken so that nerves are not over-stretched, as there is a risk that they may be damaged.

9.1.1 Nerve Cells

The nervous system is complex in structure and function but it only contains two principle kinds of cells: neurons (nerve cells) and neuroglia (support cells).

9.1.1.1 Neurons: Impulse conducting nerve cells

Neurons are the main cells of the nervous system. Neurons are responsible for most of the special functions attributed to the nervous system such as sensing, thinking, remembering, controlling muscular activity, and regulating glandular secretions.

Neurons are able to conduct electrochemical impulses. They have a main cell body, containing a nucleus, and an axon (long branched process). Neurons are usually covered and insulated by a myelin sheath [Section 9.1.1.2].

9.1.1.2 Neuroglia: nervous system support cells

The myelin sheath that surrounds nerves is an insulating phospholipid layer, which is enveloped by cells known as oligodendrocytes in the central nervous system (CNS), and Schwann cells in the peripheral nervous system (PNS). Other specialised cells include the microglia, which are the small scavenger cells of the brain and spinal cord.

9.1.2 Classification of Neurons

There are several types of neurons (nerve cells). These include sensory (afferent) neurons and motor (efferent) neurons, interneurons, somatic neurons and visceral neurons.

9.1.2.1 Afferent (sensory) neurons

Afferent (sensory) neurons conduct impulses from receptors such as those in the skin to the central nervous system (CNS). Afferent neurons or sensory neurons can receive nerve impulses from either the sensory-somatic nervous system [Section 9.2.2.1] or from the autonomic nervous system [Section 9.2.2.2].

9.1.2.2 Efferent (motor) neurons

Efferent (motor) neurons conduct impulses from the CNS to the effector organs (eg muscles or organs). Efferent or motor neurons can receive nerve impulses from either the sensory-somatic nervous system [Section 9.2.2.1] or from the autonomic nervous system [Section 9.2.2.2].

9.1.2.3 Interneurons

Interneurons exist between the afferent and efferent neurons and can be excitatory (stimulate a muscle to activate or tense) or inhibitory (stimulate a muscle to relax).

9.1.2.4 Visceral neurons

Visceral neurons are neurons in organs with hollow cavities. Visceral neurons can be either afferent (sensory) or efferent (motor).

9.1.2.5 Somatic neurons

Somatic neurons are nerves cells conveying information to and from the skin, fascia and musculoskeletal systems. Somatic neurons can be either afferent (sensory) or efferent (motor).

9.1.3 Synapses: Junctions between Neurons

Synapses are functional junctions between two neurons, or between a neuron and an effector, such as a muscle or a gland. Synapses may be electrical or chemical in nature.

9.1.3.1 Chemical synapse Communication: Neurotransmitters

Chemical synapse communication is facilitated by neurotransmitters, which are chemicals released by the pre-synaptic membrane that interact with receptors on the post-synaptic membrane where they may either inhibit or excite electrical activity of the post-synaptic membrane. The most common neurotransmitters in the body are acetylcholine (ACh), adrenalin and noradrenaline.

9.1.3.2 Electrical synapse Communication

Electrical synapse communication between neurons moves directly from one cell to the next. Electrical synapse communication allows faster conduction and synchronicity than chemical synapses.

9.1.4 Neuromuscular Junctions: Nerves Communicating with Muscles

Neuromuscular junctions (NMJs) are the joining of nerves to muscles. NMJs are chemical synapses between the motor nerve axon terminal and the muscle cell motor end plate. Acetylcholine (ACh) a neurotransmitter, changes the permeability of the muscle cell to calcium, which initiates activation of a muscle cell.

9.1.5 Neurophysiology

Electrical synapse communication [Section 9.1.3.2] in neurons spreads directly from one cell to another, thus allowing faster conduction and synchronicity than chemical synapse communication [Section 9.1.3.2]. Electrical synapse communication depends on two basic properties of neuronal plasma (cell) membranes (phospholipid bilayer):
* The value of the resting membrane potential (RMP), which is the electrical voltage across membranes.
* The state of the ion channels or pores in the membranes, which may be either open or closed.

An action potential (AP) is the electrical impulse or signal that travels down the neuron. It is a wave of negativity that self-propagates along the membrane of a neuron or muscle fibre (cell). The refractory period is the period after an AP is generated when a second AP cannot be initiated even with a strong stimulus. This is when the membrane is repolarising. Local anaesthetics work by preventing the opening of voltage-gated ion channels so that impulses cannot pass up the neuron.

The conduction speed of nerve impulses is determined by the following:
* The amount of myelin sheathing (myelin increases conduction speed since it acts as an electrical insulator);
* The fibre diameter (larger diameter fibres have increased speed of conduction);
* The temperature (increased temperature increases speed).

9.1.6 Regeneration of Nervous Tissue

Nervous tissue has a very limited ability to repair. In the central nervous system (CNS) [Section 9.2.1] there is little to no repair of damaged neurons as scar tissue is a physical barrier to regeneration. In the peripheral nervous system (PNS) [Section 9.2.1] regeneration may occur via collateral sprouting branches of nerves finding their way to distal denervated segments using an intact myelin sheath as its guide. Surgical reattachment may also enhance regrowth of nerves.

9.2 ORGANISATION OF THE NERVOUS SYSTEM

The nervous system is an electrochemical communication system that runs throughout the entire body. Information is transported along nerves and through the body by neurotransmitter molecules, which sometimes resemble and can behave as hormones or immunotransmitters, and which can liaise and communicate with the endocrine and immune systems [Section 11.1.4].

9.2.1 Main Structural Components of the Nervous System

The nervous system is physically divided into 2 main parts:

- **The central nervous system (CNS)** includes the brain (cerebrum, brainstem, and cerebellum) and spinal cord.
- **The peripheral nervous system (PNS)** includes the cranial nerves (12 pairs), spinal nerves (sensory and motor), and the autonomic nervous system (ANS).

9.2.2 Main Functional Components of the Nervous system

The nervous system is functionally divided into two main parts: the sensory-somatic nervous system (SNS), which is under conscious control, and the autonomic nervous system (ANS), which is generally under unconscious control.

9.2.2.1 The sensory-somatic nervous system (SNS)

The sensory-somatic nervous system (SNS) is that part of the nervous system which is generally considered to be under voluntary control. This includes all the nerves, which control all the muscles that we can voluntarily move. However, in reality most people can only control a small percentage of the muscular potential unless they have done years of training in *yoga*, dance or some other whole body oriented physical system.

The SNS includes the sensory neurons that convey information from the skin and special sense receptors mainly in the head, the body wall and in the extremities to the CNS. The SNS also includes the motor neurons that convey information from the CNS to the skeletal muscles.

9.2.2.2 The autonomic nervous system (ANS)

The autonomic nervous system (ANS), structurally part of the peripheral nervous system (PNS), contains nerves dedicated to visceral activity and glandular secretion. It is divided into three parts:

- The sympathetic nervous system (SPNS) [Section 9.5.1]
- The parasympathetic nervous system (PSNS) [Section 9.5.2]
- The enteric nervous system (ENS) [Section 9.5.3]

The ANS includes the sensory neurons that convey information from receptors primarily in the viscera (hollow organs) to the CNS, and motor neurons that convey information from the CNS to the viscera.

9.3 CENTRAL NERVOUS SYSTEM

9.3.1 The Brain

9.3.1.1 Cerebral hemispheres

A pair of cerebral hemispheres makes up the largest area of the brain. They consist of an outer grey cortex (nuclei), and inner white matter (tracts of axons). The cerebral hemispheres are divided into lobes related to the cranial bones covering them. All areas of the cortex are involved in memory.

The **lobes of the cortex** have different functions as follows:

- **Frontal lobe**: reasoning, abstract thinking, aggression, sexual behaviour, olfaction (smell), speech, and voluntary motor movement.
- **Parietal lobe**: sensory areas, taste, language, abstract reasoning (maths).
- **Temporal lobe**: language interpretation, auditory (hearing), memory.
- **Occipital lobe**: visual area.
- **Limbic lobe**: emotions - love, anger, aggression, compulsion.

Structurally both cerebral hemispheres are similar. Functionally, the left cerebral hemisphere performs mathematical, analytical and verbal functions, while the right cerebral hemisphere performs visual, spatial and musical functions.

9.3.1.2 Meninges

The meninges are three fibrous coverings around the brain and spinal cord. The dura mater is the tough outer layer close to the bone. The arachnoid mater sits flush with the dura mater and has spidery like processes. The pia mater adheres to the spinal cord and brain.

9.3.1.3 Subcortex

The subcortex sits below the cortex and consists of white matter, basal ganglia (nuclei) and ventricles.

9.3.1.3.1 Ventricles
Ventricles are cavities within the brain that produce 400-500 ml/day of cerebrospinal fluid (CSF), which functions to cushion the brain and spinal cord and to provide nutrition. CSF fills the subarachnoid space (between the arachnoid and pia mater), and is then reabsorbed into the bloodstream.

9.3.1.3.2 Basal ganglia
Basal ganglia constitute the main coordinating centre of the brain. These nuclei are involved in planning, initiation, maintenance and termination of habitual or automatic movements like walking. They are instrumental in maintaining muscle tone and programming sequential postural movements.

Diseases of the basal ganglia include Parkinsons disease, a disease characterised by rigidity and resting tremors due to a lack of the neurotransmitter dopamine, resulting in an increase in basal ganglia (BG) output which in turn inhibits the motor cortex. A disease with the opposite effect is Tourettes syndrome which is an overproduction of dopamine resulting in decreased BG output and over-stimulation of the cortex, characterised by tics, very fast thinking and movement and uncontrolled utterances.

9.3.1.3.3 White matter
White matter has tracts (bundles of axons) travelling in three directions. The corpus callosum connects the left and right cerebral hemispheres. The association tracts connect anterior and posterior parts of the cerebral hemispheres and the projection tracts through the internal capsule are the ascending and descending tracts connecting the brain with the rest of the body.

9.3.1.4 Diencephalon

The diencephalon sits between the cerebral hemispheres and consists of the thalamus, hypothalamus, and pineal gland.

9.3.1.4.1 Thalamus
The thalamus is a relay station for sensory impulses to the cerebral cortex from the brainstem, cerebellum, and association fibres. It functions (i) to integrate sensory information to an appropriate motor and emotional response and (ii) to maintain and regulate awareness (conscious state). It consists of six nuclei: dealing with (i) hearing, (ii) vision, (iii) taste, touch, temperature, pain and vibration, (iv) voluntary motor, (v) arousal, and (vi) emotions and memory.

9.3.1.4.2 Hypothalamus [Section 11.1.3.1]
The hypothalamus regulates homeostasis of the visceral system; regulates body temperature, the drive to eat, and is associated with rage and aggression.

9.3.1.4.3 Pineal Gland [Section 11.1.3.3]
The pineal gland is the only unpaired structure in the brain. It produces melatonin, a pigment-enhancing hormone that is related to body rhythms. Melatonin production is stimulated by darkness. The pineal gland has many functions that are not yet fully understood but which are directly affected by *yoga* and meditation.

9.3.1.5 Brainstem

The brainstem consists of the midbrain, pons and medulla.

> **Midbrain**: The midbrain contains tracts connecting the upper brain and spinal cord; tracts from the thalamus, midbrain and medulla to the cerebellum; centres for involuntary visual (blink, pupil dilation) and auditory reflexes.
>
> **Pons**: The pons has transverse fibres connecting the left and right cerebellum and longitudinal fibres of the ascending sensory and descending motor tracts.
>
> **Medulla**: The medulla contains control centres for the respiratory system and cardiovascular system.

9.3.1.6 Cerebellum

The cerebellum is connected to the brainstem but separated from the cerebrum by dura mater. The function of the cerebellum is to compare intended movements with what movement is actually happening, and to give corrective feedback if necessary. It regulates posture, balance, muscle tone and fine movement. The cerebellum is involved in acquisition of skill. As a movement pattern is repeated and requires less feedback correction, it becomes a predictive movement, that is, a response can be produced based on prior learning (feed-forward response) like walking. Diseases of the cerebellum result in a loss of: automation; smooth movements; balance; and predictive ability, which cause an increase in sway on walking, the need for a larger base of support, speech slurring, over/under shooting, and intention tremor.

9.3.2. Spinal Cord

The spinal cord begins at the foramen magnum of the skull and ends at the vertebral level L1, L2 as the conus medullaris, from which the cauda equina (horses tail) of nerves descends. The spinal cord is shorter than the vertebral column, and lumbar punctures (CSF samples) and epidural anaesthetics must be below L2 to avoid damage to the spinal cord. There are 31 pairs of spinal nerves coming off the spinal cord. The inside of the spinal cord, as seen in a transverse section, consists of central grey nuclei in an H shape. The dorsal horns contain incoming sensory nerves; the ventral horns contain outgoing motor nerves. Lateral horns are present only in the thoracic and upper lumber regions and contain nerves to the autonomic nervous system (ANS).

9.3.2.1 Internal anatomy of the spinal cord

Ascending spinal cord tracts are sensory pathways (carry sensory information) to the thalamus, cerebral cortex and cerebellar cortex. Nervous impulses for pain, temperature and coarse touch travel in the spinothalamic tracts, which cross the midline in the spinal cord. Information on fine touch, pressure, proprioception and vibration travel in the dorsal column tracts. The gracile tract carries lower limb information and is situated medially and the cuneate tract carries upper limb information and is situated laterally.

> **Descending spinal cord tracts** are motor pathways (carry motor information) that descend from the cerebral cortex to the skeletal muscles along the corticospinal tract. Extrapyramidal tracts include all other descending motor tracts.

9.3.2.1 Damage to the Spinal cord

Damage to the spinal cord is very serious. If a person with suspected spinal cord compromise or cauda equina compromise wants to do a *yoga* class, the teacher would be prudent to recommend a hospital instead.

Spinal cord Compromise results from compression of the spinal cord. Symptoms may include:
*   Non-dermatomal (not to do with skin sensation) bilateral (both sides of the body) neurological (nervous system problems) symptoms
*   Ataxia (unsteadiness of gait).

Cauda Equina Compromise results from compression of the cauda equina and may have the following symptoms:
*   Alterations in bladder, bowel or sexual function
*   Altered sensation in a saddle distribution (the region around the perineum buttocks and inner thighs)
*   Pain made worse with movement or a Valsalva manouvre, which involves making *ha-mula bandha* (contracting the lower abdomen) and *ha-uddiyaya bandha* (contracting the chest) after holding the breath in.

The peripheral nervous system (PNS) is a collection of axons of sensory neurons and motor neurons arising directly from the spinal cord and going to the extremities. Axons are like the tail processes of neurons and may be up to one metre in length.

9.4.1 Cranial Nerves and Spinal Nerves
9.4.1.1 Spinal nerves and nerve roots

Spinal nerves and nerve roots can be compressed by degenerative joint disease, degenerative disc disease, cysts or tumours and can lead to sensory, motor and reflex loss. Dorsal rami of spinal nerves supply the back muscles and skin. Ventral rami of spinal nerves in the thoracic T2-T12 go directly to the body structures they supply. All other ventral rami form networks called plexuses (braid), by joining with adjacent ventral rami.

9.4.1.2 Nerve plexuses

The main nerve plexuses are the cervical plexus, brachial plexus, lumbar plexus and sacral plexus.

9.4.1.2.1 Cervical plexus
The cervical plexus is formed by ventral rami of C1-C5. It supplies the skin, muscles of the head, neck and upper shoulders and gives rise to the phrenic nerve of the diaphragm.

9.4.1.2.2 Brachial plexus
The brachial plexus formed by ventral rami of C5-C8, and T1, passes over the first rib under the clavicle and enters the axilla. It supplies the shoulder and upper limb. Four important nerves arise. These are shown in Table 9.1. The radial nerve can be tensioned (stretched) in *atanu puritat mudra* . The

median nerve can be tensioned (stretched) in *kloman mudra* and *bukka puritat mudra*

. The ulnar nerve can be tensioned (stretched) in *buddizuddi mudra* and

anumukha puritat mudra [Figures 9.1 - 9.5].

Table 9.1 Nerves of the brachial plexus and effects of damage to them [Section 9.4.1.2.2]

NERVE	ACTIONS OF NERVE	EFFECTS OF NERVE LESION
Musculocutaneous	Arm & forearm flexors	Sensory loss & pain to lateral forearm; poor or absent biceps jerk reflex; motor deficit of elbow flexors with elbow fully supinated (biceps & brachialis)
Radial	Posterior arm & forearm extensors	Sensory loss, pain & motor loss around the thumb; poor or absent biceps jerk reflex; motor deficit of elbow, wrist & finger extensors; wrist drop
Median	Anterior forearm flexors & palm flexors	Sensory loss in lateral palm; pain in thumb, index and middle fingers to forearm; Carpal tunnel syndrome
Ulna	Anteromedial forearm & palm	Sensory loss, pain & motor loss around the fourth and fifth fingers and medial palm;difficulty abducting & adducting fingers; claw hand

9.4.1.2.3 Lumbar plexus
The lumbar plexus is formed by the ventral rami of spinal nerves L1-L4. The lumbar plexus supplies the anterolateral abdominal wall, external genitals and lower limb via the femoral nerve. Femoral nerve lesions may result in pain and sensory loss in the anterior thigh and medial leg, loss of the knee-jerk reflex and motor deficit to the knee extensors.

The sacral plexus is formed from ventral rami of spinal nerves L4, L5, S1-S4, is situated in front of the sacrum, and supplies the buttocks, perineum, and lower extremity. The sciatic nerve arises from the sacral plexus

The sciatic nerve is the largest nerve in the body. It arises from L4 - S3 and is comprised of two nerves: (i) the tibial nerve (L4-S3) goes to the back of the leg and (ii) common peroneal nerve (L4-S2) goes to the front of the leg. Injury to the common peroneal nerve may lead to pain in the buttock and down the back of the leg, loss of sensation over the anterior leg and foot and motor deficits in the lateral hamstrings and ankle dorsiflexors and evertors. Injury to the tibial nerve is often painless but may lead to loss of sensation in the sole of the foot and motor deficits in the medial hamstrings and ankle plantarflexors and invertors. Injury to the sciatic nerve can be caused by herniated discs, dislocated hip, osteoarthritis of the lumbar spine, pressure from the uterus during pregnancy, improperly administered gluteal intramuscular injection and muscle spasm.

9.4.1.3 Myotomes

A myotome is a group of muscles primarily innervated by the motor fibers of a single nerve root or spinal nerve. Selections of muscles that can be used to test the myotomes of the upper and lower limb are shown in Table 9.2.

Table 9.2 Myotomes of upper and lower limbs: Main muscles used for assessment of spinal nerves [Section 9.4.1.3]

Spinal nerve	Muscles Innervated (Not all listed)	Main Actions of Muscles Listed	Reflexes
C1-C2		Neck flexion	
C3		Neck side flexion	
C4	Trapezius	Shoulder elevation	
C5	Deltoid	Arm abduction	Biceps jerk
C6	Biceps brachii	Elbow flexion	Biceps jerk
C7	Triceps brachii	Elbow extension	Triceps jerk
C8	Extensor pollicis longus	Thumb extension	
C8	Flexor digitorum profundus	Flexion of interphalangeal joints	
T1	Intrinsic action of fingers	Flexion of MCPs extension of IPs	
L1			No myotome
L2	Iliopsoas	Hip flexion	
L3	Quadriceps	Knee extension	Knee jerk reflex
L4	Tibialis anterior	Dorsiflexion & inversion	
L5	Extensor hallucis longus	Big toe extension	
S1	Gastrocnemius	Ankle plantarflexion	Ankle jerk reflex
S1	Peroneus longus & brevis	Eversion	Ankle jerk reflex
S2	Flexor digitorum longus	Toe flexion	

9.4.1.4 Dermatomes

A dermatome is a specific area of skin primarily innervated by the motor fibers of a single nerve root or spinal nerve. Dermatomes sometimes overlap. They reflect cutaneous (skin) pain and pain referred to skin from nerve root irritation or visceral pain. C1 has no dermatome because there is no sensory root. Knowledge of the dermatomes can supplement information obtained from the myotomes to assess which segment of the spinal cord or which spinal nerve is malfunctioning. Good dermatome maps and myotome maps are easily available on the internet (eg http://www.apparelyzed.com/myo-dermatomes.html).

9.4.1.5 Spinal nerve or nerve root (SN/NR) compromise

Spinal nerve roots branch out from each side of the spinal cord and then join to form the spinal nerves, which pass through openings between the spinal bones (vertebrae) and then form branches that extend throughout the body. Each spinal nerve is attached to the spinal cord by two nerve roots. Spinal nerves or nerve roots can be occasionally trapped due to improper movements during daily activity and also in a *hatha yoga* practice especially when strength is not balanced with flexibility and someone tries to bend their back excessively while not maintaining a grip of relevant *bandhas* (muscle co-activations).

- **Possible causes of SN/NR compromise include**:
  o Mechanical compromise of the nerve leading to <u>intraneural oedema</u> (swelling inside nerve sheath) that causes pressure on the <u>axons</u>
  o Compromise of the <u>blood vessels</u> associated with the SN/NR
  o <u>Traction</u> injuries.

- **Symptoms of SN/NR compromise include**:
  o Pain in a <u>dermatomal distribution</u>
  o Radiating or extending pain from the <u>lumbar spine</u> past the buttocks; or pain referred from the <u>cervical spine</u> past the shoulder
  o Altered sensation in the upper or lower limb (eg anaesthesia)
  o Limb pain that may be related to a <u>lumbar spine</u> or <u>cervical spine</u> condition.

- **Testing of a SN/NR compromise**:
  o If a SN/NR compromise or any other serious neurological problem is suspected the person with the symptoms should be referred to a physiotherapist or doctor for a full neurological assessment which would include tests for <u>myotomes</u>, <u>dermatomes</u> and <u>reflexes</u>.

Implications of a positive neurological test (ie weak muscles unilaterally) include a possible compromise of a <u>spinal nerve</u> or <u>nerve root</u>.

9.4.2 Reflexes

A <u>reflex</u> is a fast response to a change (stimulus) in the internal or external environment and is an attempt to quickly restore <u>homeostasis</u> (a state of equilibrium in the body).

A <u>reflex arc</u> is the most basic conduction pathway through the <u>nervous system</u>, connecting a <u>receptor</u> with an <u>effector</u>. It consists of (i) a <u>receptor</u>, (ii) a <u>sensory neuron</u>, (iii) an <u>integrating centre</u> in the CNS, (iv) a <u>motor neuron</u>, and (v) an <u>effector</u>.

9.4.2.1 Myotatic (stretch) reflex

The <u>myotatic (stretch) reflex</u> is a feedback mechanism to control muscle length. A slight stretch of muscle activates <u>receptors</u> in the muscle called <u>muscle spindles</u> that monitor change in length of a muscle. This generates a nerve <u>action potential</u> to the <u>spinal cord</u>, where the <u>sensory neuron</u> <u>synapses</u> with the <u>motor neuron</u> in the <u>anterior grey horn</u>. The <u>motor neuron</u> projects to the same muscle as the muscle spindle, causing the muscle to contract. For example, the <u>patella tendon reflex</u> is initiated by tapping the <u>patella tendon</u>. This tendon is attached to the <u>quadriceps</u> muscle and the tapping generates a slight stretching of the muscle. This triggers the <u>stretch reflex activation</u>, causing the lower leg to kick forward.

9.4.2.2 Reciprocal inhibition reflex

Reciprocal reflex inhibition is when the antagonistic muscle opposing the agonist muscle activation relaxes as the stretched muscle contracts during the stretch reflex. This is what triggers the hamstrings to relax during the patella tendon reflex.

9.4.2.3 Inverse myotatic reflex (tendon reflex)

The <u>inverse myotatic reflex</u>, also known as the <u>tendon reflex</u>, is a feedback mechanism to control muscle <u>tension</u>. It has been believed that <u>receptors</u> called <u>golgi tendon organs</u> (GTOs) in the tendon that lie near the <u>musculotendinous junction</u> respond to changes in <u>tension</u> caused by <u>passive muscle stretching</u> or <u>muscle activation</u>. An increase in <u>tension</u> stimulates the GTO to send <u>nerve impulses</u> to the <u>spinal cord</u> along a <u>sensory neuron</u>. The <u>sensory neuron</u> <u>synapses</u> with an <u>inhibitory interneuron</u>, which then <u>synapses</u> with and inhibits the <u>motor neuron</u> that innervates the muscle of the GTO. This results in relaxation of the muscle, which protects the tendon, and muscle from damage due to excessive <u>tension</u>. There is also a <u>synapse</u> onto an excitatory <u>interneuron</u> that results in <u>activation</u> of the <u>antagonist</u> muscle (reciprocal innervation again!). However, although the <u>reflex</u> relaxation phenomenon definitely occurs after a stretch has been held for some time, or if the muscle being stretched is <u>activated</u>, this commonly accepted theory regarding the GTOs may still be flawed [Alter, 1996].

9.4.2.4 Flexor and crossed extensor reflex

The <u>flexor and crossed extensor reflex</u> is a contralateral <u>reflex arc</u> that results in the <u>activation</u> of four <u>reflex</u> arcs. When you step on a sharp object for example the leg is flexed (flexor <u>reflex</u> excited and extensors inhibited) and the contralateral leg goes into <u>extension</u> (extensor <u>reflex</u> excited and flexors inhibited) to maintain balance.

9.4.3 Sensory receptors: Neuronal Circuits for Processing Information

Input to the nervous system is provided by various types of sensory receptors. These include proprioceptors that detect joint position [Section 9.4.3.1], nociceptors that perceive tissue damage [Section 9.4.3.2], chemoreceptors that sense carbon dioxide concentrations [Section 9.4.3.3], baroreceptors that detect changes in pressure [Section 9.4.3.4], photoreceptors that detect changes in light [Section 9.6.1], hair cells that detect sound [Section 9.6.2], and maculae and crista which detect balance [Section 9.6.3].

9.4.3.1 Proprioceptors: Sensing balance and positioning:

Proprioception is the receipt of information from muscles, tendons and the labyrinth of the inner ear that enables the brain to determine the position and movements of the various parts of the body. Proprioceptors are receptors located in muscles, tendons and joints that send information to the brain regarding body position and movements.

9.4.3.2 Nociceptors: Perceiving tissue damage:

Nociception is the process that involves the detection of tissue damage (transduction), the transmission of the nociceptive information along the peripheral nerves and through the spinal cord, and its modulation. Nociceptors are free nerve endings involved in nociception.

Pain is an unpleasant sensory and emotional experience associated with actual or potential tissue damage, or described in terms of such damage. Pain is a phenomenon of the brain. Technically, it does not exist until the cerebral cortex receives information via the nervous system from sites of actual or perceived pain. This information, however, is not pain itself but may lead to the experience of pain. It is information evoked by noxious stimuli, and the process by which it is detected and transmitted which is referred to as nociception. Acute pain [Section 1.8.1] is pain arising in the first few days following tissue damage that is associated with tissue repair and with inflammation [Section 10.2.3.1.]. Chronic pain [Section 1.8.1] is pain persisting longer than the tissue damage causing the pain would take to heal. Neurogenic pain is pain caused by nociceptive activity within nerves themselves. Psychogenic pain is chronic pain for which health providers cannot find adequate biological cause. It exists when there is a discrepancy between pain behaviour and observable tissue damage to explain that behaviour. Referred pain is pain from deep structures perceived as arising from a surface area remote from its actual origin. The area where the pain is felt is innervated by the same spinal segment as the deep structure.

Endorphins and enkephalins are a class of neurotransmitter molecules that have analgesic (pain relieving) properties. Endorphins are released into the bloodstream and have a role in providing analgesia during major stress. Enkephalins are present at various sites in the nervous system, where the inhibitory influences they exert inhibit pain perception or block nociceptive transmission.

Pain gate control theory: This states there is a neural gate that can be relatively open or closed modulating incoming nociceptive signals before the brain experiences them as pain. Pain gate control depends on:
- Amount of activity in the pain fibres
- Amount of activity in other peripheral nerve fibres
- Messages descending from the brain

Conditions that open the pain gate:
- Physical conditions such as:
  - Extent of injury
  - Inappropriate levels of activity
- Emotional conditions such as:
  - Stress
  - Depression
- Mental conditions such as:
  - Focus on pain
  - Boredom due to little involvement in life

Conditions that close the pain gate:
- Physical conditions such as:
  - Counter-stimulation
  - Heat, massage, exercise ☐ *Yoga*
- Emotional conditions such as:
  - Positive emotions
  - Relaxation and rest ☐ *Yoga*
- Mental conditions such as:
  - Intense concentration
  - Life involvement ☐ *Yoga*

Hence, *yoga* can be useful to reduce pain on physical, mental and emotional levels.

9.4.3.3 Chemoreceptors: Sensing chemical concentrations [Sections 8.1.6.2]

Chemoreceptors are chemo-sensitive cells, which are sensitive to oxygen insufficiency, carbon dioxide excess or hydrogen ion excess. Chemoreceptors transmit nervous signals to the respiratory centre of the brain to help regulate respiratory activity. The largest numbers of chemoreceptors are in the carotid bodies, which are located bilaterally in the bifurcations of the common carotid arteries. There are also many chemoreceptors in the aortic bodies located in the arch of the aorta, and there are a few chemoreceptors associated with the arteries of the thoracic and abdominal regions. There are also chemo-sensitive cells in the respiratory centre of the brain [Guyton, 1991].

An increase in carbon dioxide levels in the blood detected by the chemoreceptors in the body and chemosensitive cells in the respiratory centre of the brain causes a moderate increase in vasodilation (blood vessel expansion) in most tissues and marked increase in vasodilation in the brain.

Chemoreceptors also respond to changes in the partial pressure of carbon dioxide in the blood. They recognise an increase in carbon dioxide as a signal that arterial blood pressure has fallen, and so they stimulate the vasomotor centre to increase blood pressure.

9.4.3.4 Baroreceptors: Sensing arterial pressure [Sections 8.1.6.1 & 9.7.6.4]

The most important mechanism for arterial pressure control is the baroreceptor reflex. This reflex is initiated by stretch receptors called baroreceptors, which are located in the walls of large arteries. A rise in arterial pressure stretches the baroreceptors and causes them to transmit signals to the central nervous system (CNS) and feedback signals are then sent back through to the autonomic nervous system (ANS) in particular to the parasympathetic nervous system, to reduce arterial pressure [Guyton, 1991]. Baroreceptors respond more to a rapidly changing pressure than to a stationary pressure. Baroreceptors reset themselves every few days to whatever pressure they are exposed. If baroreceptors are unable, through the ANS and CNS, to rebalance from an increase in blood pressure, then the baroreceptors will cease to be stimulated and the higher blood pressure will be recognised as normal blood pressure.

9.5 AUTONOMIC NERVOUS SYSTEM

The autonomic nervous system (ANS), which is part of the peripheral nervous system, usually operates without conscious control. However, some advanced *hatha yoga* practitioners have demonstrated a control over the ANS. The ANS is regulated by the hypothalamus and medulla, which receive input from the emotions (limbic system), and the many senses which include smell, and taste, temperature, pressure, blood chemical levels, etc. Input from visceral sensory (afferent) neurons comes from chemoreceptors in blood, mechanoreceptors in organ walls and baroreceptors in blood vessels detecting stretch. Output via autonomic visceral motor (efferent) neurons regulates smooth muscle, cardiac muscle and glands. This effects pupil size, blood vessel dilation, heart rate, gastrointestinal movement and gland secretion.

The three main branches of the ANS are the sympathetic nervous system [Section 9.5.1], the parasympathetic nervous system [Section 9.5.2] and the enteric nervous system [Section 9.5.3]. The main effects of the sympathetic nervous system, the parasympathetic nervous system are shown in Table 9.3.

9.5.1 Sympathetic Nervous System

The sympathetic nervous system is most stimulated during the so-called flight or fight response. The sympathetic nervous system arises from T1-L2 (thoracolumbar outflow). Ganglia are remote from the organ and close to the central nervous system (CNS). Each preganglionic fibre synapses with many postganglionic fibres; thus divergence to many visceral effectors occurs. Distribution of the sympathetic nervous system is throughout the body.

9.5.2 Parasympathetic Nervous System

The parasympathetic nervous system is mainly in control in the normal relaxed state. This can be thought of as the rest and digest response. The parasympathetic nervous system arises from the cranium and from S2-S4 (cranio-sacral outflow). Ganglia are close to or within the effector organ. No divergence occurs. Distribution of the parasympathetic nervous system is to the head, viscera of the thorax, abdomen, and pelvis.

Table 9.3 Effects of sympathetic and parasympathetic nervous systems [Section 9.5]

BODY REGION	SYMPATHETIC NERVOUS SYSTEM [Section 9.5.1]	PARASYMPATHETIC NERVOUS SYSTEM [Section 9.5.2]
Heart	Increased heart rate	Decreased heart rate
Eyes (Iris)	Pupil dilation (expansion)	Pupil constriction
Salivary glands	Saliva production reduced	Saliva production increased
Oral/Nasal mucosa	Mucous production decreased	Mucous production increased
Skin	Vasoconstriction, sweating, piloerection	
Liver	Increased conversion of glycogen to glucose	
Stomach	Peristalsis reduced	Gastric juice secreted; motility increased
Intestines	Contraction of sphincters of the digestive system → Decrease in intestinal motility (constipation)	Relaxation of sphincters, increase in peristalsis of digestive system → Increase in intestinal motility
Kidney	Decreased urine production	Increased urine production
Bladder	Relaxation of bladder wall	Contraction of bladder wall (urination)
Lung	Bronchial tubes dilated (relaxed)	Bronchial tubes constricted

9.5.3 Enteric Nervous System

The enteric nervous system is the most recently discovered branch of the autonomic nervous system (ANS) and forms an important part of the nervous control of the digestive system and the processes that regulates the assimilation of food. It is at least as large as the other parts of the ANS and it contains as many neurons as the spinal cord.

The principal components of the enteric nervous system are two networks or plexuses of neurons, the myenteric plexus and the submucous plexus both of which are embedded in the wall of the digestive tract and extend from esophageus to anus.

The enteric nervous system has a vast array of neurotransmitters. It can and does function autonomously, but normal digestive function involves communication with the central nervous system.

While some scientists consider the enteric nervous system as a third division of the autonomic nervous system, some scientists think of the enteric NS as the enteric brain, quite distinct from the central nervous system and peripheral nervous system, with a mind of its own. The enteric nervous system has many structures and chemicals similar to those of the brain. It has sensory neurons and motor neurons, information processing circuits, and glial cells. It uses the major neurotransmitters: dopamine, serotonin, acetylcholine, nitric oxide and noradrenaline. It even has benzodiazepines, chemicals of the family of psychoactive drugs that includes Valium and Xanax. Like the spinal cord, the enteric nervous system transmits and processes messages.

9.6 SPECIAL SENSES

Special senses include vision (ophthalmic), hearing (auditory), equilibrium (vestibular), smell (olfaction), taste (gustation). The special senses allow us to detect specific changes in the environment.

9.6.1 The Visual System

Related structures include the eyeball, optic nerve, accessory structures (eyebrows, eyelids, eyelashes, extrinsic eye muscles and lacrimal apparatus) and the brain. The primary visual area in the brain is in the occipital lobe.

The lacrimal gland produces 1 ml/day of tears, a watery solution containing salts, some mucous and a bactericidal enzyme called lysosome. Tears are spread over the eyeball by blinking and cleared away by evaporation or through the lacrimal canals and into the nose. Their function is to clean, lubricate and moisten the eyeball.

Six extrinsic eye muscles coordinate to move the eyes together, smoothly and precisely in all directions, they are superior rectus (elevation), inferior rectus (depression), medial rectus (adduction), lateral rectus (abduction), inferior oblique (left rotation) and superior oblique (right rotation).

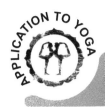

No 9.1 Gazing at particular points during some *yoga* postures (*dristhi*) can increase the stretch

The extrinsic eye muscles have fascial connections to the neck muscle. Therefore, when the eyes are moved the neck muscles will undergo some reflex activation and slightly increase their level of stretch. This is particularly useful to use in twisting postures. When you twist your neck to the right, for example, the stretch can be increased if you also turn your eyes to the right.

The eyeballs important structures include:
* **Cornea**: transparent, avascular, fibrous coat where most refraction of light occurs.
* **Sclera**: tough connective tissue, white of the eye, maintains shape of the eye and provides site for muscle attachment.
* **Iris**: coloured part of the eye, regulates light entering the eye by the sphincter pupillage muscle (pupil enlarges, under sympathetic nervous sytem control) and the radial pupillae muscle (pupil contracts, under parasympathetic nervous sytem control).
* **Lens**: avascular, transparent, refractive media responsible for focussing image on the retina by altering shape when adjustments for distance need to be made. Cataracts are due to build up of proteins making the lens opaque.
* **Aqueous humour**: watery fluid that refracts light, provides nutrition and maintains intraocular pressure. Glaucoma is a build up of pressure due to blockage in drainage that causes retina degeneration and blindness.
* **Retina**: receives light at the back of the eye and converts it into nerve impulses that go to the brain via the optic nerve. The optic nerve leaves the eyeball at the optic disc, together with the retinal artery and vein.
* **Photoreceptors (rods and cones)**: transduce (convert) light energy into receptor potentials. Rods are important for black and white vision and dim light. Cones are important for colour vision and sharpness in bright light.
* **Intrinsic eye muscles**: include the iris muscles and the ciliary muscle which when contracted relaxes the lens and vice versa.

Image formation on the retina involves refraction of light rays by the cornea and lens, accommodation of the lens by increasing in its curvature for near vision and a constriction of the pupil to prevent light rays from entering the eye through the periphery of the lens. Convergence of the eyeballs means they move medially so they are both directed toward an object being viewed.

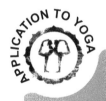

No 9.2 Gazing at particular points during a *yoga* practice (*dristhi*) can reduce input to the brain and improve meditation

The optic nerve is the largest nervous input entering the brain apart from the spinal cord itself. Therefore, a more restful and meditative *yoga* practice can be obtained when the eyes are kept as still as possible throughout the *yoga* practice. *Dristhis* or gazing points can be used in every pose. The simplest places to gaze are at a point on the floor for ease of balance, and at the tip of the nose to keep the forehead relaxed. More difficult gazing points include the centre of the forehead, which can make some people very tense, and the sky which makes balancing very difficult.

9.6.2 The Auditory System
Sound waves enter the external auditory canal, strike the tympanic membrane, pass through the ossicles, strike the oval window, set up waves in the perilymph, strike the vestibular membrane and scala tympani, increase pressure in the endolymph, strike the basilar membrane and stimulate hairs on the spiral organ of Corti. Hair cells (auditory receptors) release neurotransmitters that initiate nerve impulses, thus converting mechanical energy into receptor potentials.

Perforated eardrum (tympanic membrane) is caused by shock waves of compressed air, eg gunshot, scuba diving, skull fractures, and acute middle ear infections.

The eustachian tube connects the nasopharynx to the middle ear and functions to equalise the pressure on both sides of the tympanic eardrum and prevent excessive painful stretch. Normally it is closed but opens when you yawn, sneeze or swallow.

The tensor tympani and stapedius muscles connect to the ossicles and contract to dampen vibrations of the ossicles resulting from large noises, thus protecting damage to the internal ear.

Conduction deafness is a reduction in signal transmission caused by a blockage in the ear canal (wax), damaged eardrum or damage to the ossicles. Sensorineural deafness is due to inner ear damage where the hairs sit flat, producing a permanent ringing sensation called tinnitus.

9.6.3 The Vestibular System
The vestibular system is located in the inner ear in the three semicircular canals (dynamic equilibrium) and the utricle and saccule (static equilibrium).

Semicircular canals sit at right angles to each other and recognise rotations of the head in different directions, by the movement of endolymph in the canals. Horizontal semicircular canals give information on rotation in the horizontal plane (spinning on a merry-go-round). Posterior semicircular canals give information on rotation in the coronal plane (cartwheels). Anterior semicircular canals give information on rotation in the sagittal plane (somersaults).

Angular semicircular acceleration causes the endolymph to flow in a direction opposite to the head rotation, past hair receptor cells in the ampulla, causing an electrical impulse to be generated and sent to the brain.

The utricle and the saccule detect head position and linear acceleration.

9.7 APPLIED ANATOMY & PHYSIOLOGY OF THE NERVOUS SYSTEM IN HATHA YOGA

In *hatha yoga*, strength, flexibility and the ability to relax can be greatly developed through understanding and applying the principles of musculoskeletal anatomy and neurophysiology. Stretching, strengthening, and relaxation in *yoga* are interdependent.

When the attachments of muscles are moved apart, there must be an awareness of the possibility that nervous tissue may be being tensioned (stretched). By taking advantage of the nerve reflexes, antagonistic (opposing) muscle groups can be simultaneously stretched, strengthened and relaxed.

9.7.1 Principles of Stretching in *Hatha Yoga*
The principles used for stretching a muscle or muscle group in *yoga* include:
1.   Use synergistic muscles to maximise the distance between proximal and distal muscle attachments.
2.   Inhibit the stretch reflex in antagonistic muscles.
3.   Use reciprocal inhibition to strengthen agonist muscles and stretch and relax antagonist muscles.
4.   Use the inverse myotatic reflex to stretch, strengthen and relax antagonistic muscles.
5.   Lengthen the antagonist side of the joint without shortening the agonist side (the stretch not squash principle).
6.   Apply principles of nerve tensioning or neural mobilisation (nerve stretching) [Section 9.7.3].

PRINCIPLE #1.   Use synergistic muscles to maximise the distance between proximal and distal muscle attachments:
*   Synergistic muscle activations can be used in *yoga* exercises to maximise the distance between the proximal and distal attachments of a muscle to be stretched; and also to take advantage of the many fascial connections between muscles,

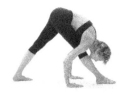

eg. a standing hamstring stretch such as *parsvottanasana*

- Use hip flexors to increase anterior pelvic tilt which increases hamstring stretches by moving hamstring proximal attachments at the ischial tuberosities, further away from their distal attachments below the knee.
- Increase the intensity of the hamstring stretch by activating stretch synergists including hip flexors, hip abductors, hip external rotators, ankle plantar flexors, ankle evertors, spinal flexors (abdominal muscles) and spinal extensors.
- After using the muscles to position the body, less effort is required to maintain the position. By softening the same muscles within the posture you can conserve energy, reduce higher than normal blood pressure and increase general levels of relaxation.

PRINCIPLE #2.   Inhibit the <u>stretch reflex</u> in antagonistic muscles:
- The stretch reflex needs to be taken into account when doing any stretch. To help inhibit the stretch reflex, which is potentially damaging when trying to stretch the following instructions can be of assistance:
- Move slowly into the stretches.
- Staying some time in each posture (eg. five long breaths or at least 20 – 30 seconds) if that posture is mainly held with passive muscles.
- Think about the stretch while doing it (i.e. focus on the stretch, where it is and how it feels) in order to inhibit the stretch reflex.
- Moving deeper into each stretch in synchrony with the exhalation in order to calm the nervous system by slowing the heart (the heart usually slows on each exhalation because of the effects of the respiratory pump [Sections 1.0.4, 8.1.2.3.2 & 8.4.1]).

PRINCIPLE #3.   Use <u>reciprocal inhibition</u> to strengthen agonist muscles and stretch and relax antagonist muscles:
- Activation of an agonist causes reflex reciprocal relaxation of the antagonist.

- EXAMPLE 1: A standing stretch of the hamstrings (knee flexors) such as *parsvottanasana*

  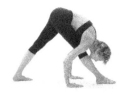 is enhanced by the activation of the quadriceps (knee extensors), which allow the hamstrings to stretch and relax even further.
  When the quadriceps are activated the knee is taken further into extension, and hamstring activity generated by the stretch reflex is minimised due to reciprocal inhibition.

- EXAMPLE 2: Actively depressing and protracting the shoulder will stretch and relax the shoulder elevators and retractors.
  When the depressors of the shoulder girdle (in particular pectoralis major and latissimus dorsi) generate tension in the shortened position they stretch the elevators and retractors of the shoulder girdle and relax these retractors and elevators by reciprocal reflex inhibition.

PRINCIPLE #4.   Use the <u>inverse myotatic reflex</u> to stretch, strengthen and relax antagonistic muscles:
- By making a muscle (the antagonist) generate tension for a short time while in a lengthened state (isometric muscle activation against resistance) the golgi tendon organ is stimulated. This causes a reflex relaxation of that muscle once it stops actively generating tension (inverse myotatic reflex). This

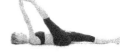

leads to an increase in the stretch, strength training for the muscle and enhanced relaxation.

- EXAMPLE 1: The supine <u>hamstring</u> stretch known as *supta padangusthasana.*
- In the supine <u>hamstring</u> stretch, if the <u>hamstring</u> that is being stretched generates <u>tension</u> in the lengthened state (i.e. an <u>isometric</u> <u>muscle activation</u> against resistance), then this enables a more relaxed lengthened state in the hamstring after the period of generating <u>tension</u>.

PRINCIPLE #5. Lengthen the antagonist side of joint without shortening the agonist side (the stretch not squash principle):

- *Yoga* teachers often observe that beginners do not so much stretch their body as squash it.
- An example of the stretch not squash principle can be seen with the simple prone, upper limb supported back <u>extension</u> exercise known in physiotherapy as a Mackenzie exercise and known in *yoga* as

bhujangasana (the cobra pose). In this exercise, a stretch may be felt in the <u>anterior</u> trunk or a squashing feeling can be experienced in the <u>posterior</u> trunk depending on how the exercise is performed. By pulling the chest forward using the arms and in particular the <u>posterior deltoid</u> muscle a stretch in <u>anterior</u> body may be experienced. However pushing down and forward with the arms and using <u>pectoralis major</u> may cause the <u>posterior</u> trunk to feel squashed.
- Similarly, in forward bending poses (<u>hip flexion</u> and <u>spinal flexion</u> exercises), depending on how the exercise is performed, there is a lengthening in the <u>posterior</u> trunk and one may feel a squashing or shortening in the <u>anterior</u> trunk. In this case, a <u>posterior pelvic tilt</u> will usually increase the stretch in the <u>posterior</u> trunk, while decreasing the stretch in the <u>anterior</u> trunk. Conversely, an <u>anterior pelvic tilt</u> will usually cause an increase in the length of the <u>anterior</u> trunk while decreasing the length of the <u>posterior</u> trunk.
- This principle can also be applied to <u>lateral flexion</u> exercises.

PRINCIPLE #6. Apply the principles of <u>nerve tensioning or neural mobilisation</u> (nerve stretching)
[See Section 9.7.3]:

- *Yoga* affects the <u>nervous system</u> as some *asanas* (static postures) and *mudras* (energy-control gestures) can apply <u>tension</u> (stretch) to specific nerves. Note that when nerves are tensioned (stretched) then usually so are <u>acupunture meridians</u> and the *yoga nadis* (subtle channels).
- The principles of <u>neural tensioning</u> or <u>neural mobilisation</u> as applied in physiotherapy can also be applied in *yoga asanas* and *mudras* to increase <u>range of movement</u> (ROM), to treat tight neural structures, and to help relax the body. For example:
  o Many *yoga* standing postures put the arms into positions similar to a physiotherapy test known as the <u>upper limb tension test</u>, which can help alleviate some people's shoulder and upper limb pain, but which can also aggravate other people's <u>nervous system</u>.

  o *Supta padanghusthasana* (supine hamstring stretch) is similar to a physiotherapy test known as the <u>straight leg raise</u> (SLR) test, which can help alleviate some people's lower back and lower limb pain, but which can also aggravate other people's <u>nervous system</u>.

  o *Uttanasana* (standing forward-bend) and other <u>spinal flexion</u> and <u>hip flexion</u> postures are similar to a physiotherapy <u>neural tension</u> test known as the <u>slump test</u>, which can help alleviate some people's spinal pain and back pain, but which can also aggravate other people's <u>nervous system</u>.

o   *Supta virasana* , *bhekasana* , *kulpha hanumanasana*
and other similar postures resemble a physiotherapy <u>neural tension</u> test known as the <u>prone knee bend</u> (PKB).

Yoga incorporates <u>neural tensioning</u> (nerve stretching), which for normal people can maintain their pain-free <u>range of movement</u> (ROM), and which for people with injuries may relieve pain by freeing nerves and increasing ROM, in a similar way that physiotherapists use <u>nerve tensioning</u> and <u>neural mobilisation</u>.

9.7.2 Relaxation in *Yoga*

Relaxation of muscles has been shown to reduce stress. The basic concepts that *yoga* uses to help relax muscles translates to a reduction of stress in the <u>brain</u>.

It is helpful and sometimes necessary to learn how to activate a muscle in order to learn how to relax it, i.e. you must be able to turn a muscle on before you are able to turn it off. *Yoga* exercises bring awareness or sensation of the body through learning how to contract or stretch the different body parts. By applying a practical understanding of <u>spinal reflexes</u>, such as the <u>stretch reflex</u> and <u>reciprocal relaxation</u>, one is able to consciously relax a muscle then further relax by <u>activation</u> of the <u>antagonist</u>.

Awareness of breath in postures helps to control <u>blood pressure</u> and to focus the mind, both of which help to reduce stress. While breathing in postures, attention should be constantly made to keep face, neck and throat relaxed, as this allows the brain to maintain an adequate supply of blood without the flow of blood to the brain being impeded by muscle tension in these parts of the face, neck or throat. While the aim of your *yoga* practice should be to remain as relaxed as possible during the practice, for most people at the end of each *yoga* practice it is important to take at least 5 – 15 minutes of relaxed sitting or supine relaxation (*Savasana*) with observation of the breath to further relax the body and brain. This relaxation is most successful if people have succeeded in getting out of their <u>brain</u> and into their body with physical practice of *asana* (static postures) and *vinyasa* (dynamic exercises) beforehand.

9.7.3 Nerve Stretching in *Yoga* (Nerve tensioning or neural mobilisation)

In this book and elsewhere, <u>nerve tensioning</u> is often referred to as nerve stretching for simplicity. However, because the actual nerve tissue is rarely stretched without potentially causing damage, the technically correct term for what is occurring during the *yoga asanas* and *mudras* discussed in this book, is <u>nerve tensioning</u> or <u>neural mobilisation</u>.

Contraindications of <u>neural mobilisation</u> or <u>nerve tensioning</u> (i.e. situations where nerve stretching should not be done) include irritable conditions, inflammation, signs of spinal cord compromise, malignancy, nerve root compression, peripheral neuropathy (disorders of the peripheral nerves), and complex regional pain syndrome (burning pain that may occur in the arm or leg after an injury or surgery).

<u>Neural mobilisation</u> (nerve stretching or neural tensioning) is a technique that was developed by David Butler in Australia [Butler, 1996]. Nerves, like all soft tissues in the body, can become restricted and tight and become a source of pain. Shortening of nerves can be due to trauma or injury, or the result of ongoing poor posture. This is often the case with neck and arm pain. <u>Neural mobilisation</u> uses specific postures that can tension neural tissues and gently stretch target nerves. Butler suggests that altered neurodynamics are the cause of many problems including headaches, and that appropriate neural mobilisation can provide relief. Studies have shown <u>neural mobilisation</u> techniques to be effective treatment for <u>carpal tunnel syndorme</u> [Tal-Akabi & Rushton, 2000], chronic lateral elbow pain with signs of nerve entrapment [Elkstrom & Holden, 2002], thoracic outlet syndrome [Mackinnon & Novak, 2002], sciatica and lower back pain [Miller, 2005]. *Hatha yoga* also has many *asanas* (static postures) and *mudras* (energy-control gestures) that can apply tension (stretch) to specific nerves [Figures 9.1 - 9.8].

Although nerve tissue has some elastic qualities and is known to be able to be elongated up to 20% before it tears, it is well understood that nerve tissue does not itself stretch much at all before it becomes non-functional. Studies have shown that after elongation of as little as 6%, nerves may have undergone sufficient mechanical deformation to have impaired electrochemical conduction [Wall et al., 1992]. After elongation 8% of intraneural blood flow is impeded which also impairs nerve function [Clarke et al., 1992]. However, during daily movements and especially during a *hatha yoga* practice neural tissue may have to elongate by up to 5 centimetres [Alter, 1996]. Elongation of neural tissue is mainly due to nerve slackness and the course of the nerves in relation to the joints, and only minimally due to elasticity in the nerve tissue itself. Nerve slackness is to do with (i) the undulating nature of the of the nerve trunk in its bed, (ii) the undulating nature of the nerve fibre bundles (<u>fasciculi</u>) in the <u>perineurium</u> (connective tissue sheath covering the fasciculi) and (iii) the undulating course of each nerve fibre in the <u>fasciculi</u> [Alter, 1996]. The course or pathway of the nerve in relation to the joints is also and important factor that protects nerves from overstretching. Most nerves traverse the flexor aspect of a joint and so are only minimally stretched when the joint is extended [Alter, 1996]. The only two important exceptions are the <u>ulnar nerve</u> which crosses the extensor aspect of the <u>elbow joint complex</u> and the <u>sciatic nerve</u> which crosses the extensor aspect of the <u>hip joint complex</u>.

1.   Brachial plexus stretches in *hatha yoga*

The <u>brachial plexus</u> is <u>tensioned</u> (stretched) with correct positioning of the <u>scapulothoracic (ST) joint</u> and the <u>glenohumeral (GH) joint</u> of the <u>shoulder joint complex</u>.

- The basic stretch of the <u>brachial plexus</u> increases (↑) with <u>shoulder (GH) abduction</u>, <u>shoulder (GH) depression</u> and <u>neck contra-lateral flexion</u>.
- There is a possible risk of over-tensioning the <u>brachial plexus</u> in, for example, in *parsva*

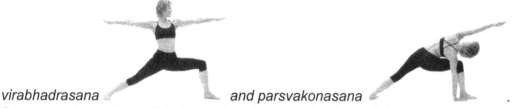

virabhadrasana   *and parsvakonasana*   .

- Other variations of <u>brachial plexus</u> stretches exist for the <u>radial nerve</u> [Figure 9.1], <u>median nerve</u> [Figures 9.2, 9.3] and <u>ulnar nerve</u> [Figures 9.4, 9.5] when the following movements are added to the basic shoulder movements above:

Radial nerve stretch [Figure 9.1]

- <u>Shoulder (ST) depression</u> and <u>retraction</u>;
- <u>Shoulder (GH) abduction</u>, <u>internal rotation</u> and (slight) <u>flexion</u>;
- <u>Elbow extension</u> and <u>pronation</u>;
- <u>Wrist flexion</u> and <u>ulnar deviation</u> (<u>wrist adduction</u>).

Figure 9.1: *Atanu puritat mudra:* <u>Tensioning</u> (stretching) of the <u>radial nerve</u> of the <u>brachial plexus</u> and the <u>large intestine acupuncture meridian</u>: Effects of *atanu puritat mudra* intensify with increasing <u>shoulder (ST) depression</u>, <u>retraction</u> and <u>internal rotation</u>; <u>shoulder (GH) abduction</u>, <u>flexion</u> and <u>internal rotation</u>; <u>elbow extension</u> and <u>pronation</u>; and <u>wrist flexion</u> and <u>ulnar deviation</u>.

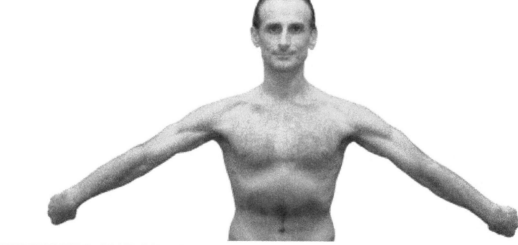

Median nerve stretches [Figures 9.2 & 9.3]

- Shoulder (ST) depression and protraction;
- Shoulder (GH) abduction, external rotation and (slight) extension;
- Elbow extension and supination [figure 9.2] **or**, pronation [figure 9.3] .
- Wrist extension and ulnar deviation [figure 9.2] **or**, radial deviation [figure 9.3] .

Figure 9.2: *Kloman mudra*: Tensioning (stretching) of the ventral aspect of the median nerve of the brachial plexus and the lung acupuncture meridian: Effects of *kloman mudra* intensify with increasing shoulder (ST) depression, protraction and external rotation; shoulder (GH) abduction, extension, and external rotation; elbow extension and supination; and wrist extension and ulnar deviation.

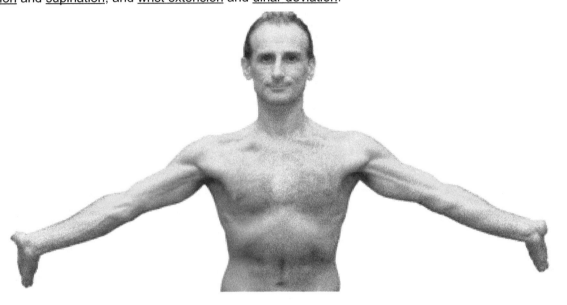

Figure 9.3: *Bukka puritat mudra*: Tensioning (stretch) of dorsal aspect of median nerve of brachial plexus and the pericardium acupuncture meridian: Effects of *bukka puritat mudra* intensify with increasing shoulder (ST) depression, protraction and external rotation; shoulder (GH) abduction, extension, and external rotation; elbow extension and pronation; wrist extension and radial deviation.

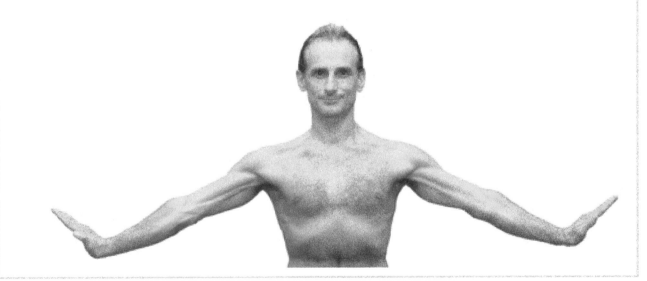

Ulnar nerve stretches [Figures 9.4 & 9.5]

- Shoulder (ST) depression and protraction;
- Shoulder (GH) abduction, external rotation [figure 9.4] **or** internal rotation [figure 9.5] and (slight) extension;
- Elbow flexion and pronation;
- Wrist extension and radial deviation (wrist abduction).

Figure 9.4: *Buddhizuddhi mudra*: Tensioning (stretching) of ventral aspect of ulnar nerve of brachial plexus; and the heart acupuncture meridian: Effects of *buddhizuddhi mudra* intensify with increasing shoulder (ST) depression, protraction and external rotation; shoulder (GH) abduction, extension, and external rotation; elbow flexion and pronation; and wrist extension and radial deviation.

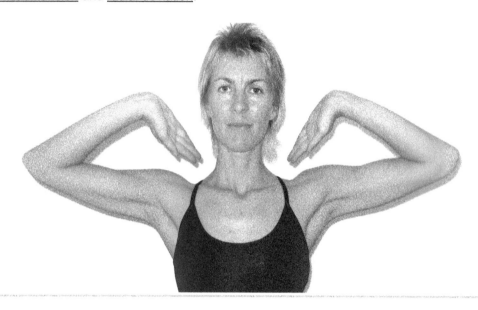

Figure 9.5: *Anumukha puritat mudra*: Tensioning (stretching) of dorsal aspect of ulnar nerve of brachial plexus and the small intestine acupuncture meridian: Effects of *anumukha puritat mudra* intensify with increasing shoulder (ST) depression, retraction and internal rotation; shoulder (GH) abduction, flexion, and internal rotation; elbow flexion and pronation; and wrist extension and radial deviation.

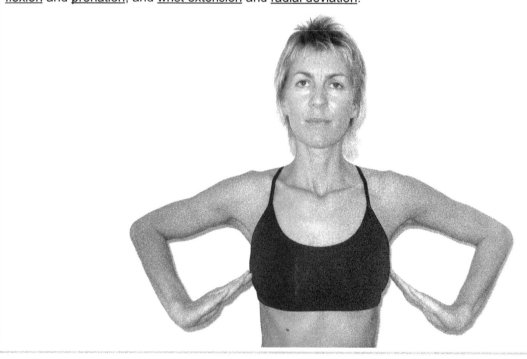

2. **Sacral plexus Stretches** [Figure 9.6]
• Tensioning of the <u>sciatic nerve</u> increases in intensity with <u>hip flexion</u>, <u>knee extension</u>, <u>ankle dorsiflexion</u>, <u>neck flexion;</u>
• There is a potential risk of <u>over-tensioning</u> (over-stretching) the <u>sciatic nerve</u> in all <u>hamstring</u> stretches;
• Impingement of the <u>sciatic nerve</u> or pain from the <u>sciatic nerve</u> may release and improve with <u>piriformis</u> and <u>gluteal</u> stretches, eg. cross-legged forward bends such as

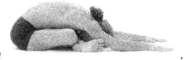

adho mukha swastikasana   .

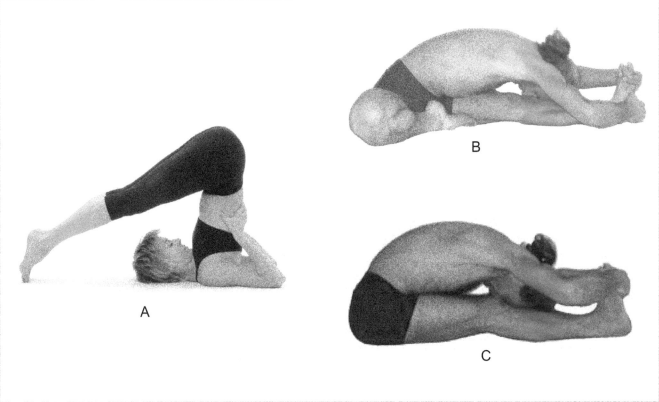

Figure 9.6: *Vasti mudra*: <u>Tensioning</u> (stretching) of the <u>sciatic nerve</u> of the <u>sacral plexus</u> and the <u>urinary bladder acupuncture meridian</u>: *vasti mudra* in (a) *halasana,* (b) *janu sirsasana and* (c) *pascimottanasana*: Effects of *vasti mudra* intensify with increasing <u>cervical spine flexion</u>, <u>thoracic spine flexion</u> and <u>lumbar spine flexion</u>; <u>hip flexion</u>; <u>knee extension</u>; and <u>ankle dorsiflexion</u> (<u>extension</u>).

3. **Femoral nerve stretches** [Figure 9.7]
• <u>Tensioning</u> of the <u>femoral nerve</u> increases in intensity with increasing <u>neck flexion</u>, <u>thoracic flexion</u> and <u>lumbar flexion</u>; <u>hip extension</u>; <u>knee flexion</u>; and <u>ankle plantarflexion</u> (<u>flexion</u>).
• There is a potential risk of <u>over-tensioning</u> (over-stretching) the <u>femoral nerve</u> in all postures that stretch

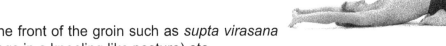

the front of the groin such as *supta virasana*   (lying back between the legs in a kneeling like posture) etc.

Figure 9.7: *Jathara mudra*: Tensioning (stretching) of the femoral nerve of the lumbar plexus and the stomach acupuncture meridian: *Jathara mudra* in
(a) *adho mukha san calanasana* with loss of effects of *jathara mudra* in
(b) *urdhva mukha san calanasana* but are replaced by tensioning of the vagus nerve at the front of the neck;
(c) *eka pada sarvangasana* (left leg in *jathara mudra* and right leg in *vasti mudra*);
(d) *urdhva mukha kulpha san calanasana*: Effects of *jathara mudra* intensify with increasing cervical spine flexion, thoracic spine flexion and lumbar spine flexion; hip extension; knee flexion and ankle plantarflexion (flexion).

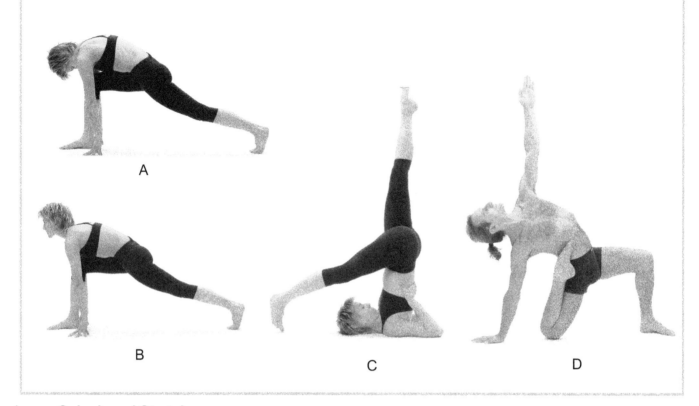

A

B

C

D

4. **Spinal cord Stretches** [Figures 9.6a & 6c]
   • Tensioning of the spinal cord increases in intensity with spinal flexion (i.e. cervical, thoracic, and lumbar flexion) and traction , hip flexion, knee extension and ankle dorsiflexion;
   • There is a potential risk of over-tensioning (over-stretching) the spinal cord in *halasana* (plough posture) [Figure 9.6a], *uttanasana* (standing straight legged forward bend) *pascimottanasana* (seated straight legged forward bend) [Figure 9.6c], etc.

5. **Vagus nerve Stretches** [Figure 9.8]
• Tensioning of the vagus nerve increases in intensity with cervical spine flexion and head extension;

• ☐ Possible risk of over-stretch in *urdhva mukha svanasana* 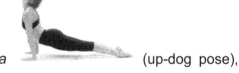 (up-dog pose),

bhujangasana (cobra pose), and other poses which incorporate the stretching of the anterior (front) of the neck as for *tha-jalandhara bandha* [Section 7.4.1.2.2].

Figure 9.8: *Garbha graha mudra in laghu vajrasana*: Tensioning (stretch) of the vagus nerve and the conception vessel acupuncture meridian. Effects of *garbha graha mudra* intensify with increasing head extension, cervical spine flexion, thoracic spine extension, lumbar spine extension; hip extension; knee flexion and ankle plantarflexion (flexion).

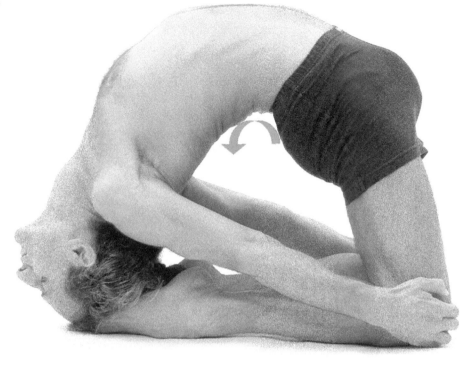

NB. EACH NEURAL TENSIONING (NERVE STRETCH) CAN BE POTENTIALLY RELEASING AND BENEFICIAL AS A TREATMENT OR, IF INAPROPRIATELY APPLIED, IT MAY BE VERY DANGEROUS AND HARMFUL TO THE NERVOUS SYSTEM.

9.7.4 Spinal Reflexes and their use in *Hatha Yoga*

Myotatic (stretch) reflex [Sections 1.7.2.2.1.1, 9.4.2.1 & 12.7.2.2.2.1]

Muscle stretch 🠒 Muscle activation

Yoga suggestions:
- Focus on stretching muscle to inhibit stretch reflex muscle activation
- Move slowly into each stretch

Reciprocal reflex [Sections 1.7.2.2.1.2, 9.4.2.2 & 12.7.2.2.2.1]

Agonist muscle activation 🠒 Antagonist muscle relaxation

Yoga Suggestions:
- Periodically contract an agonist to further relax the antagonist,
- eg. tighten quadriceps in hamstring stretch
- eg. tighten shoulder depressors to relax shoulder elevators
- eg. tighten hip extensors to relax hip flexors while lunging

Inverse myotatic reflex [Sections 1.7.2.2.3.1, 9.4.2.3 & 12.7.2.2.2.1]

Muscle stretch or tension 🠒 Muscle relaxation

Yoga Suggestions:
- Sustain a stretch until relaxation takes place
- Deepen postures on exhale, hold still on inhale
- Use contract and relax method of working on muscle against resistance for a period, i.e. utilise Proprioceptive Neuromuscular Facilitation (PNF)

9.7.5 Relationship Between the Nasal cycle, the Autonomic Nervous System, and Cerebral Hemispheric Dominance

The nasal cycle relates to the alternating nature of breathing through different nostrils throughout the day to automatically regulate temperature and metabolism. The sympathetic and parasympathetic branches of the autonomic nervous system (ANS) [Section 9.5] regulate the nasal cycle. The nasal cycle is also linked to the sidedness of the right and left cerebral hemispheres [Section 9.3.1.1] of the brain.

Electrical studies on the brain reveal a correlation between cerebral hemispheric dominance and the nasal cycle [Shannahoff-Khalsa, 1993]. Other related studies have shown that breathing through the right nostril is related to activation of the sympathetic nervous system, while breathing through the left nostril is related to the activation of the parasympathetic nervous system [Haight & Cole, 1989; Mohan & Eccles, 1989 Backen, 1990; Stancák & Kuna, 1994;Schiff & Rump, 1995]. These studies have demonstrated that people who are chronic right-nostril breathers (due to congenital or accidental blockage of the left nostril) tend to:

- Sleep less than most people,
- Experience more positive emotions than most people,
- Have a tendency to be hotter than most people, and
- Tend to get stressed more easily.

Studies have also shown that people who are chronic left nostril breathers (due to congenital or accidental blockage of the right nostril) tend to:
- Sleep more than most people,
- Experience less positive emotions than most people,
- Have a tendency to be colder than most people, and
- Tend not to get stressed so easily.

9.7.5.1 Applications of the nasal cycle to *nadis, asanas and pranayama*

Science is only beginning to understand the links between the nostrils, the nasal cycle, the two halves of the autonomic nervous system (ANS) (i.e. the sympathetic nervous system and the parasympathetic nervous system), the left and right cerebral hemispheres of the brain, and body posture. *Yogic* science has incorporated this type of knowledge for millennia. However, most of the *yogic* information about this subject has either been lost, or is not being taught by those who know about it. The right nostril represents the external terminus of the *pingala nadi*, which is a subtle channel that can heat and stimulate the body through the sympathetic nervous system. The left nostril represents the external terminus of the *ida nadi*, which is a subtle channel that can cool and calm the body and which is related to the parasympathetic nervous system.

Posture can also affect the lateralisation of the nervous system in the same manner that the nasal cycle affects the parasympathetic and sympathetic chains of the ANS. Postural asymmetries between the lateral halves of the body will cause the patent cavity of the nasal airway to change sides [Haight & Cole, 1989; Backen, 1990]. In addition, unilateral muscle activation is correlated with contralateral cerebral hemisphere activation [Schiff & Rump, 1995]. *Yoga* practitioners should work with *asana* (postural) and *vinyasa* (movement) practice to discover the asymmetries in the body and then work towards correcting what is abnormal and try to understand the cause of the asymmetry. Take note of the natural asymmetry in the body (resulting from organ sidedness etc.) and notice how this affects the functioning of the whole body [Appendix B]. Each asymmetry in the body reflects some sort of imbalance between the sympathetic nervous system and parasympathetic nervous system. It is well known in *yogic* and scientific circles, for example, that compression of the left underarm with a *yoga danda* (a rod or staff), or even with a strong *ha-amsa bandha* [Section 2.5.1.6, Appendix C] will cause the radial pulse of that arm to slow or stop while closing the nostril on the same side, and opening the nostril on the opposite side.

Breathing through the more efficient or dominant nostril is associated with increased activation of the contralateral (opposite) cerebral hemisphere, and with improved performance on cognitive tasks, which reflect the functions of that hemisphere [Shannahoff-Khalsa, 1993]. There is a similar relationship between nasal efficiency and emotional functions of the cerebral hemispheres. Following left nostril forced breathing, subjects report a more negative emotional state, score higher on an anxiety test, and tell stories that are more negative in emotional tone [Schiff & Rump, 1995].

Breathing through the left nostril stimulates the parasympathetic nervous system and movement of *prana* through *ida nadi*, while breathing through the right nostril stimulates the sympathetic nervous system and movement of *prana* through *pingala nadi*. *Yoga* practitioners are advised to work with *nadi sodhana pranayama* (alternate nostril breathing) and gently manipulate the pressure of the fingers over the nose so the breath length and volume is the same on both sides of the nose. Other useful practices are *surya bhedana pranayama* (inhaling through right nostril only, and stimulating *pingala nadi*), which stimulates the sympathetic nervous system and significantly heats the body, and *candra bhedana pranayama* (inhaling through left nostril only, and stimulating *ida nadi*), which stimulates the parasympathetic nervous system and significantly cools the body, and calms it down. Research has indicated that *surya bhedana pranayama* and *candra bhedana pranayama* have a balancing effect on the functional activity of the left and right hemisphere [Stancák & Kuna, 1994]. Care should be taken when experimenting with these *pranayamas*, especially *candra bhedana pranayama,* as one's emotional state can also be affected [Schiff & Rump, 1995].

9.7.6 Effects of *Pranayama* (Breath-control) on the Nervous system

Pranayama (breath-control) can significantly affect the nervous system. The way one breathes can vary tremendously. The effects of the various types of breathing on the nervous system and the emotions can be dramatic.

Natural breathing [Section 9.7.6.1] is the natural flow of one's breath as it would be without interference. Observance of natural breathing is the first step in *pranayama*. When one is passive, natural breathing is generally minimal in sound, depth, and volume. The effects of natural breathing on the nervous system are discussed below.

Hyperventilation [Section 9.7.6.2, Table 8.1.1] is a type of breathing that increases minute ventilation (the amount of air taken in per minute), relative to the amount breathed during natural breathing, either by increasing the volume or depth of each breath and/or increasing the rate or speed of the breath. The effects of hyperventilation on the nervous system are discussed below.

Hypoventilation [Section 9.7.6.3, Table 8.1.1] is a type of breathing that decreases minute ventilation (the amount of air taken in per minute), relative to the amount one breathes during natural breathing, either by decreasing the volume or depth of each breath and/or decreasing the rate or speed of one's breath. The effects of hypoventilation on the nervous system are discussed below.

Regulation of the breath can also be done by emphasising the natural pauses at the end of inhalation and exhalation [Section 9.7.6.4]. The natural pause or voluntary retention of the breath (*kumbhaka*) after an inhalation is called *antara* (internal) *kumbhaka*. The natural pause or voluntary retention of the breath after an exhalation is called *bahya* (external) *kumbhaka*.

Application of the *bandhas* [Sections 1.7.3 & 7.5.1] during *kumbhaka* can have significant effects on the nervous system. The application of *ha-mula bandha* after inhalation retention has been well researched by scientists who refer to this practice as the Valsalva manoeuvre [Section 7.4.1.1.1.2].

After the advanced *yoga* practitioner has explored the various types inhalation (*puraka*), exhalation (*recaka*) and breath-retention (*kumbhaka*), they eventually return to a very special type of natural breathing that is so minimal in sound and volume that it is almost imperceptible. This state is called *kevala kumbhaka* [Section 9.7.6.1] [Devananda, 1987].

Some of these effects of the various types of breathing are described below [Sections 9.7.6.1-4] and elsewhere in these notes [Sections 8.4 & 10.3].

EXTREME CAUTION IS ADVISED WHEN ALTERING THE NATURAL FLOW OF BREATHING OR RETAINING THE BREATH, AND ESPECIALLY IF INCORPORATING THE USE OF THE *BANDHAS* WITH BREATH-RETENTION.

9.7.6.1 Effects of natural breathing on the nervous system

Once a person has established a practice of the most basic *vinyasas* (dynamic exercises) and *asanas* (static postures) of a *hatha yoga* practice, then a concurrent *pranayama* (breath-control) practice can be introduced. At the most simple level a student should be directed to observe natural breathing, i.e. the natural flow of the breath.

Natural breathing is the type of breathing that people tend to do while sitting quietly in meditation, or reading etc. When passive, a healthy person's breath is generally silent, shallow and little (reduced minute ventilation). Many people adopt the erroneous action of making the sound of *ujjayi pranayama* so loud that it creates excess tension in the throat and may actually cause a reflex nasal congestion. Studies have shown that the inspiratory and expiratory airflow through the nostrils can cause reflex nasal congestion [Mohan & Eccles, 1989]. Therefore, although you should be able to listen to the sound of your own breath in *ujjayi pranayama*, if it is it so loud that someone else can hear it also then it will probably be causing inward tension, and maybe even causing nasal congestion.

As one gets more experienced in *pranayama* and learns to further observe the natural flow of quiet breathing, a paradox arises. The paradox is that the act of observing natural breathing (try to do natural breathing while reading this) causes the very nature of the breath to change. When carefully observing natural breathing, the breath tends to become much finer, and tends to become a type of hypoventilation. Natural breathing will slow the heart and therefore decrease sympathetic nervous system stimulation, while increasing parasympathetic nervous system stimulation. With continued observance of natural breathing when sitting or lying quietly, the practitioner can approach a state described in the texts as *kevala kumbhaka*, which is like a long breath-retention that is not planned. The inhalations and exhalations in *kevala kumbhaka* are so silent, small in volume and so infrequent that a state of non-breathing is approached. In the *Yoga Sutras of Patanjali* it says *yogah citta vrtti nirodhah* – yoga involves the stilling of the fluctuations of the mind [Iyengar, 1993]. In the *Hatha Yoga Pradipika of Swatmarama* it says he who restrains the breath restrains also the workings of the mind [Devananda, 1987], which is almost the same as what is said in the *Yoga Sutras of Patanjali* but in the opposite way. When *kevala kumbhaka* is approached the mind is very calm and rested, and a true stilling of the fluctuations of the mind (*vrttis*) can been established by stilling the fluctuations in the breath.

9.7.6.2 Effects of hyperventilation on the nervous system

Hyperventilation [Section 8.2.9.4.1, Table 8.1] is breathing more than the body thinks it needs at that time. It may be achieved with or without holding the breath but will occur more easily if the breath is not held in or held out. Many of the breathing exercises taught in *yoga* classes lead to hyperventilation. Even those exercises which do involve holding the breath will tend to cause hyperventilation as many teachers encourage deep breathing, but few practitioners can safely hold full lungs long enough, or breathe deeply slow enough, to breathe less than the normal minute ventilation.

Hyperventilation has some benefits. Hyperventilation trains the muscles of the chest and abdomen to increase the rate and depth of the breath. This causes an increase in body heat, which can facilitate joint mobility. The increased chest expansion during inhalation in hyperventilation not only enhances the inhalation, but also teaches *tha-uddiyana bandha* while maintaining *ha-mula bandha* [Section 1.7.3 & 7.3.1, Figures 7.9 & 8.1, Appendix C]. The rapid compression of chest and abdomen during exhalation in hyperventilation not only enhances the exhalation, but also teaches *ha-uddiyana bandha* and *ha-mula bandha* [Section 1.7.3 & 7.3.1, Figures 7.9 & 8.1, Appendix C]. In addition, hyperventilation causes the depletion of carbon dioxide, which results in the body becoming more alkaline because of respiratory alkalosis [Sections 9.7.6.3, 9.7.6.4, 10.3; Table 8.1.1]. The major positive effect of an alkaline system is that it also makes the synovial fluid more liquid and thus increases flexibility in the same way that heat does. The major clinical effect of alkalosis (an over-alkaline system) is over-excitability of the nervous system, which affects both the central nervous system (CNS) and peripheral nervous system [Guyton, 1991]. High levels of alkalinity in the bloodstream and body fluids can make the nervous system hypersensitive, which can manifest as joint pain, allergies, skin rashes and emotional disturbances. The major negative effect of respiratory alkalosis is that chemoreceptors in the carotid arteries and also those in the bronchial tubes detect the reduction in carbon dioxide levels and cause vasoconstriction and bronchoconstriction, which reduce the flow of blood and air to the brain and lungs respectively. Hyperventilation also tends to speed the heartbeat and therefore increases sympathetic nervous system stimulation, and decreases parasympathetic nervous system stimulation.

9.7.6.3 Effects of hypoventilation on the nervous system

Hypoventilation [Section 8.2.9.4.2, Table 8.1.2] is breathing less than the body thinks it needs at that time. Hypoventilation may be achieved with deep or shallow breathing, fast or slow breathing, and with or without holding the breath. However, hypoventilation will occur most easily if the breathing involves complete exhalations with only small volume inhalations, is slow in speed, and is either held in or out or preferably both [Section 9.7.6.4]. It is usually only the experienced *yogic* practitioner who can achieve real hypoventilation and generate a respiratory acidosis by increasing the levels of carbon dioxide and carbonic acid in the blood. The major clinical effect of acidosis (an over-acidic system) is de-sensitisation of the nervous system, which affects both the central nervous system and peripheral nervous system [Guyton, 1991]. Obviously extreme hypoventilation and extreme respiratory acidosis can kill someone. However, mild hypoventilation has quite a few benefits especially for the *yoga* practitioner. Hypoventilation tends to slow the heartbeat and therefore decreases sympathetic nervous system stimulation, and increases parasympathetic nervous system stimulation. Mild hypoventilation tends to leave the body in a more neutral balanced state compared to hyperventilation, which tends to result in a respiratory alkalosis [Sections 9.7.6.2, 9.7.6.4, 10.3; Table 8.1.1]. Someone who is able to hypoventilate can hold their breath for a relatively long time and therefore apply the *bandhas* in much better fashion, both using inhalation retention and exhalation retention [Section 9.7.6.4]. In addition, if one is able to generate a mild respiratory acidosis using hypoventilation with complete exhalations, small volume inhalations, slow speed, and holding the breath both in and out [Section 9.7.6.4], then one can easily derive the benefits of living on the traditional *yogic phalari* diet of fruit, salad and vegetables [Section 10.3]. In the *Yogayajnavalkya Samhita,* one of the oldest texts on *hatha yoga* [Desikachar, 2000], it says that those who can do *kevala kumbhaka pranayama,* which is essentially no noticeable breathing (hypoventilation), will have mastery over hunger [*Yogayajnavalkya Samhita* Verses VI.60-VI.64]. Conversely, a practitioner can usually only sustain a practice with hypoventilation, which generates a respiratory acidosis, if they have a lifestyle, diet and thought pattern which tends to generate a metabolic alkalosis to compensate for it. Finally, one of the most consistent findings in the many studies of meditation was the presence of some sort of hypoventilation which was associated with coherent synchronous brain wave patterns [Section 9.8.1].

Many people tend to hypoventilate in everyday life, but any positive benefits are lost because they usually never make complete exhalations, which require the complete application of *ha-mula bandha* and *ha-uddiyana bandha*. If hypoventilation is not achieved through complete exhalations and small volumes of air during inhalations, then it may confer several disadvantages. Complete exhalations rid the lungs of any stale air. Most people in everyday life breathe only small volumes (shallow tidal breathing) but in every breath have about half a lung of stale air. Complete exhalations also generate body heat, which helps mobilise synovial fluids and the joints since a complete exhalation requires application of *ha-mula bandha* and *ha-uddiyana bandha*. Most people in everyday life do not generate any body heat as they breathe, therefore their body remains stiff. Conversely, those who hyperventilate can derive flexibility, by increasing the fluidity of their synovial fluids, and hence their flexibility, by alkalising their system with breathing (which also helps mobilise synovial fluids), and perhaps also by heating their body with *bandhas* involved with forced deep breathing.

Take note that it is very easy to hyperventilate, and generate a temporary alkalosis, but is not so easy to hypoventilate and generate a respiratory acidosis. Consider the following: Natural breathing involves approximately 500 ml of air per breath and about 12 breaths per minute for a normal young adult man. Therefore, minute ventilation is 6000 ml per minute. A full inhalation, the vital capacity, is about 4600 for young adult man. Hence, for such a person to hypoventilate at rest it would involve breathing less than 6000 ml per minute, which may be achieved with 1.3 full breaths per minute, or about one breath every 45 seconds. For the average person breathing like this during a *yoga* practice is not possible to do. Therefore, for most people deep breathing will lead to hyperventilation and hence alkalosis. An alternative and more achievable way of not hyperventilating during a practice is to not take full lungs of air but rather take either one 1500 ml breath every 15 seconds or one 500 ml breath every 5 seconds - which is of course tidal breathing.

9.7.6.4 Effects of *kumbhaka* (breath-retention) on the nervous system

Research has shown that the beginner practitioner of *pranayama* has an increased <u>minute ventilation</u> [Section 8.2.9.4] and greater tendency towards <u>hyperventilation</u> [Karambelkar *et al*,.1982]. Beginner practitioners of *pranayama* also tend to finish their practice in a state of mild <u>respiratory alkalosis</u> due to their increased <u>carbon dioxide</u> output. <u>Alkalosis</u> leads to an over-excitability of the <u>nervous system</u> [Guyton, 1991]. People who <u>hyperventilate</u> in their practice of *asana* or *pranayama* often find that the resultant <u>respiratory alkalosis</u> leaves them very hungry [Sections 8.4.3, 9.7.6.2, 10.3; Table 8.1.1]. Since most food is <u>acidic</u> in nature, it tends to ground or balance people who have become light-headed or hypersensitive because of <u>alkalosis</u>.

Conversely, published research has shown that the experienced practitioner of *pranayama* tends to have a decreased <u>minute ventilation</u> [Section 8.2.9.4] and greater tendency towards <u>hypoventilation</u> [Karambelkar *et al*,.1982]. Hence, experienced practitioners of *pranayama* tend to finish their practice in a slightly <u>acidic</u> state due to their decreased output and increased retention of <u>carbon dioxide</u>. Experienced practitioners who can practise *asana* or *pranayama* in such a way as to <u>hypoventilate</u> (breathe less, and hold their breath longer), often find that their resultant mild <u>respiratory acidosis</u> leaves them satiated, and not at all hungry. Since most heavy food leaves an <u>acidic residue</u> in the blood after digestion, especially food containing significant protein, it becomes unappealing to ingest food that creates a more <u>acidic</u> internal condition after breathing in a way which has already lead to a mildly <u>acidic</u> condition, as such behaviour would leave the <u>nervous system</u> in a very de-sensitised condition. Instead the advanced practitioner who tends to <u>hypoventilate</u> during *pranayama* is able to balance their pH levels and their <u>nervous system</u> after their practice with an <u>alkaline</u> lifestyle, which allows them to include more fresh fruit, salad and vegetables in their diet, and not be as dependant on high protein and highly processed foods, which have many long-term problems [Section 10.3]. A lack of hunger or excessive hunger straight after finishing a *yoga* practice or any exercise may be indicative of <u>acid-alkaline</u> levels generated by the type of breathing performed during the exercise. Part of the reason why cigarette smokers crave food when they initially give up is because they are dependent on the <u>acidity</u> given to them through smoking and then seek that <u>acidity</u> in food. Conversely, smokers often tend to forget to eat as they have no craving for extra levels of <u>acid</u> since they have enough already.

When the <u>heart</u> speeds up this is associated with an increase in <u>sympathetic nervous system</u> stimulation, and conversely, when the <u>heart</u> slows this is associated with an increase in <u>parasympathetic nervous system</u> stimulation. The speed of the <u>heart</u> can be observed to change significantly through the controlled breath cycles of *Ujjayi pranayama* with *kumbhaka* (<u>breath-retention</u>). It may be assumed that the <u>heart</u> speed reflects and is reflected by the level of <u>sympathetic nervous system</u> versus <u>parasympathetic nervous system</u> stimulation. At the start of the <u>inhalation retention</u> the heartbeat is seen to increase immediately after inhalation ceases and this is probably associated with transient <u>sympathetic nervous system</u> stimulation. Presumably, this increase is due to the effects of the <u>respiratory pump</u> [Section 8.1.2.3.2] and in particular, the suction-like effects of the *tha-uddiyana bandha* [Section 7.4.1.3.1] used to expand the chest on inhale. After a few moments of <u>breath-retention</u>, the heartbeat slows, perhaps partly due to the cessation of effects of the <u>respiratory pump</u> and perhaps due to an increase in <u>intra-thoracic pressure</u> (ITP) causing <u>baroreceptors</u> to register an increase in <u>blood pressure</u> and stimulate <u>parasympathetic</u> output. Towards the end of a <u>breath-retention</u> the heartbeat is seen to increase again and this increase is presumably due an increase in <u>carbon dioxide</u> levels registering with the <u>chemoreceptors</u>, which then stimulate <u>sympathetic</u> output in order to increase blood flow to the <u>brain</u>.

If <u>breath-retention</u> (breath-holding) is preceded by <u>hyperventilation</u> one can notice the effects of pH on the body in a pronounced fashion. A period of controlled <u>hyperventilation</u> (increased breathing) will lead to decreased <u>carbon dioxide</u> levels in the body associated with decreased <u>carbonic acid</u> in the blood, and hence increased <u>alkalinity</u>. Immediately after ceasing <u>hyperventilation</u> and beginning <u>inhalation retention</u> there may be a sense of light-headedness, perhaps tingling in the fingers, even some <u>nausea</u>, which are typical effects of mild <u>alkalosis</u> on the <u>nervous system</u>. After a period of 10–20 seconds the <u>carbon dioxide</u> levels increase sufficiently to balance this transient <u>alkalosis</u> and a feeling of wellness ensues for some time. When <u>breath-retention</u> (breath-holding) is preceded by <u>hyperventilation</u> the breath is able to be retained inside for a period that is significantly longer than a <u>breath retention</u> not preceded by <u>hyperventilation</u>.

9.7.6.5 Effects of using *bandhas* during *kumbhaka* (breath-retention) on the nervous system

Bandhas are essentially maintained as <u>co-activations</u> of <u>antagonistic</u> (opposing) muscles [Section 1.7.3]. <u>Isometric</u> muscle activity greater than 25% of the maximum possible muscle activity tends to cause an increase in <u>blood pressure</u> [Section 12.3.2]. Although the situation can be modified by intelligent use of *ha-* and *tha- bandhas*, in general, use of the *bandhas* especially when the breath is held (*kumbhaka*) will cause an increase in <u>blood pressure</u>. If <u>blood pressure</u> increases then this will be sensed by <u>baroreceptors</u> [Sections 8.1.6.1 & 9.4.3.4], which will lead to <u>parasympathetic nervous system</u> output being stimulated to slow the <u>heart rate</u> and thus reduce <u>blood pressure</u>. Note that <u>baroreceptors</u> respond more to a rapidly changing pressure than to a stationary pressure. Therefore, the combination of *kumbhaka* (<u>breath-retention</u>), *bandha* (muscle <u>co-activation</u>), and *vinyasa* (movement or dynamic exercise) is an extremely potent way of affecting the <u>blood pressure</u> and its <u>nervous system</u> control. Since <u>baroreceptors</u> reset themselves every few days to whatever pressure they are exposed, one must take care that the use of *bandhas* in a practice does not lead to a long-term increase in <u>blood pressure</u>. One must be able to totally relax the entire body immediately if the practice is stopped suddenly, be able to maintain the key counter-*bandhas* (soft face, neck and throat) [Section 1.7.3.6] throughout the practice, and especially be able to balance the application of each *ha-bandha* with a subsequent *tha-bandha*.

Recent research has demonstrated that a certain amount of control over the <u>autonomic nervous system</u> is possible using the <u>Valsalva manoeuvre</u> [Piha, 1995; Smith *et al*,.1996]. Since the <u>Valsalva manoeuvre</u> is an attempt at forced exhalation with a closed glottis, which is essentially the same as activating a *ha-mula bandha* and *ha-uddiyana bandha* after holding the breath in [Section 7.4.1.1.1.2], it can be concluded that these *bandhas* can affect the <u>autonomic nervous system</u> in a similar way.

A note of caution needs to be emphasised. Do not do any <u>breath-retention</u> work with strong *bandha* work without the guidance of an experienced teacher. Many experienced *yoga* practitioners have demonstrated their ability to control their <u>heart rate</u> and even stop the pulse and <u>heart</u> beating, but it requires many years of experience, much preparation and skilful instruction. One should note that the <u>Valsalva manoeuvre</u>, which is essentially identical to *ha-mula bandha* and *ha-uddiyana bandha* performed during *antara kumbhaka* (inhalation retention), has been associated with cardiac arrhythmias and rarely, sudden death [Sperry, 1994].

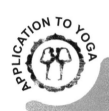

No 9.3 Use your diaphragm to breathe into the abdomen to help you relax and balance your nervous system

The <u>diaphragm</u> (and breathing in general) is often thought of as the bridge between body and mind because it can be controlled by the conscious mind (which relates to the <u>somatic</u> nervous system) and the unconscious mind (which relates more to the <u>autonomic</u> nervous system). Breathing <u>diaphragmatically</u> (<u>abdominal</u> breathing) can reestablish the natural balance between your <u>parasymphathetic</u> nervous system (the 'relaxation response') and your <u>sympathetic</u> nervous system (the 'flight or fight response'). Natural breathing or controlled <u>diaphragmatic</u> breathing can calm nerves, balance emotions, and enhance the functioning of the body systems that are under <u>autonomic</u> (automatic) control such as those to do with digestion, reproductive health, immunity and healing.

9.8 EFFECT OF THE MEDITATIVE PRACTICES ON THE NERVOUS SYSTEM

The meditative practices of *yoga* can be thought of as the last four stages of the *astanga yoga* system, *Pratayahara* (<u>meditative sense-control</u>), *Dharana* (<u>meditative concentration</u>), *Dhyana* (<u>meditative contemplation</u>), and *Samadhi* (<u>meditative absorption</u>).

Meditation is a Western term for a highly evolved process that uses various techniques of relaxation, <u>meditative sense-control</u>, <u>meditative concentration</u>, <u>meditative contemplation</u>, and visualisation to control the mind, its thoughts and its emotions, until a state of clear, blissful, mental silence can be attained. Advanced *yogins* can even control the physiological functions of the body during <u>meditative states</u>.

9.8.1 Physiological effects of Meditation

There have been many studies on meditation, but relatively few consistent effects are demonstrated between studies. The reason may be that, according to the ancient *yogic* texts, there are many types of meditative states possible, yet modern scientific literature tries to group meditation as one thing. There are at least three distinct meditative states defined in the *Patanjali-yoga-sutra* [Iyengar, 1993], seventeen meditative states according to the *Yoga-yajnavalkya-samhita* [Desikachar, 2000] and even more if one includes the many stages of *Samadhi* (meditative absorption). In addition, there are many approaches to achieve these meditative states. The *yogin* can meditate using any posture. The meditation can be static or dynamic, done with or without breath-control (*Pranayama*), and anything can be used as an object for meditation.

Jevning *et al.* [1996] have subjectively described meditation as a very relaxed but at the same time, a very alert state. Lazar *et al.* [2000] describe meditation as a conscious mental process that induces a set of integrated physiologic changes termed the relaxation response. Jevning *et al.* [1992] called meditation a wakeful hypo-metabolic integrated response. However, studies of certain *Tantric* [Corby et al., 1978], *Buddhist* [Benson et al., 1990] and *Taoist* meditations [Peng et al., 1999] demonstrate stimulation of autonomic nervous activity.

The most consistent findings in the many studies of meditation was the presence of some sort of hypoventilation [Wolkove et al., 1984; Sudsuang et al., 1991; Peng et al., 1999], and coherent synchronous brain wave patterns [Badawi et al., 1984; Arambula et al., 2001; Travis & Pearson, 2000; Travis, 2001] distinct from that of ordinary waking, hypnosis or sleep [Hewitt, 1983]. However, various studies of meditation have reported the presence of levels of coherent brain wave patterns in the delta [Stigsby et al., 1981], theta [Kubota et al., 2001], alpha [Dillbeck & Bronson, 1981, Aftanas & Golocheikine, 2001], and beta [Benson et al., 1990; Sim & Tsol, 1992] ranges. For various reasons, foremost being the subjective nature of meditation, it is not always possible to determine which of the meditative practices are being examined in each scientific paper.

Other reported physiological effects of meditation include: muscle relaxation [Patel & North, 1975; Narayu et al., 1990], lowered blood pressure [Wenneberg et al., 1997; Barnes et al., 1999; 2001], reduced heart rate, increased cardiac output [Dillbeck & Orme-Johnson, 1987], increased cerebral flow, reduction of CO_2 generation by muscle [Kesterson & Clinch, 1989], decreased sensitivity to carbon dioxide [Wolkove et al., 1984], reduced oxygen consumption [Wilson et al., 1987], increased galvanic skin resistance, decreased spontaneous electrodermal response, increased sensory perception and attentiveness [Brown et al., 1984], and decreased reaction times [Sudsuang et al, 1991]. Meditation training may also reduce the lactate response to exercise more effectively than simple relaxation does [Solberg et al., 2000].

Reported metabolic effects of meditation include: Increased blood pH during meditation but decreased arterial pH afterwards, resulting in a mild metabolic acidosis, decreased plasma lactate, changes of glucose metabolism pattern [Herzog et al., 1990], decreased adrenocortical activity just after 30 minutes of meditation and long-term decreased cortisol secretion [Sudsuang et al, 1991], changes in the secretion and release of several pituitary hormones [MacLean et al., 1997], increased concentrations of molecules thought to play an important role in learning and memory [Travis & Orme-Johnson, 1989] and increased levels of melatonin [Masion et al., 1995; Tooley et al., 2000], which probably promotes analgesia and reduces stress and insomnia [Elias & Wilson 1995; Harte et al., 1995].

Experienced meditators show higher plasma melatonin levels in the period immediately following meditation compared with the same period at the same time on a control night. Therefore, meditation can affect plasma melatonin levels. Facilitation of higher physiological melatonin levels at appropriate times of day might be one avenue through which the claimed health promoting effects of meditation occur [Tooley *et al.*, 2000]. Melatonin has many reported health benefits, including anti-ageing effects, anti-cancer properties [Masion et al., 1995], and immune system enhancing effects [Maestroni, 2001]. Increased melatonin levels produced in association with meditation may help to explain why many meditators do not require much sleep.

9.8.2 Types of Meditative Practices

There are many types of meditation. *Buddhist* monks are reported to have thousands of meditative techniques [Yeshe, 1999]. Each meditative technique can be done with or without breath-control (*Pranayama*), and can be a starting point to move into all the meditative states. All these meditations can progress to the ultimate state of meditative absorption (*Samadhi*) where the breath is not controlled but is in the state of *kevala-kumbhaka*, which is prolonged hypoventilation with breathing so minimal that it appears as apnoea (no breathing).

The <u>meditative state</u> can be achieved in any static posture and during movement. Most of the studies on meditation have mainly focused on <u>meditative states</u> obtained in seated or supine positions. Only a few studies have described <u>meditative states</u> in other *yoga* postures [Junker & Dworkis, 1986; Kamei et al., 2001]. Styles of *Taoist yoga* including *Tai-chi* and *qi-gong* have been described as dynamic meditations [Liu et al., 1990; Jin, 1992].

Seated <u>meditative practices</u> can be done with sheer willpower alone, but for many people it is quite difficult to sit still and just be with one's self, let alone concentrate or contemplate anything. The *yogic* texts recommend new *yogins* to work initially with <u>physical exercises</u> (*Asana*) and <u>breath-control</u> (*Pranayama*), then work with the physical *yoga* approaches to the meditative practices and finally progress to the seated <u>meditative practices</u>.

The inverted postures of *viparita karani mudra* [Figure 12.3] can be used as a preparation for <u>meditative practices</u> or as a meditative practice itself. *Viparita karani mudra* promotes <u>hypoventilation</u>, which is associated with the <u>coherent synchronous brain wave patterns</u> seen in <u>meditative states</u> [Badawi et al., 1984; Arambula et al., 2001; Travis & Pearson, 2000; Travis, 2001]. Hence, *viparita karani mudra* prepares the *yogin* for seated <u>meditative practices</u>, and is traditionally practised just before seated meditation.

The *Yoga-yajnavalkya-samhita* states that the last four stages of *astanga yoga* are the inner or <u>meditative practices</u> [Mohan, 2000]. Although it is possible to enter a <u>meditative state</u> with no preparation, as do those who practise styles of non-physical *yoga*, this is not possible for most people. The first four limbs of *astanga yoga* prepare the *yogin* for the <u>meditative state</u>. The ethical disciplines (*Yama* and *Niyama*) are an ongoing mental preparation for the *yogin* that involve restraints such as non-violence and non-attachment. Physical exercises (*Asana*) prepare the body physically to comfortably sit for meditation. Breath-control (*Pranayama*) helps to focus the mind, sensitise the <u>nervous system</u>, and can act as a bridge between the gross body and the more subtle mind. Breath-control can be used to initiate any of the <u>meditative practices</u>, which are the last four stages of *astanga yoga*.

The *Patanjali-yoga-sutra* essentially describes *yoga* as *citta vrtti nirodha*, which is the ultimate *raja yoga* <u>meditative state</u> when the fluctuations (*vrtti*) of the mind (*citta*) are stilled (*nirodha*) [Iyengar, 1993]. In scientific terms, this can be interpreted and seen as <u>coherent synchronous brain wave patterns</u>. The *Hatha yoga-pradipika* describes *yoga* as *prana vrtti nirodha*, which is the ultimate *hatha yoga* <u>meditative state</u> in which the fluctuations (*vrtti*) of the breath (*prana*) are stilled (*nirodha*) [Vishnu-Devananda, 1987]. In scientific terms, this can be interpreted as <u>hypoventilation</u> (long slow breathing, minimal breathing or breath-suspension).

The ancient *yoga* texts are clear in stating that *citta* (mind or consciousness) and *prana* (essential life force in the breath) move as one, and are always together in the body [Iyengar, 1993]. If *yoga* is stillness in mind and *yoga* is stillness in breath, then when there is stillness in mind there should be stillness in breath and vice versa. There are therefore essentially two approaches to achieve *yoga* and reach a <u>meditative state</u>, the *raja yoga* approach and the *hatha yoga* approach. These two approaches lead to a <u>meditative state</u> that is physiologically similar in terms of <u>brain wave patterns</u> and physiological responses.

In the *raja yoga* approach, which mainly uses the <u>meditative practices</u> of <u>non physical *yoga*</u>, the *yogin* stills the mind, generating <u>coherent synchronous brain wave patterns</u> [Corby et al., 1978; Aftanas & Golocheikine, 2001]. The body then responds with *kevala kumbhaka*, a state of <u>hypoventilation</u> in which the breath is almost imperceptible or spontaneously absent [Farrow & Herbert, 1982; Badawi *et al.*, 1984; Gallois, 1984; Travis & Wallace, 1997]. In the *hatha yoga* approach <u>physical *yoga*</u> (<u>physical exercises</u> and <u>breath-control</u>) is used to bring a stillness to the breath which is seen as some form of <u>hypoventilation</u> [Stanescu et al., 1981; Miyamura et al., 2002]. The mind then responds with a calmness that is associated with the presence of <u>coherent synchronous brain wave patterns</u> [Hebert & Lehmann, 1977; Stancak et al., 1993; Arambula *et al*, 2001].

Note however, that both the *hatha yoga* and *raja yoga* approaches *to astanga yoga* allow all the <u>meditative practices</u> to be done with or without <u>breath-control</u> (*Pranayama*). Therefore, the meditative practices can be examined in terms of a <u>physical *yoga*</u> approach similar to the main focus of *hatha yoga* and non physical *yoga* approach similar to the main focus of *raja yoga*.

9.8.2.1 Meditative states derived through a physical *yoga* approach

The four meditative practices of *astanga yoga* can be obtained with physical *yoga*. In the physical *yoga* approach the *yogin* can use physical exercises (*Asana*) or breath-control (*Pranayama*) to still the fluctuations of the breath in order to still the fluctuations in the mind.

The *Yoga-yajnavalkya-samhita* describes meditative sense-control (*Pratayahara*) as an initial period of sensory awareness, which is considered an external (*bahya*) process, followed by a period of sensory withdrawal, an internal (*abhyantara*) process [Desikachar, 1998]. In *bahya-pratayahara,* the *yogin* creates a heightened sensory awareness that is very useful for helping to unify body and mind in the present moment. This helps calm the mind by moving the *yogins* attention away from the problems of everyday life. Pure mental processes can achieve *bahya-pratayahara*, and many meditators attempt to do this. However, in order to help stimulate the nervous system to a heightened state of sensory awareness the *yogin* can practise breath-control (*Pranayama*) involving some hyperventilation (increased breathing). Hyperventilation alkalises the blood, which sensitises the nervous system and brings the *yogin* into a state of heightened awareness. The *yogin* can then be extremely receptive to what is happening in the body at that time, and can develop the ability to sense and examine injuries or medical conditions. Methods for solving problems in the body are easier to devise when a heightened state of awareness makes those problems more obvious. Once the *yogin* has had a chance for self-examination in a state of heightened awareness, the second or internal form of *Pratayahara* can begin.

The second form of *Pratayahara* is an internal (*abhyantara*) process. In *abhyantara-pratayahara,* the *yogin* begins the process of dissociating or withdrawing from the senses. Experienced *yogins* can withdraw from their senses spontaneously. However, three forms of *Pranayama* involving hypoventilation (reduced breathing) can facilitate sensory withdrawal (*abhyantara-pratayahara*) and the remaining meditative states of concentration (*Dharana*), contemplation (*Dhyana*) and absorption (*Samadhi*).

There are essentially three types of breath-control (*Pranayama*) that can be used to still the fluctuations in the breath, in order to still the fluctuations in the mind. Most people can gently attempt all three of these methods of breath-control (*Pranayama*). However, to be successful in calming the nervous system rather than stimulating it, the result in all three techniques should be hypoventilation (reduced breathing), which leads to a mild acidosis and calms the nervous system [Guyton, 1991]. The best methods of breath-control (*Pranayama*) for creating a meditative state are those that involve conscious [Arambula et al., 2001; Miyamura et al., 2002] or unconscious hypoventilation [Vempati & Telles, 2002]. Probably the greatest paradox in people's perception of *yoga* is that they think that *yoga* is about breathing, whereas in fact the *yogin* strives to use as little air as possible in breathing (hypoventilation). In the same way as a car is considered more efficient if it can run on less fuel the *yogin* aspires to function with less air. The three methods of breath-control (*Pranayama*) that can promote hypoventilation and help in developing a meditative state are:

- Respiratory suspension (breath-holding)
- Long slow deep breathing
- Minimal breathing

The first method of breath-control (*Pranayama*) that is useful for developing a meditative state is to hold the breath in (*antara-kumbhaka*) or hold the breath out (*bahya-kumbhaka*) as long as possible. Complete breath-retention definitely stops the fluctuations of the breath and this is when the ancient texts say the fluctuations of the mind cease also. Brain wave studies on advanced meditators demonstrate novel brain wave patterns that suggest a quietened but alert mental state during periods of breath-suspension [Farrow & Herbert, 1982; Gallois, 1984; Badawi et al., 1984].

The second method of breath-control (*Pranayama*) that is useful for developing a meditative state is long slow deep breathing. Following studies of an experienced *kundalini-yogin,* Arambula *et al.* [2001] suggested that a shift in breathing patterns to long slow breathing contributes to the development of synchronous alpha brain wave activity. If breathing can be done very slowly with no strain, even as slow as one complete breath per minute, and the exhalations are especially emphasised, the parasympathetic nervous system is activated and the <u>heart rate</u> slows [Zeier, 1984]. If breathing is very slow there is little perceptible movement in the chest or <u>abdomen</u>, and the mind then becomes calm. Using this type of breathing for meditation is also best for advanced *yogins* who have mastered the art of <u>breath-control</u> (*Pranayama*).

The third method of <u>breath-control</u> (*Pranayama*) that is useful for developing a <u>meditative state</u> involves <u>hypoventilation</u> with minimal breathing. Minimal breathing involves making very small, almost imperceptible breaths with no noticeable breath-sound and hardly any movement in the chest or <u>abdomen</u>. Minimal breathing is quite accessible to most people practising in a non-strenuous way such as simple sitting. It is the type of breathing that the practitioners of most meditation traditions will unconsciously do [Sudsuang *et al.*, 1991]. Eventually minimal breathing develops into what the texts refer to as *kevala-kumbhaka,* which is described in the *yogic* texts as the perfect state of non-breathing where the fluctuations in the breath have ceased [Pranavananda, 1992]. The presence of *kevala-kumbhaka* is regarded a sign that the *yogin* has reached the ultimate state of <u>meditative absorption</u> (*Samadhi*). Several clinical trials have demonstrated that during meditation with minimal breathing there are often times when the breath spontaneously and often unconsciously stops [Farrow & Herbert, 1982; Badawi *et al.*, 1984].

In *Taoist yoga*, such as *qi-gong*, minimal breathing is called *qi*-breath (energy breath) and *kevala-kumbhaka* is referred to as resting-breath. These two types of <u>breath-control</u> are thought to be the best for both the physical exercises and meditative practices of *Taoist yoga* [Liu, 1991].

9.8.2.2 Meditative states derived through a non physical *yoga* approach

In the <u>non physical *yoga*</u> approach to the *astanga yoga* <u>meditative states</u>, many techniques can still the fluctuations of the mind. Each of these techniques initially focuses on one of the meditative stages of the *astanga yoga*, but can then potentially take the practitioner through all the stages of *astanga yoga* to the ultimate state of <u>meditative absorption</u> (*Samadhi*).

9.8.2.2.1 The non physical *yoga* approach to *Pratayahara* (meditative sense-control)

Meditative sense-control (*Pratayahara*) is practised in the popular Zen *Buddhist* techniques of mindfulness meditation [Sun *et al.*, 2002] and Vipassana meditation [Hart, 1987]. Relaxation techniques such as the supine *yoga-nidra* [Satyananda, 1996], which evoke the relaxation response [Lazar et al., 2000] can also be considered to be techniques of <u>meditative sense-control</u> (*Pratayahara*). These techniques involve observing all the sensations, pleasant and painful, coming from one's posture, breathing, thoughts, and feelings, without judging or trying to change them. Meditative sense-control can be useful in the treatment of people facing pain and illness. It is possible to control pain and discomfort through techniques of <u>meditative sense-control</u> such as mindfulness meditation [Sun *et al.*, 2002]. In a randomised controlled trial of mindfulness meditation, which is a type of *jnana yoga* (*yoga* of self-knowledge), participants reduced their psychological symptomatology and increased the sense of control in their life [Astin, 1997].

9.8.2.2.2 The non physical *yoga* approach to *Dharana* (meditative concentration)

The *raja yoga*-style meditative technique known as <u>meditative concentration</u> (*Dharana*) [Delmonte, 1989] involves simply concentrating on one thing, or nothing, while being still. Brain wave studies comparing concentrative and non-concentrative *Taoist* meditation suggest that theta <u>brain wave</u> rhythms are related to <u>meditative concentration</u> [Pan et al., 1994]. Studies on Zen meditation showed increased theta <u>brain wave</u> activity on an electroencelograph (EEG), reflecting mental concentration as well as relief from anxiety [Kubota et al., 2001]. Dunn et al. [1999] have shown that <u>meditative concentration</u> (*Dharana*) produces a unique physiological state that is separate to the unique physiological state produced by mindfulness meditation, which is a type of *Pratayahara*.

9.8.2.2.3 The non physical *yoga* approach to *Dhyana* (meditative contemplation)

Dhyana has been translated as <u>meditative contemplation</u>. It is possible to contemplate on anything. A devotional <u>meditative contemplation</u> is a type of *bhakti yoga*. <u>Meditative contemplations</u> on a sound or on an image are types of *mantra yoga* and *yantra yoga* respectively. These practices require tremendous concentration; hence, *mantra yoga* and *yantra yoga* are combinations of *Dharana* and *Dhyana*. In fact, *Dhyana* (contemplation) requires *Dharana* (concentration) as a pre-requisite.

9.8.2.2.3.1 *Mantra yoga*

Mantra yoga is a popular method of meditation that uses chanting of sounds and phrases to induce a meditative state. Chanting can be done audibly as a type of breath-control (*Pranayama*) or mentally, with or without breath-control. Types of *mantra yoga* are used in *Vedic*, *Tantric* and *Buddhist* meditative practices, and are used in the devotional practices of Christians, Muslims, Jews and tribal cultures around the world. *Yogins* can chant *mantras* aloud or recite them mentally during exhalation, but can also recite them mentally during inhalation and inhalation retention. Chanting is a practice that develops the left side of the brain because it involves a type of aural visualisation to remember the chant. The ability to chant may be enhanced by breathing through the right nostril, which stimulates the left side of the brain.

In a study by Bernardi et al. [2001b], it was found that both rosary prayer (recitation of the *Ave Maria* in Latin) and *mantra* caused synchronous increases in cardiovascular rhythms when recited aloud six times a minute. Baroreflex sensitivity also increased significantly. The imposed breath-control (*Pranayama*) pattern of six breaths per minute induced favourable psychological and possibly physiological effects [Bernardi et al., 2001b].

Following a clinical trial of seven experienced meditators it was deduced that *mantra* meditation (mental chanting of OM) caused an increase in mental alertness and relaxation (as shown by the reduced heart rate) [Telles *et al.*, 1995]. *Mantra* meditation was found to be more effective at reducing anxiety than either relaxation techniques [Dilbeck, 1977] or meditative concentration [Eppley & Adams, 1989]. This may be related to the fact that relaxation techniques often involve some type of sense-control (*Pratayahara*), which is the fifth out of eight stages of *astanga yoga*; and meditative concentration (*Dharana*) is the sixth out of eight stages of *astanga yoga*. However, *mantra* meditations are part of *Dhyana,* which is the seventh stage of *astanga yoga*. *Dhyana* is usually translated as contemplation in *Vedic* texts, but in *Tantric* texts, *Dhyana* is translated as visualisation. The practice of mentally chanting is a type of visualisation (visualising a sound). The *Patanjali-yoga-sutra* implies that there is a sequential progression in the eight stages of *astanga yoga*. Therefore, to be practising at the seventh stage of *astanga yoga* (*Dhyana*) implies that the fifth and sixth stages are already present. Hence, it is to be expected that *mantra* meditation, a type of *Dhyana*, has a more potent effect than concentration or relaxation techniques alone.

Mantra meditation has been associated with the generation of coherent alpha [Travis, 2001] and theta waves [Aftanas & Golocheikine, 2001]. Studies on memory show a strong relationship between alpha wave power and memory performance during memorizing words [Vogt et al., 1998] and significant theta synchronization during the recognition of words [Klimesch et al., 1997]. Mental chanting involves memory and recognition of words; hence it is understandable why chanting is such a powerful technique for bringing about a meditative state. This may represent evidence in support of studies reporting that meditation improves one's memory [Atwood & Maltin, 1991]. Similar brain wave patterns as seen during meditation are also apparent during important stages of sleep [Sei & Morita, 1996; Benca et al., 1999; Cantero et al., 1999; et al., 2001]. This may support Krishnamacharyas often-quoted statement that *yoga* and meditation can replace sleep [Desikachar, 1998].

Transcendental meditation (TM)

Mantra yoga is the basis of Transcendental meditation (TM), which has been very well studied. Most of the scientific literature on meditation is derived from TM. However, most of the scientific papers on TM are published by a university owned by the TM organisation, making the claims made in these papers regarding the efficacy of TM seem self-serving, even though many are reported as randomised controlled studies.

Based on the results of many physiological experiments on TM, Jevning *et al.* [1992] hypothesize that meditation is an integrated response with peripheral circulatory and metabolic changes subserving increased central nervous activity. During TM, there is increased cardiac output, probable increased cerebral blood flow, apparent cessation of carbon dioxide generation by muscle, fivefold increase in the blood plasma antidiuretic hormone arginine vasopressin (AVP) and coherent synchronous brain wave patterns [Jevning et al., 1992; 1996]. It was found that TM increased the exercise tolerance in patients with coronary artery disease [Zamarra et al., 1996].

In an extensive study of a single advanced TM meditator, pure consciousness experiences were associated with periods of spontaneous breath suspension, reduced heart rate, high basal skin resistance, stable phasic skin resistance, markedly reduced mean respiration rate, reduced mean minute ventilation (hypoventilation), reduced mean metabolic rate and statistically consistent coherent synchronous brain wave patterns [Farrow & Herbert, 1982].

9.8.2.2.3.2 *Yantra yoga*

Yantra yoga is essentially a type of *Dhyana* (<u>meditative contemplation</u>), which involves mental or physical gazing at an image or a design. In *Tantric* texts *Dhyana* is translated as visualisation. *Yantras* are images that are either focused on visually with eyes open, or visualised internally. Types of *yantra yoga* are used in *Vedic*, *Tantric*, *Buddhist* and *Taoist* <u>meditative practices</u>. Internal and external visualisation techniques can induce <u>brain wave patterns</u>, with the characteristic alpha and theta waves specific to the <u>meditative state</u> [von Stein & Sarnthein, 2000]. Visualisation is a practice that develops the right side of the <u>brain</u>. The ability to visualise may be enhanced by breathing through the left nostril, which stimulates the right side of the <u>brain</u>.

9.8.2.2.3.3 *Laya yoga*

Laya yoga, considered an intermediate between *hatha yoga* and *raja yoga*, uses an advanced combination of *Pranayama* (<u>breath-control</u>), *mantra yoga* (chanting) and *yantra yoga* (visualisation). In *laya yoga, cakras* (energy centres of the body) are visualised and sounds associated with these *cakras* are mentally chanted. In conjunction with advanced <u>breath-control</u> (*Pranayama*), this practice culminates in *kundalini yoga* in which dormant energies are said to be awakened in the <u>spine</u>. Peng *et al.* [1999] studied traditional forms of *kundalini-tantra* meditation and reported extremely prominent <u>heart rate</u> oscillations associated with slow breathing.

Benson *et al.* [1990] studied three *Tibetan* monks practising a type of *laya yoga,* and found that these experienced meditators could raise their metabolic rate by 61% or lower it by 64% at will, and that their <u>brain wave patterns</u> showed a marked asymmetry in alpha and beta activity between the hemispheres with increased beta activity.

Another study of *Tantric* meditation [Corby et al., 1978] showed that proficient meditators increased <u>autonomic nervous system</u> (ANS) activation during meditation while inexperienced meditators demonstrated ANS during relaxation. During meditation, proficient meditators demonstrated increased alpha and theta <u>brain wave patterns</u>, but there was minimal evidence of sleep [Corby et al., 1978].

The findings of Peng *et al.* [1999], Benson et al. [1990], and Corby *et al.* [1978] challenge the notion of meditation as only being an autonomically quiescent state. Similar patterns of <u>coherent synchronous brain waves</u> have been seen in several other meditation studies [Arambula et al., 2001; Travis, 2001; Aftanas & Golocheikine, 2001].

9.8.3 Effects of the Meditative Practices

9.8.3.1 Beneficial effects of meditation

The reported psychological effects of meditation used as a therapy are not based on properly randomised and controlled trials, and placebo comparisons for meditation are problematic. Atwood and Maltin [1991] described how meditation helps to develop patience and to be aware of a problem before attempting to solve it, promoting a non-judgmental attitude. It helps people to be comfortable with ambiguity, ignorance and uncertainty. Meditators learn to recognise and trust their inner nature and wisdom. Meditation fosters the recognition of personal responsibility.

Reports claim that meditation helps improve memory [Atwood & Maltin, 1991], increases vigour [Kutz et al., 1985a, b], and enhances compassion, acceptance and tolerance to self and others [Dua & Swinden, 1992]. Shapiro [1992] found that 88% of subjects reported greater happiness and joy, positive thinking, increased self-confidence, effectiveness (getting things done), and better problem-solving skills [Dillbeck & Vesely, 1986]. Other reported beneficial effects include greater control of feelings, more relaxation, greater resilience [Scheler, 1992] and increased life expectancy [Wallace et al., 1982; Alexander et al., 1989].

9.8.3.2 Adverse effects and dangers of seated meditation

Many people are not initially suitable or do not have the predisposition for a static, seated meditative practice. Adverse effects of static, seated meditation described in the literature include: anxiety, panic, tension, boredom, pain, confusion, disorientation, decreased motivation, impaired sense of reality, feeling spaced out, depression, increased negativity, being more judgmental, feeling addicted to meditation, uncomfortable kinaesthetic sensations, dissociation, feelings of guilt, symptoms of psychosis, grandiosity, elation, destructive behaviour, suicidal feelings, defencelessness, fear, anger, apprehension and despair [Kutz et al., 1985a,b; Craven, 1989; Shapiro, 1992]. Many of these problems have been associated with the practice of transcendental meditation (TM)

[Perez-De-Albeniz & Holmes, 2000].

Zuroff and Schwarz [1980] did a two-year follow-up of a controlled experiment comparing the effects of TM with muscle relaxation. They concluded that TM is not universally beneficial as only some subjects (15%-20%) enjoyed the practice enough, or found it useful enough to maintain it.

Ancient texts such as the *Patanjali-yoga-sutra* are clear that the eight steps of *astanga yoga* should be followed in some sequence. It is safer for most people to practise physical yoga, including simple relaxation, first, then once established in these, progress to the meditative practices [Iyengar, 1993, Mohan 2000].

In a controlled clinical trial by Wood [1993] comparing the effects of relaxation, visualization (*Dhyana*), and physical yoga (physical exercises and breath-control), normal volunteers found that physical yoga produced a significantly greater increase in perceptions of mental and physical energy and feelings of alertness and enthusiasm than the other two procedures. Relaxation and visualization made subjects more sleepy and sluggish than physical yoga, and visualization made them less content than physical yoga and more upset than relaxation. Wood [1993] thus found that a simple, easy to learn, 30 minute program of physical yoga that could be practised even by the elderly, had a markedly invigorating effect on perceptions of both mental and physical energy and increased high positive mood in the participants.

9.8.4 Dynamic Meditative Practices
The results of a study comparing the isometric squeeze-relaxation technique with meditation suggest that isometric squeeze-relaxation may be more appropriate for individuals who have difficulty focusing, and meditation for those who already possess well-developed relaxation skills at a trait level [Weinstein & Smith, 1992]. The *hatha yoga* styles derived from the teachings of Sivananda and his main students usually conclude the *yogic* physical exercises with an isometric squeeze relaxation as a preparation for the supine relaxation (*savasana*) which is then usually followed by a static seated meditation. In contrast, the *hatha yoga* styles derived from Krishnamacharya's main students incorporate activation and relaxation of specific muscles during most postures. This is especially so in the *Iyengar yoga* style. In addition, because there is generally a flowing movement (*vinyasa*) between each posture, especially in the styles of Patabhi Jois and Desikachar, muscles are obliged to be active for the period they are needed to bring the body in or out of a posture, and can then relax briefly in each pose to some extent.

To maintain the process of activating and relaxing muscles throughout a dynamic practice in a manner that provides the best effect on each of the body systems requires constant attention that mimics the mental state of meditation. In fact it is possible to achieve all the meditative states mentioned so far during a dynamic meditative practice. For many people, a dynamic meditation, especially one in which there are challenges that help maintain focus such as balancing on one leg, is far more engaging than a passive, sitting meditation. Perhaps the reason for the recent international trend towards dynamic styles of *hatha yoga* as a form of exercise and meditative practice is related to the sedentary nature of most people's lives. After sitting at a desk or in front of a computer all day, the thought of sitting to meditate is not appealing for most people. However, the idea of a dynamic meditation such as one offered in many *hatha yoga* styles has become very popular in recent times. The popularity of styles such as power *yoga*, a type of *astanga vinyasa yoga*, is evidenced by its regular mention in the popular press (eg. cover story Time Magazine) [Corliss, 2001]. A dynamic *hatha yoga* meditative style practice can engage the mind, stimulate circulation and breathing, massage glands and internal organs, energise and heat the body, all while flowing in and out of various stretching and strengthening postures at various speeds. Moving meditations, such as *yogic siddhi* flying [Orme-Johnson & Gelderloos,1988], *qi-gong* [Pan et al., 1994] and dynamic *hatha yoga* [Junker & Dworkis, 1986; Kamei et al., 2000] have all been shown to create coherent synchronous brain wave patterns, similar to those seen in many of the studies of static meditation [Travis, 2001]. It may therefore be possible for even a newer *yoga* practitioner to meditate while moving through a series of *hatha yoga* postures with eyes open [Junker & Dworkis, 1986].

****

Chapter Breakdown

****

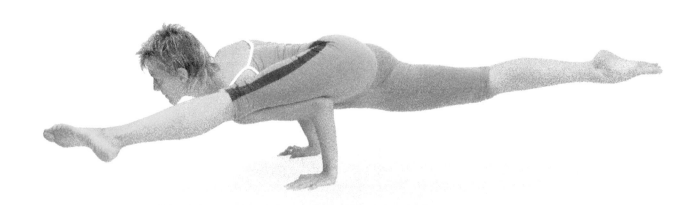

**Bianca Machliss with elbows massaging the organs of digestion in *Eka Pada Mayura Koundinyasana*.
Photo courtesy of Alejandro Rolandi.**

10.0 INTRODUCTION TO APPLIED ANATOMY & PHYSIOLOGY OF THE DIGESTIVE SYSTEM, IMMUNE SYSTEM AND NUTRITION IN *HATHA YOGA*

The body can process food best when the digestive system is functioning properly. Nutrients must be well absorbed and wastes correctly eliminated. Good absorption of nutrients and elimination of wastes will promote the healthy functioning of the immune system. If diet is poor, or if the digestive processes are hampered by excess life-stress or incorrect lifestyle habits, the health of the digestive system will suffer, and consequently the health of the immune system will also be affected.

Hatha yoga asanas (static postures) *vinyasas* (dynamic exercises) and *pranayamas* (breathing exercises) can affect the digestion and absorption of food by stimulating circulation and by mechanically massaging the gastrointestinal tract.

Pranayama (the breathing component of *hatha yoga*) can also affect digestion especially with the use of the *bandhas* (internal muscular locks defined anatomically as the co-activation of opposing muscle groups around joint complexes) [Sections 1.7.3 & 7.5.1].

Similarly, the type of *pranayama* (for example fast, slow, deep or shallow) that can be practised will be determined, to an extent, by what food is eaten. This is because metabolism of ingested food will lead to a particular acid-base level in the blood and in the body, which must be then balanced by the respiratory system. The respiratory system can alter the pH of the blood by retaining or expelling carbon dioxide in order to change the levels of carbonic acid in the blood [Section 8.4.4]. If we generate an acid pH from the metabolism of the food we eat (metabolic acidosis), we then automatically begin to breathe in such a way as to decrease acid levels and therefore blow off carbon dioxide with hyperventilation, which creates a respiratory alkalosis. Conversely, if the food we eat leads to an alkaline state in the body after it has been metabolised (metabolic alkalosis) then we will tend to breathe in a way as to retain carbon dioxide by hypoventilation, and generate a respiratory acidosis.

10.1 THE DIGESTIVE SYSTEM

Food is processed through the digestive system by (i) ingestion, (ii) movements (ie peristalsis), (iii) mechanical, chemical and enzymatic digestion, (iv) absorption, and, (v) defecation.

Digestive Organs and Structures are divided into two main groups:
* **Gastrointestinal (GI) tract**, which is a continuous tube-like structure from the mouth through the pharynx, to oesophagus, to stomach to small intestine, to large intestine, to rectum, and finally to anus.
* **Accessory structures**, which include the teeth, tongue, salivary glands, liver, gall bladder, and pancreas.

10.1.1 Salivary Glands
The salivary glands secrete an amylase called ptyalin, an enzyme which starts the chemical digestion of complex carbohydrates. The complex carbohydrates are broken down to single simple sugars which can then be used by the cells of the body after they are transported to the blood. Saliva helps lubricate food. Salivation is entirely under parasympathetic nervous system control.

10.1.2 Oesophagus
The oesophagus is a collapsible, muscular tube that connects the pharynx at the back of the mouth and throat to the stomach.

10.1.3 Stomach
The stomach is a muscular bulging of the digestive tract that begins at the bottom of the oesophagus and ends at the pyloric sphincter. The stomach walls secrete hydrochloric acid (HCl) and enzymes called proteases for the initial breakdown of proteins. Special features of the stomach for digestion include rugae (folds or wrinkles in the stomach wall which increase surface area) and mucous forming glands. Mechanical digestion in the stomach consists of muscular waves generated by a three-layered muscular wall designed for efficient mechanical movement.

Chemical digestion in the stomach is mainly the conversion of proteins into <u>peptides</u> (short chains of <u>amino acids</u>) by the actions of <u>hydrochloric acid</u> (HCl) and the <u>enzyme</u> <u>pepsin</u>. Regulation of the <u>gastric secretions</u> is by nervous and hormonal mechanisms. Absorption of nutrients in the stomach is limited to some water, certain electrolytes (salts), drugs and alcohol.

The stomach secretes the <u>enzyme</u> <u>rennin</u>, which functions to coagulate <u>casein</u> (a major milk protein) and make it accessible to <u>hydrochloric acid</u> and <u>enzyme</u> breakdown. <u>Rennin</u> is only present in young mammals. **Casein protein, which comprises 80% of all milk protein, is therefore not well digested in adults.**

10.1.4 Small intestine
The <u>small intestine</u> extends from the <u>pyloric sphincter</u> to the <u>ileocecal sphincter</u>. It is divided into the <u>duodenum</u>, <u>jejunum</u>, and <u>ileum</u>. Many secretory glands, villi, and folds increase the surface area of the interior walls of the <u>small intestine</u> and make it highly adapted for the efficient digestion of food and absorption of nutrients.

Intestinal and <u>pancreatic enzymes</u> break down:
- <u>Complex carbohydrates</u> (essentially chains of sugar molecules) like <u>starch</u>, into shorter carbohydrate chains then into single sugars such as <u>glucose</u>
- <u>Proteins</u> (long chains of <u>amino acids</u>) into shorter peptides (short chains of <u>amino acids</u>)
- <u>Peptides</u> into individual <u>amino acids</u>
- <u>Triglycerides</u> into <u>fatty acids</u> and <u>monoglycerides</u>
- <u>Nucleotides</u> to <u>pentoses</u> and <u>nitrogenous bases.</u>

Absorption of nutrients in the <u>small intestine</u> involves the movement of digestion products of the <u>gastrointestinal tract</u> into the blood or lymph through the <u>intestinal villi</u>.

10.1.5 Large Intestine
The <u>large intestine</u> extends from the <u>ileocecal sphincter</u> to the <u>anus</u>, and divides into the <u>caecum, colon</u> (ascending, transverse and descending), <u>rectum</u> and <u>anal canal</u>. Water, electrolytes and vitamins can be absorbed into the blood through the walls of the large and small intestines.

10.1.5.1 Bacterial digestion of food

Digestion of food is completed in the <u>large intestine</u> mainly by bacterial action. Some of the bacteria living and feeding from the intestine are beneficial to us and are often referred to as friendly or good bacteria. Other bacteria living and feeding from the intestine are not beneficial to our heath are often referred to as unfriendly or bad bacteria.

10.1.5.2 Friendly or good bacteria in the large intestine

The so-called friendly bacteria are generally <u>aerobic</u> (ie require the presence of <u>oxygen</u> to survive). These bacteria often synthesise certain vitamins and other substances that may be absorbed from the intestines to be beneficial for us. Some authors suggest that bacterially synthesied <u>vitamin B12</u> may also be absorbed from the intestines in this way, possibly explaining why so many vegans over the world do not suffer from <u>vitamin B12</u> deficiency.

10.1.5.3 Unfriendly or bad bacteria in the large intestine

The so-called unfriendly bacteria are predominantly <u>anaerobic</u> (ie they thrive best in the absence of <u>oxygen</u>). These bacteria synthesise many chemicals and gases, which we may absorb and which act as poisons that bind to receptor sites on our body cells. By binding to cellular receptor sites these bacterial poisons block either important enzymatic pathways and processes or block the receptor sites for <u>neurotransmitters</u>, hormones, or <u>immunotransmitters</u>. This can affect our moods and emotional states, our energy levels, and our ability to stay healthy and recover from injury or illness.

10.1.6 Rectum
The <u>rectum</u> consists of the last part of the <u>large intestine</u>. The <u>rectum</u> terminates with the <u>anus</u>. The <u>rectum</u> contains <u>faeces</u>, which consists of water, inorganic salts, epithelial cells, bacteria and undigested foods.

10.1.7 Liver
The <u>liver</u> has left and right lobes with a caudate and quadrate lobe associated with the right lobe. Lobes are made up of <u>liver</u> cells (<u>reticulocytes</u> and <u>reticuloendothelial cells</u>), sinusoids, and a central vein.

10.1.7.1 Functions of the liver

The liver is known to have more than 500 functions, including:
(i)   Carbohydrate metabolism
(ii)   Lipid metabolism
(iii)   Protein metabolism
(iv)   Detoxification of drugs, hormones and chemicals introduced into the body
(v)   Excretion of bilirubin (breakdown product of red blood cells) into bile
(vi)   Synthesis of bile salts
(vii)   Storage of glycogen, vitamins and minerals
(viii) Phagocytosis
(ix)   Activation of vitamin D

10.1.7.2 Production of bile

Hepatocytes (specialised liver cells) produce bile (1 litre per day). Bile consists mostly of water and bile salts, cholesterol, lecithin and bilirubin. Bile is partially an excretion product and partially a digestive secretion. Bile plays an important role in the breakdown of fat. Cholesterol is made soluble by bile salts and lecithin.

10.1.8 Gallbladder

The gallbladder is a sac, located in a fossa on the visceral surface of the liver, which functions to store and concentrate bile. Bile is secreted into the common bile duct via the influence of the enzyme cholycystokinin (CCK).

10.1.9 Pancreas

The pancreas is connected to the duodenum via the pancreatic duct, and the pancreatic accessory duct. The pancreas has two types of cells:

- **Pancreatic islet cells** that secrete hormones such as insulin, which lowers blood glucose by stimulating transport of glucose to cells [Table 11.1]

- **Pancreatic acini cells** that secrete pancreatic juice, which contains enzymes such as:
  o   pancreatic amylase that digests complex carbohydrates like starch
  o   trypsin, chymotrypsin, and carboxypeptidase that digest proteins
  o   pancreatic lipase that digest fats or triglycerides
  o   ribonuclease and deoxyribonuclease that digest nucleic acids [Section 11.3.4] such as deoxyribonucleic acid (DNA) and ribonucleic acid (RNA).

10.2 THE IMMUNE SYSTEM

The immune system, which includes cells of the thymus, lymph nodes, spleen and bone marrow, is one of the most complex systems in the body, second only to the nervous system [Chapter 9]. The immune system uses the lymphatic and circulatory systems as its highways through the body.

The immune system is highly interactive with itself and other systems in the body, which allows it to attack what is foreign and to preserve what is self in normal situations. A healthy diet can support the immune system, as can a reasonable amount of yoga or other exercise. If diet or lifestyle (including exercise and yoga) is inadequate in supporting the immune system, the immune system may fail to recognise self and dangerous autoimmune diseases may arise.

Relatively low levels of stress, as generated with non-aggressive hatha yoga and other exercises, have been shown to help the immune system to function better. Relatively high levels of stress such as those generated by a more aggressive and stimulating hatha yoga practices may actually be detrimental to the immune system.

An appropriate diet that supports the immune system is one that balances with lifestyle, and takes into account the type of exercise and breathing practised. To practise a lot of hatha yoga throughout life, it is necessary to balance with diet to support the type of asana (postures and exercises) and pranayama (breath-control) [Section 10.3]. For example, a person who tends to hyperventilate (breathe more air than they really need) during their practice will tend to crave and require a relatively acidic or high protein diet to balance the alkalinity generated by their breathing. If, however, a person tends to hypoventilate (breathe less air than they feel they would like to) then they will tend to crave and require a relatively alkaline or low protein diet to balance the relative acidity generated by their breathing. There is not really a right or wrong way to breathe, exercise or eat, but what is required more than anything is the **balance between breathing, exercising and eating**.

10.2.1 The Lymphatic System

The lymphatic system functions to return tissue fluid to the vascular (blood) system; and to contribute lymphocytes (immune system cells) and antibodies to the blood, as part of the defence systems of the body.

The lymphatic system is a one-way drainage system from the periphery to the heart that consists of lymphatic vessels, lymphatic organs, lymph nodes and diffuse lymphatic tissue. It functions to drain interstitial fluid, transport dietary fats and protect against invasion by non-specific defences and specific immune responses.

10.2.1.1 Lymphatic vessels

Lymphatic capillaries are blind-ended vessels beginning in the periphery which are larger and more porous than blood capillaries. Some lymphatic vessels are similar in structure to veins but with thinner walls. They have little elastic tissue and not a lot of smooth muscle. There is not much muscular help in propelling fluid along lymph vessels towards the heart, hence the presence of many one-way valves, which look like bumps in the walls of these ducts. Two main lymphatic ducts, the thoracic duct and right lymphatic duct contain appreciable amounts of smooth muscle and drain into the subclavian veins near the heart. Lymph flow is relatively slow and sporadic (approximately 1-2 ml/min). It is aided and regulated by:

(i)   Continuous production of lymph which pushes fluid forward (hydrostatic pressure)
(ii)   Musculoskeletal pump and respiratory pump, which also help to reduce swelling
(iii)   One-way flow valves which prevent back flow
(iv)   Contractions of smooth muscle in right lymphatic and thoracic ducts

10.2.2 Immune system Organs and Cells

10.2.2.1 Lymph nodes

Lymph nodes are small oval structures located along the course of principle lymphatic vessels. Lymph nodes are filled with lymph fluid (lymph) and lymphocytes. Lymph nodes are encapsulated by a connective tissue capsule. They are the sites of proliferation of plasma cells and T cells. The function of lymph nodes is to filter lymph and contribute lymphocytes to it.

Inside lymph nodes, lymphocytes act as macrophages to filter out lymph fluid. Lymph fluid enters each lymph node via a number of afferent (entering) lymphatic vessels. Lymph fluid leaves each lymph node through a larger single efferent (departing) vessel. After leaving a lymph node, the lymph fluid is cleaner but carries more lymphocytes. The lymph fluid eventually goes back into the circulatory system.

10.2.2.2 Tonsils

The tonsils are large aggregations of lymphatic nodules embedded in mucous membranes.

10.2.2.3 Spleen

The spleen is the largest aggregation of lymphatic tissue in the body. It is the site of B cell proliferation into plasma cells, phagocytosis of bacteria and worn out red blood cells, and the storage of blood.

10.2.2.4 Thymus gland

The thymus lies between the sternum (breast bone) and the large blood vessels above the heart. It is the site of T cell maturation.

10.2.3 Natural and Acquired Immunity

10.2.3.1 Non-specific resistance to disease

Resistance is the ability to ward off disease. Susceptibility is the lack of resistance.

Non-specific resistance refers to a wide range of body responses against a wide range of pathogens. Non-specific resistance includes:

- **Mechanical factors** [Section 10.2.3.1.1]
- **Chemical factors** [Section 10.2.3.1.2]
- **Antimicrobial substances** [Section 10.2.3.1.3]
- **Natural killer cells** [Section 10.2.3.1.4]
- **Phagocytosis** [Section 10.2.3.1.5]
- **Inflammation** [Section 10.2.3.1.6]
- **Fever** [Section 10.2.3.1.7]

10.2.3.1.1 Mechanical resistance to disease: skin and mucous membranes

Mechanical resistance to disease includes the protective effects of skin, mucous membranes (mucosa), nasal hairs and vomiting. When a host encounters a bacterial antigen (a non-self particle), viral antigen, or chemical antigen, the first line of defence is the skin and the mucous membranes.

Body openings such as the gastroinstestinal (GI) tract, genitourinary (GU) tract and respiratory tract are protected from antigenic attack by the mucosa which secretes powerful protein-digesting enzymes and antibodies which can immobilise and/or destroy invading antigens.

10.2.3.1.2 Chemical resistance to disease

Chemical resistance to disease includes the protective effects of stomach acid destroying dangerous organic and inorganic material when swallowed. Both mechanical and chemical barriers block the initial attempts of microbes and foreign substances to penetrate the body and cause disease.

10.2.3.1.3 Antimicrobial resistance to disease: skin and mucous membranes

Antimicrobial substances such as interferon and the complement system provide a second line of defence should microbes penetrate the skin and mucous membranes.

Interferons are produced by body cells that have been infected by viruses. They induce uninfected cells to synthesise antiviral proteins that inhibit intracellular viral replication in uninfected cells.

The **complement system** constitutes a group of at least 20 normally inactive proteins found in serum that forms a component of non-specific resistance and immunity by bringing about microbial cytolysis (cell membrane disruption), opsonisation (coating of the microbe to promote phagocytosis), and inflammation.

10.2.3.1.4 Natural killer (NK) cell resistance to disease

Natural killer (NK) cells are a population of lymphocytes that have the ability to destroy a large variety of infectious microbes plus certain spontaneously arising tumours. Their mode of action is unclear yet, but it is known that they also secrete interferon.

10.2.3.1.5 Phagocytosis

Phagocytosis is a process in which cells called phagocytes ingest particulate matter, especially the ingestion and destruction of microbes, cell debris, and other foreign matter. There are two main types of phagocytes: neutrophils and macrophages.

Neutrophils are short lived and make up 60% of white blood cells. They can squeeze through capillary walls to patrol tissue and are released in large numbers during infection.

Macrophages live longer than neutrophils and travel in blood as monocytes. They are found in organs such as lungs, liver, kidney, spleen and lymph nodes and cut up pathogens to display antigens which trigger an immune response.

10.2.3.1.6 Inflammation

Inflammation is a localised, protective response to tissue injury designed to destroy, dilute, or wall off the infecting agent or injured tissue. It is characterised by:

(i) **Redness**
(ii) **Pain** (generally acute pain)
(iii) **Heat**
(iv) **Swelling**
(v) **Loss of function** (not always)

Since inflammation is one of the body's non-specific internal defence systems, the inflammatory response of a tissue to a cut is the same as the response to a burn, radiation, or bacterial or viral invasion. Three basic stages in inflammation are:

      (i)   Vasodilation and increased permeability of blood vessels
      (ii)   Phagocyte migration
      (iii)   Repair.

Vasodilation is an increase in the diameter of blood vessels, which allows more blood to flow through the damaged area. Increased permeability permits defensive mediators in the blood, such as antibodies, phagocytes and clotting factors, to enter the injured area.

Phagocytes appear on the scene within an hour after the inflammatory process begins. Neutrophils arrive first then monocytes arrive a few hours later and transform into wandering macrophages that augment the phagocytic activity of fixed macrophages.

10.2.3.1.7 Fever

Fever intensifies the effects of interferons, inhibits the growth of some microbes, and speeds up many body reactions which aid repair.

10.2.3.2 Specific resistance to disease: Immunity

Specific resistance involves the production of a specific lymphocyte or antibody against a specific antigen. This is called immunity. Antigens are chemical substances that, when introduced into the body, are recognised as foreign by antigen receptors. Antibodies are proteins that combine specifically with the antigens that triggered their production.

10.2.3.2.1 Types of immune response

10.2.3.2.1.1 Cell-mediated immunity (CMI)

Cell-mediated immunity (CMI) refers to the destruction of antigens by T cells (which are derived from stem cells in bone marrow, but which mature in the thymus gland). In CMI response, an antigen is recognised, specific T cells proliferate and differentiate into effector cells, and the antigen is eliminated.

10.2.3.2.1.2 Antibody-mediated (humeral) immunity (AMI)

AMI refers to the destruction of antigens by antibodies. Antibodies are synthesised by transformed B cells called plasma cells, which are derived from stem cells in bone marrow.

10.2.3.2.2 Immunological memory

Immunisation against certain microbes is possible because memory B cells and memory T cells remain after the primary response to an antigen. The secondary response provides protection should the microbe enter the body again.

Cancer cells may display tumour-specific antigens and are often destroyed by the body's immune system (immunological surveillance) [Section 10.2.3.2.3].

With advancing age, the immune system tends to function less effectively. A person's diet also has a significant impact on the health and functioning of the immune system.

10.2.3.2.3 Human Leucocyte Antigen (HLA) system

The human immune system has a number of alternative mechanisms that allow the body to determine self from non-self so that foreign proteins from bacteria, viruses, etc. can be recognised, destroyed, and eliminated. The Human Leucocyte Antigen (HLA) system is probably the most complex of these mechanisms. This system, which was first discovered when it was found that tissue from one human could not be grafted to another without rejection, functions to initiate an immune response against parasites, bacteria and viruses [Lunven, 1999].

All body cells manufacture HLA proteins, whose function is to bind short peptides (protein fragments) and display them on the cell surface. Most of the peptides are derived from the body's own proteins (self-peptides). However, when a virus or bacteria infect the body, the HLA molecules pick up peptides derived from broken-down proteins of the virus or bacteria and present them to T-lymphocytes. The purpose of T-lymphocytes is to continually scan the surfaces of other cells to recognise foreign peptides while ignoring self-peptides [Lunven, 1999].

Initially a T-cell receptor recognises a foreign peptide. Then, a complex series of steps is executed which ultimately destroys the cell presenting the foreign peptide. Then the living viruses or bacteria in the body which also have peptide sequences similar to those which were presented will also be recognised and destroyed. When the HLA system loses the ability to recognise self (self-peptides) from non-self (foreign peptides), the T-lymphocytes attack the body's own tissue, resulting in what is known as an autoimmune disease (eg, coeliac disease, insulin dependant diabetes melitis (IDDM), multiple sclerosis, dermatitis herpetiformis, ankylosing spondylitis, etc.) [Section 10.2.4.2] [Lunven, 1999].

10.2.4 Immunosuppressive Diseases

10.2.4.1 Acquired immune deficiency syndrome (AIDS)

Acquired immune deficiency syndrome (AIDS) is supposedly caused by the human immunodeficiency virus (HIV), which is speculated to slowly destroy the T4 lymphocyte population [Section 10.2.3.2.3] and render the victim susceptible to a range of other opportunistic diseases.

10.2.4.2 Autoimmune diseases

Autoimmune diseases are thought to occur when self-tolerance breaks down. The immune system fails to recognise self-antigens and attacks them. Diseases that are believed to have an autoimmune cause include rheumatoid arthritis (RA) [Section 1.5.4.1], systemic lupus erythematous (SLE) and multiple sclerosis (MS) [Section 10.2.3.2.3].

10.3 NUTRITION & DIET FOR PRACTITIONERS OF *HATHA YOGA*

Diet and *hatha yoga* are integrally related. While it is not necessary to improve diet to practise *hatha yoga* and receive benefits from it, a healthy diet may make the practice of *hatha yoga* much easier. Similarly, the properly applied techniques of *hatha yoga* may benefit a person with a weak digestive or immune system, and may allow a person with a poor diet to digest and absorb food better and to some extent compensate for the poorness of their diet. However, the best results in terms of health, flexibility, strength and the ability to reach focused mental states with *hatha yoga* may be achieved when both diet and *hatha yoga* are managed together. The serious aspirant of *hatha yoga* must address his or her diet if they wish to really make progress with their practice. A special internal physiology is needed in order to achieve the necessary strength, flexibility, and movement of *prana* (vital energy) through the *nadis* (subtle channels) and circulatory systems in order to allow the efficient transport of information and energy through the body. A slightly more alkaline internal pH than is considered normal (mild metabolic alkalosis) should be developed and fostered through modification of diet, lifestyle and thought, which allows the prolonged breath retentions (hypoventilation) required for nearly all advanced *hatha yoga* practices.

A gradual change towards the classical *hatha yoga diet* (a low protein vegetarian diet with an emphasis on alkalising fresh fruit, salads, sprouted grains, and steamed vegetables) in combination with an appropriate *pranayama* (breath-control) practice may help to:
i.   Improve the flexibility of the joints, muscles, skin, and other tissues
ii.   Improve the strength of the bones and muscles
iii.   Improve the circulation
iv.   Improve the breathing (in particular the ability to retain the breath)
v.   Improve the generation and transport of energy in the body
vi.   Stabilise the nervous system
vii.   Improve the functioning of the immune system.

In short, a gradual change towards the classical *hatha yoga diet* may improve the ability to practise *hatha yoga*. *Hatha yoga asanas* (static postures), *vinyasas* (dynamic exercises) and *pranayamas* (breathing exercises) can affect the digestion of food and the absorption and metabolism of nutrients in several ways. *Hatha yoga* techniques can help to:
i.   Improve the digestion of food
ii.   Improve the absorption of nutrients
iii.   Improve the elimination of wastes
iv.   Increase the mobilisation of fat
v.   Minimise the need for food
vi.   Increase or decrease appetite according to need
vii.   Improve diet
viii.   Improve the functioning of the immune system.

Hatha yoga can affect the digestive system and immune system as well as metabolic physiology in several ways. *Hatha yoga asanas* and *pranayamas* and their associated *ha-bandhas* (compressive internal locks) and *tha-bandhas* (expansive internal locks) [Section 1.7.3.4] can be used to stimulate the digestive system by mechanically massaging the gastrointestinal (GI) tract with physical compression and expansion of the lower trunk and spine. *Hatha yoga asanas* can massage the GI tract with forward bending and backward bending postures, twisting postures, side-bending postures, and also through the reversal of the flow of gravity in the inverted or semi-inverted postures (*viparita karani*). *Hatha yoga asanas, vinyasas,* and their associated *ha-* and *tha-bandhas* can also affect the absorption of nutrients by cells over the entire body by stimulating circulation.

Hatha yoga asanas, pranayamas and their associated *mudras* (gestures) can be used to stimulate the nervous system regulators of the digestive system, immune system and endocrine system. The activity of the digestive system can be enhanced by stimulation of the parasympathetic nervous system (PNS) [Section 10.1.1] using *pranayama.* This can be done by either prolonging exhalation [Section 8.4.4], or by using left nostril breathing as in *candra sodhana pranayama* [Section 9.7.5]. Also, the nerves of the PNS may be stimulated by the *mudras* (gestures) of *nadi hatha yoga* [Section 1.7.2] which may tension (stretch) nerves such as the vagus nerve which is an important regulator of the PNS [Section 9.7.3].

Hatha yoga pranayamas can significantly alter the pH (acid-alkaline levels) of the blood and thereby influence many of the body's metabolic pathways. The rate and depth of breathing can also significantly affect things such as joint flexibility, and intra-cranial blood pressure.

IMPORTANT NOTE ON POTENTIAL CHANGES IN DIET: **Strict adherence to the classical *hatha* yoga diet (a low protein vegetarian diet with an emphasis on alkalising fresh fruit, salads, sprouted grains, and steamed vegetables) is only safe and sustainable for extended periods if the following requirements are met:**

1. **The transition from a more regular diet to the classical *hatha* yoga diet must be a slow process of adaptation where both the body's physiology and the mind gradually learn to adjust.**
2. ***Pranayama* (breath-control) practised on its own or with *asana* (static postures) and *vinyasas* (dynamic exercises) must ideally reduce minute ventilation (the amount of air breathed in per minute). This will increase the amount of carbon dioxide retained in the body and hence increase the amounts of carbonic acid in the blood in order to counter the alkalising effects of the classical *hatha* yoga diet.**

The main danger with alkalosis (excess of alkali in the body) is that the nervous system becomes hypersensitive. Hyperventilation leads to temporary alkalosis, which can cause or contribute to asthma, dizziness, fainting, headaches, unsteadiness, paraesthesia, skin rashes, excessive appetite, nervous sensitivity and emotional instability [Section 12.7.1.2.1.2]. Similarly, it is relatively common that people who switch to a fruitarian diet develop allergies and become emotionaly ungrounded. Such extreme diet is only safely sustainable with very slow adaptation; and it should be supported by a sound theoretical and practical understanding of internal physiology and *pranayama*, allowing easy retention of the breath using only a relatively low amount of air per minute. It should only be attempted with the guidance of a very experienced teacher.

10.3.1 Main Types of Nutrients in Food

The main food types the body deals with are
1. Carbohydrates (including simple sugars and starches)
2. Proteins (including simple amino acids, structural proteins, and enzymes)
3. Fats (including simple fats, compound fats, and derived fats like cholesterol).

These nutrients are present in most foods in various amounts. However, if one group is dominant in the food, the food is labelled as that type. For example, rice contains significant amounts of both carbohydrate and protein, but it contains relatively more carbohydrate. Therefore, rice is labelled a carbohydrate food and hence some people believe that it does not contain protein. Even a simple fruit such as an orange, which is mainly thought of as containing carbohydrate only (fruit sugar), also has at least 14 proteins.

10.3.1.1 Carbohydrates

Carbohydrates are composed of carbon (C), oxygen (O), and hydrogen (H), or as the name suggests, carbohydrates are composed of carbon and water (H_2O). Carbohydrates have the general formula $C_6H_{12}O_6$.

10.3.1.1.1 Simple carbohydrates

Simple carbohydrates are sugars. The simplest sugars consist of only one unit and include glucose and fructose. Glucose is the body's primary energy fuel, and therefore the concentration of glucose in blood needs to be regulated. Glucose is absorbed directly into the blood from the digestive system. The presence of excess glucose in the blood triggers the release of the hormone insulin from the pancreas, which causes an uptake of glucose into the cells. A rapid increase in blood glucose concentration is often followed by an insulin-induced removal of excess glucose from the blood known as hypoglycaemia, which feels like a light-headed weakness. Hypoglycaemia gives you a craving for more sweet food, which is one reason why sweet desserts are such a popular follow-up to most conventional meals. Fructose, on the other hand, as the main sugar in fruit is unable to be used immediately in the blood. This sugar must be first processed by the liver, which converts it via the enzyme fructose 1-phosphate into a precursor of glucose that cells can then use.

10.3.1.1.2 Complex carbohydrates

Complex carbohydrates like starch consist of long chains of simple sugars such as glucose. Complex carbohydrates are present in starch-containing foods such as rice, wheat and other grains, and starchy vegetables such as potatoes. The main digestion of starch takes place in the mouth with a salivary gland amylase enzyme called ptyalin, an acid-sensitive enzyme. People with weak digestion should not mix complex carbohydrates with acidic tasting foods, as this will deactivate the ptyalin. Mixing complex carbohydrates with protein foods may lead to poor digestion because the protein will stimulate the production of stomach hydrochloric acid, which will deactivate the ptyalin and inhibit the digestion of the complex carbohydrates. It is also the reason why chewing is so important, as most of the digestion of complex carbohydrates should take place in the mouth. With adequate chewing (60 to 70 chews per mouthful), foods like bread and rice will taste sweet (which for most people, never happens!).

10.3.1.2 Proteins

Proteins consist of long chains of amino acids. The body must breakdown the proteins to their subunit amino acid parts so that they can be used by body cells.

10.3.1.2.1 Amino acids

Amino acids can be synthesised within the body from simple precursors such as glucose. Some amino acids are not usually made by the human body, but may be supplied by some of the bacteria living within the human digestive tract. Amino acids not usually made by the human body are referred to as essential amino acids.

For nearly everyone, a small amount of essential amino acids needs to be obtained from the diet to maintain normal health. In a healthy body, free of accumulated waste and toxins, the required amounts of all the essential amino acids which the body can not synthesise by itself can be supplied by an adequate amount and variety of herbs, sprouted grains, vegetables and fruits. The provisos are that:

- The body has to adapt slowly to such a diet or it will react adversely on many levels
- The body must be already free of accumulated waste and toxins
- No new toxic substances are being put into the body or being generated inside the body.

10.3.1.3 Fats

Fats (more correctly termed lipids) include fats which are solid at room temperature, and oils which are liquid at room temperature. Fats contain the same structural elements as carbohydrates except the atoms are linked in significantly different ways. Fats are the major source of stored energy for the body, they cushion and protect the major organs and they act as an insulator, preserving body heat. Fats can be classified into three groups: (i) simple fats; (ii) compound fats; (iii) derived fats.

Simple fats consist primarily of triglycerides. Triglycerides consist of a glycerol molecule with three fatty acid chains attached to it. Triglycerides account for more than 95% of all fat in the body. Fatty acids are chains of carbon which give fats their unique flavor and texture. They differ by the number of carbon atoms (short chain, medium chain or long chain fatty acids) and the bonding of carbons and arrangement of hydrogens along carbon chain (saturated, monounsaturated or polyunsaturated fatty acids).

Fatty acids serve a number of important functions. Fatty acids are:

- used as components of cells and membranes, eg certain long-chain fatty acids
- digested to provide energy (calories), eg particularly short-chain fatty acids
- digested to provide essential fatty acids, eg linoleic acid and alpha-linolenic acid.

Compound fats are formed from simple fats combined with additional chemicals. The most important compound fats are lipoproteins, which are molecules composed of protein, triglycerides and cholesterol.

Derived fats are made up of simple fats and compound fats but they dont contain fatty acids. The best example of this kind of fat is cholesterol, which is present only in foods from animal sources.

All fats (lipids) have high caloric density, yielding 9 kilocalories per gram, regardless of length of carbon chain and saturation. This is more than twice that of carbohydrates and protein, which yield only 4 kilocalories per gram.

Relatively small amounts of fat are needed for a healthy person to maintain good health. The biggest danger lies in eating fat that has been cooked or heated. Many studies from as early as the 1950s have clearly linked eating heated fat (including heated essential fatty acids and cholesterol) as a high risk factor for cancer. Therefore, never cook in oil, and avoid all heated oils.

10.3.1.3.1 Fat that is good to eat

Probably the best vegetarian low protein sources of fat that do not have to be processed are avocado and coconut. There is ample good fat in avocado and it makes an excellent replacement for oils with vegetables and salads, and a replacement for butter on bread (if bread is still eaten). Coconut fat is also good but it is best fresh. All grains have essential fats that are usually altered or damaged if the grains are cooked, but which are made easily available when the grains are sprouted. Many herbs and vegetables also contain significant percentages of fat. Even lettuce has 9% of its entire solid portion as fat, including essential fatty acids such as linoleic acid [Section 10.3.1.3.2].

The dangers of eating fat in the form of oil are that oils require processing, and stored oils tend to go rancid. Processing oil or any food may change or damage a food and make it poisonous. In addition, the processing usually involves toxic chemicals, traces of which may be found in the final product. However, probably the best oils to use, if you use them, are organic extra virgin cold pressed olive oil and coconut oil.

10.3.1.3.2 Essential fatty acids

Essential fatty acids cannot be synthesised by the body and need to be obtained from the diet. They can be converted to compounds that are very important in the central nervous system, and elsewhere in the body. There are two types of essential fatty acids: omega-3 and omega-6. In food, alpha-linolenic acid is the major omega-3 fatty acid, and linoleic acid is the major omega-6 fatty acid [Ogilvie, 2001].

Comparison of Dietary Fats [adapted from Ogilvie, 2001]
- Table shows proportions (%) of <u>fatty acids</u> (saturated, polyunsaturated and monounsaturated) making up total fat composition of various fats and oils.
- The oils/fats have been listed in order of increasing saturated fat content.

NAME OF FAT/OIL	SATURATED	POLYUNSATURATED		MONOUNSATURATED
		Linoleic Acid (Omega 6)	Alpha-Linolenic Acid (Omega 3)	
Canola Oil	7	22	10	61
Hempseed	8	55	25	12
Flaxseed Oil	10	17	55	18
Safflower Oil	10	76	trace	14
Sunflower Oil	12	71	1	16
Corn Oil	13	57	1	29
Olive Oil	15	9	1	75
Soybean Oil	15	54	8	23
Peanut Oil	19	33	trace	48
Cottonseed Oil	27	54	trace	19
Lard	43	9	1	47
Beef Tallow	48	2	1	49
Palm Oil	51	10	trace	39
Butterfat	68	3	1	28
Coconut Oil	91	2	0	7

10.3.1.3.3 Trans fatty acids

<u>Trans fatty acids</u> are <u>unsaturated fatty acids</u> that contain at least one double bond in the trans configuration. <u>Trans fatty acids</u> are high in margarines and hydrogenated oils but are present in many of the processed foods the average Australian or American eats. These fats are known to interfere with <u>omega-3 fatty acid</u> absorption and are now beginning to be recognised as perhaps the most disease-promoting of any of the fats. A report from the US National Academy of Sciences found that <u>trans fatty acids</u> promotes heart disease and have concluded that the only safe intake of <u>trans fatty acids</u> is zero.

Anything that is fried, even vegetables, has <u>trans fatty acids</u> and the potent cancer-causing substance <u>acrylamide</u>. <u>Acrylamide</u>, a white, odourless, but potentially carcinogenic (cancer-causing), chemical, has been found in many common foods such as potato chips, French fries, bread, rice and cereals. <u>Acrylamide</u> has also been shown to cause cancer and neurotoxic effects in animal studies and damage to the <u>nervous system</u> in humans who were exposed to the chemical at work.

10.3.1.3.4 Derived fats: cholesterol

The most well known derived fat is <u>cholesterol</u>, which is a sterol (steroid alcohol) derived from <u>simple </u>fats and <u>compound </u>fats. <u>Cholesterol</u> contains no <u>fatty acids</u>, but still exhibits some of the characteristics of fat. <u>Cholesterol</u> is only synthesised in animals. It is present in all animal cells and is either consumed in foods (exogenous <u>cholesterol</u>) or synthesised within the animal (human) cells.

<u>Cholesterol</u> is used in the building of <u>cell membranes</u>, the synthesis of <u>vitamin D</u>, the <u>nervous system</u>, the synthesis of hormones, and for the formation of the bile <u>secretions</u> that emulsify fat during digestion.

<u>Cholesterol</u> is packaged in a soluble coating, which allows it to be easily and safely transported through the body. The soluble coating is disrupted with cooking which renders the <u>cholesterol</u> a danger to the body.

The richest source of <u>cholesterol</u> in foods is in egg yolks. <u>Cholesterol</u> is also present in significant quantities in all meat, especially red meats and organ meats, shellfish, and dairy products. There is no <u>cholesterol</u> in any foods of plant origin. Some vegetable oils, like coconut and palm oil, are high in <u>saturated fat</u>, which can raise blood cholesterol, but these oils still do not contain any dietary <u>cholesterol</u>.

10.3.2 Problems Resulting from Ingesting an Excess of the Main Food Types

Probably the biggest problem of most Western diets is excess. People generally eat too much food. Some foods are definitely healthier than others, and certain excesses have their own specific dangers as described below, but it has been repeatedly shown in experiments on mice and other animals for decades that lifespan is prolonged by reduced calorific intake of all foods.

10.3.2.1 Carbohydrates: Problems resulting from eating excess carbohydrates

10.3.2.1.1 Problems with excess sugar

The main fruit sugar, fructose, goes to the liver and is converted to glucose before it can be used by the cells. This is in contrast to many other simple sugars, such as glucose itself, which go directly to the blood, resulting in an imbalance in the blood insulin levels which can lead to hypoglycaemia and diabetes. *Excess sugar is either converted to fat or is digested by bacteria in the digestive tract*.

10.3.2.1.2 Problems with excess complex carbohydrates

Excess complex carbohydrates are fermented or become mechanical blocking agents. Most sources of complex carbohydrates such as grains also contain high levels of phytates, which are chemical agents that inhibit digestive enzymes. Phytates are not destroyed in the cooking process. *Excess carbohydrate is either converted to fat or is digested by bacteria in the digestive tract*.

10.3.2.2 Proteins: Problems resulting from eating excess protein

10.3.2.2.1 Problems with excess amino acids

If there are excess free amino acids in the body, they are de-aminated and converted to simpler molecules such as sugars and uric acid. Excess uric acid is the main cause of gout, and contributes to all other diseases of acid-alkali imbalance eg osteoporosis and dental caries.

10.3.2.2.2 Problems with eating excess complex protein

If protein is mal-combined or taken in excess, it may be left only partially digested. The partially digested food particles may be small enough to enter the bloodstream but too large to enter cells or be eliminated by the kidneys. Such partial digestion-products of proteins may act as mechanical blocking agents of various body systems including the skin (leading to pimples, acne, boils, skin rashes, etc). *Excess protein is either converted to fat or is digested by bacteria in the digestive tract.*

10.3.2.2.3 Problems with high protein diets

The recommended daily allowance of protein each day is 30-90 grams per day. The average Australian or American eats up to 150–300 grams per day. Most of the high protein food ingested in the West is some form of meat. Most Western people's diets have far too much protein for adult bodies. There are two main problems with excess protein. These are:

- Excess dietary protein leads to an increased level of acid in the body which can leach calcium from the bones and teeth [Section 10.3.4] and lead to such problems as osteoporosis, arthritis, dental caries, gout, kidney stones, arteriosclerosis etc.

- Excess protein is either converted to sugar and fat or is fermented (putrefied by internal anaerobic bacteria). Much of the smell that comes out of people when they exercise is due to the improper decomposition of excess protein by internal anaerobic bacteria.

10.3.2.3 Fats: Problems resulting from eating excess fat

10.3.2.3.1 Problems with eating excess simple fats

Fat is usually always eaten in excess. Fat inhibits gastric secretions, and therefore inhibits the digestion of proteins. Fat increases endogenous cholesterol synthesis. An increase in blood fat levels is a well-established risk indicator for coronary heart disease. Fat increases ketone levels, which causes liver damage.

10.3.2.3.2 Problems with eating excess cholesterol

When cooked the soluble coating of cholesterol is destroyed and it then deposits on the walls of blood vessels (atherosclerosis). Cholesterol has a negative effect on the immune system by paralysing macrophages.

Cooking cholesterol is exceptionally deleterious to health. This is shown by research revealing that in animal models, oxidised fats, oils and cholesterol induce higher levels of arterial plaque than do the corresponding non-oxidised fats, oils and cholesterol. In addition, in tests where high-cholesterol diets were given to rabbits, the consumption of scrambled or baked eggs produced increases in serum cholesterol of 6-7 times the pre-existing levels, while fried or hard-boiled eggs raised levels by 10-14 times [Tu, 1999].

10.3.2.3.3 Problems with eating excess polyunsaturated fat

Avoid margarine and all polyunsaturated fats. Polyunsaturated fat (eg in margarine) was for some time said to be good for you because it was seen to lead to a decrease in blood cholesterol. However, it was found that the level of cholesterol in the blood decreased only because polyunsaturated fat causes cholesterol to be taken up by the blood vessel walls, and leads to a hardening of the arterial walls (atherosclerosis).

Polyunsaturated fat has been shown to increase the cholesterol in the liver, which leads to gall stones. Polyunsaturated fat has also been shown to decrease the bacterial synthesis of B vitamins, increase the body's requirement for vitamin E and decrease the body's ability to absorb calcium.

10.3.2.3.4 Lipotoxaemia: excess fat in the bloodstream

When the blood becomes saturated with fat, a condition referred to as lipotoxemia results. Fat can retard the cells of the immune system and increase the body's requirement for certain vitamins. Lipotoxaemia is linked with various types of cancer and potentially leads to atherosclerosis (a hardening of the arteries), which is the precursor of heart attacks, strokes, and deep vein thrombosis.

10.3.3 Problems Arising from Traditional Diets

Although traditional diets allow people to live long enough to bring up children, most people never die of old age as such. Death that is not by accident is usually linked to lifestyle and very commonly linked with the conventional diet. The main problems associated with most conventional diets are outlined below [Section 10.3.3.1]. Problems related to specific foods are also discussed [Section 10.3.3.2].

10.3.3.1 Main problems with conventional eating

What most people eat today has become so much part of our culture that it is very hard for even the nutritionist to really say whether something is good or bad for a person. Most of the eating done in the developed world is centred around social interaction. Whereas in the rest of the world the diet is dependant on the availability of the food in a particular area.

In addition, there are many variables that can change the way a particular food or diet will affect the body. Food may be poorly digested for a number of reasons [Section 10.3.3.1.1]. Partially digested food may enter the blood stream and affect the immune system [Sections 10.3.3.1.2 & 10.3.6]. Food residues may act as a mechanical obstruction to the absorption of nutrients and the elimination of wastes [Section 10.3.3.1.3]. Carbohydrates may be fermented [Section 10.3.3.1.4]. Proteins may be putrefied by intestinal bacteria [Section 10.3.3.1.5]. Cooked food often undergoes chemical changes [Section 10.3.3.1.6]. Processed foods have been altered significantly and have many dangerous additives [Section 10.3.3.1.7]. Most medicines and pharmaceuticals, and many health foods, including vitamin and mineral supplements may be hazardous to health [Section 10.3.3.1.8]. Most non-organic and some organic vegetables and fruits are laden with dangerous pesticide residues, and have been altered by irradiation and/or genetic manipulation [Section 10.3.3.1.9]. Social commitments and advertising propaganda encourage us to eat unhealthy foods [Section 10.3.3.1.10].

10.3.3.1.1 Poor digestion of food due to physiological or emotional reasons

Unless food is fully digested, it cannot be utilised by the cells of the body. Complete digestion of complex carbohydrates like starch, which are essentially chains of simple sugars, involves the breakdown of complex carbohydrates into single sugar molecules. Complete digestion of protein is the breakdown of long chains of amino acids (proteins) into single amino acids. Only single amino acids and single simple sugars can be absorbed and utilised by the body's cells. Food can often remain undigested or be only partially digested for several reasons:

• Poor food combining
• Eating too quickly or overeating
• Excess dilution of digestive enzymes with liquids consumed close to or at the time of eating
• Eating while emotionally unstable or when the sympathetic nervous system is overactive and the parasympathetic nervous system is underactive
• Poor digestive enzyme activity

10.3.3.1.2 Partially digested food may enter the blood stream and disturb the immune system

The cells of the body cannot use partially digested food that has entered the blood stream [Section 10.3.3.1.2]. Therefore, partially digested food has to be removed by the immune system or be filtered out by the kidneys. If these conventional routes of elimination are not available or are already overloaded, then partially digested food that has entered the bloodstream may evoke an allergic reaction, or an autoimmune reaction of some sort [Sections 10.2.3.2.3 & 10.3.3.2.1]. Partially digested food may also be excreted through the skin as some sort of pimple or boil etc. Partially digested food stuffs such as short chains of sugars, amino acids or fats may result from the incomplete digestion of complex carbohydrates, proteins or fats respectively.

10.3.3.1.3 Adhesive properties of certain foods lead to production of an impermeable plastic- concrete lining in the intestines

Most adults who have been examined have a thick layer on the inside of their intestines, which is the result of years of glue-like foods such as bread and milk. Flour (starch) and water make very good glue and is a common element in most human diets. Similarly, casein, the major protein in milk, which is not well digested in adults due to the lack of rennin [Section 10.3.3.2], is sold commercially as glue.

The combination of these and other glue-like substances that we either eat or are produced by the bacteria inside us lead to a thick impermeable layer on the inside of the intestines. This layer, which lines most people's intestines, resembles tough semi-elastic, plastic-concrete pipeline.

The plastic-concrete lining of our intestines inhibits the absorption of nutrients into the blood, inhibits the elimination of wastes from the blood to the intestines and inhibits or completely prevents peristalsis (the natural movement of food along the gut). The intestinal lumen becomes very narrow in some parts due to the blockage created by this plastic-concrete lining, and much distended with diverticula in other parts.

The removal of this so-called plastic-concrete pipeline lining the intestine may be achieved through

a combination of a cleansing diet, modified fasting, and *yogic* exercises, including *viparita karani*

[Section 12.7.1.3.3.2], *pranayama* 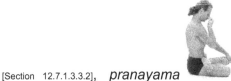 [Sections 8.4.1.3 & 9.7.5.1], *bandhas* [Section 1.7.3, Appendix C],

mudras 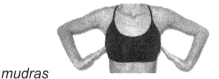 [Section 9.7.3], and in particular *kriyas* (*yogic* cleansing processes),

such as *nauli* 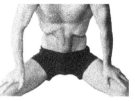 [Section 12.7.1.3.2] and *lauliki* [Sections 10.3.10.3 & 12.7.1.3.2].

When eliminated from the body, this plastic-concrete pipeline can be palpated with gloves and indeed is very tough yet semi-elastic like plastic concrete. It may be up to a metre long with the same shape as the intestines it lined. Bernard Jenson has taken graphic photographs of this type of plastic-concrete-pipeline-effect that can be seen in his excellent book, *Tissue Cleansing Through Bowel Management* [Jenson, 1981].

10.3.3.1.4 Bacterial fermentation of carbohydrates can create unpleasant effects in the body

When carbohydrates are passed through the digestive system too quickly or mal-digested due to overeating, incorrect food combining or ill health, the microorganisms that inhabit the intestines degrade undigested carbohydrates into gases (usually carbon dioxide) and alcohols (usually ethanol). This can lead to cramping, bloating, flatus and social problems! [Section 10.3.5.1]

10.3.3.1.5 Bacterial fermentation of proteins (putrefaction) can produce dangerous chemicals in the body
[Section 10.3.5.2]

Putrefaction refers to the decomposition of proteins by anaerobic organisms [Wimmera, 1979]. When proteins are pushed through the digestive system too quickly or mal-digested due to overeating, incorrect food combining or ill health, the microorganisms which inhabit the intestines degrade undigested food into potent gases, eg hydrogen sulphide (rotten egg gas) and poisonous chemicals, eg putrescine and cadaverine.

10.3.3.1.6 Cooking food may significantly alter its chemical structure

A well-known problem with cooking food is the destruction of vitamins and accessible minerals. A less known, but more significant, problem of cooking food is that of denaturation (inactivation/destruction) of nearly all the enzymes that occur naturally in fresh foods which can assist in the digestion of those foods.

Another problem is that when food is heated or cooked, the chemical structures can be altered due to a series of reactions, known as Maillard reactions, taking place between proteins and carbohydrates. Maillard reactions occur during storage at room temperature, as well as during cooking. These reactions accelerate as temperature increases. This is possible in virtually all foods as nearly all foods contain both proteins and carbohydrates.

Cooked meat contains less Maillard molecules than foods high in protein and carbohydrate, such as milk that has been heated under the same conditions. However, Maillard molecules are the precursor of carcinogenic (cancer causing) compounds called heterocyclic amines found in high-temperature grilled meat and fish. Mutagens in meat are usually produced in the crust during frying, broiling, and baking. Another important source of Maillard molecules is meat extracts, consumed as gravies and meat bouillons. Mutagenicity increases with temperature and with cooking time [Tu, 1999].

Cooking can also increase levels of the carcinogen acrylamide in foods. Acrylamide [Section 10.3.1.3.2] has been found particularly in high carbohydrate foods cooked at high temperatures. This includes processed bread, other grain products and potatoes.

10.3.3.1.7 Processed foods have been altered significantly and have many dangerous additives

Almost all processed foods have some sort of additive, in the form of flavouring, colouring, and preservatives. In some countries, like Australia, what has been added is noted on the packet. However, many of the chemical agents used to process the foods remain in trace amounts in the final product. Legally, if a substance is present in less than a certain amount, it does not have to be included on the label. There is good evidence available that clearly demonstrates that many common food additives including NutraSweet (aspartame), monosodium glutamate (MSG), and hydrolysed vegetable protein (HVP) have potent mutagenic (mutation causing) and carcinogenic (cancer causing) properties, and may significantly affect emotional state, mental state and well being. The safety of many commonly used food additives has never really been checked [Clark, 1999; Hollingsworth, 2000].

10.3.3.1.8 Most medicines, pharmaceuticals, and many so-called health foods, including vitamin and mineral supplements may be hazardous to health

Most medicines and pharmaceuticals, and many so-called health foods, are significantly processed and therefore have many dangerous additives and chemicals that are not even listed in the ingredients. There are generally enough vitamins and minerals in fresh food. Organic foods are by far more preferable and should be eaten wherever possible. Supplements may help in some cases but often just add to the working load on the body's eliminative organs. In addition, many but not all vitamin and mineral supplements may not be absorbed as they come from sources that the body is unable to process. Also, many, but not all, supplements contain trace amounts of dangerous chemical residues because of the process of manufacturing. The best food supplements are those that are made by you, such as fresh-pressed wheat grass juice.

10.3.3.1.9 Most non-organic and some organic vegetables and fruits are laden with dangerous pesticide residues, and have been altered by irradiation and/or genetic manipulation

Pesticide residues are present in significant quantities in all non-organic foods. These chemicals are known to have mutagenic (mutation causing) and carcinogenic (cancer causing) properties and should be avoided where possible [Clark, 1999]. The pesticides chlordane and heptachlor cause cancer, harm the immune system and are endocrine system disruptors [Cohen, 2001].

Food irradiation is increasingly prevalent. Avoid irradiated foods wherever possible as they contain radiolytic products that include formaldehyde and benzene which are known carcinogens [Hollingsworth, 2000]. Genetic manipulation of food is a relatively recent innovation so the dangers are not yet so evident. Possible dangers include: allergic responses reactions to novel proteins produced from genetically modified genes, and increased toxicity from unexpected enhanced natural plant toxins.

Organic food has been shown to contain more vitamins and minerals than non-organic food. It also contains far less hormones, fertilisers and pesticide residues. In addition, growing your own food and sprouting seeds at home ensures a regular supply of more healthy food than can be bought in most shops.

It is generally believed that fruits and vegetables contain little to no vitamin B12. This is invariably the case with non-organic fruits and vegetables but is probably not the case for organic fruits and vegetables. Organic produce tends to harbour greater levels of microorganisms, and therefore has a relatively short shelf-life compared to non-organic produce. These microorganisms often synthesise vitamin B12 which may be assimilated when the vegetables are eaten.

10.3.3.1.10 Social commitments and advertising propaganda encourage us to eat unhealthy foods

The food industry is a global multi-billion-dollar business. A lot of very elaborate advertising from food companies tries to convince the public to buy and eat food that is not necessarily good for them. An example is the well-known idea of Five Main Food Groups where dairy products and meats have such a high place of importance. This concept was developed in the 1950s by the meat and dairy industries. More unbiased research has shown that there should be much more emphasis on fresh fruit and vegetables but large companies do not profit from this information being given out.

Another important example is genetically engineered soybeans, which are promoted as a health food, without declaring they are genetically manipulated. Even organic soybeans are legally allowed to contain up to 10% genetically altered seed in the United States! Genetic engineering of foods has many potential health risks by itself [Section 10.3.3.1.9]. However, there are many problems with all soy produce [Section 10.3.3.2.4]. Large multinational companies have planted soy crops over significant portions of the United States. It is essential for the financial future of these companies to convince people that soy foods are good to eat, even if is not healthy at all.

10.3.3.2 The main problems with commonly used foods

The dangers of eating common foods such as meat [Sections 10.3.2.2.3 & 10.3.3.1.6] and eggs [Section 10.3.3.2.2] have been discussed at length elsewhere in this and in other texts. Suffice to say meat and eggs are very acid forming, and generally are not conducive to the traditional yogic lifestyle. The problems of more common foods, which are not usually thought of as being dangerous to health, are discussed below. This includes the problems associated with the consumption of bread [Section 10.3.3.2.1], legumes [Section 10.3.3.2.2], dairy products [Section 10.3.3.2.3], soy products [Section 10.3.3.2.4], and salty foods [Section 10.3.3.2.5].

10.3.3.2.1 Problems with bread and other processed complex carbohydrates

Bread and other processed complex carbohydrates form the staple diet of many cultures. Although not generally thought of as being unhealthy, excess of these foods may cause significant health problems. In addition, reduction or elimination of these foods from the diet may make the practice of *hatha yoga* much easier [Section 10.3.4.1, Table 10.1 Note 17].

Bread and other processed complex carbohydrates contain many anti-nutrients, which include chemical inhibitors of digestion called phytates. Other anti-nutrients include, molecular-mimicking proteins, protease inhibitors and alpha-amylase inhibitors, all of which adversely affect our digestive system and our immune system.

Phytic acid has the potential to bind calcium, zinc, iron and other minerals, thereby reducing their availability in the body. Binding of these important minerals by phytic acid can impair bone growth and metabolism. Research has implicated zinc deficiency as a result of excessive cereal grain consumption in retarding skeletal growth including cases of hypo-gonadal dwarfism seen in modern-day Iran. In addition, complex formation of phytic acid with proteins may inhibit the enzymatic digestion of the protein. Phytate-related deficiencies of iron and zinc occur in many populations that subsist on unleavened wholegrain bread and rely on it as a primary source of these minerals. There are other anti-nutrients in cereal grains that directly impair vitamin D metabolism [Lunven, 1999].

No human can live on a diet composed entirely of cereal grains since they contain no Vitamin C. When cereal grain calories reach 50% or more of the daily caloric intake, humans suffer severe health consequences, hence the pellagra and berri-berri outbreaks of the last few hundred years. Additionally, not only in humans, but in virtually every animal model studied (dog, rat, guinea pig, baboon, etc.), high cereal grain consumption promotes and induces rickets (a bone-deforming disease) and osteomalacia (a condition characterised by softening of the bones).

Much evidence has been accumulated implicating cereal grains in the autoimmune process. There is substantial evidence (both epidemiological and clinical) showing the role cereal grains may play in the aetiology of such diverse autoimmune diseases as multiple sclerosis (MS), insulin-dependent diabetes mellitus (IDDM), rheumatoid arthritis, Sjogrens syndrome, dermatitis herpetiformis and IgA nephropathy. Wheat can wreak havoc with the immune system. Wheat contains peptide sequences (short protein molecules) which often are only partially digested but are small enough to enter the blood stream. These peptide sequences resemble a wide variety of the body's tissue peptide sequences and hence induce autoimmune disease via the process of molecular mimicry. Macrophages ingest the circulating partially digested wheat proteins. HLA molecules [Section 10.2.3.3.] within the macrophage then present amino-acid sequences of the fragmented peptide to circulating T-lymphocytes, which multiply and attack the partially digested wheat proteins, but they also attack any other self-antigen which has a similar amino-acid sequence, ie they attack the body's own tissues [Cordain, 1999].

Cereal-free, legume-free, dairy-free, and yeast-free diets potentially have therapeutic benefit in many autoimmune related disorders via their ability to reduce gut permeability and decrease the exogenous antigenic load both from pathogenic bacteria and from potentially self-mimicking dietary peptides [Cordain, 1999].

Both in cereals and legumes there are alpha-amylase inhibitors (inhibitors of starch-degrading enzymes). Primarily in legumes, but also in cereals, there are trypsin inhibitors (inhibitors of protein-degrading enzymes). These inhibitors are not fully denatured (destroyed) by normal cooking processes and may represent as much as 1% of wheat flour. In addition, because of their thermostability, these inhibitors persist through bread-baking, and occur in large amounts in the centre of loaves [Liener, 1994].

Both cereal grains and legumes [Section 10.3.3.2.3] contain lectins that bind intestinal epithelial cells and change the permeability characteristics of these intestinal cells. Lectins cause an increase of the translocation of gut bacteria, increased overgrowth of gut bacteria, as well as a change in the gut flora. In addition, lectins cause increased expression of intracellular adhesion molecules in lymphocytes that allows bacterial immune complexes to move from the gut to the affected tissue. Additionally, cereal and legume lectins increase lymphocytic expression of common inflammatory chemicals that are known promoters of autoimmune disease.

One of the major problems with most complex carbohydrates (bread, rice etc) is their easy conversion to glucose (and other simple sugars). Increased blood glucose leads to decreased Vitamin C which depresses the immune system. Increased blood glucose also promotes the growth of cancer because cancer cells can only metabolise anaerobically and for this glucose is the perfect fuel.

The hormone insulin is produced in response to increased levels of blood glucose. The main role of insulin is to stimulate body cells to take up glucose. When levels of insulin become elevated the cells commonly develop insulin resistance, ie the cells no longer respond to insulin. This results in mature onset diabetes, in which there is an excess of sugar in the blood. In some cases this can develop into insulin deficient diabetes where insulin is no longer produced at all.

Important markers for a long lifespan are known to be reduced blood glucose and reduced blood insulin levels. Insulin has many roles and so hyperinsulinaemia (excess blood insulin) can have many devastating effects in the body. Insulin mediates blood lipids (fats). Increased levels of insulin promote increased levels of fat in the blood, that can also cause increases in blood clotting (thromboses), plaque build up and numerous other problems of the cardiovascular system.

Insulin is mitogenic (causes cell division), so increased levels of insulin also increases the risk of cancer. Insulin also causes a decrease in nitric oxide [Section 12.7.1.2, Applications to Yoga 12.2] which is a vasodilator (expands blood vessel diameters). Therefore, hyperinsulinaemia (excess insulin) due to insulin resistance also causes increased blood pressure.

Insulin resistance causes the excretion from the body of magnesium, which is a muscle relaxant. Therefore muscle tension in the body increases and blood pressure is further increased. Reduced levels of magnesium further complicate the problem and increase insulin resistance because magnesium is needed for insulin to work properly. Also, magnesium is needed to make insulin, therefore eventually there is no insulin at all.

Insulin resistance also causes the excretion of calcium which leads to increased levels of osteoporosis, atherosclerosis and arthritis. The lack of calcium also causes retention of sodium which leads to increased blood pressure (BP), and increase in the activity of the sympathetic nervous system, increased stress and decreased levels of immunity.

When blood glucose is not being properly utilised as a fuel, as in cases of insulin resistance, protein from muscle mass becomes a fuel source. This depletes muscle mass and causes an increase in oxidation and glycation. Glycation is the binding of a protein molecule to a glucose molecule resulting in the formation of damaged, nonfunctioning structures. Glycation alters protein structure and decreases biological activity. Glycated proteins, also known as advanced glycated end-products (AGEs), are very toxic. They accumulate in affected tissue and are reliable markers of disease. Many age-related diseases such as arthritis, chronic inflammation, atherosclerosis, cataract and neurological impairment are at least partially attributable to glycation.

10.3.3.2.2 Problems with legumes, beans and peanuts

As with grain consumption, there are hunter-gatherers who have been documented eating legumes. However, in most cases, the legumes are cooked or the tender, early sprouts are eaten raw rather than the mature pod. Some legumes in their raw state are less toxic than others. However, most legumes in their mature state are non-digestible and/or toxic to most mammals when eaten in even moderate quantities. Interested readers are referred to:

- Implications of anti-nutritional components in soybean foods. [Liener, 1994]
- Anti-nutritional and toxic factors in food legumes: a review. [Gupta, 1987]
- Food poisoning from raw red kidney beans. [Noah et al., 1980]
- The toxicity of phaseolus vulgaris lectins: Nitrogen balance and immunochemical studies. [Pusztai et al., 1981].

These references summarise the basics about legume indigestibility/toxicity; however, there are hundreds, if not thousands, of citations documenting the anti-nutritional properties of legumes. Legumes contain a wide variety of anti-nutrient compounds that influence multiple tissues and systems. Normal cooking procedures do not always eliminate these anti-nutrients. Beans contain many indigestible carbohydrates such as raffinose. These compounds can be fermented by intestinal bacteria and cause gas.

Legume starch contains trypsin inhibitors, which inactivate native pancreatic trypsin and retard the digestion of protein. In animal models, this was shown to cause pancreatic enlargement by increasing pancreatic cholecystokinin levels.

10.3.3.2.3 Problems with milk and dairy products

Although milk was recommended in some old *hatha yoga* texts, many advanced *yoga* practitioners would not drink it. In addition, many of the problems of milk are significantly enhanced today because of the presence of large amounts of antibiotics, pesticides, hormones and other chemicals either added directly to the milk or fed to cows. Furthermore, the milk most people drink is generally pasteurised (cooked). Heating a complex mixture of carbohydrates, proteins and fats such as milk, induces many chemical changes to take place. Heating the fat in milk will, as in the heating of all fats, lead to the production of carcinogens (cancer-causing chemicals). In addition, heating carbohydrates and proteins together may cause them to chemically bind and significantly alter their structure and function in the body [Section 10.3.3.1.6].

The way milk is manufactured today creates many potential problems. The information below comes from many scientific studies. Some studies are only partially referenced with the journal where information was taken. In such cases, and when no reference is cited for a statement, assume that the information has come from the excellent and well referenced 600-page website of Robert Cohen which details the scientific studies done on the deleterious effects of milk (http://www.notmilk.com).

If milk is still an important part of your diet, then some compromises and alternatives are available. It is believed that goat's milk is thought to be better than cow's milk. Fresh, unpasteurised, unhomogenised milk is usually better than pasteurised and homogenised milk. Fermented milks (eg kefir, yoghurt) are probably better than unfermented milk. Other safe alternatives to animal millk include nut and seed milks (eg fresh almond milk) but not soy milk.

Glue-like effects of milk

One of the reputed benefits of milk is its high protein content. Casein protein, which comprises 80% of all milk protein, is not well digested in adults due to the lack of the enzyme rennin. During early childhood, the stomach secretes rennin to coagulate casein in order to make it accessible to hydrochloric acid and enzymatic breakdown. Casein is used in the production of plastics, and sold commercially as a very strong glue that binds wood to wood, and glues labels to bottles. Therefore, in the human body most milk protein (casein) remains undigested or only partially digested in adult humans and is subsequently either degraded or putrefied by bacteria [Section 10.3.3.1.5] or will remain in the body as a strong glue that will contribute to the plastic-concrete pipeline effect [Section 10.3.3.1.3].

Most people are unable to digest milk sugar

A significant portion of the worlds population is unable to digest lactose (the major sugar in milk) due to a lack of the enzyme lactase. Lactose intolerance affects 75% of the world's population, including most Asian and African people. Symptoms include bloating, flatulence, abdominal pain and diarrhoea. Chronic diarrhoea is the most common gastrointestinal symptom of intolerance of cow's milk among children [Capano et al., 1984].

Milk consumption contributes to osteoporosis

American women have been consuming an average of two pounds of milk per day for their entire lives, yet thirty million American women have osteoporosis. Drinking milk does not prevent bone loss. Ingesting too much protein accelerates bone loss. In order to absorb calcium, the body needs comparable amounts of another mineral element, magnesium. Milk and dairy products contain only small amounts of magnesium.

Magnesium is the centre atom of chlorophyll, which is the green pigment in plants that functions as part of light harvesting complex, but which is structurally almost identical to haem in blood. One of the best sources of easily absorbable calcium is leafy green vegetables.

Countries shown to have the highest rates of osteoporosis, such as the United States, England, and Sweden, consume the most milk. Conversely, China and Japan, where people eat much less protein and dairy food, have low rates of osteoporosis [Nutrition Action Healthletter, June, 1993].

Osteoporosis is caused by a number of things, one of the most important being excessive dietary protein. Dietary protein increases levels of acid in the blood, which is neutralised by calcium mobilised (taken or leached) from the skeleton. Increasing protein intake by 100% may cause calcium loss to double [Journal of Nutrition, 1981; 3 111].

An important 12-year Harvard University study of 77,761 women [Feskanich et al.,1997] found that women consuming greater amounts of calcium from dairy foods had significantly increased risks of hip fractures, while no increase in fracture risk was observed for the same levels of calcium from non-dairy sources. According to the study, women who drank two or more glasses of milk per day had 145% greater risk of hip fracture when compared with women consuming one glass or less per week.

In a Sydney-based study in 1990–1991, it was found that consumption of dairy products, particularly at age 20 years, was associated with an increased risk of hip fracture in old age. It was also shown that the metabolism of dietary protein causes increased urinary excretion of calcium [Cumming & Klineberg, 1994].

Cow's milk growth hormone encourages growth of human cancer cells

The most powerful growth hormone produced in a cow's body is identical to the most powerful growth hormone in the human body [Martin, 2003]. That hormone, insulin-like growth factor (IGF) is present in cow's milk and has been repeatedly identified as the key factor in the growth and proliferation of breast, prostate and lung cancers.

Pasteurisation of milk does not kill all bacteria

At the first sign of heat treatment (pasteurisation), many bacteria in milk form spores. When the milk cools, spores re-emerge into their original bacterial forms. Mycobacterium paratuberculosis is a bacterium found in many of America's dairy herds and 100% of Crohne's disease patients. These bacteria are not destroyed by pasteurisation and cross the species barrier from cow to human.

Listeria organisms are excreted in cow's milk. These organisms can escape pasteurisation, grow well in a refrigerator and are ingested by consumers [Dalton, 1997].

Curing alone may not be a sufficient pathogen control step to eliminate Salmonella, Listeria, and Escherichia coli from cheese. A drop of sour milk may contain more than 50 million bacteria.

Milk consumption contributes to childhood infections

The Chief of Paediatrics at Johns Hopkins Medical School (Frank Oski) and America's most famous paediatrician, Benjamin Spock, agreed upon the same treatment for childhood ear infections. Both physicians recommended a protocol in which all milk and dairy products should be eliminated from the diets of all children.

Milk consumption contributes to diabetes

More than 20 well-documented studies have prompted one researcher to write that the link between milk and juvenile diabetes is very solid [Diabetes Care Journal, 1974]. This is especially the case with pasteurised milk, where lactose is converted to beta-lactose, which is more rapidly processed.

Milk consumption contributes to obesity and heart disease

According to USDA figures, each day, the average American eats just 5 ounces of meat and chicken containing saturated fat and cholesterol, and 29.2 ounces of milk and dairy products. Saturated bovine fat contained in milk, cheese, ice-cream and other dairy products has been identified as the single most causative factor of America's obesity epidemic, and the link to heart disease being America's number-one killer.

A Survey of Mortality Rates and Food Consumption Statistics of 24 Countries, [Medical Hypothesis 7:907-918, 1981] stated that milk and milk products gave the highest correlation coefficient to heart disease, while sugar, animal proteins and animal fats came in second, third and fourth respectively.

The British medical journal, *The Lancet,* published findings that more patients who had suffered a myocardial infarction had elevated levels of antibodies against milk proteins than was found in a comparable group of patients without coronary heart disease [Davies, 1980].

Most milk contains carcinogenic growth factors due to cows being treated with genetically engineered growth hormones

In the United States, cows are usually treated with genetically engineered bovine growth hormone and they produce milk that has been proven to result in increased amounts of insulin-like growth factor, a hormone identified as the key role player in fuelling the growth of human breast cancer, prostate cancer, lung cancer and colon cancer.

Milk protein consumption contributes to anaemia (low iron content in blood)

Cow's milk proteins can cause blood loss from the intestinal tract, reduce the body's supply of iron, and cause anaemia [Journal of Paediatrics].

Most milk contains high levels of pesticides, dioxins and other poisons

Dioxins are highly toxic by-products of industrial processes including chemical and municipal waste incineration. These compounds penetrate the environment via air, water and soil and are incorporated in food chains. The level of dioxin in a single serving of vanilla ice-cream tested was almost 200 times greater than the safe daily dose.

In 1988 America's Food and Drug Administration (FDA) did a survey of milk samples from grocery stores in 10 cities found that 73% of the samples contained pesticide residues. More than 2,200 samples of cow's milk were tested in India, and 85% of the samples contained pesticide levels above human tolerance limits.

The pesticides chlordane and heptachlor cause cancer, harm the immune system and are endocrine system disruptors. Dairy cattle in Oahu were fed pineapple leaves containing heptachlor residues. As a result, the local milk and dairy supply remained contaminated for years.

Milk contains somatic cells, which are dead red and white blood cells from the cow. Another name for somatic cells is pus cells. America's FDA sets the legal standard for the allowable number of pus cells that can be sold in milk. One litre of American milk may contain no more than 750 million pus cells.

Milk consumption implicated in Sudden Infant Death Syndrome (SIDS)

British medical journal, *The Lancet,* has stated that hypersensitivity to milk is implicated as a cause of Sudden Infant Death Syndrome (SIDS). Those infants who died of SIDS expressed inappropriate or inflammatory responses suggesting violent allergic reactions to a foreign protein. Lung tissue and cells showed responses similar to bronchial wall inflammation in asthma. Those who consumed cow's milk were fourteen times more likely to die from diarrhoea-related complications and four times more likely to die of pneumonia than were breast-fed babies. Intolerance and allergy to cow's milk products may be a factor in SIDS.

About 80 % of cows that are producing milk are pregnant and are synthesising hormones continuously, and these hormones are naturally going into their milk for their calves to drink. Progesterone breaks down into androgens, which have been implicated as a factor in the development of acne. Hormones found in cow's milk include: oestradiol, oestriol, progesterone, prolactin and oxytocin.

Milk contains many hormones that disturb the endocrine system

In a review of the known bioactive hormones [Section 11.1.2.] and growth factors in milk [Grosvenor, 1992] it is stated that there are many hormones in cow's milk that invariably affect our endocrine system. Each sip of cow's milk contains:

- Pituitary hormones (PRL, GH, TSH, FSH, LH, ACTH Oxytocin),
- Hypothalamic hormones (TRH, LHRH, somatostatin, PRL-inhibiting factor, PRL-releasing factor, GnRH, GRH)
- Pancreatic hormones
- Thyroid hormones
- Parathyroid hormones
- Adrenal hormones
- Gonadal hormones
- Steroid hormones (estradiol, estriol, progesterone, testosterone, 17-Ketosteroids, Corticosterone, Vitamin D)
- Gut hormones (vasoactive intestinal peptide, bombasine, cholecystokinin, gastrin, gastrin inhibitory peptide, pancreatic peptide, substance P, neurotendinal)

10.3.3.2.4 Problems with soybean products

Soybeans and their products (soy milk, tofu, tempeh, soy sauce soy burgers etc) are best avoided. Many people (especially the companies who have invested so much time and money into soybeans and their production) advocate the use of soybean products because of their health benefits. However, Sheehan [1998b] states that he is unconvinced that the long history of apparent safe use of soy products could provide confidence that they are indeed without risk. Soy may definitely contain some beneficial substances, but much evidence accumulated over the last few decades strongly suggests many of the substances in soybeans and soybean products are deleterious to health. Many scientific articles are available discussing possible dangers of soy products. Following is some of the information available from reputable scientific journals indicating the dangers of soybean products, and some of the copious information on this subject available on the Internet. Statements that are not fully referenced may be verified from any of the more recent review articles available on the subject.

Deleterious effects of soy produce on hormone levels and the endocrine system

Soy products include phytoestrogens, which are chemicals that mimic the actions of the hormone oestrogen but do not perform exactly the same functions. Phytoestrogens are therefore capable of leading to an imbalance of hormones, which in women may predispose them to cancer, and which in men may lead to a depression of male sexual characteristics.

There is abundant evidence that some of the isoflavones found in soy, including genistein and equol, demonstrate toxicity in oestrogen sensitive tissues and in the thyroid. Genistein is clearly estrogenic; it possesses the chemical structural features necessary for estrogenic activity [Miksicek, 1998].

Soy genistein could be a risk factor for a number of oestrogen-associated diseases [Sheehan 1998a]. It may be that no dose of soy protein isolate is without risk; the extent of risk is simply a function of dose [Sheehan 1998a].

Deleterious effecys of soy produce on the brain and nervous system

Some of the chemicals present in soybeans have been shown to bind to receptor sites in the brain and may be the cause of significant neural problems including suspected intelligence loss from vascular dementia.

A thirty-year study of Japanese Americans suggests that regular consumption of tofu over many years in middle life may have an adverse influence on brain ageing, manifest as accelerated atrophy, cognitive decline, and a lowering of the threshold for the clinical manifestations of Alzheimer's disease [White et al., 1996a, 1996b]. This prospective study followed the histories of 7,000 men and showed that Alzheimer's disease prevalence in Hawaiian men was similar to European-ancestry Americans and to Japanese [White et al., 1996a]. In contrast, vascular dementia prevalence is similar in Hawaii and Japan and both are higher than in European-ancestry Americans. This suggests that common ancestry or environmental factors in Japan and Hawaii are responsible for the higher prevalence of vascular dementia in these locations. Subsequently, this same group showed a significant dose-dependent risk (up to 2.4 fold) for development of vascular dementia and brain atrophy from consumption of tofu, a soy product rich in isoflavones [White, et al., 1996b].

Given that oestrogens are important for maintenance of brain function in women; that the male brain contains aromatase, the enzyme that converts testosterone to oestradiol; and that isoflavones inhibit this enzymatic activity [Irvine, 1998], there is a mechanistic basis for the human findings suggesting that soy (tofu) phytoestrogens causes vascular dementia [Sheehan, 1998b].

Deleterious effects of soy produce on the male reproductive system

Research has shown that animals fed a soy-free diet had significantly larger testes than controls fed a soy-containing diet [Atanassova et al. 2000]. The continuous presence of soy in an animal diet retarded sperm development and resulted in lifelong alterations in body weight, testes weight and hormone (FSH) levels [Atanassova et al. 2000]. This has significant implications for all studies of male reproductive development and function. Phytoestrogens in soy produce are potential endocrine system disruptors in males and affect the function of the male sex glands [Santti et al., 1998].

The incidence of development disorders of the male reproductive tract has more than doubled in the past 30–50 years, while sperm counts have declined by about half. The increasing incidence of reproductive abnormalities in the human male may be related to increased oestrogen exposure. Some of this exposure may come from dietary based phytoestrogens [Sharpe & Skakkebaek 1993].

Deleterious effects of soy produce on the female reproductive system

Women receiving soy supplements show menstrual cycle disturbances, including an increased oestradiol level in the follicular phase [Setchell, et al., 1997] [Section 11.3.2.7].

An important study done at Cambridge University [Cassidy et al., 1994] has demonstrated that even modest doses of soy (60 g per day for one month) had an unambiguous biological effect on menstrual cycle length and the hormones that trigger ovulation. The menstrual cycle was lengthened by 1½ days and the two main ovulation hormones were reduced to a half (FSH) and a third (LH) of their levels before the soy diet was started [Tables 11.1 & 11.2, Sections 11.1 & 11.3]. This means that the soy isoflavones are biologically active in humans at dietary levels. Hence, these pre-menopausal women were on the soy diet for 30 days, yet it took up to three months for the effects to wear off.

Woodhams [1995] suggests that over eons of progressive development the soybean has evolved as the most suitable way for the soy plant to reproduce itself. It may well be that the evolutionary advantage that the phytoestrogens confer on soybeans is their ability to adversely affect the reproductive health of their predators. The phytoestrogens in subterranean clover are certainly capable of causing permanent infertility in some sheep [Braden et al. 1967]. Although the short-term oestrogenic effects of these isoflavones in sheep were reversible, prolonged grazing resulted in the infertility syndrome that became known as clover disease and led to permanent histological changes to the uterus and ovaries [Setchell, 1985]. The fertility of other animals such as quail [Leopald, 1976], and cheetahs [Setchell et al. 1987] is also negatively affected by phytoestrogens.

Significant toxicity of certain compounds in soybeans

Soy contains several naturally occurring compounds that are toxic to humans and animals. A list of these compounds is given at the Soy Online Service (www.soyonlineservice.co.nz). The soy toxins that the Soy Online Service has concerns about include protease inhibitors, phytic acid, soy lectins (or haemagglutinins), nitrosamines, manganese concentrations and the mysterious soyatoxin. Soyatoxin is a recently discovered naturally occurring toxic chemical occurring in soybeans [Vasconcelos et al., 1996].

Probably the best known of the soy toxins are the protease inhibitors, which are enzymes that break down proteins for use by the body. In the rat, high levels of exposure to protease inhibitors (such as that found in raw soy flour) cause pancreatic cancer whereas moderate levels cause the rat pancreas to be more susceptible to cancer-causing agents. It is prudent therefore, that when preparing soy foods, such as boiled or roasted soybeans or soy milk, to ensure that they are adequately heated.

Soybeans have a very high level of phytates [Mohamed et al., 1986]. Phytates are good metal chelating agents and are particularly adept at binding metals in their so-called divalent state, such as calcium (Ca^{2+}), copper (Cu^{2+}), iron (Fe^{2+}), manganese (Mn^{2+}) and zinc (Zn^{2+}). If metals are bound up in a phytate-complex, they are less available to the body for nutritive purposes (ie is less bio-available). The development of iron deficiency due to excess dietary phytate levels may have an independent direct action on brain function [Hallberg, 1989].

Soyatoxin has been shown to produce dyspnoea (difficulty in breathing), tonic-clonic convulsions (a seizure involving the entire body), and flaccid paralysis prior to death in intra-peritoneally injected mice.

Nitrosamines, which are among the most carcinogenic compounds in existence, are not naturally occurring in soybeans but form during processing of soy products by the reaction of nitrite with amines. Consumers of soy protein isolate could be exposed daily to levels of nitrosamines that are 35 times greater than the government established safe limit.

Negative effects of soy produce on the behaviour of children

Research ongoing for a decade at two University of California campuses affirms that <u>manganese</u> in soy infant formula currently on shelves permits an estimated safe <u>manganese</u> dose of about 120 times the amount found in breastmilk, which may damage the infant brain and trigger aberrant behaviour in adolescents [Goodman, 2000].

Deleterious effects of soy produce on the immune system

A retrospective analysis by Fort *et al* [1990] documents the association of soy formula given to infants and <u>autoimmune</u> <u>thyroid</u> disease. <u>Isoflavones</u> in soybeans are inhibitors of the <u>thyroid peroxidase</u>, which makes T3 and T4. Inhibition can be expected to generate <u>thyroid</u> abnormalities, including goitre and <u>autoimmune</u> <u>thyroiditis</u>.

There are significant reports of <u>goitrogenic</u> effects from soy consumption in human infants [Chorazy et al., 1995] and adults [Ishizuki, et al., 1991].

Carcinogenic effects of soybean compounds

There exists a significant body of animal data that demonstrates <u>goitrogenic</u> and even <u>carcinogenic</u> effects of soy products [Kimura et al., 1976]. Several recent studies [Dees et al., 1997; Hsieh et al., 1998; McMichael-Phillips et al. 1998] have shown that certain <u>phytoestrogens</u> present in soy products are <u>carcinogenic</u>. In one study from the University of Illinois [Allred et al., 2001] dietary <u>genistin</u> resulted in an increased tumour growth rate and cell proliferation similar to that observed with <u>genistein</u>. The remaining mice were switched to diets free of <u>genistin</u> and <u>genistein</u>. Removal of the <u>isoflavones</u> from the diet resulted in tumour regression. In summary, <u>genistin</u>, like <u>genistein</u>, may act as an <u>oestrogen</u> agonist to increase proliferation of <u>oestrogen-dependent</u> breast cancer cells, and on its removal, tumours regress [Allred et al., 2001]. This represents clear information that soy protein isolates containing increasing concentrations of <u>genistein</u> stimulate the growth of <u>oestrogen-dependent</u> breast cancer cells <u>in vivo</u> in a dose-dependent manner.

Deleterious effects of soy produce on infants

Fort *et al* [1990] reports of a doubling of risk for <u>autoimmune</u> <u>thyroid</u> disease in children who had received soy formulas as infants compared to infants receiving other forms of milk.

The serum levels of <u>isoflavones</u> in infants receiving soy formula are about five times higher than in women receiving soy supplements who show <u>menstrual cycle</u> disturbances, including an increased <u>oestradiol</u> level in the follicular phase [Setchell, et al., 1997].

While soymilks for infant feeding are common, potential implications of long term exposure to <u>phytoestrogens</u> that are present in soy-milk appears to have been overlooked and their situation could be considered analogous to sheep grazing on clover containing <u>isoflavones</u> that became permanently infertile [Setchell 1985].

Additional problems with soybeans and soy produce

If soy consumers follow the advice of *PROTEIN TECHNOLOGIES INTERNATIONAL* (manufacturers of isolated soy protein) and consume 100 grams of soy protein per day, their daily <u>genistein</u> intake could easily exceed 200 milligrams per day. This level of <u>genistein</u> intake should definitely be avoided. For comparison, it should be noted that Japanese males consume, on average, less than 10 milligrams of <u>genistein</u> per day [Fukutake et al., 1996].

Many vegetarians in the USA, Europe and Australasia would think nothing of consuming 8 ounces (about 220 grams) of tofu and a couple of glasses of soy milk per day, two or three times a week. However, this is well in excess of what Asians typically consume. A survey of 1,242 men and 3,596 women in Japan estimated the amount of soy protein consumed from these sources was about 8 grams per day for men and 7 grams per day for women [Nagata et al., 1998].

Other problems associated with soy products include the high level of genetic engineering that has affected much of the soy in the world; and significant amounts of aluminium residues in most processed soy products, which is believed to be a significant contributor to <u>Alzheimer's disease</u>. As well as obvious soy foods like tofu, soymilk and miso, and other soy products such as <u>isolated soy</u> protein (ISP) and <u>soy protein concentrate</u> (SPC), very many processed foods contain soy, some examples available from the SOY ONLINE SERVICE at <u>http://www.soyonlineservice.co.nz</u> are:

Biscuits	Breads	Vegetarian burgers
Cakes	Crackers	Bakery products
Pastries	Meat substitutes	Pancakes
Chicken nuggets	Legume meal	Fish fingers
Pies	Meat extenders	Hydrolysed vegetable protein (HVP)
Yoghurt	Breakfast cereals	Sausages
Soups	Baby foods	Doughnuts
Vegetarian meats	Sandwich spreads	Baby rusks
Pet Foods	Animal feeds	Textured vegetable protein (TVP)

The SOY ONLINE SERVICE further reports that soy is one of the most allergenic foods in modern diets. Soy has been shown to contain at least 30 allergenic proteins.

10.3.3.2.5 Salt: Dangers of additional salt in the diet

There is definitely enough natural salt in a natural diet to satisfy the body's metabolic needs. No added salt may be required if living off natural unprocessed food. If processed foods are included in the diet, however, there is evidence to suggest that some added sea salt may be of benefit to the metabolism. Nevertheless salt is an inhibitor of many enzymes, especially if given in excess. Excess salt inflames the stomach. Excess salt causes uric acid retention. Excess salt may aggravate premenstrual tension. Excess salt causes oestrogen to bind more water leading to hypertension, greater bloating at certain times during the menstrual cycle, and evidence suggests that this leads to the production of cellulite. The question is, how much is excess salt? Some authors suggest that some salt is even good to take when drinking water and other authors suggest that the requirement for salt increases the more cereal grain food eaten.

Excess salt is also thought to increase blood pressure, and is associated with asthma, stomach and naso-pharyngeal cancer, calcium loss and increased stroke mortality independent of the effect on blood pressure.

Excess salt may also cause increased calcium excretion [Nordin k. 1993] and loss of bone mass [Devine et al. 1995]. Because the kidneys excrete calcium with sodium [Nordin et al. 1993], high levels of dietary sodium are now generally recognised to be the single greatest dietary risk factor for osteoporosis [Matkovic et al. 1995; Devine et al. 1995; Cappuccio 1996]. It seems, then, that the excess salt intake in many Western diets is seen as normal.

10.3.3.2.6 Foods that disturb concentration, meditation and balance

According to the Chinese Buddhist monks and many other people who meditate and/or do a lot of *yoga*, avoid garlic, onions, shallots, spring onions, leek, and all excessive spicy foods as these are too stimulating and will make it difficult to concentrate or meditate. Even balancing on one leg is often more difficult after these foods have been ingested in significant quantity.

10.3.4 Acid-alkali Balance

The acid and alkali (base) levels of the blood, and the fluids of the intracellular spaces needs to be maintained at a pH of about 7.4 (slightly alkaline) [Section 10.3.4.1, Note 1]. The reasons for maintaining a homeostasis (sameness) of this pH, and the way the body regulates this pH are described in Table 10.1. The main reason the pH must be regulated in this way is to maintain an electrochemical potential difference between each cell's central Nucleus (pH ~5.0), and peripheral Cytoplasm (pH ~8.0). This electrochemical potential difference is essentially the **Life Force** of each cell.

The body needs to maintain a constant pH level of about pH 7.4 (slightly more alkaline than water) in the blood to:

- Help keep the electrochemical potential difference between the nucleus of a cell and the cytoplasm (electricity or life force of each cell) [Figure 10.1]
- Maintain proper enzyme function
- Maintain the integrity of the structural proteins which give cells their shape
- Help keep the synovial fluid (for joint lubrication) in a fluid state (the fluid is more viscous in the presence of acids).

Table 10.1 Effects of acidic and alkaline states of the blood and intracellular fluids

EFFECTS OF BLOOD PH LEVELS (ACID OR ALKALI) [1] ON THE BODY SYSTEMS	ACIDIC[2] Blood & Body Fluids	ALKALINE[3] Blood & Body Fluids
BLOOD CHEMISTRY: pH of Blood & Body Fluids (N.B. Acid pH is low while Alkaline pH is high)	↓ pH (Decreased pH)	↑ pH (Increased pH)
NERVOUS SYSTEM: Sensitivity of the nervous system [6]	↓ Sensitivity of nervous system	↑ Sensitivity of nervous system
CARDIOPULMONARY SYSTEM: Ability to tolerate Carbon Dioxide (which converts to Carbonic acid) in the Body [7]	↓ Tolerance to CO_2	↑ Tolerance to CO_2
→ Ventilation (Average Litres of Air Breathed per Minute) [8]	↑ Ventilation	↓ Ventilation
→ Maximum Length of Breath Retention (holding) [9]	↓ Retention	↑ Retention
□ Dilation (expansion) of Arteries to Brain & Body [10]	↑ Arterial Dilation	↓ Arterial Dilation
→ Blood Flow to Brain & Body [11]	↑ Blood Flow	↓ Blood Flow
□ Dilation of Bronchioles (Expansion or Widening of Air Channels to Lungs) [12]	↑ Bronchiole Dilation	↓ Bronchiole Dilation
→ Air Flow to Alveoli (Lungs) [13]	↑	↓
→ Effort Required for Breathing [14]	↓	↑
MUSCULOSKELETAL SYSTEM: Viscosity (thickness) of Synovial Fluid in Joints [15]	↑	↓
→ Joint Flexibility [16]	↓ Joint Flexibility	↑ Joint Flexibility
RENAL (KIDNEY) SYSTEM: Work for the Kidneys to Filter the Blood [17]	↑ Work for Kidneys	↓ Work for Kidneys
CELL BIOCHEMISTRY: Life Force of each cell (Electrochemical Potential Difference between Nucleus & Cytoplasm) [18]	↓ Life Force of cells	↑ Life Force of cells
→ Oxygen Supply to Cells [19]	↑ Oxygen to Cells	↓ Oxygen to Cells
→ Nutrient Transport to Cells [20]	↑ Nutrients to Cells	↓ Nutrients to Cells
→ Removal of Wastes from Cells [21]	↑ Waste Removal	↓ Waste Removal
→ Calcium Leaching from Bones & Teeth to Neutralise Acid in Blood & Intracellular Fluids [22]	↑ Calcium Leaching	↓ Calcium Leaching
□ Probability of Osteoporosis (Brittle Bones) [23]	↑ Osteoporosis	↓ Osteoporosis
□ Probability of Dental Caries (Tooth Decay) [24]	↑ Dental Caries	↓ Dental Caries
□ Formation of Insoluble Calcium Complexes, from Calcium Binding to Acid residues [25]	↑ Formation of Insoluble Calcium Complexes	↓ Formation of Insoluble Calcium Complexes
→ Probability of Arthritis [26]	↑ Arthritis	↓ Arthritis
→ Probability of Atherosclerosis [27]	↑ Atherosclerosis	↓ Atherosclerosis
→ Tolerance to Metabolic Acids (eg Lactic Acid) [28]	↓ Tolerance to Metabolic Acids	↑ Tolerance to Metabolic Acids
□ Capacity to do Anaerobic Work or Exercise [29]	↓ Capacity to do Anaerobic Work	↑ Capacity to do Anaerobic Work

Figure 10.1 Cellular pH and its effect on the electrochemical energy of the Life Force of a cell.
A normal cell has a central nucleus that is <u>acidic</u> (pH ~5.0), and an outer cytoplasm that is <u>alkaline</u> (pH ~8.0). Like in the battery of a car, electrochemical current or electricity flows between the two compartments while their pH remains sufficiently different. The normal flow of electrons from one compartment to the next can be thought of as the life force of the cell. If the pH of the blood (normally pH 7.4) reduces and becomes more acid, cytoplasm pH also reduces, and the electrical flow between nucleus and cytoplasm also reduces. Once there is no potential difference between nucleus and cytoplasm, cell death occurs. The body has many mechanisms to prevent any significant change in blood pH.

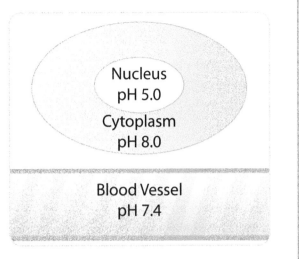

Nucleus
pH 5.0

Cytoplasm
pH 8.0

Blood Vessel
pH 7.4

10.3.4.1 Effects of acid and alkali states in the blood and intracellular fluids on the body systems

[Including Notes # for Table 10.1]

The effects of <u>acid</u> and <u>alkali</u> states in the blood and intracellular fluids on each of the body systems is outlined in Table 10.1.

Acid-alkali (pH) levels [Table 10.1 Note # 1]

<u>Acid-alkali</u> (pH) levels are measured in terms of pH, which is a measure of the amount of <u>hydrogen ions</u> (H⁺) in a solution. When the <u>hydrogen ion concentration</u> of a solution increases, the solution is said to become more <u>acidic</u>. Conversely, when the <u>hydrogen ion concentration</u> of a solution decreases, the solution is said to become less <u>acidic</u> and more <u>alkaline</u>. pH is a logarithmic measurement, so pH of 7.0 is actually a <u>hydrogen ion concentration</u> of 10^{-7} moles per litre (moles/l) [Appendix D] which is the same as water (H_2O). pH can also be thought of as the inverse of the concentration of <u>hydroxide ions</u> (OH⁻). When <u>hydroxide ion concentration</u> increases, the solution is said to become more <u>basic</u> or <u>alkaline</u>. Water (H_2O) is said to be neutral (neither <u>acid</u> nor <u>alkali</u>) because it has the same amount of H⁺ and OH⁻. (Note that H⁺ + OH⁻ = H_2O). Hence, a solution with pH of 6 is more <u>acid</u> than water as it has 10 times more <u>hydrogen ions</u> than water. A solution with a pH of 8 has 10 times less <u>hydrogen ions</u> than water and 10 times more <u>hydroxide ions</u> than water therefore it is <u>alkaline</u>.

<u>Acid-alkali</u> (pH) levels in the blood and tissue fluids are affected and regulated by <u>metabolic factors</u> (diet and exercise) and <u>respiratory factors</u> (breathing), and mental factors (our thoughts and attitudes). <u>Acid-alkali</u> (pH) levels are regulated by:

- How we breathe (ie the depth and speed of each in and out breath and the length of the pauses between the inhalation and exhalation)
- What we breathe (ie the freshness of the air or the level of pollution)
- The food that we eat and how it is processed in the body.

The most significant effect on <u>blood pH</u> and <u>body fluid pH</u> comes from the food that we eat. Each type of food will, after its digestion, leave a residue in the blood which is either <u>acid</u>, <u>alkaline</u>, or neutral.

Acidic body systems [Table 10.1 Note # 2]

An <u>acid</u> system is defined here to be where the internal environment of the body (especially the blood and intracellular fluids) tends to be in a more <u>acidic</u> state than the normal <u>blood pH</u> of ~7.4 (less than pH 7.4). This state is termed <u>acidosis</u>, when the pH is always below about pH 7.0.

Alkaline body systems [Table 10.1 Note # 3]

An alkaline system is defined here to be one where the internal environment of the body (especially the blood and intracellular fluids) tends to be in a more alkaline state than the normal blood pH of ~7.4 (greater than pH 7.4). This state is termed alkalosis when the pH is always above pH 7.4.

Normal (~neutral) body systems

A neutral body system is defined here as one where the internal environment of the body (especially the blood and intracellular fluids) tends to be easily maintained at normal blood pH of ~7.4 (which is actually slightly alkaline). In other words, the normal pH is easily maintained in blood pH about 7.4 without having to overwork the kidneys or draw upon the body's calcium reserves stored in the bones and teeth.

Acidic diet [Table 10.1 Note # 4]

The diet which leaves the greatest amount of acid residues in the blood and which tends to leave the body systems in a more acidic state is a diet which is high in protein (especially animal protein) and complex carbohydrates and is processed. Foods that tend to leave a primarily acidic residue in the blood following digestion include:

- Meats (including chicken, fish and other sea animals)
- Eggs
- Grains (with millet and buckwheat being the least acidic)
- Nuts (with almonds being the least acidic)
- Cheeses and most processed dairy products
- Soybeans, lentils, peanuts and other legumes
- Heated or rancid oils (and all food cooked in oil)
- Most medicines
- Food additives such as preservatives and colourings and many other substances that are not even listed on the labelling of processed foods because government regulations deem them to be insignificant in quantity, but which nevertheless have been shown to affect the body.

Alkaline Diet [Table 10.1 Note # 5]

The diet which leaves the greatest amount of alkaline residues in the blood and which tends to leave the body systems in a more alkaline state is one that is low in protein, low in complex carbohydrates, and is unprocessed. This type of diet is ideally fresh, organic, vegan food. Foods that tend to leave a primarily alkaline residue in the blood following digestion include:

- Fruits (uncooked)
- Fruit juices (fresh)
- Vegetable juices (fresh)
- Sprouted seeds and grains (uncooked)
- Salad leaves and fresh herbs (uncooked)
- Vegetables (fresh and lightly steamed)
- Almonds, buckwheat and millet are sometimes said to be slightly alkaline forming by some authors.

Acid-alkali effects on the nervous system [Table 10.1 Note # 6]

The nervous system becomes less sensitive in conditions where the pH is lower than the normal of 7.3 (ie excess acidic residues in the bloodstream and in the intracellular fluids). Conversely, the nervous system becomes more sensitive (even hypersensitive) in conditions where the pH is higher than the normal of 7.3 (ie excess alkaline residues in the blood stream and in the intracellular fluids). In conditions of extreme acidity, for example after prolonged intense exercise, the pH has been recorded to be as low as pH 6.8. When the pH is this low however, nausea, headache, dizziness and often pain in the muscle groups being used, may result [McArdle et al., 1991, p288].

Acid-alkali effects on the cardiopulmonary system [Table 10.1 Note # 7]

Carbon dioxide (CO_2) converts to carbonic acid in the blood stream. The pH of the blood must be kept at about pH 7.4. Therefore, the body is more able to deal with CO_2 in an alkaline body system, and less able to deal with CO_2 in an acidic body system.

Minute ventilation [Table 10.1 Note # 8]

Minute ventilation is defined to be the average litres of air breathed per minute (l/min), or volume of air breathed per minute is a product of the average number of breaths taken each minute times the average amount of air in each breath. The average person at rest takes about 12 breaths (br) per minute (min) with each breath being about 500 millilitres (ml). Therefore, the average person breathes 6 litres per minute at rest (12 br/min X 500 ml/br = 6000 ml/min). A person with a body system that tends to be more acidic tends to breathe more than the average in order to expel CO_2 and thus reduce the levels of carbonic acid.

Breath retention (breath holding) [Table 10.1 Note # 9]

Since breath retention causes an increase in CO_2, which converts to carbonic acid in the blood stream, a person with an acid system tends to have a reduced ability to hold the breath, while the same individual with an alkaline system tends to have an increased ability to hold the breath.

Vascular chemoreceptors [Table 10.1 Notes # 10 & 11]

Chemoreceptors throughout the body are able to sense high concentrations of CO_2 or carbonic acid in the blood and use this as a signal to dilate (expand) the blood vessels in order to increase blood flow, especially to the brain [Guyton, 1991]. Hence, a common side effect of hyperventilation is a dizziness resulting from lack of oxygen to the brain.

Respiratory chemoreceptors [Table 10.1 Notes # 12 & 13]

Receptors in the respiratory system are able to sense high concentrations of CO_2 in the lungs and use this as a signal to dilate (expand) the bronchioles in order to increase air flow to the lungs. Hence, a common side effect of hyperventilation (over-breathing) in people who are prone to asthma, is an asthma attack or some symptoms of shortness of breath or wheezing.

Effort of breathing [Table 10.1 Note # 14]

When the bronchioles are dilated, or expanded in diameter, the effort required for breathing is reduced. This is the case when there is a higher level of CO_2.

Acid-alkali effects on the musculoskeletal system [Table 10.1 Notes # 15 & 16]

It is well known that most substances in the bloodstream, whether normal or pathological, easily enter the joint cavity [Moore, 1985]. Therefore, the pH of the blood rapidly affects the pH of the synovial fluid in the joints, around tendons and around bursae. Synovial fluid becomes more viscous in acid conditions and less viscous in alkaline conditions. Hence, an alkaline diet leaves the joints more flexible in everyday life. A temporary alkalinity can be also brought to the body with hyperventilation (relatively fast and deep breathing) which tends to rid the blood of CO_2 and therefore also of carbonic acid. This makes your joints temporarily more flexible. This is the reason why many traditional yoga styles begin their practice with something like surya namaskar (salute to the sun) which involves relatively fast and deep breathing

Acid-alkali effects on the renal system [Table 10.1 Note # 17]

An acidic diet puts a strain on the kidneys, which is the final place that regulates the acid-alkali levels in the body. In conditions of excess acid (more common than excess alkali) the kidneys will excrete hydrogen ions and ammonia into the urine while trying to reabsorb alkaline substances such as hydroxide ions (OH⁻).

Acid-alkali effects on cell biochemistry [Table 10.1 Note # 18]

Figure 10.1 explains why the life force of each cell is depleted with an acid diet.

Circulation to the cells [Table 10.1 Notes # 19-21]

Circulation of blood to the cells is reduced with an acidic diet for several reasons. These reasons include:

*   Reduction in the electrochemical potential (life force) of the cells, which assists in the transport of substances across the cell membranes.
*   Thickening of blood from waste products of the acid diet which are often bound and neutralised by minerals such as calcium, leaving insoluble substances that thicken the blood and impede blood flow.
*   Lipotoxaemia resulting from excess fat in the blood.

Homeostasis

The acidic or alkaline state left in the body after eating food has to be corrected (neutralised) for the body to function normally. For most people, the food eaten leaves an acidic residue in the blood (a lower pH value than the normal pH of 7.4). Normal pH has to be restored either by:

- Eliminating the acidic residues using the kidneys mainly.
- Increasing the rate and/or the depth of the breath (hyperventilation) in order to blow off extra carbon dioxide and thereby reduce the blood levels of carbonic acid in order to decrease the acid levels of the blood (increasing pH).
- Neutralising the acid residues of food in the blood with the body's calcium reserves.

Calcium leaching from bones and teeth [Table 10.1 Notes # 22-27]

Calcium is a good neutraliser of acid residues and there is a plentiful supply in the bones and the teeth. Many studies have shown that acid residues in the blood are often neutralised by leaching calcium from the bones and teeth [Section 10.8]. This neutralisation process leads to the production of insoluble salts, which are difficult to eliminate from the body and often end up lodging in joints (leading to arthritic conditions) or being taken up by blood vessels (atherosclerosis).

Structural proteins and enzymes [Table 10.1 Notes # 30-31]

Structural proteins and enzymes are designed to optimally function at one ideal pH. Therefore, to place an excessive acidic load on the body can compromise the integrity of structural proteins and impair the functioning of many enzymes.

Limited aerobic capacity [Table 10.1 Notes # 28-29]

With a predominantly acidic diet, the body has more difficulty dealing with the products of anaerobic metabolism, in particular lactic acid. Therefore an acidic diet limits the anaerobic capacity of the body.

10.3.4.2 Diseases caused by acid-alkali imbalances

The acidic or alkaline state left in the body after eating food has to be corrected and or neutralised for the body to function normally. This is referred to as the process of homeostasis. Normal pH has to be restored either by:

- Neutralising the acid residues of food in the blood with the body's calcium reserves. This may lead to many diseases including osteoporosis, dental caries, arthritis, atherosclerosis, and gout.
- Increasing the rate and/or the depth of the breath (hyperventilation) in order to blow off extra carbon dioxide and thereby reduce the blood levels of carbonic acid in order to decrease the acid levels of the blood (increasing pH), which may cause breathlessness or asthma problems.
- Eliminating the acidic residues using the kidneys mainly, which may eventually lead to kidney stones, and eventually perhaps kidney failure.

Osteoporosis

Osteoporosis is a very common brittle bone disease caused by leaching of calcium from the bones to neutralise the acid residues. Due to the processes of pasteurisation, homogenisation and other factors, most of the calcium in milk is in the bound salt form of calcium oxalate and is unavailable for use by the body. Significant amounts of organic calcium are available from leafy green vegetables (eg parsley), fresh dates, and other fruits.

Dental caries

Dental caries or tooth decay is a very common problem occurring due to brittle, porous teeth that have been leached of calcium in order to neutralise acidic residues.

Arthritis

When calcium from the bones and teeth or from the diet binds to acid residues of food in order to neutralise them, insoluble salts may be produced that lodge in the joint spaces and contribute to arthritic conditions.

Atherosclerosis

Atherosclerosis occurs when cholesterol and calcium salts (which form when calcium binds to acid residues of food in order to neutralise their action) are taken up by blood vessel walls making them hard and inflexible. This process is stimulated by the presence of polyunsaturated fats.

The effects of <u>acid</u> and <u>alkali</u> diets, and the resultant <u>acid</u> and <u>alkali</u> states in the blood on the <u>body systems</u>, are outlined in Table 10.1. Some of the references for this material are further detailed in Section 10.3.4.

10.3.5 Digestion and Mal-digestion of Food

If food is not properly digested (mal-digestion), whole arrays of problems arise including the <u>fermentation</u> of excess carbohydrates, <u>putrefaction</u> of excess proteins and improper breakdown of fats.

10.3.5.1 Digestion of foods containing complex carbohydrates

<u>Complex carbohydrates</u> are long linked chains of sugar molecules. Foods generally referred to as <u>complex carbohydrates</u>, include starch foods such as wheat (in bread or pasta), rice, potatoes, etc. They also contain significant amounts of other foodstuffs such as protein. <u>Complex carbohydrates</u> can either undergo **normal digestion** [Table 10.2], or **mal-digestion** (partial digestion and <u>fermentation</u> leading to <u>indigestion</u>) [Table 10.3].

Table 10.2 Normal digestion of complex carbohydrates

In ideal conditions complex carbohydrates may be digested in the mouth by the salivary amylase ptyalin or in the small intestine by pancreatic amylase to leave (A) simple sugars (B) acidic residues of miineral complexes and (C) digestive inhibitors:

- (A) SIMPLE SUGARS: eg glucose, galactose, fructose; which may be converted to:
  o **Energy** plus **carbon dioxide** and **water ($ATP + CO_2 + H_2O$)**; or
  o **Building blocks** eg amino acids for synthesising structural molecules; or
  o **Fat**: excess carbohydrate is usually converted to fat.

- (B) ACID RESIDUES OF MINERAL COMPLEXES: [Table 10.1] When most complex carbohydrates are digested and enter the blood stream they leave an acid ash or mineral residue in the blood which increases the acid levels of the blood (ie decreases the pH), which leads to:

  o **Low pH (acid) in blood** [Table 10.1] causing calcium to be leached from the bones and teeth in order to neutralise the acid in the blood, which leads to:
    - **Osteoporosis** (brittle bones due to calcium leaching from the bones to neutralise the acid in the blood).

    - **Dental caries** (decayed teeth due to calcium leaching from the teeth to neutralise the acid in the blood).

    - **Arthritis** (pain and stiffness in joints due to insoluble acid-bound calcium complexes, formed as a result of the neutralisation of the acid pH in the blood, lodging in the joint spaces).

    - **Atherosclerosis** (hardening of the arterial walls due to the insoluble acid-bound calcium complexes being absorbed into the arterial walls. NB this happens more in the presence of polyunsaturated fat).

    - **Cell death** (due to increased acid in blood crossing cell walls and leading to a reduction in the potential difference, or electrical gradient (or life force), between nucleus (normally acid) and cytoplasm (normally alkaline) of the cells leading to a loss.

- (C) DIGESTIVE INHIBITORS: enzymatic or chemical inhibitors of digestion are present in most seeds and grains in order to protect these seeds from being prematurely eaten by animals or microorganisms.
  o **Enzymatic inhibitors of digestion**, which are inactivated or destroyed by cooking
  o **Chemical inhibitors of digestion** (eg phytates), which are not destroyed by cooking but can be inactivated in the sprouting process that seeds and grains may undergo.

Table 10.3 Mal-digestion of complex carbohydrates

In non ideal conditions, such as during illness or emotional states, after overeating or mal-combining of food, or in the presence of digestive inhibitors (above); complex carbohydrates are either only partially digested or broken down, or remain undigested and not broken down at all. Undigested or partially digested complex carbohydrates act as (A) mechanical blocking agents in the body and are subject to microbial (B) fermentation unless they are rapidly moved out of the intestines. If partially digested complex carbohydrates enter the bloodstream they may act to give (C) food allergies.

- (A) MECHANICAL BLOCKING AGENTS: Undigested or partially digested complex carbohydrates may act as mechanical blocking agents in the intestines. Partially digested complex carbohydrates may also be able to cross the intestinal wall and act as mechanical blocking agents in other channels through the body, such as the blood and lymph and vessels and the kidney tubules.
  - o **Mechanical blockage of the intestinal tract**: this may be due to:
    - **Physical obstruction** from the undigested food mass, which may become fermented (below).
    - **Adhesive properties of starch**: Starch (eg flour) plus water creates a type of glue which can block the intestinal tract or cover the intestinal walls leading to:
      - **Mal-absorption of nutrients** from the intestine through the intestinal walls to the bloodstream, and
      - **Poor elimination of wastes** from the bloodstream through the intestinal walls to the bloodstream, and
      - **Poor elimination of wastes** from the bloodstream for the intestinal walls to the intestines
  - o **Mechanical blockage in the rest of the body**: Partial breakdown products of complex carbohydrates may cross the intestinal tract into the bloodstream leading to:
    - **Blockage of blood vessels** leading to:
      - **Blood pressure increase**
      - **Circulation decrease**
    - **Intracellular blockage** (since partial breakdown products of complex carbohydrates are not usually absorbed by cells, they remain in the intracellular spaces), causing:
      - **Mal-absorption of nutrients** from the intracellular spaces through the cell walls to the inside (cytoplasm) of the cell, and
      - **Poor elimination of wastes** from the inside of the cells through the cell walls to the intracellular spaces

- (B) FERMENTATION: if complex carbohydrates are not rapidly processed in the intestinal tract by the body, then they are used as food by microorganisms that are always present in the intestinal tract. The products of microbial degradation of complex carbohydrates, known as fermentation, are (i) gas, (ii) alcohol, and more (iii) microorganisms.
  - o **(i) Gas**, usually carbon dioxide (CO_2), leads to
    - **Bloating**, or a feeling of fullness with discomfort
    - **Bowel distension**, leading to
      - **Assimilation** of food being decreased
      - **Energy supply** depleted
      - **Bowels rupture risk** increased
    - **Anoxia**: lack of oxygen due to presence of other gases in particular carbon di-oxide, leading to:
      - **Anaerobic bacteria** increase in number
      - **Aerobic bacteria** decrease in number
      - **Embarrassing noises** coming out of the body leading to:
        - o **Social problems**

  - o **(ii) Alcohol**, usually ethyl alcohol, which can cause
    - **Nausea**
    - **Headache**
    - **Dehydration**
    - **Over-stimulation**
    - **Memory loss**
    - **Liver damage**

- o **(iii) Microorganisms**: Microorganisms multiply as they digest the complex carbohydrates. This leads to:
  - **Intestinal blockage** caused by mass and volume of the growing microorganisms
  - **Poisonous wastes** produced by certain microorganisms
  - **Increased levels of infection**
  - **Nutrient loss** caused by the microorganisms using the nutrients for their own growth.
  - **Displacement of normal healthy microorganisms**, which are mainly aerobic bacteria.

- **(C)** FOOD ALLERGIES: Partial breakdown products of complex carbohydrates are often not recognised by the immune system as being foreign to the body. This is because starches and other complex carbohydrates are often fed to young children before they have their teeth and therefore before they have enzymes like ptyalin in the saliva which help digest starch. Since the immune system does not fully integrate itself until about the age of five, partial breakdown products of food may not be recognised as foreign by the immune system and not be removed even in adulthood. When these partial breakdown products build up in sufficient quantities enough to disrupt the internal environment of the body and they are not stopped by the immune system they manifest as the symptoms of an allergic reaction, which may be thought of as the body's last line of defence. Symptoms of an allergic response to mal-digestion of complex carbohydrates may include:
  - o Boils
  - o Rashes
  - o Asthma
  - o Pimples
  - o Eczema
  - o Dermatitis
  - o Disturbed immune system
  - o Neurological disorders
  - o Physiological disorders
  - o Immune system dysfunction

10.3.5.2 Digestion of foods containing proteins

Proteins are long linked chains of amino acid molecules. Foods generally referred to as protein foods are named thus because they contain large amounts of proteins. Protein foods include most animal products such as meat, fish, chicken, eggs, dairy products, etc. and vegetable products such as soybeans and their derivatives, and most nuts. Protein foods can either undergo **normal digestion** [Table 10.4], or **mal-digestion** (partial digestion and putrefaction (fermentation of proteins) leading to indigestion) [Table 10.1].

Table 10.4 Normal digestion of proteins

In ideal conditions protein foods may be fully broken down to (A) amino acids. If in excess, the amino acids are broken down further leaving (B) acidic residues in the bloodstream:

- **(A)** AMINO ACIDS: eg Tryptophan, Tyrosine, Cysteine etc.; which may used in the following ways:
  - o **Combined to make new proteins:** The amino acids can be rebuilt into new proteins which may be either:
    - **Structural proteins** or
    - **Enzymes**
  - o **Broken down to make sugar and ammonia**
    - **Sugar** which gets converted to:
      - **Energy + CO_2 + H_2O**
    - **Ammonia** which:
      - **Is a toxic poison**
      - **Gets converted to uric acid** which:
        - o Lodges in joints and causes gout
      - **Causes neurological problems**
  - o **Converted to Fat**

- **(B)** ACID RESIDUES OF PROTEIN DIGESTION: [Table 10.1] When there is excess protein in the body, it is broken down to amino acids which, when in excess, are then broken down to smaller molecules that leave an acid residue in the blood following digestion, leading to:
  - o **Low pH (acid) in blood** [Table 10.1] which leads to calcium being leached from the bones and teeth in order to neutralise the acid the blood, which leads to:
    - **Osteoporosis** (brittle bones due to calcium leaching)
    - **Dental caries** (decayed teeth due to calcium leaching)
    - **Arthritis** (pain and stiffness in joints)
    - **Atherosclerosis** (hardening of the arterial walls)
    - **Cell death**

Table 10.5 Mal-digestion of proteins

In non-ideal conditions, such as during illness or emotional states, after overeating or mal-combining of food, or in the presence of digestive inhibitors (for example ingested fat); proteins are either only partially digested or broken down, or remain undigested and not broken down at all. Undigested or partially digested proteins act as (a) mechanical blocking agents in the body and are subject to microbial, (b) putrefaction (fermentation of proteins) unless they are rapidly moved out of the intestines. If partially digested proteins enter the bloodstream they may act to give (c) food allergies.

- (A) MECHANICAL BLOCKING AGENTS: Undigested or partially digested proteins may act as (i) mechanical blocking agents in the intestinal tract. Partially digested proteins consisting of a string of amino acids of varying length may also be able to cross the intestinal wall and act as (ii) mechanical blocking agents in the rest of the body, such as blood and lymph and vessels, kidney tubules, joint spaces, and intracellular spaces.

    o **(i) Mechanical blockage of the intestinal tract**: this may be due to:
        - **Physical obstruction** from the undigested food mass, which may undergo putrefaction (fermentation of proteins by bacteria, see below)

        - **Adhesive properties of casein protein**: Casein (the main protein in dairy products) plus water creates a type of glue which can block the intestinal tract or cover the intestinal walls leading to:
            - **Mal-absorption of nutrients** from the intestine through the intestinal walls to the bloodstream.
            - **Poor elimination of wastes** from the bloodstream for the intestinal walls to the intestines.

    o **(ii) Mechanical blockage in the rest of the body**: Partial breakdown products of proteins may cross the intestinal tract into the bloodstream leading to:
        - **Blockage of blood vessels** leading to:
            - **Blood pressure increases**
            - **Circulation decreases**

        - **Intracellular blockage** (since partial breakdown products of proteins are not usually absorbed by cells, they remain in the intracellular spaces), causing:
            - **Mal absorption of nutrients** from the intracellular spaces through the cell walls to the inside (cytoplasm) of the cell.
            - **Poor elimination of wastes** from the inside of the cells through the cell walls to the intracellular spaces.

- (B) FERMENTATION (Putrefaction): if proteins are not rapidly processed in the intestinal tract by the body, they are used as food by microorganisms that are always present in the intestinal tract. The products of microbial degradation of proteins, known as putrefaction, are (i) toxic gases, (ii) poisonous chemicals, and more (iii) microorganisms of an undesirable nature

    o **(i) Toxic Gases**: such as hydrogen sulphide (rotten egg gas), leads to:
        - **Bloating**, or a feeling of fullness with discomfort
        - **Bowel distension**, leading to:
            - **Assimilation** of food ability decreased
            - **Energy supply** depleted
            - **Bowel rupture risk** increased
        - **Anoxia**: lack of oxygen due to presence of other gases in particular carbon dioxide, leading to:
            - **Anaerobic bacteria** increase in number
            - **Aerobic bacteria** decrease in number
        - **Foul smells** coming out of the body leading to:
            - **Social problems**

    o **(ii) Poisonous chemicals** such as putrescine and cadaverine, which can cause:
        - **Nausea**
        - **Headache**
        - **Overstimulation of nerves**
        - **Hormonal changes**
        - **Disturbance of emotional states**
        - **Memory loss**
        - **Liver damage**

- o **(iii) Microorganisms of an undesirable nature**: Microorganisms multiply as they digest the proteins. This leads to:
  - **Intestinal blockage** caused by the shear mass and volume of the growing microorganisms
  - **Poisonous wastes** produced by certain microorganisms
  - **Increased levels of infection**
  - **Nutrient loss** caused by the microorganisms using the nutrients for their own growth.
  - **Displacement of normal healthy microorganisms**, which are mainly aerobic bacteria, with unfriendly anaerobic bacteria.

- **(C) FOOD ALLERGIES**: This is similar to the mal-digestion of complex carbohydrates, but tends to be worse since proteins tend to have more toxic breakdown products than complex carbohydrates. Partial breakdown products of proteins are often not recognised by the immune system as being foreign to the body, since these substances were presented to the body in early childhood when the immune system had not fully integrated itself. As in the case of mal-digested complex carbohydrates, an allergic reaction to partial breakdown products of protein which are not recognised as foreign by the immune system can manifest in many ways including:
  - o Boils
  - o Rashes
  - o Asthma
  - o Pimples
  - o Excema
  - o Dermatitis
  - o Disturbed immune system
  - o Neurological disorders
  - o Immune system dysfunction
  - o Physiological disorders

10.3.5.3 Digestion of foods containing fats

Unheated fats:
- Are only needed in small amounts for:
  - o Cell membrane synthesis
  - o Hormones synthesis.

Heated fats may have:
- Denatured molecular structure
- Altered chemical properties
- Carcinogenic (cancer causing) properties

Excess fat:
- Inhibits gastric secretions which inhibits the digestion of protein
- Increases ketone levels which contributes to liver damage

Cholesterol:
- Is synthesised in animals only (humans also make enough of their own):
  - o For use in the nervous system
  - o For the production of certain hormones.
- Is denatured by cooking, since its soluble coating is disrupted or destroyed, and it becomes insoluble.
- Deposits in blood vessel walls once it has been denatured by cooking, leading to atherosclerosis.
- Paralyses macrophages (scavengers of the immune system) which:
  - o Inhibits the functioning of the immune system in general.

10.3.6 Effects of Nutrition on the Immune system

Studies that discuss the effect of nutrition on the <u>immune system</u> are many. Below are a few points regarding some vitamins and minerals.

- **Zinc:** Deficiency leads to impaired <u>antibody mediated immunity</u> (AMI) and <u>cell mediated immunity</u> (CMI) responses [Section 10.2.3.2.1]. Zinc supplementation causes <u>immunostimulation</u>. <u>Zinc</u> has been reported to improve the depressed <u>immune system</u> of aged animals. According to an article published in the medical journal *The Lancet* in 1991, men who ejaculate more than five times a day risk severe immune deficiency diseases from the <u>zinc</u> loss alone. Hence the *yogic* concept of minimising sperm loss may be seen to have a rational scientific basis.

- **Iron:** Deficiency leads to impaired AMI and CMI responses; similarly, <u>iron</u> overload also impairs immune responses and may be responsible for some diseases.

- **Copper:** Deficiency depresses the <u>immune system</u>, whereas supplementation has been reported to enhance <u>immunocompetence</u>.

- **Selenium:** Deficiency results in depressed AMI and CMI responses. Supplementation is reported to be <u>immunostimulatory</u> and may be of assistance in protecting against malaria.

- **Vitamin A:** Deficiency decreases AMI response. <u>Vitamin A</u> supplementation increases <u>cytotoxic</u> (cell-killing) responses to <u>T cells</u>, <u>natural killer cells</u> [Section 10.2.3.1.4] and <u>macrophages</u>.

- **Vitamin C:** Supplementation enhances CMI response but not the AMI response.

- **Vitamin E:** Deficiency is rare, but supplementation is reported to have an <u>immunostimulatory</u> effect. This may be related to the effects of <u>vitamin E</u> as an antioxidant.

10.3.7 Feeding Young Children

Children, especially infants, require high amounts of good clean, unheated fats and proteins. The best source of fats come from avocado and fresh unheated coconut (young green coconuts, and coconut oil). Some of the best proteins come from uncooked sprouted grains and seeds, such as the young sprouts (two or three days old) of buckwheat and lentil.

Nut and seed milks and nut and seed butters are also a good source of protein once the child is old enough to have them and possible <u>allergic reactions</u> are excluded. Nut and seed milks can be blended with fruit and vegetables to make rich creamy (non-dairy) sauces for dipping vegetables into and delicious smoothies.

Children who are untainted with artificial foods usually know what is best for them to eat. Young kids often like sweet mushy foods which reflects their natural desire for fresh, ripe fruit but this can often be confused with a sometimes socially or drug-induced effect of other sweet mushy foods such as chocolate, custard, and cakes. Also popular with children are crispy foods but it is important not to give them processed crispy foods and instead create your own crispy food snacks. Using an oven or a dessicator to dry combinations of seeds, nuts, fruits and vegetables is one way of creating healthy snack foods.

<u>Amylases</u> (<u>enzymes</u>) for the digesting of <u>starch</u> are not present in substantial amounts in either the mouth [Section 10.1.1] or in the <u>small intestine</u> [Section 10.1.1] and pancreas [Section 10.1.1] in children until well after the formation of teeth. <u>Salivary amylase</u> does not reach adult levels until 19 months. <u>Pancreatic amylase</u> is very low ($1•6\%$ of the adult level at birth) until four months and does not increase until the end of the first year, with mature levels only reached by the fifth year [Gillard et al. 1983]. Therefore one of the worst foods for infants is rice cereal and other foods containing <u>complex carbohydrates</u>, as these foods are not correctly digested at all and may lead to <u>digestive system</u> disturbances such as <u>diarrhoea</u>, promote the growth of unhealthy bacteria and adversely affect the <u>immune system</u>, perhaps causing allergies in later life.

The immune system of children

The <u>immune system</u> of children is not fully developed until the child is about five years old. Any food which is ingested but not digested properly, thus creating partial breakdown products that may enter the bloodstream, may disturb the developing <u>immune system</u>. Partial breakdown products of foods are often small enough to enter the blood stream but are too large or inappropriate to be used by the cells. The immature <u>immune system</u> may respond to partial breakdown products of foods, by incorrectly labelling them as self. Then in later life these breakdown products will not be suitably removed from the body. The body will believe the partial breakdown products belong in the body and instead they will remain to perhaps cause allergic reactions which may manifest in many ways including boils, rashes, asthma, pimples, eczema, dermatitis and food intolerances. Mal-digested partial breakdown products of complex carbohydrates (such as those contained in rice cereals) are probably the most problematic of foods for the developing immune system.

10.3.8 *Yogic* Diets

The most commonly recommended yogic diet in ancient *yoga* texts such as the *Hatha Yoga Pradipika*, the *Gheranda Samhita* and the *Siva Samhita* is the *Sattvic diet,* which is considered pure food. In most places in India, this is generally regarded to be a lacto-vegetarian diet, which includes nuts and grains. When available however and for special occasions the *Phalari diet* is adopted. The *phalari* diet is mainly fruit with some cooked root vegetables. This is generally considered a much higher yogic diet. Many aspirants in India and elsewhere have also spent long periods eating almost nothing or only drinking fluids, and even breatharianism (living only on air and sunlight!) is still considered by some *yogis* to be a valid diet, which may be survived on indefinitely if an advanced *yogi* is ready for it.

A realistic attainable *yogic* diet for the West that may be gradually adapted to over some years provided there is an associated *pranayama* (hypoventilation) practice [Section 10.3.10.3] is a diet of:
- Fresh fruit and vegetable juices
- Fresh whole fruit
- Sprouted salads
- Steamed vegetables.

Such a diet takes time, even years to comfortably adjust to, both mentally as well as physically, but when it is achieved for some time, the level of basic health and vitality is unsurpassed. Studies done on this and similar diets are presented in Section 10.3.9.

The *Tantric Yoga* philosophy on diet is slightly different. Although the basic diet is the same as in the traditional *yoga* diet, it is believed that, as the gastric fire increases (ie your ability to digest and or safely process food), it is possible to eat almost anything (including animal products, alcohol, and even drugs and poisons). Complete awareness and full knowledge of potential side effects of the food is present, yet with complete control of the autonomic nervous system and internal physiology, no harm results from eating such food. Note that such control has been demonstrated by only a few rare individuals who can also perform feats such as alter the speed of the heart and even stop the heart for some time.

10.3.9 Scientific Research on Diets Similar to the Yogic Diets

The articles cited and summarised in this chapter are all published scientific studies that support the information presented in this chapter. This is only a small selection of many hundreds of scientific articles available. Abstracts of all such articles are available on the Internet with a MEDLINE search.

10.3.9.1 Studies on people living on an uncooked vegan diet (living food diet)

Vegans who were following a strict, uncooked vegan diet (living food diet) were studied [Rauma et al., 1995]. The calculated dietary antioxidant intakes by the vegans, expressed as percentages of the US recommended dietary allowances (RDA), were as follows: 305% of Vitamin C, 247% of vitamin A, 313% of vitamin E, 92% of zinc, 120% of copper, and 49% of selenium. Compared with omnivores assessed in these trials, the vegans had significantly higher blood concentrations of beta-carotene, Vitamin C, and vitamin E, as well as higher erythrocyte superoxide dismutase activity. These experiments suggest that the living food diet provides significantly more dietary antioxidants than does a cooked, omnivorous diet, and that long-term adherents of this diet have a better antioxidant status than omnivorous control subjects.

10.3.9.2 Studies on vegans

McCarty [1999] notes that, since amino acids modulate the secretion of both the hormones insulin and glucagon, the composition of dietary protein therefore has the potential to influence the balance of glucagon and insulin activity. Many vegan proteins, are higher in non-essential amino acids than most animal-derived food proteins, and as a result should favour glucagon production. McCarty points out that vegans tend to have low serum lipids, lean physiques, shorter stature, later puberty, and decreased risk for certain prominent cancers. Low-fat vegan diets may be especially protective in regard to cancers linked to insulin resistance, namely, breast and colon cancer, as well as prostate cancer. Conversely, the high IGF-I activity associated with heavy ingestion of animal products may be largely responsible for the epidemic of Western cancers in wealthy societies. Vegans are also likely to have a decreased risk of cancer due to their higher intake of phytochemicals. In addition, low-fat vegan diets coupled with exercise training has been shown to lead to a regression of coronary stenoses; such regimens also tend to markedly improve diabetic control and lower elevated blood pressure. Risk of many other degenerative disorders may also be decreased in vegans.

10.3.9.3 Studies on vegan children

Suzuki [1995] determined that the vitamin B12 status of a group of vegan children aged 7 to 14 was the same as vitamin B12 status of an age-matched omnivorous control group. The vegans diets included brown rice and 2-4 g of nori (dried seaweed which contains vitamin B12) each day. Suzuki concluded that the consumption of nori might keep vegans from suffering B12 deficiency.

In a study by Sanders and Purves [1981], the nutritional status of 23 vegan children between one and five years was assessed using anthropometric and dietary criteria. All of the children had been breastfed for at least the first six months of life and in most cases well into the second year. It was concluded that, provided sufficient care is taken, a vegan diet could meet the nutritional requirements of the preschool child.

10.3.9.4 Studies comparing cooked versus uncooked food

In a study on the effects of eating an uncooked vegetable diet for 1 week in a group of volunteers suffering from a variety of chronic illnesses [Hänninen et al., 1992], a control group ate the same food but cooked for 2 minutes in a microwave oven. After one week on the regimen, both groups showed a decrease in serum protein, urea, and cholesterol. Blood glucose and alanine aminotransferase (ALAT) activity increased in both groups, although all within the normal range. Serum tocopherol (vitamin E) and retinol (vitamin A) increased only in the group eating the uncooked diet. In both groups urinary sodium dropped drastically without a significant change in potassium.

10.3.9.5 Studies on the levels of toxins such as dioxins in various food types

A comparison of various diets found that a vegan diet showed the lowest level of dioxins. Food of animal origin, particularly dairy products, meat, and fish, was identified as the primary immediate source of dioxins and other toxic chemicals [Schecter et al. 1997].

10.3.9.6 Studies on the effects of low-calorie, low-fat diets

In numerous animal experiments, a diet low in calories, low in fat and nutrient-dense, conforms to that which has promoted health, retarded ageing, and extended maximum life span. The eight residents of Biosphere 2 (a 3.15 acre artificial ecosystem that is energetically open but materially closed, with air, water, and organic material being recycled) who had been living on a low calorie, low-fat diet for six months had experienced significant, reductions in cholesterol and blood pressure [Walford, Harris, & Gunion 1992].

10.3.9.7 Studies on the effect of vegan diets on rheumatoid arthritis, obesity and heart disease

In controlled experiments, [Peltonen et al, 1997] it was found that when rheumatoid arthritis (RA) patients were fed living food, in the form of an uncooked vegan diet rich in lactobacilli, the faecal flora was altered and this change was associated with improvement in the arthritis. In another controlled dietary study on rheumatoid arthritis [Kjeldsen-Kragh et al.,1991] it was found that fasting followed by a vegan diet was an effective treatment.

After a controlled dietary experiment [Key et al. 1990] it was concluded that a vegan diet causes a substantial increase in sex hormone binding globulin (SHBG) which is a plasma protein found in mammals that regulates the bioavailability of sex steroids. Botwood et al. [1995] have shown that in women SHBG concentrations are negatively correlated with the amount of body fat. Serum SHBG concentrations are inversely correlated with both fasting and glucose-stimulated insulin levels, and insulin has been shown to have a direct inhibitory effect on SHBG synthesis and secretion by cultured cells. Therefore, obese women may benefit in terms of weight reduction by adopting a vegan diet.

Sanders, Ellis, and Dickerson [1978] compared the fats in the cells of vegans and omnivore controls. It was concluded that a vegan-type diet might be the diet of choice in the treatment of ischemic heart disease, angina pectoris, and certain hyperlipidemias.

In a study by Lindahl *et al* [1984] 29 patients who had suffered from essential hypertension for an average of eight years, all receiving long-term medication for hypertension, were subject to therapy with vegan food for one year. In almost all cases, medication was withdrawn or drastically reduced. There was a significant decrease in systolic and diastolic blood pressure.

In a similar study by Lindahl *et al* [1985] 35 patients who had suffered from bronchial asthma for an average of 12 years, all receiving long-term medication, 20 including cortisone, were subject to therapy with vegan food for one year. In almost all cases, medication was withdrawn or drastically reduced. There was a significant decrease in asthma symptoms.

10.3.9.8 Studies on effects of diets on blood calcium and acid-alkaline levels in blood and bone

Dwyer *et al* [1985] conducted acid-alkaline ash calculations for 7 days worth of omnivore, lacto-ovo, and vegan diets. Vegetarian diets were significantly more alkaline than the omnivore diets, and vegan diets were more alkaline than lacto-ovo-vegetarian diets.

Parfitt [1987] found that, in order to maintain adequate calcium levels in the blood, the body's remodelling system that regulates bone mass sacrifices bone in order to obtain its calcium.

Marsh *et al* [1988] found that the amount and type of dietary protein affects bone mineral loss after the menopause. After 10 years of studying 1,600 women, those who had followed the lacto-ovo-vegetarian diet for at least 20 years had only 18% less bone mineral by age 80 whereas closely paired omnivores had 35% less bone mineral. In addition, the self-selected weighed food intake showed no statistical difference in nutrient intakes but a difference in the acid-alkaline formation of diet.

The effect of supplementing a basal diet containing 697 mg calcium daily (17.4 mmol/d) with an additional 900 mg calcium daily from milk, calcium chloride, or a calcium carbonate preparation was examined in eight adult males during a 56-d metabolic balance study. Lewis *et al* [1989] found that the ingestion of the milk or calcium supplements had no overall effect on calcium retention by these subjects because the milk and supplements depressed absorption of calcium in the gut and fractional tubular re-absorption of calcium in the kidneys.

Grigorov and Sineok [1982] studied the acid-alkaline balance in rats and found that with growing age there was a rising trend towards a decrease in blood pH due to a declining reliability of the organism's buffer systems and a diminished reserve capacity of the regulatory mechanisms of the acid-alkaline balance. While a diet of animal fats and proteins produced metabolic acidosis, a carbohydrate diet produced metabolic alkalosis [Grigorov & Sineok, 1982].

Cook *et al* [1996] did experiments on cats and found that, given a choice of diet, cats avoided high protein diets in an attempt to maintain acid-alkaline homeostasis.

Giannini *et al* [1998] found that people with calcium stones and hypercalciuria (high levels of calcium in the blood) had low blood pH and a disordered bone metabolism and bone loss. Excessive acid, of dietary origin, was suggested as the cause.

Bushings *et al* [1997] found that metabolic acidosis induces the resorption of cultured bone, resulting in a net efflux of calcium (Ca) from the bone and an apparent loss of mineral potassium (K).

New *et al* [1997] compared current and past dietary intake and bone-mineral density between 994 healthy pre-menopausal women aged 45-49. In women with higher intakes of zinc, magnesium, potassium and fibre, bone mineral density was significantly higher. Bone mineral density was lower in women reporting a low intake of milk and fruit in early adulthood than in women with a medium or high intake. New *et al.* [1997] suggested that high, long-term intake of these nutrients may be important to bone health, possibly because of their beneficial effect on acid-alkaline balance.

10.3.10 *Hatha Yoga* for the Immune system and the Digestive System

Hatha *yoga* for the <u>immune system</u> and <u>digestive system</u> has to incorporate not just the *asanas*, which do have a definite role, but also the *pranayamas, bandhas, mudras* and *kriyas*.

10.3.10.1 *Hatha Yoga* for the immune system

Hatha yoga for the <u>immune system</u> is less to do with the actual postures performed but more to do with the attitude and intent of the *yoga* practice. The two most important aspects of the body to concentrate on in order to support the <u>immune system</u> are the <u>circulatory system</u> and <u>nervous system</u>. The way you practise can profoundly affect the outcomes for both the <u>circulatory system</u> and <u>nervous system</u> and, therefore, also the <u>immune system</u>. For example, <u>muscle activations</u> can range from extreme hardness with maximum <u>muscle activation</u> or extreme softness with the muscles as relaxed as possible for the posture to still be performed safely; the breathing work can have infinite variation; and the length of time in each pose will also affect the results.

BKS Iyengar [2000] outlines a series of mainly passive supported postures that he has found to enhance the flow of blood and assist in the health of the <u>immune system</u>. He has also included a series of postures that may assist to relieve the symptoms of <u>Acquired Immune Deficiency Syndrome</u> (AIDS).

Many studies have shown that mild stimulation of the <u>sympathetic nervous system</u> (SNS) that stimulates the secretion of the hormone <u>adrenaline</u> in relatively low blood concentrations is beneficial for the <u>immune system</u>. However, intense stimulation of the SNS that activates the secretion of the <u>adrenaline</u> in relatively high blood concentrations leads to a depression of the <u>immune system</u>. *Hatha yoga* practice with a balance between intensity of *pranayama* and *asana* work may lead to the type of stimulation that supports rather than inhibits the <u>immune system</u>. Assessing whether this has been achieved is best done in a case-by-case subjective manner. Physical indicators of a *hatha yoga* practice that mildly stimulates the SNS to enhance the <u>immune system</u> may include:
- Mild sweat with uniform body heat throughout the practice
- A feeling of balanced and even calmness after the practice

Physical indicators of a *hatha yoga* practice that under-stimulates the SNS without enhancing the <u>immune system</u> may include:
- No change in body heat
- No change in feeling after the practice.

In opposition to this, physical indicators of a *hatha yoga* practice that over-stimulates the SNS and thus may depress the <u>immune system</u> may include:
- Profuse sweating during the practice
- A feeling that the nerves have been jarred at the end of the practice
- Emotional instability at the end of the practice.

10.3.10.2 The use of the *bandhas* in the regulation of the diet

When *bandhas* are applied and incorporated into daily *yoga* practice [Figure 10.2], and maintained during every breath, the effects on eating are generally twofold:
1. The appetite is generally suppressed for at least some time after the practice finishes.
2. The food that you are eventually drawn to eating after a prolonged period of practising *hatha yoga,* with the *bandhas* maintained throughout each posture and each breath, tends to be more <u>alkaline</u> in nature than your previous diet. That is, the food tends to be generally lighter in calories, higher in water content, and contains reduced amounts of protein and <u>complex carbohydrates</u> compared to your previous diet.

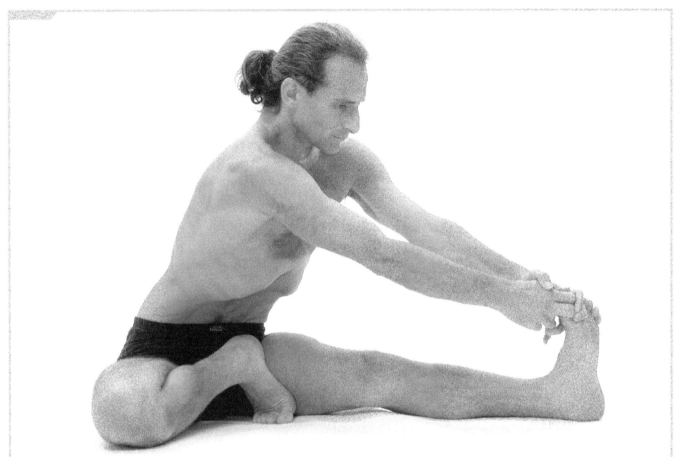

Figure 10.2: *Bhaga maha mudra* with *uddiyana* and *mula bandha*: Regular practice of *bandhas* and *mudras* in a *hatha yoga* practice help to suppress the appetite

10.3.10.3 Appetite is generally suppressed for some time after a practice where *bandhas* are maintained with hypoventilation

Appetite tends to be reduced after a practice where the *bandhas* are applied throughout each breath and in every posture. This is partly due to the central root lock (*mula bandha*) causing a contraction around the stomach and the other organs of digestion. The compression around the abdomen tends to push energy away from the organs of digestion. Fermentation and putrefaction are less likely to occur in the cavities of the digestive organs when they have become small and compressed by the pressure imposed by abdominal muscle contractions of a *ha-mula bandha* [eg Figure 10.2]. In addition, the electrochemical signals of the parasympathetic nervous system, which generally are sent to the stomach to stimulate the appetite, will also be suppressed. This suppression of the parasympathetic input is partly caused by the pushing away effect of *ha-mula bandha* but also due to the abdominal muscle tension created by the *ha-mula bandha* stimulating the sympathetic nervous system, which suppresses the appetite. Finally, if *tha-uddiyana bandha* [eg Figure 10.2] and the other *tha-bandhas* (expansive *bandhas*) in the rest of the body are maintained throughout the practice, then energy in the form of oxygenated blood and nutrients will be pulled from the centre of the body and the organs of digestion towards the periphery. At the same time, the compressive force generated by the abdominal muscles in *ha-mula bandha* is pushing the blood and nutrients away from the centre of the body. The body is therefore left feeling charged. This originates from the *prana* (life-force) in the breath that is drawn to the chest then upper abdomen with the *tha-uddiyana bandha* on the inhale and then directed from the body's centre to its periphery.

If, alternatively, the abdomen is kept soft and expanded throughout a *hatha yoga* practice then the reverse of the above will happen. Energy and the requirement for food will be drawn towards the relatively low pressure expanded abdominal centre, and the organs of digestion. A craving for food is more likely to occur after (or even sometimes during) the *yoga* practice. Nutrients will no longer be pushed from the centre and pulled to the periphery so a feeling of lethargy may ensue and a craving for food is more likely to occur after (or even sometimes during) the *yoga* practice. Finally, often the urge to eat is usually not one of genuine hunger but a genuine need to help move <u>fermenting</u> and <u>putrefying</u> food residues from the stomach and through the <u>gastrointestinal tract</u>. Therefore, we often eat to help push the stale or rotting food from our bowels with fresh <u>unfermented</u> food. A similar pushing effect may be obtained by using the pushing effect of the <u>spinal flexor</u> and <u>spinal extensor</u> muscles in *mula bandha*.

One tends to be more content with more light and fresh food after a practice where *bandhas* are maintained with hypoventilation

A *yoga* practice in which *ha-mula bandha* and *tha-uddiyana bandha* are maintained throughout each in-breath and out-breath [eg Figure 10.2] , tends to reduce the amount of air that is taken into the <u>lungs</u> per minute. With the abdomen drawn inwards, as in *ha-mula bandha*, the diaphragm cannot move as far down (caudally) as it can when the abdomen is fully relaxed. In addition, when the inhalation takes place with the chest already at its maximum expansion as in *tha-uddiyana bandha*, and the abdomen at its maximum muscular compression as in *ha-mula bandha*, the maximum inspiratory volume of air is only small relative to the maximum lung capacity when no *bandhas* are applied before the inspiration begins. Prolonged breathing in this manner is a type of hypoventilation that tends to lead to a build up of CO_2 in the body and hence a build up of <u>carbonic acid</u>. The resulting <u>respiratory acidosis</u> then has to be balanced by a <u>metabolic alkalosis</u>. The easiest way to balance <u>acidity</u> in the body via the metabolism is through an <u>alkalising</u> diet of light fresh foods or to remain free of food for some time after practice, which is exactly what is recommended in all the classical *yoga* texts.

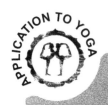

No 10.1 Use your diaphragm to breathe into the abdomen to help the digestive system and immune system function better

Breathing into the abdomen (diaphragmatic breathing) stimulates the parasympathetic nervous system, which controls the digestive and immune systems. Therefore, on a neurological level, diaphragmatic breathing helps digestion of food as well recovery from disease and illness, and the healing of injuries.

Also on a neurological level, the natural activity (contraction) of the diaphragm (the main muscle of abdominal inhalation) can help digestive and immune system function by reciprocally relaxing or inhibiting the muscles of forced abdominal exhalation that pull the navel to the spine. Exhaling fully by drawing the navel to the spine is great for emptying the lungs, massaging the internal organs, and pushing 'stale blood and other fluids' out of them. However, keeping the navel to the spine and not relaxing the muscles that do this on inhalation by breathing diaphragmatically is a common chronic practice in many people. This erroneous practice tends to keep pressure on the internal organs of digestion and immunity and prevent the entry of fresh blood into these organs.

On a physical level, breathing naturally into the abdomen when it is firmed by posture or natural activities such as relaxed walking (provided the navel has not been drawn closer to the spine) helps digestion and immunity because the internal organs involved are massaged (compressed) as the diaphragm actively moves away from the chest into the abdomen on inhalation, and then released and relaxed (expanded) as the diaphragm passively moves towards the chest and away from the abdomen on exhalation.

****

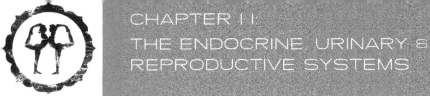
Chapter Breakdown

****

11.0 INTRODUCTION TO THE APPLIED ANATOMY & PHYSIOLOGY OF THE ENDOCRINE, URINARY & REPRODUCTIVE SYSTEMS IN *HATHA YOGA*

Hatha yoga for the endocrine system focuses around the major *cakras* or *yogic* psycho-energetic centres. Each of these esoteric energy centres is reputed to correspond anatomically to a nerve plexus and an endocrine gland.

Hatha yoga for the urinary system focuses on static postures (*asanas*) and dynamic exercises (*vinyasas*) which can enhance circulation to the urinary system. *Asanas* and *vinyasas* can also bring strength, flexibility and control to the muscles of the perineum, pelvic floor, lower abdomen, lower back, inner thighs and buttocks. These muscles have fascial connections to the organs of the urinary system. When these muscles are activated they pull (exert forces) on the urinary system organs which help to physically massage and stimulate them. In addition, appropriately applied *asanas, vinyasas, bandhas* (internal locks)*, mudras* (energy-control gestures and exercises) and *pranayamas* (breath-control exercises) can affect the nervous system control of the urinary system, stimulate acupuncture meridians affecting this body system and assist the flow of *prana* (subtle energy) and *citta* (consciousness) through the *nadis* (subtle channels). Thus *mula bandha* is a useful practice for the health of the urinary system.

In a similar fashion *hatha yoga* can effectively work on the male and female reproductive systems. The male reproductive system can generally be addressed as for the urinary system with an emphasis on *mula bandha* practice. However, *hatha yoga* for the female reproductive system is far more complex in that it has to take into account a woman's age and current physiological state, eg prepubescent, menstruation, pregnancy or menopause. A good reference is the work of Geeta Iyengar's [1983] book *Yoga: a Gem for Women*.

11.1. THE ENDOCRINE SYSTEM

11.1.1 Endocrine and Exocrine Glands

11.1.1.1 Exocrine glands
Exocrine glands secrete their products through ducts into body cavities or onto body surfaces.

11.1.1.2 Endocrine glands
Endocrine glands secrete hormones into the blood.

11.1.1.3 Endocrine system
The endocrine system consists of endocrine glands and several organs that contain endocrine tissue.

11.1.1.4 Homeostasis
Homeostasis is the consistency of the body's internal environment. The endocrine system uses hormones, while the nervous system uses nerve impulses to control homeostasis.

11.1.2 Hormones
Hormones are chemical messengers. They are secretions of endocrine tissue that alter the physiological activity of target cells in the body. Hormones are chemically classified as steroids, amines, proteins, or eicosanoids. Water-soluble protein hormones circulate freely in the blood, while the fat-soluble protein hormones are attached to transport proteins.

Hormones only affect specific target cells that have receptors to recognise and bind to a particular hormone. Receptor numbers may increase or decrease (up-regulation or down-regulation respectively). Up-regulation and down-regulation forms the basis of the physiological mechanisms for the addictions to many drugs such as heroin or morphine. It is for the same reason that some people may get addicted to certain exercise regimes if they generate endorphins (endogenous morphine).

11.1.2.1 Effects of hormones

- Hormones help regulate metabolism, energy balance, and the chemical composition and volume of the extracellular fluid throughout the internal environment.
- Hormones help regulate the control of smooth muscle and cardiac muscle fibres, secretion by the glands and certain activities of the immune system.
- Hormones play an important role in growth, development and reproduction.

11.1.3 Major Endocrine Glands

The major endocrine glands and their secretions are described in Table 11.1.

11.1.3.1 Hypothalamus[Table 11.1]

The hypothalamus is a small region between the lobes of the thalamus in the brain; it is the primary link between the endocrine system and the nervous system.

11.1.3.2 Pituitary gland [Table 11.1]

The pituitary gland is a pea-sized structure attached to the hypothalamus. The posterior pituitary, which stores and secretes oxytocin and antidiuretic hormone (ADH), contains the axons of about 5000 neurons whose cell bodies are located in the hypothalamus, which is where oxytocin and ADH are actually produced. The anterior pituitary is the main endocrine portion that produces and secretes the other main pituitary hormones.

11.1.3.3 Pineal gland [Table 11.1]

The pineal gland has only recently begun to be understood by medical science. It is attached to the roof of the third ventricle of the brain. Melatonin, an important secretion of the pineal gland is stimulated by darkness. Melatonin affects circadian cycles (daily rhythms), and therefore also affects the timing and release of many other hormones.

Melatonin is a potent antioxidant. It can prevent both the initiation and promotion of cancer and plays an important role in the immune system. Melatonin induces activated T cells to release opioid peptides with immune-enhancing and anti-stress properties. These peptides cross-react and bind specifically to thymus gland receptors.

Deep sleep and meditation produce melatonin under certain conditions [Tooley et al., 2000]. Melatonin is produced in greater quantities when there is some stimulation of parasympathetic nervous system [Section 9.5.2], and when feeling calm. The practice of *nadi sodhana pranayama* [Figure 8.1] (alternate nostril breathing) allows a practitioner to readily modify the levels of melatonin.

Abbreviations used in Table 11.1: H = hormone; RH = releasing hormone; IH = inhibiting hormone; SH = stimulating hormone.

Table 11.1 Endocrine organs or tissues: their major hormones and important actions
Abbreviations: H = Hormone; RH = Releasing hormone; SH = Stimulating hormone

ENDOCRINE ORGAN/TISSUE	HORMONE	ACTION
Hypothalamus	1. Corticotropin-RH 2. Gonadotropin-RH. (GnRH) 3. Growth hormone RH 4. Somatostatin 5. Prolactin-IH 6. Prolactin-RH 7. Thyrotropin-RH	1. Increases ACTH production 2. Increases FSH & LH secretion 3. Increases GH secretion 4. Decreases GH secretion 5. Decreases PR secretion 6. Increases PR secretion 7. Increases TSH secretion
Pituitary gland	1. Adrenocorticotropic H (ACTH) 2. Follicle stimulating H (FSH) 3. Growth H (GH) 4. Lutenizing H (LH) 5. Prolactin (PR) 6. Thyroid SH (TSH) 7. Melanocyte SH (MSH) 8. Antidiuretic H (ADH) 9. Oxytocin	1. Secretion of adrenal hormones. 2. Oogenesis; spermatogenesis; regulation of menstruation. 3. Anabolism, growth & development. 4. Oogenesis; spermatogenesis; regulation of menstruation. 5. Milk production. 6. Production & secretion of thyroid hormones. 7. Functions not well understood. 8. Water reabsorption. 9. Milk letdown; uterine contraction.

Gland/Tissue	Hormone(s)	Function(s)
Pineal gland	1. Melatonin	1. Regulation of circadian (daily) rhythms; effects on the brain, reproductive system, & secretion of other hormones; production of melatonin is stimulated by darkness, states of meditation and the *yoga* practices of *nadi sodhana pranayama* (and more powerfully – *candra bhedana pranayama*) and *trataka* (light gazing).
Thyroid gland	1. Calcitonin 2. Thyroxine	1. Increases bone deposition of calcium; decreases plasma calcium. 2. Regulates metabolism, growth, development, & activity of the nervous system.
Parathyroid glands	1. Parathormone	1. Increases blood calcium, decreases blood phosphate.
Thymus gland	1. Thymosin & other hormones	1. Stimulates maturation of T cells; possibly retard the aging process.
Adrenal glands	1. Aldosterone 2. Androgens 3. Cortisol 4. Adrenalin & Noradrenaline	1. Increases sodium retention & potassium excretion. 2. Stimulates sexual drive & hair growth in females. 3. Regulates metabolism; resists stress; & counters inflammatory response. 4. Produces effects that mimic the sympathetic nervous system during stress.
Kidney tissue	1. Calcitriol (active form of vitamin D produced in the skin) 2. Erythropoietin	1. Aids absorption of calcium from foods; regulates concentrations of calcium & phosphate in body fluids. 2. Stimulates red blood cell production in bone marrow.
Testes	1. Testosterone 2. Inhibin	1. Develops & maintains male sexual characteristics; regulate spermatogenensis; stimulates descent of the testes before birth. 2. Inhibits secretion of FSH to control sperm production.
Ovaries	1. Oestradiol & Progesterone 2. Inhibin	1. Develops & maintains female sexual characteristics, including development of mammary glands & uterus; regulates menstrual cycle [Table 11.2]. 2. Inhibit secretion of FSH towards the end the menstrual cycle.
Placenta	1. Human chorionic gonadotropin 2. Human placental lactogen 3. Relaxin 4. Oestrogen 5. Progesterone	1. Maintains corpus luteum during pregnancy. 2. Prepares for lactation; supports foetal bone growth. 3. Relaxes pubic symphysis & helps dilate the uterine cervix near the end of pregnancy. 4. Maintains uterine lining; stimulates breasts. 5. Stimulates breasts; inhibits uterine contraction.
Stomach tissue	1. Gastrin 2. Motilin	1. Increases gastric secretions; increases stomach motility. 2. Increases stomach motility.
Heart (atrium)	1. Atrial natriuretic hormone	1. Regulates solute and water loss by the kidney.

Most tissues	1. Prostaglandins	1. Increases inflammation; stimulates uterine contraction.
Duodenal tissue	1. Cholecystokinin (CCK). (secretion is stimulated by the presence of fats & proteins) 2. Gastric inhibitory peptide (GIP) 3. Secretin	1. Contraction of gall bladder; increases pancreatic enzyme secretion; inhibits gastric emptying; stimulates secretion and motility in the small intestine; induces satiety. 2. Inhibits stomach motility and release of gastric juices; stimulates release of insulin. 3. Causes the stomach to produce pepsin, the liver to make bile, and the pancreas to produce alkaline secretions; inhibits gastric juice secretion & gastrin release; and inhibits gastric emptying; stimulated by high acid levels in the intestine.
Pancreas	1. Glucagon 2. Insulin 3. Somatostatin 4. Pancreatic polypeptide	1. Raises blood glucose by increased breakdown of glycogen to glucose in liver, and increased conversion of other nutrients to glucose in liver. 2. Lowers blood glucose by stimulating transport of glucose to cells, conversion of glucose to glycogen, & decreased synthesis of glucose from other nutrients; also increases lipogenesis (fat production) & protein synthesis 3. Inhibits secretion of insulin and glucagon. 4. Regulates release of pancreatic digestive enzymes.

11.1.3.4 Thyroid gland [Table 11.1]

The thyroid gland is located just below the larynx, weighing about 30g, with lateral lobes on either side of the trachea and an anterior mass joining them. The thyroid gland receives about 80-120ml/min of blood and collects and contains most of the iodide in the body that it uses to synthesise thyroid hormones. Thyroid hormones regulate:

• Basal metabolic rate
• Cellular metabolism
• Growth and development.

11.1.3.5 Parathyroid glands [Table 11.1]

The parathyroid glands are small round masses of tissue embedded on the posterior surfaces of the lateral lobes of the thyroid gland. The parathyroid glands function to regulate calcium (increases) and phosphate (decreases) homeostasis in the blood.

11.1.3.6 Thymus gland [Table 11.1]

The thymus gland is a bi-lobed organ, located in the mediastinum, posterior to the sternum and between the lungs. It plays an essential role in the immune system (maturation of T lymphocytes), hence it is a major link between the endocrine system and the immune system.

11.1.3.7 Pancreas [Table 11.1]

The pancreas is attached to the first loop of the duodenum as it leaves the stomach. This is both an endocrine gland and an exocrine gland.

11.1.3.8 Adrenal glands [Table 11.1]

The paired adrenal glands are attached to the superior portion of each kidney. They consist of an outer, larger, adrenal cortex that produces steroid hormones such as aldosterone, cortisol and certain androgens and an inner, smaller, adrenal medulla that produces the catecholamines, adrenaline and noradrenaline.

11.1.3.9 Gonads [Table 11.1]

Gonads are the gamete-producing organs. Gametes are the sex cells. Female gonads are the ovaries, and male gonads are the testes [Section 11.3]. Both gonads produce hormones that affect the whole body.

11.1.3.10 Other endocrine tissues [Table 11.1]

Probably every tissue in the body will eventually be shown to secrete some hormones. All cells capable of undergoing an inflammatory response may secrete prostaglandin hormones. The gastrointestinal (GI) tract secretes many hormones to do with the digestion and absorption of food. The atria of the heart secrete a hormone that helps control blood pressure. The kidneys secrete erythropoietin, a hormone that stimulates red blood cell production. The skin produces vitamin D, which acts as a hormone controlling the homeostasis of calcium and phosphate.

11.1.4 Relationship Between the Endocrine, Nervous and Immune Systems

Until recently, these three body systems were thought of as being independent, but in the last twenty years it has become increasingly apparent that these three systems interact and communicate with each other.

11.1.4.1 Psychoneuroimmunology (PNI)

Psychoneuroimmunology (PNI) is the study of the inter-relationships between the three body-mind systems that serve as communication networks in the orchestration of homeostasis, which are the endocrine, nervous and immune systems.

Interactions between the endocrine system, nervous system and immune system include the following:

- Hormones such as insulin [Section 10.3.3.2.1] have been shown to act like neurotransmitters in the brain.
- The nerves of the gastro-intestinal (GI) tract are so complex that they have been designated as a third element of the autonomic nervous system, called the enteric nervous system (ENS) [Section 9.5.3] which has been shown to respond to the neurotransmitter effects of many GI hormones and other hormones.
- Nerve endings in the spleen and the thymus have been shown to have a synapse-like relationship [Section 9.1.3] with lymphocytes [Section 10.2].
- Chemical mediators synthesised and secreted by cells of the immune system [Section 10.2] (immunotransmitters) have been shown to function like neurotransmitters [Section 9.1.3.1] in some places and like hormones in other places.
- Neurotransmitters have been found in immune tissue such as bone marrow.
- Cortisol (an adrenal hormone which increases with stress) has been shown to inhibit cells of the immune system. Cortisol has also been shown to be increased in people who are depressed.
- At low concentrations adrenaline has been shown to stimulate the immune system.
- Small protein hormones called cytokines are secreted by many types of white blood cells and also by brain cells. This suggests a communication between the immune system (white blood cells) the nervous system (brain) and the endocrine system (cytokine hormones).

There is a growing body of evidence suggesting that thoughts and emotions that people generate have a direct influence on the state of their major body systems and hence their overall health.

11.2 THE URINARY SYSTEM

The urinary system (in particular the kidney) is central to the process of elimination in the body. Other important organs of elimination are the lungs, skin and gastrointestinal (GI) tract. The urinary system consists of two kidneys, two ureters, one urinary bladder and the urethra.

11.2.1 Kidneys

Location of the kidneys

The kidneys are attached to the posterior abdominal wall between the levels of T12 and L3 vertebrae.

External and internal organisation of the kidneys

Each kidney is enclosed and protected by a renal capsule, adipose capsule and renal fascia. Internally the kidneys have an outer cortex and an inner medulla.

Function of the kidneys

The function of the kidney is to regulate: (a) the volume and composition of the blood; (b) blood pressure; (c) blood plasma pH; and (c) some aspects of metabolism. Kidneys receive about 1.1 litres/minute of blood flow (20% of cardiac output).

Functional unit of the kidneys: The nephron

The functional unit of the kidney is the renal tubule or nephron. There are millions of nephrons in each kidney and each nephron produces a very small amount of urine. The nephron consists of a renal corpuscle (glomerulus and glomerular capsule) and a renal tubule.

Function of the nephrons

Nephrons function as a primary route by which metabolic end products such as urea, uric acid, creatinine, ammonia, phosphate and sulphate leave the body. Nephrons maintain homeostasis (equilibrium or constant conditions) of body fluid volume and solute composition by balancing urinary excretion with dietary intake of water and ions of minerals such as chlorine, sodium, potassium and calcium. The nephrons control blood plasma pH.

Blood enters the kidneys via the renal artery and leaves via the renal vein. The nephrons form urine by glomerular filtration of blood, tubular reabsorption of useful substances and tubular secretion of unwanted substances. The glomerular capsule filters most substances in the blood. The exception is blood cells and proteins, which are not filtered. Chemicals not needed are discharged into the urine by tubular secretion. Included for discharge are ions (potassium, hydrogen, and ammonium), nitrogenous wastes (urea, creatine) and certain drugs.

Urine

Urine is the end product of a process in which about 200 litres/day of a protein free filtrate of blood passes through tiny tubular structures that modify its composition, reducing its volume by reabsorption to about 1% to make urine (about 1-2 ml/min). Urine contains many substances that can still be useful for the body. Urine is a sterile, antiseptic fluid. It is the excess nutrients, metabolites and water from the blood plasma.

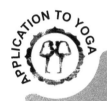

No 11.1 Amaroli: the *yogic* practice of drinking your own urine may be of great benefit

Various types of auto-urine therapy are possible. The main component of urine, called urea, is used in many cosmetics as it is recognised as being one of the best moisturisers available. Your own urine may be used topically to clean certain infections of the skin. It can even be used very successfully for ear and eye infections. Drinking your own urine has reputedly many health benefits especially for the immune system. Many studies have been published over the last 100 years that document the efficacy of auto-urine therapy. Much information is also available on the internet.

(*See http://www.geocities.com/Athens/Ithaca/9012/amaroli.htm#Resources*)

11.2.2 Ureters

The ureters are tubular structures at the rear of the peritoneal cavity (abdominal cavity) that transport urine from the renal pelvis to the urinary bladder mainly by peristalsis.

11.2.3 Urinary Bladder

The urinary bladder is located posterior to the pubic symphysis. Its function is to store the urine prior to micturition (urination). Lack of control over micturition is called incontinence; failure to void urine completely or normally is called retention.

11.2.4 Urethra

The urethra is the tube leading from the floor of the urinary bladder and functioning to discharge urine from the body.

11.3 THE REPRODUCTIVE SYSTEM

Reproduction is the process by which new individuals of a species are produced and the genetic material is passed from one generation to another.

Reproductive organs are (i) gonads, which produce gametes (sex cells); (ii) ducts, which transport and store gametes; and (iii) accessory sex glands, which produce material that supports the gametes.

11.3.1 Male Reproductive System

The male reproductive system includes the testes, the scrotum, the male duct system and the accessory sex glands:

11.3.1.1 Testes (gonads)

The testes are oval-shaped glands (gonads) in the scrotum, which contain seminiferous tubules where sperm are made (spermatogenesis), and where testosterone is produced. Testosterone, the most important male hormone, controls the growth, development, and maintenance of sex organs; stimulates bone growth, protein anabolism and sperm maturation and stimulates the development of male secondary characteristics.

11.3.1.2 Scrotum

The scrotum is an outpouching of the abdomen supporting the testes, which regulate their temperature by activation and relaxation of the cremaster muscle.

11.3.1.3 Male duct system

The male duct system includes the:
- **Seminiferous tubules** where sperm production takes place
- **Ductus epididymis** the site of sperm maturation and storage
- **Ductus (vas) deferens** which stores sperm and propels them to the urethra for ejaculation
- **Ejaculatory ducts** which forms from the union of the ducts from the seminal vesicles and the ductus (vas) deferens, and which eject spermatozoa into the **Prostatic urethra**.

11.3.1.4 Accessory sex glands

Semen is a mixture of spermatozoa (mature sperm cells) and secretions from the three accessory glands:
(i)   **Seminal vesicles** (alkaline secretion to neutralise acidity of male urethra and female vagina, constitutes 60% of semen and helps in sperm viability).
(ii)   **Prostate gland** (slightly acid secretion that contributes to sperm motility).
(iii)   **Bulbourethral glands** (alkaline mucous secretion for lubrication).

11.3.1.5 Penis

The penis is the male organ of copulation. It achieves erection by the expansion of its blood sinuses under the influence of sexual excitation.

11.3.2 Female Reproductive System

The female reproduction system includes the ovaries, uterine tubes (fallopian tubes), uterus, vagina, vulva and mammary glands.

11.3.2.1 Ovaries (gonads)

The ovaries are situated in the upper pelvic cavity on either side of the uterus; they produce secondary oocytes (AKA gametes, ova, or eggs) by the process of oogenesis and discharge them (ovulation). The ovaries secrete hormones such as oestrogens, progesterones, inhibin and relaxin.

11.3.2.2 Uterine tubes (fallopian tubes)

The fallopian tubes transport ova from the ovaries to the uterus by the action of cilia (small hairs) and peristaltic contractions of the tube walls.

11.3.2.3 Uterus

The uterus has the size and shape of an inverted pear; functions in menstruation, transportation of spermatozoa, implantation of a fertilised ovum, development of a foetus during pregnancy and labour.

Table 11.2 Phases of the female reproductive cycle

Abbreviations: LH = Luteinising hormone; FSH = Follicle stimulating hormone

DAYS	OVARY (OVARIAN CYCLE)	UTERUS (MENSTRUAL CYCLE)	HORMONE LEVELS
1 to 4	**Follicular phase begins**: corpus luteum degenerates; several follicles begin to mature.	**Menstrual phase**: outer layer of endometrium sheds after oestradiol and progesterone levels fall.	Oestradiol, progesterone, FSH and LH levels all low.
5 to 13	**Follicular phase continues**: FSH stimulates follicle maturation.	**Proliferative phase**: endometrium regrows	Oestradiol rising; Progesterone low; FSH & LH rise sharply; Oestradiol falls after follicle ovulates.
14	**Ovulatory phase**: surge of LH causes ovulation.	Increased cervical mucous which is thin, watery & clear, but can stretch 12-15 cm; basal body temperature increases by 0.2-0.4°C; cervix opens, rises & becomes softer; occasional ovarian pain (lasting from a few hours to a few days).	Oestradiol falls after follicle ovulates.
15 to 28	**Luteal phase**: corpus luteum secretes oestradiol & progesterone.	**Secretory phase**: endometrium thickens in readiness for implantation & secretes uterine milk.	Oestradiol & progesterone high; FSH & LH low.

11.3.2.4 Vagina

The vagina functions as:
(i)   a passageway for spermatozoa and the menstrual flow
(ii)   receptacle of the penis during sexual intercourse
(iii)   the lower portion of the birth canal (and so is capable of considerable distension).

11.3.2.5 Vulva

The vulva is the female external genitals and consists of the mons pubis, labia major and labia minor, clitoris, vestibule, vaginal orifice and urethral orifice, hymen, bulb of the vestibule and the paraurethral gland, greater vestibular gland and lesser vestibular gland.

11.3.2.6 Mammary glands

The mammary glands are modified sweat glands over the pectoralis major muscles whose function is to synthesise, secrete, and eject milk (lactation) and whose development is dependent on oestrogen and progesterone. Milk secretion is mainly due to the hormone prolactin and milk ejection is stimulated by the hormone oxytocin.

11.3.2.7 Female reproductive cycle [Table 11.2]

The function of the menstrual cycle (average length 28 days; normal range 21-35 days) is to prepare the inner layer of the uterus (endometrium) each month for the reception of the fertilised egg. The menstrual cycle and ovarian cycle are controlled by gonadotropin releasing hormone (GnRH) from the , which stimulates the release of follicle stimulating hormone (FSH) and luteinizing hormone (LH) by the anterior pituitary gland.

11.3.3 Development
11.3.3.1 Development during pregnancy

Pregnancy starts with fertilisation, which is the penetration of the secondary oocyte by a sperm cell to form a zygote and the subsequent union of sperm and ovum nuclei.

11.3.3.2 Embryonic development

During embryonic growth the primary germ layers (ectoderm, mesoderm and endoderm, which all form tissues in the developing organism) and the embryonic membranes (the yolk sac, amnion, chorion, and allantois) are formed.

Foetal and maternal materials (eg gases, nutrients, drugs and alcohol) are exchanged through the placenta. Most microorganisms cannot cross the placenta but certain viruses (eg HIV and the viruses causing German measles, chicken pox, and polio) are able to pass through the placenta.

11.3.3.3 Gestation

Gestation is the period that the foetus is carried in the uterus. It lasts about 266 days after fertilisation.

11.3.3.4 Maternal changes during pregnancy

During gestation, several important anatomical and physiological changes take place in the mother. These include:
- Anatomical changes, such as a massive increase in the size of the uterus, which nearly fills the abdominal cavity by the end of pregnancy, and which may exert considerable pressure on all the abdominal organs.
- Physiological changes induced by maternal and placental hormones, such as weight gain due to foetus, amniotic fluid, placenta, uterine enlargement, increased body water, increased storage of proteins, fats and minerals.

Other changes during pregnancy include:
- Breast enlargement
- Lower back pain due to increased lordosis
- Cardiopulmonary changes such as increases in lung tidal volume
- Heart stroke volume and heart rate
- Increase in appetite
- Decease in gastrointestinal (GI) tract motility which may result in constipation
- Changes in skin pigmentation
- Changes in the reproductive system such as increased vascularity of the vulva and increased vascularity and pliability of the vagina

11.3.3.5 Foetal changes

During pregnancy, the foetus is totally dependent on the mother. At birth, important changes must take place in the respiratory system and the cardiovascular system in order for the baby to become independent.

11.3.4 Inheritance

The major biochemical involved in inheritance is deoxyribonucleic acid (DNA). DNA is a nucleic acid that is in the shape of a double helix constructed of two long strands of nucleotides consisting of one of four nitrogenous bases designated A, G, C, or T. Encoded in the DNA is genetic information that is passed from one generation to the next as inheritance.

The two strands of the DNA double helix are complementary; one dictates the structure of the other. An A on one strand must always be paired with a T on the other strand. Similarly a G on one strand must always be paired with a C on the other strand. This principle forms the basis of replication of DNA and hence the basis of inheritance.

11.4 APPLIED ANATOMY & PHYSIOLOGY OF THE ENDOCRINE, URINARY & REPRODUCTIVE SYSTEMS IN HATHA YOGA

11.4.1 Applied Physiology of the Endocrine System in *Hatha Yoga*

Efficient circulation is essential for health because it enhances the delivery of nutrients and the removal of metabolic wastes from each of the body cells, but in *yoga* terms, it has one more function that is essential. Efficient circulation enhances communication between cells via the transportation of biochemical signals such as hormones, neurotransmitters and immunotransmitters.

The newly emerging field of psychoneuroimmunology [Maier *et al.*, 1994] considers these biochemical signals to be at the core of our thinking process, therefore their transport can be thought of as the physiological basis for the mobilisation of consciousness throughout the body. Psychoneuroimmunology is the study of the interrelationships between psychological, neuroendocrine and immunological parameters and is concerned with how these relationships may affect an individual's health.

Substantial evidence indicates that exercise is associated with improvements in mental health, neuroendocrine, and immune functioning [La Perriere *et al.*, 1994]. *Yoga* and psychoneuroimmunology are both holistic approaches to health. Ward [1995] discusses the close relationship between psychoneuroimmunology, meditation and holistic medicine.

11.4.1.1 Interrelationship between endocrine, nervous, urinary and reproductive systems, *cakras* and acupuncture

Hatha yoga work for the endocrine system focuses around the major *cakras* (pronounced charkras) or *yogic* psychic centres. Each of these esoteric energy centres corresponds anatomically to a nerve plexus and an endocrine gland [Saraswati, 1985; Motoyama, 1993] [Table 11.4].

Yoga teaches that the vital energy of the body or life force, which is referred to as *prana,* is absorbed through the body from the universe through energy centres called *cakras*. Motoyama [1993] has done many experiments that give scientific support to the ancient *yogic* belief in the physical existence of the seven to ten main *cakras* and their close connection with corresponding parts of the nervous system and endocrine system. Table 11.3 shows the relationships between the *cakras*, the endocrine system, nervous system, urinary system, reproductive system and emotional states. This information is derived from Swami Satyananda Saraswati's [1985] classic book *Kundalini Tantra* which refers to Motoyama's work in some detail and from Motoyama's [1993] work entitled *A Study of Yoga from Eastern and Western Medical Viewpoints – Control of Body and Mind through the Activation of Prana*.

Table 11.3 Relationship between the eight main *cakras*, the nervous system and the endocrine system [Adapted from Maheshwarananda, 2004; Raman, 1998 & Saraswati, 1985]

CAKRA	PHYSICAL LOCATION	FUNCTION	NERVOUS SYSTEM	ENDOCRINE SYSTEM
MULADHARA	Perineum; cervix	Control of the element earth nourishment, absorption, elimination, control of sexual energy	Sacrococcygeal plexus, inferior hypogastric plexus, coeliac plexus	Gonads (testes or ovaries)
SVADISTHANA	Coccyx	Control of the element water and smell	Pelvic plexus, hypogastric plexus	Adrenal glands
MANIPURA	Behind the navel	Control of the element fire	Gastric plexus, solar plexus	Pancreas
ANAHATA	Behind the heart	Control of the element air	Cardiac plexus	Thymus gland
VISHUDDHI	Behind the throat	Control of the element ether Mastery leads to distinct fluid & clear speech	Cervical, pharangeal larangeal, carotid plexus	Thyroid gland
AJNA	Centre of forehead	The activation of joy. and knowledge	Cavernous plexus, thalamus Medulla oblongata	Pituitary gland
BINDU	Back of the head beneath the cowlick	Calming the emotions	Hypothalmus	Hypothalmus
SAHASRARA	Crown of Head	Harmonious functioning of all parts of the brain	Hypothalamic pituitary plexus, Cerebrum (brain)	Pineal gland

Motoyama's [1993] research provides evidence indicating that the Indian system of *cakras* (subtle energy centres) and *nadis* (energy channels) is related to the acupuncture meridian system. He asserts that these are essentially the same systems and they are related to the various body systems [Table 11.4].

The *cakras* need to be opened sequentially from the base *cakra* upwards. This can be encouraged by learning to move one vertebra at a time from the base of the spine (L4-L5) upwards and by using complete breathing (Section 8.4.6).

11.4.2 Applied Anatomy and Physiology of the Urinary System in *Hatha Yoga*

Research on the effects of *hatha yoga* on the urinary system is very limited. Therefore a thorough analysis of this subject is beyond the scope of this book. However, experienced *yoga* teachers routinely prescribe *hatha yoga* for the urinary system and it is predominantly centred on application of the central *bandhas*, muscular, postural and gravitational stimulation of the the region of the kidneys and stimulation of the nerves and acupuncture meridians pertaining to this body system.

A regular and gentle practice of *mula bandha* [Sections 1.7.3 & 7.4.1] throughout life can help improve the health of the urinary system. *Mula bandha* is a *yogic* muscular lock that involves a subtle activation of muscles of the perineum, the lower abdominal muscles especially transversus abdominis and the lower back extensors especially multifidus.

Table 11.4 Relationship between *cakras*, body systems and acupuncture meridians

CAKRA	RELATED BODY SYSTEMS	RELATED ACUPUNCTURE MERIDIANS
MULADHARA SVADISTHANA	Urinary and reproductive systems	Kidney, urinary bladder, small intestine, liver and triple heater
MANIPURA	Digestive system	Liver, gall bladder, stomach, spleen, large intestine and small intestine
ANAHATA	Circulatory system	Heart, heart constrictor and small intestine
VISHUDDHI	Respiratory system	Lung, heart constrictor and large intestine
AJNA BINDU SAHASRARA	Central nervous system	Urinary bladder, small intestine, governor vessel and conception vessel

Since the fibres of the perineum connect in part to fibres of the anal musculature as well as the fibres of gluteus maximus, and since gluteus maximus connects with the lower back extensors and the lower abdominal muscles, tensing the perineum can stimulate myotatic (stretch) reflex activation of the lower back extensors and the lower abdominal muscles. The *yoga* emphasis on strengthening the pelvic floor with *mula bandha* has additional benefits for sexual health, perinatal health and incontinence.

Yoga teachers regularly report that *hatha yoga* can be of tremendous assistance to the kidneys. It is widely believed that postures such as backward bending (spinal extension) postures, twisting (spinal axial rotation) postures and side-bending (lateral flexion) postures can massage the kidneys and significantly improve their function.

11.4.3 Applied anatomy and physiology of the reproductive system in *Hatha Yoga*

Hatha yoga for the reproductive systems obviously differs for male and female *yoga* practitioners. In addition there is also a lot of variety in the type of practices a woman should do at various stages of her life, for example during menstruation and during pregnancy.

11.4.3.1 *Hatha yoga* for the male reproductive system

Scientific research on the effects of *hatha yoga* on the male reproductive system is very limited. Therefore a thorough analysis of this subject is beyond the scope of this book. However, experienced *yoga* teachers routinely prescribe *hatha yoga* for the male reproductive system which emphasises *mula bandha* (especially the aspect of *mula bandha* related to the perineum) [Sections 4.4.9 & 7.4.1.1], *asvini mudra* (controlled contraction and expansion of the anal sphincter muscles) and *vajroli mudra* (control of the sphincter urethrae muscle that stops the male urinating).

Mula bandha should be practised throughout one's *yoga* practice with a gentle emphasis on activating the muscles of the perineum just before the exhalation begins. *Asvini mudra* can be practised as an exercise alone but a more powerful practice can be done with an exhalation retention and *uddiyana bandha* ideally while performing an forward bending *asana* such as *pascimottanasana*. *Vajroli mudra* can be eventually practised in a similar way to *asvini mudra* but in the beginning it is very difficult to differentiate between *mula bandha*, *asvini mudra* and *vajroli mudra* so a useful exercise for some people is to practise *vajroli mudra* while urinating in order to stop and start the flow of urine at will.

According to B.K.S. Iyengar in *Light on Yoga* [1966] a possible sequence of postures for advanced *yoga* practitioners that may assist men to prevent and perhaps treat impotence, spermaturia, sterility or prostrate problems can be as shown in Figure 11.1. Mr Iyengar presents a far simpler sequence in *Yoga: the Path to Holistic Health* [2001], which is far more practical and accessible for less experienced practitioners and for people who are physically limited. Both the simple male reproductive system sequence shown shown in *Yoga: the Path to Holistic Health* [2001] and especially the advanced sequence shown in Figure 11.1 have an emphasis

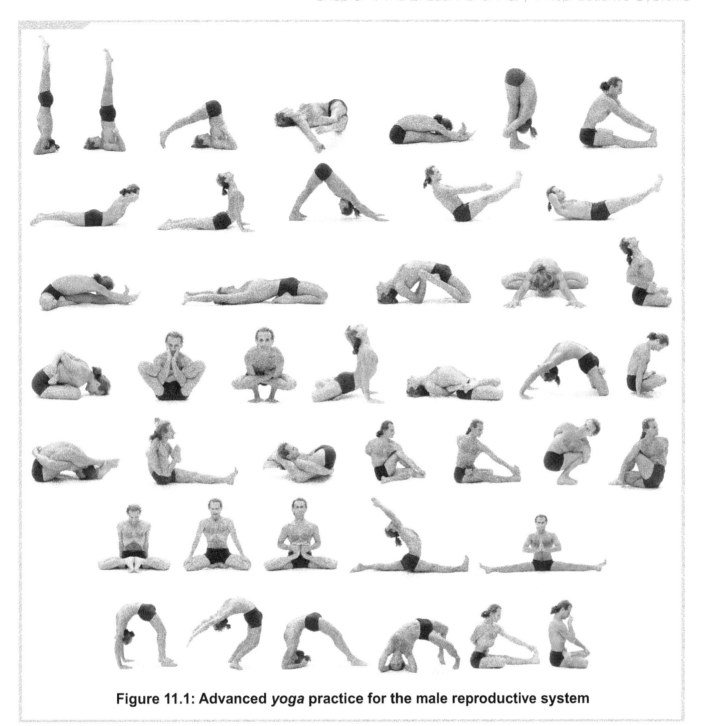

Figure 11.1: Advanced *yoga* practice for the male reproductive system

on activating and stretching the muscles and tissues in the region around the pelvis, using a combination of forward bending (spinal flexion), twisting (spinal axial rotation), backward bending (spinal extension), hip opening and inverted postures. All these types of postures change the forces acting on the region around the perineum and the male reproductive organs. Activation or stretching of the muscles in these regions pulls on fascial connections to the organs of the male reproductive system. When these muscles are activated they pull on the male reproductive system organs which help to physically massage and stimulate them. In addition, appropriately applied *asanas, vinyasas, bandhas, mudras* and *pranayamas* can affect the nervous system control of the male reproductive system, stimulate acupuncture meridians affecting this body system and assist in the flow of *prana* (subtle energy) and *citta* (consciousness) through the *nadis* (subtle channels). The sequence shown in Figure 11.1 concludes with a *pranayama* practice which includes *nadi sodhana pranayama* (alternate nostril breathing) to balance the nervous system.

11.4.3.2 *Hatha yoga* for the female reproductive system

There are no scientific papers currently available on the effects of *hatha yoga* on the <u>female reproductive system</u>. However, there is a vast amount of literature available on how conventional exercise may influence the normal <u>menstrual cycle</u> [DeCree, 1998]. It is known that premenarchal training may have the effect of delaying the onset of menses in some girls and in postmenarchal woman, strenuous exercise can definitely alter bleeding patterns usually resulting in reversible <u>oligomenorrhea</u> (infrequent menstruation) progressing toward <u>amenorrhea</u> (absence of menstrual bleeding) as the exercise increases [Hale, 1983; Bullen *et al*, 1985]. This is not the case for everyone, however, and other factors such as percentage of body fat, stress, diet, and energy drain also play a role. It is usually observed that menses resumes its pre-exercise pattern after a period of rest. Most research suggests that oxygen consumption, heart rate and perceived exertion during exercise are not

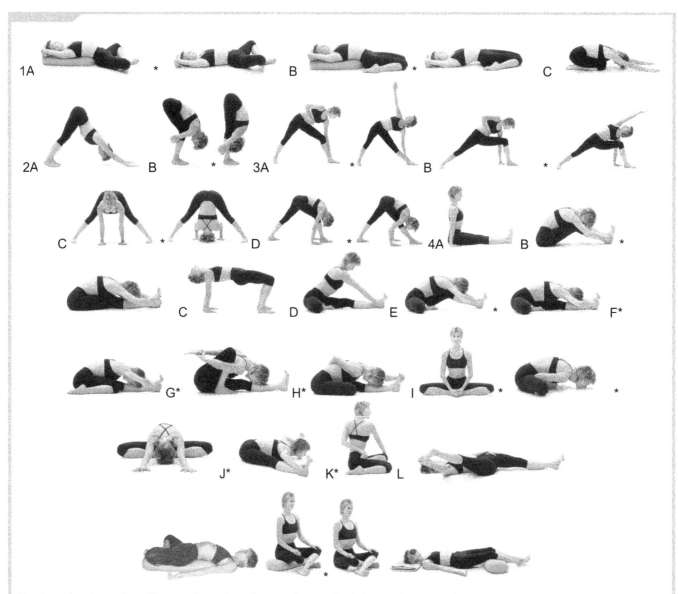

Numbers denote sections. Postures in each section may be practised alternately or one after the other. Not all postures in each section need to be attempted in each practice. Choose only those poses in each section for which you have the time and energy.

Standing postures (2A-B & 3A-D) are optional during menstruation. Some teachers discourage them completely but without them many less flexible or more stressed people find it difficult to do the more passive postures that come later in the sequence. If standing poses are practised at this time they should be practised gently, for a short time only and with supporting props (eg. chairs, bolsters or the wall) if required.

* = more difficult or optional versions of postures;

Beginners should not attempt this sequence without supervision from a qualified instructor;

Caution: Most of the poses shown here need to be specifically modified and simplified for the individual, especially if there are any pre-existing musculoskeletal problems or medical conditions.

Do not attempt this sequence unless you have attended classes where these postures were taught.

Figure 11.2: Menstrual sequence for experienced *yoga* practitioners

affected by the menstrual cycle, but several studies report a higher cardiovascular strain during moderate exercise in the mid-luteal phase [Table 11.2] of the menstrual cycle [Janse de Jonge, 2003]. It has also been shown that, for women and girls, the dangers of excessively rigorous exercise regimens can include disturbances in reproductive function as well as a negative impact on bone density [Greene, 1999].

11.4.3.2.1 *Hatha yoga* during menstruation

Hatha yoga can resemble conventional exercise and even strenuous exercise but it can also be significantly different in many ways. Therefore, opinion varies as to what women should do with respect to *yoga* during menstruation.

Although there are no scientific studies to verify it, the general consensus is that inversions such as *sirsasana* (headstand) and *sarvangasana* (shoulderstand) are not to be practised during the time of menstruation. The reason most commonly given is that inversions reverse the flow of gravity and cause the retention of the menstrual blood, exactly opposite to what nature is intending. Clinical evidence in *yoga* classes has led to the common belief (perhaps justified) that those who do practise inversions during menstruation may be more prone to such problems as ovarian cysts.

Some *yoga* traditions believe that no *hatha yoga* postures at all should be done during the first three days of menstruation while others believe it is okay to do a gentle or passive practice as outlined in Figure 11.2. Some research suggests that women who do not exercise at least a bit during their menses have greater levels of pain at this time [Hightower, 1997] and also have impaired concentration and behavioural changes [Aganoff & Boyle , 1994]. The practice sequence shown in Figure 11.2 consists mainly of forward bending (spinal flexion) postures, gentle chest opening (thoracic spine extension), passive backward bending (lumbar spine extension) postures and postures that gently stretch the hips and pelvic region. This practice sequence is based on information from Geeta Iyengar's book *Yoga: A Gem for Women* [1983] and B.K.S. Iyengar's *Yoga: The Path to Holistic Health* [2001]. Depending on a person's level of flexibility, each posture can be performed with the use of props

 (bolsters, blankets, etc.) (generally easier) or without the use of props (harder*).

11.4.3.2.2 *Hatha yoga* during pregnancy

The following notes are precautions and suggestions for teachers and students on how pregnant women should approach a yoga practice:
- When teaching or practising prenatal *yoga* one should always consider the mother's personal state and needs and always err on the side of caution. For every posture or exercise given, check with the mother-to-be (yourself if you are pregnant) if it feels okay.
- Note that there are two possible types of prenatal *yoga* students. Those that have never done *yoga* before they got pregnant and those that have done *yoga* at some level.
- Pregnant women who have not done *yoga* before their pregnancy should attend special prenatal classes for people who have not done *yoga* before. These classes should be very gentle. Postures, stretching, strengthenig, movements and breathing should not be forced. Emphasis should be on relaxation and getting the student to rediscover her changing body on a day to day basis.
- It is unwise to accept pregnant non-*yoga* practitioners into general open level *yoga* classes, especially late in pregnancy. **NB most of the postures shown in Figure 11.3 are not suitable for someone who has not done *yoga* before their pregnancy commenced**
- For even the experienced practitioner it is wise not to practice new or difficult postures during pregnancy, instead modify and simplify familiar ones (See easy and hard * versions of postures in Figure 11.3).
- During pregnancy the hormone relaxin is released to soften connective tissues to allow the pubic symphysis to open wider for childbirth. Relaxin also affects connective tissue throughout the body making it dangerous to over-stretch. Therefore during pregnancy one should also focus on strengthening. Ankles are particularly easy to sprain during pregnancy so strengthening the ankle evertors is prudent [Sections 6.2.3 & 6.6.5; Applications to Yoga 6.4].
- A trochanter belt (to support the pelvis) may be needed if the pubic symphysis [Section 4.2.3] becomes unstable during pregnancy due to the presence of the hormone relaxin. In such cases the *yoga* practiced should be very gentle and one-legged balance postures should be avoided.

- Beware of lying on the back (supine) especially in the later stages of pregnancy (note the asterix * which denotes difficulty for some people next to supine postures in Figure 11.3). In supine postures the weight of the baby can occlude blood flow leading to <u>hypoxia</u> (below normal levels of <u>oxygen</u>) in the baby due to compression of the descending <u>aorta</u> and <u>hypoxia</u> for the mother due to compression of the <u>ascending vena cava</u>. However, the final position of comfort should usually be the mother's choice.
- Some women will get back pain just because of the position of the baby, eg. the baby's <u>spine</u> is resting on the mother's <u>spine</u>. The only position of comfort for a mother in this situation may be with <u>abdomen</u> prone

hanging in postures such as *prasarita padottanasana* .
- Beware of abortive acupuncture points. For example, the acupuncture point <u>large intestine 4</u>, located between the thumb and first finger on the dorsal hand, is sometimes recommended for <u>headache</u> in non-pregnant individuals but can induce abortion during <u>pregnancy</u>. Abortive acupuncture points may also be found on the inner calf near the <u>medial</u> <u>anterior</u> aspect of the tibia. Therefore do not do postures

such as *kulpha simhasana* in which the ankles are crossed over each other with pressure on the acupuncture points <u>Spleen 6</u> and <u>Spleen 9</u> which can induce abortion.
- Encourage a gentle practice of *mula bandha* throughout the <u>pregnancy</u> for:
    - The relief and/or prevention of lower back pain
    - The ease of relaxation during labour
    - The ease of learning to strengthen after labour
- Practise and teach <u>posterior pelvic tilting</u> [Section 4.2.4.1] (tuck the tail bone under) in supine postures

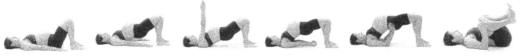 with *mula bandha*

and also in the lunge position .
- Arm strengthening is an important part of a prenatal practice. Especially focus on <u>triceps</u> (use wall push ups), <u>biceps</u> and shoulder muscles.

- Use interlocked and extended arm positions 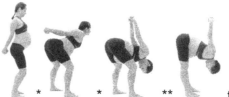 to compensate for extra weight anteriorly
- The use of inversions such as headstand and shoulderstand for prenatal *yoga* practitioners is a contentious issue amongst many *yoga* teachers and health practitioners. Evidence for or against the use of inversions during pregnancy tends to be anecdotal. Some therapists are adamant that inversions should not be done during pregnancy, but many experienced *yoga* teachers including Geeta Iyengar [1983] advocate the use of these inversions for experienced students and say they are of great benefit. However, if headstand and shoulderstand were not mastered before pregnancy they should not be attempted during pregnancy. The final decision as to whether or not to practice inversions, and till how late in pregnancy to practice them should be left up to the discretion of the experienced practitioner who is pregnant. Generally inversions are safer with support. It is good to always have a wall behind you during headstand. Many experienced *yoga* practitioners have safely practiced headstand throughout their pregnancy and have reported that it relieved backache, replenished energy and could ease the varicose veins that are often present during pregnancy. Shoulderstand, is generally more difficult to practice during pregnancy because of the undesirable abdominal strain that some people require to get in and out of the posture (unless they are helped into the posture by someone else or unless they have always been very strong, light and flexible). Therefore, most experienced *yoga* practitioners do not find shoulderstand comfortable during pregnancy

except perhaps at the start of the second trimester. Shoulderstand may be made easier with the correct support of blankets under the shoulders and the support of a wall for the feet or can be modified to just have the feet resting up a wall as demonstrated in Figure 11.3. Geeta Iyengar stresses that if breathing becomes heavy then inverted practices should be stopped. In other words unless the inversions feel very easy and safe to do, then don't do them.

- Beware of over stretching, especially with very flexible women (eg. dancers).
- Avoid constipation by having an emphasis on healthy diet with large amounts of water and fibre content.

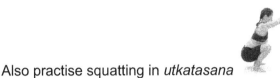

Also practise squatting in *utkatasana* and *malasana* for easier defecation, and perhaps for childbirth.

- For teachers who have not practised *yoga* while being pregnant, carefully try practising *yoga* right after eating a big meal. The type of *yoga* practice that feels okay for a non-pregnant person who has just eaten a lot of food may well be ideal for pregnant women.

General Guide for *Yoga* Practitioners during Pregnancy

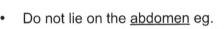

- Do not lie on the <u>abdomen</u> eg.
- Avoid compressing the abdominal region with excessive <u>tension</u> of the <u>abdominal muscles</u> eg.

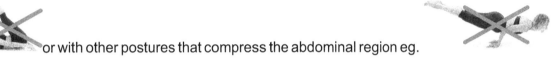or with other postures that compress the abdominal region eg.

- When your legs are straight then stand and sit with feet and knees at least hip width apart;

eg. do not stand or sit with knees together eg.

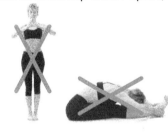

- Do not do postures which compress the groin eg 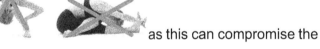 as this can compromise the <u>femoral nerve</u> and femoral <u>artery.</u>

- Avoid strong twisting around the lower trunk and <u>abdomen</u> eg. 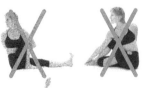 ; instead gently

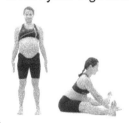

twist from the upper back and shoulders eg.
- Lying on the back may become uncomfortable in the latter part of <u>pregnancy</u>, at that time rest lying on the side with a bolster or rolled blankets between the thighs and knees and use a pillow for the head

eg.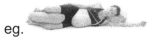

Figure 11.3: Synergy Style Prenatal Sequence for experienced *yoga* practitioners

(Modelled by Vitoria Borg-Oliver, 39 weeks pregnant with Amalia, who was born at home 6 days later on 18th March 2004)

Introductory Dynamic Sequence (1 breath per pose, or more if you need; * = harder optional postures)

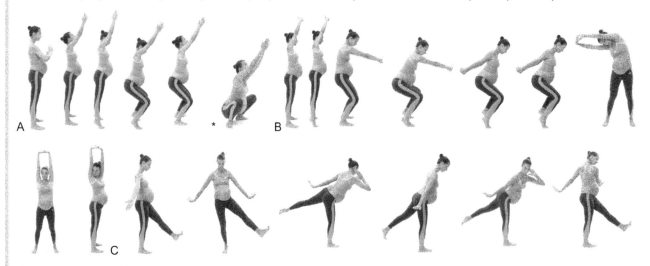

Candra Namaskar (Salute to the moon (1 breath per pose, or more if you need; * = harder optional postures)

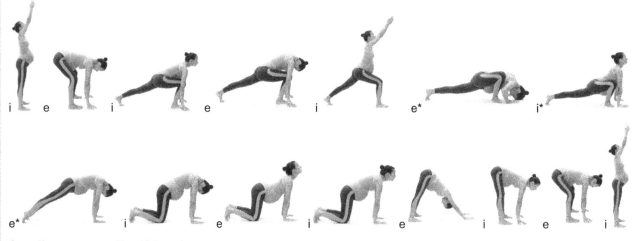

Standing postures (5 – 10 breaths per pose; choose 1 or more postures from each Section)

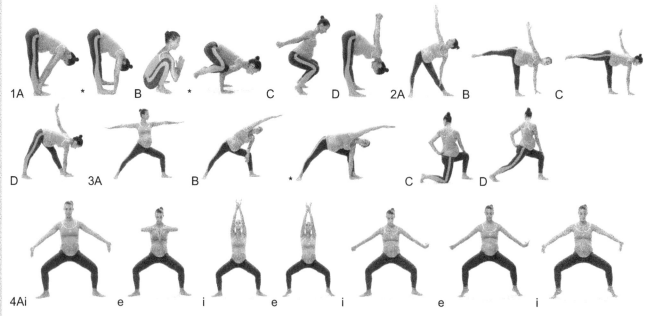

IMPORTANT NOTE: DO NOT ATTEMPT THIS SEQUENCE UNLESS YOU HAVE ATTENDED CLASSES WHERE THESE POSTURES WERE TAUGHT AND DO NOT ATTEMPT A POSTURE UNLESS YOU HAVE MASTERED IT BEFORE YOU WERE PREGNANT.

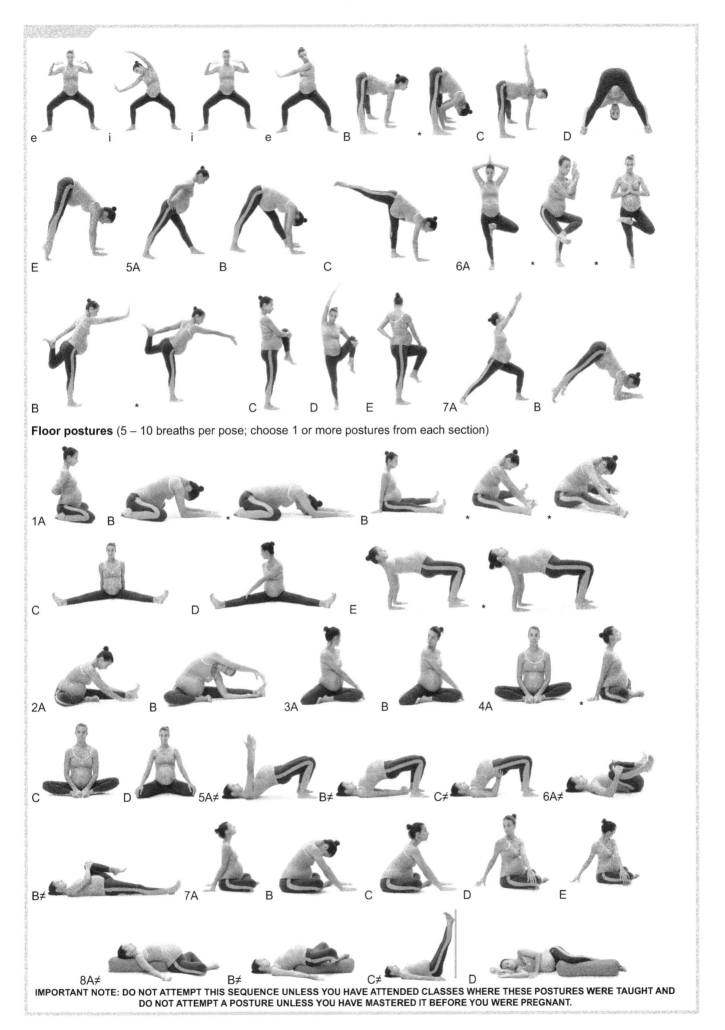

e i i e B * C D

E 5A B C 6A * *

B * C D E 7A B

Floor postures (5 – 10 breaths per pose; choose 1 or more postures from each section)

1A B * B * *

C D E *

2A B 3A B 4A *

C D 5A≠ B≠ C≠ 6A≠

B≠ 7A B C D E

8A≠ B≠ C≠ D

IMPORTANT NOTE: DO NOT ATTEMPT THIS SEQUENCE UNLESS YOU HAVE ATTENDED CLASSES WHERE THESE POSTURES WERE TAUGHT AND DO NOT ATTEMPT A POSTURE UNLESS YOU HAVE MASTERED IT BEFORE YOU WERE PREGNANT.

347

- Avoid retaining the breath in or out for more than the natural few seconds without strain; do not practise

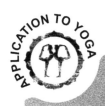

  uddiyana bandha after <u>exhalation retention</u>   i.e. do not draw the <u>abdomen</u> inwards by expanding the chest after holding the breath out.
- Modify all postures so they feel comfortable for you.
- Your body is changing every day so be receptive to the changes and adjust your practice accordingly.
- Do not over-stretch, but rather maintain some strength and cardiovascular fitness; the body is naturally softening at this time due to the hormone relaxin and it is easy to damage ligaments if you overstretch them.
- Practise *bhramari* (the humming breath) regularly as this has been shown to be excellent during <u>pregnancy</u> as it stimulates the production of the important <u>neurotransmitter</u> <u>nitric oxide</u> in the sinuses of the skull which has positive effects for the <u>reproductive system</u>, <u>immune system</u> and <u>nervous system</u> [Application to *yoga* 12.2].
- Stay relaxed in the face, neck and throat at all times.

APPLICATION TO YOGA

No 11.2 Use your diaphragm to breathe into your abdomen to help your reproductive health

Breathing into the <u>abdomen</u> (<u>diaphragmatic</u> breathing) helps regulate the <u>autonomic nervous system</u>, which controls the <u>reproductive system</u> and the <u>endocrine system</u>. Therefore, on a neurological level, <u>diaphragmatic</u> breathing helps in sexual health, fertility, menstrual cycle regularity, sexual hormone control, prostate health and other activities of the reproductive system.

Also on a neurological level, the natural activity (<u>contraction</u>) of the <u>diaphragm</u> (the main muscle of <u>abdominal</u> inhalation) can help the <u>reproductive system</u> by reciprocally relaxing or inhibiting the muscles of forced <u>abdominal</u> exhalation that pull the navel to the spine. Exhaling fully by drawing the navel to the spine is great for emptying the lungs, massaging the internal organs, and pushing 'stale blood and other fluids' out of them. However, keeping the navel to the spine and not relaxing the muscles that do this on inhalation by breathing <u>diaphragmatically</u> is a common chronic practice in many people. This erroneous practice tends to keep pressure on the internal organs of reproduction and prevent the entry of fresh blood into these organs.

On a physical level, breathing into the <u>abdomen</u> when it is firmed by posture or natural activities such as relaxed walking (provided the navel has not been drawn closer to the spine) helps sexual function because the internal organs involved are massaged (compressed) as the <u>diaphragm</u> actively moves away from the chest into the <u>abdomen</u> on inhalation, and then released and relaxed (expanded) as the <u>diaphragm</u> passively moves towards the chest and away from the <u>abdomen</u> on exhalation.

****

Notes for Figure 11.3: Prenatal *yoga* sequence for experienced *yoga* practitioners who are healthy and fit (not for beginners in *yoga* who have become pregnant).

- Numbers denote sections. Postures in each section may be practised alternately or one after the other. Not all postures in each section need to be attempted in each practice. Choose only those that you have the time and energy for.

- ≠ = These supine postures and any postures lying on the back may become uncomfortable or may cause dizziness in the latter part of pregnancy for some mothers and should in such cases be avoided.

- * = more difficult or optional versions of postures.

- **Note** that the model in this sequence was an experienced *yoga* practitioner before she got pregnant.

- Beginners should not attempt this sequence without supervision from a qualified instructor.

- **Caution:** Most of the poses shown on this sheet need to be specifically modified and simplified for the individual, especially if there are any pre-existing musculoskeletal problems or medical conditions, or any of the contraindications described in Section 11.4.3.2.2.

- **IMPORTANT NOTE: DO NOT ATTEMPT THIS SEQUENCE UNLESS YOU HAVE ATTENDED CLASSES WHERE THESE POSTURES WERE TAUGHT AND DO NOT ATTEMPT A POSTURE UNLESS YOU HAVE MASTERED IT BEFORE YOU WERE PREGNANT.**

Chapter Breakdown

****

12.0 INTRODUCTION TO EXERCISE PHYSIOLOGY & *YOGIC* PHYSIOLOGY

This chapter outlines some of the basic principles of exercise physiology. Exercise physiology and Western concepts of physiology are then compared and contrasted with *yogic* physiology and related Eastern concepts. *Hatha yoga* practices are described and discussed in terms of both Western exercise physiology and Eastern *yogic* physiology.

Among the most important principles of exercise physiology to remember when developing a *hatha yoga* practice are the concepts of specificity of training and Wolff's law. The term 'specificity of training' means practicing the same task that one wants to improve. The outcomes of training are therefore directly related to the activity employed as a training practice. Hence, if you want to develop a yoga practice that will support a functional activity, you may choose special yoga postures that most resemble the activity of your preference. An example of this is described for gait or walking in Section 12.6. Wolff's Law says that the physical effort or force you exert upon a tissue (eg bone tissue) will stimulate or provoke a change in that tissue which will be directed by your effort. So plan your practice and direct your efforts intelligently, achieve the results you are working towards.

Yogic physiology is based on a different set of principles and underlying assumptions to Western physiology. *Yogic* physiology is related to the science of *ayurveda* [Tables 12.3 & 12.4]. Although Western exercise physiology and *yogic* physiology can be compared [Table 12.2], the two should initially be studied separately before it is possible to compare them rationally. An understanding of both Western exercise physiology and *yogic* physiology, and the ability to relate the two together is an important step towards safely progressing in a *hatha yoga* practice.

12.1 EXERCISE PHYSIOLOGY

12.1.1 Energy in the Body
12.1.1.1 Units of Energy: Calories and Joules
The most common unit measure of energy is the calorie (1 calorie = 4.2 joules). A calorie is the amount of heat energy needed to increase the temperature of 1g of water by 1°C. About 100 calories is used in running a mile in six minutes 30 seconds, and 0.5 kg body fat is equivalent to 3,800 calories (16,250 kJ).

12.1.1.2 ATP: Primary energy carrying molecule in the body
For the human body to function it requires energy. Energy for activity is provided to the muscles in the form of an energy rich molecule called adenosine triphosphate (ATP).

12.1.2 Energy Systems of the Body [Table 12.1]
The method by which the body generates energy depends on the intensity and duration of activity. There are three major energy-producing systems in the body. These are: the aerobic system, which requires oxygen and is used in extended activities such as jogging or cycling; and two anaerobic systems, which function in the absence of oxygen, and which are used for high intensity exercises such as sprinting and weight lifting.

12.1.2.1 Anaerobic metabolism: anaerobic energy production
Anaerobic means in the absence of oxygen. There are two distinct systems that function in the absence of oxygen for the production of energy for activities requiring sudden bursts of movement such as jumping or sprinting.

12.1.2.1.1 Lactate system: anaerobic metabolism of glucose
The lactate system derives energy from ATP produced in anaerobic metabolism, which involves metabolic processes that occur without oxygen. The degradation of one glucose molecule leads to the production of two molecules of ATP plus lactic acid.

Table 12.1: Energy-producing systems of the body

	ANAEROBIC METABOLISM: ANAEROBIC ENERGY-PRODUCING SYSTEMS		AEROBIC METABOLISM: AEROBIC ENERGY-PRODUCING SYSTEM
	PHOSPHATE SYSTEM	LACTATE SYSTEM	
INTENSITY OF EFFORT REQUIRED	Very high; intensity 95 - 100% of maximum effort,	High intensity; 60 - 90% of maximum effort	Low intensity; Up to 60% of maximum effort
DURATION	Lasts for 10 seconds of explosive activity	At 95% max it lasts for ☐ 30 seconds, at 60% max it lasts for ☐ 30 minutes.	At low intensity there is no time limit.
FUEL	Phosphocreatine	Carbohydrate in the form of muscle glycogen & blood glucose.	Carbohydrates, fat & protein.
WASTE PRODUCT	None	Lactic acid	Carbon dioxide & water.
ATP PRODUCED	0	2 molecules of ATP per unit glucose used	36 – 38 molecules of ATP per unit glucose used
RECOVERY TIME	50% energy source is available after 30 seconds, 100% is available after 2 minutes.	Fatigue will start at 35-40 seconds of activity, exhaustion at 55-60 seconds. Once produced, lactate takes 45-60 minutes to be removed from the system.	Recover when food stores are replaced
ACTIVITIES	Short repetitive bursts of activity	400m sprint	Walking, swimming, jogging, dancing etc.

Lactic acid is a partial breakdown product of glucose as a result of anaerobic metabolism. Lactic acid accumulation in the body is toxic. Lactic acid adversely affects muscle function and leads to feelings of discomfort and nausea. It is thought that 90% of lactic acid is removed within one hour of its production and its removal is enhanced by light exercise.

12.1.2.1.2 Phosphate system: cellular supplies of high-energy phosphates
The phosphate system derives energy directly from cellular supplies of high-energy phosphate molecules such as ATP and phosphocreatine that are stored in muscle tissue. There are no residual toxic waste products resulting from the phosphate system, but cellular supplies of these molecules are very limited.

12.1.2.2 Aerobic metabolism: metabolism of glucose in the presence of oxygen

The aerobic energy production system uses energy derived from aerobic metabolism, which is the complete degradation of glucose in the presence of oxygen to carbon dioxide and water. Aerobic systems generate 36-38 molecules of ATP per glucose molecule degraded.

12.2 MUSCLE PHYSIOLOGY

The main physiological factors influencing the performance of skeletal muscle are muscle strength, muscle size (atrophy or hypertrophy), and muscle fatigue.

12.2.1 Muscle Fibre Types
Muscle fibres are usually classified into two main groups:

12.2.1.1 Slow twitch (ST) fibres
Slow twitch (ST) fibres have slow muscle activation and relaxation rates and are activated during aerobic endurance activities. ST fibres appear red due to large supplies of intracellular myoglobin, and their high capillary content.

12.2.1.2 Fast twitch (FT) fibres

Fast twitch (FT) fibres have fast muscle activation and relaxation rates and are activated during anaerobic, fast, explosive activities. FT fibres appear white because of their low levels of myoglobin, and their low capillary content. All fibres of a particular motor unit are of the same type, and all human skeletal muscles contain a mixture of types in varying distributions.

Elite athletes at extreme ends of the spectrum can have a predominance of fibre type in particular muscles. ST fibres tend to predominate in the quadriceps femoris of long distance runners, while FT fibres tend to predominate in the quadriceps femoris of sprinters.

12.2.2 Muscle Response to Training

Fast twitch (FT) fibres respond to strength training by increasing in size more than slow twitch (ST) fibres do. Hence, sprinters and weight lifters tend to develop increased muscle bulk while endurance athletes tend to be quite lean.

The ratio of fibre types appears largely to be genetically determined. Research has shown that, through training, some FT fibres can take on ST fibre characteristics. This suggests that it may be possible for a sprinter to develop their endurance capacity, since they have a high FT/ST ratio; but it is more difficult (if not impossible) to change ST to FT fibres through training.

12.2.3 Muscle Strength

The major determinant of muscle strength is the cross-sectional area of the muscle. However, an increase in muscle strength does not necessarily mean an increase in muscle size.

Other factors that determine muscle strength include internal muscle architecture, limb length, joint structure, and neural factors such as motor unit recruitment (how much of a muscle is activated by a nerve impulse).

Muscle Atrophy is muscle-wasting occurring as a result of disuse, immobilisation, trauma, disease or starvation [Section 12.4].

12.2.4 Muscle Fatigue

Muscle Fatigue is defined as the failure to sustain a given force or power resulting from impairment in the chain of command for muscle activation.

Fatigue may be central (due to lack of motivation) or peripheral in origin.
Causes of peripheral fatigue include:
*   Metabolic disturbances, eg lactic acid build up, which is thought to lead to fatigue by reducing cellular pH and thus inhibiting enzymes involved in muscle activation
*   Electrophysiological disturbances like failure of nerve function or neuromuscular transmission
*   Chronic fatigue and pain syndromes
*   Respiratory inadequacy
*   Effects of age

12.2.5. Theories of Muscle Soreness and Cramping

Muscle soreness: The reasons for muscle soreness, which may occur 24-48 hours after exercise, are not fully understood. Several theories have been proposed. The most satisfactory explanation is the:
*   **Connective tissue theory**: This says that the soreness is due to minute tears in the muscle's inelastic components (connective tissue) which occur in the eccentric phase of muscle activation.

Other, less satisfactory, explanations include:
*   **Lactic acid accumulation theory**: This may explain the short term soreness felt immediately post exercise, but since 95% of lactic acid is removed within the first hour post exercise, it does not explain the longer term post exercise soreness.
*   **Muscle micro-tear theory**: This says that the soreness is due to micro-tears in muscle fibres following unaccustomed movement. However, evidence of muscle cell membrane disruption, such as increased extracellular creatine kinase (the enzyme which breaks down phosphocreatine), exists even in the absence of pain.
*   **Pressure theory**: This has little scientific support, but suggests that post exercise inflammatory chemicals such as histamines build up in the muscles and cause pressure and thus pain.
*   **Spasm theory**: Postulates that a decrease in blood flow caused by some exercises results in the production of a pain producing substance called substance P, which stimulates nerve endings causing spasms which in turn cause further pain.

Muscle cramping has, at present, no satisfactory explanation.

12.2.6 Types of Muscle Activation

- Muscle activations can either be **static** (isometric) or **dynamic** (isotonic or isokinetic)
- **Isometric**: muscle develops tension without changing length of the muscle fibre
- **Isotonic**: muscle develops tension while changing length of the muscle fibre
- **Concentric**: muscle develops tension while shortening
- **Eccentric**: muscle develops tension while lengthening
- **Isokinetic**: maximum tension developed throughout the full range of movement (ROM) (usually requires computer enhanced weight-training machines – but can be included in intelligent *yoga* [See Applications to *yoga* 1.16]).

12.3 ENHANCING MUSCLE PERFORMANCE

12.3.1 Specificity of Training

The specificity principle simply states that to become better at a particular exercise or skill, you must perform that exercise or skill. This training response has been shown to be highly specific. What you practise in your training is exactly what you improve at most and what you do not practise you do not neccessarily improve in (even if you may practise other tasks which appear similar). Training has been shown to be specific for:

i)   Type of muscle activation
ii)   Velocity of limb movement
iii) Angle of the joint
iv)   Type of exercise
v)   Range of joint movement
vi)   Body posture.

Specificity of training is also partially due to the effects of gravity and the effects of the skill factor (neural and physiological effects).

Muscles are only strengthened in a very specific manner. It has been shown that strength training may only strengthen a muscle through the range in which the muscle is actually trained. Traditional strength training techniques often only exercise a muscle through a limited range of motion (ROM). This can also cause a decrease in muscle length and its elastic nature, therefore increasing risk of injury and reducing the effectiveness of the exercise. *Yoga* postures which activate muscles through full ROM enhance the elastic qualities of muscle (improving the stretch-shorten cycle) and muscle strength through ROM. Therefore, many extreme *yoga* postures such as the *urdhva yoga dandasana* series

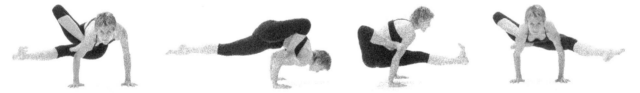

and most of the postures shown in Figures 11.1 and 12.5 are excellent to help improve muscle strength and flexibility and reduce risk of injury at other times, provided they are practiced safely. Most of these advanced postures are a delicate balance between strength and flexibility. However, activation of any muscle at the end of ROM when in a lengthened position (which is the case in many advanced postures) is potentially dangerous and must therefore be done with full concentration and care.

12.3.2 Optimal Training Load

The optimal training load can be defined as the sustainable amount of training required to give the maximum improvement in the fitness level being targeted, while giving the minimum risk of injury.

Dynamic exercise

For the best training response, the optimal training load for dynamic exercise is sub-maximal (between 3-RM and 9-RM).

A one-repetition-maximum (1-RM) is defined to be the maximum effort (or weight) a person can make (or lift) for a particular exercise once only. Therefore, a 10-RM exercise is precisely defined to be one that can only be repeated 10 times at a stretch (not 9 or 11) before fatigue.

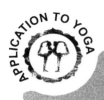

No 12.1 There are an optimum number of times to repeat each *asana* or *vinyasa* to achieve a maximum training effect

Intelligent use of *hatha yoga vinyasas* (dynamic *yoga* exercises) takes advantage of well-established research that shows the optimal training load for dynamic exercise is between 3-RM and 9-RM. A *yoga* exercise needs to be performed with a personal level of difficulty so that it can only be repeated between 3 to 9 times before it can no longer be repeated. For example if the *surya namaskar* ...

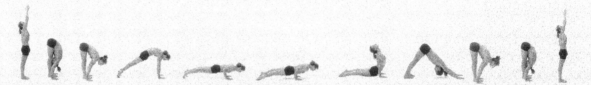

...(Salute to the Sun) that you practise can easily be performed 20 times then the way you are doing it may be too easy to give you a significant training improvement. Increasing the difficulty of this or other *yoga* exercises can be achieved in several ways:

(i) By maintaining a tighter activation of all the body musculature throughout the exercise

(ii) By slowing down or speeding up the exercise depending on which is more effective

(iii) By moving through a greater joint range of motion during the *vinyasa* (eg by further flexing and extending the shoulders, elbows, hips, knees etc).

Once the exercise is hard enough that it can only be performed between a minimum of 3 and a maximum of 9 times before you can no longer repeat it (without resting), then the optimal training load has been found and the greatest improvements in dynamic strength can be obtained.

Isometric exercise

For isometric exercise the optimal training intensity is also sub-maximal. One study in which training was done with 3 sets of ten 5 second isometric muscle activations at 25%, 50% or 100% of maximal, showed that 50% of maximal produced better strength increases than 25% or 100% of maximal.

In isometric muscle activations of greater than 15-20% of maximal effort, blood flow through working muscles is increasingly impaired as the activating muscle fibres compress or collapse blood vessels. Reduced blood flow, due to the occluded blood vessels, leads to the following problems:

i) A decreased supply of oxygen to the muscle tissue which necessitates a greater percentage of the energy to be produced by anaerobic means.

ii) A decreased ability to remove heat, and metabolic waste products, such as lactic acid, that are produced by the anaerobically working muscle tissue.

iii) A net increase in total peripheral resistance, which results in larger increases in arterial blood pressure than are seen in dynamic exercise. This makes strong isometric exercise potentially harmful for people with cardiovascular problems.

Eccentric contractions are thought to place greater stress on muscle tissue than concentric muscle activations. Therefore, some researchers suggest that training with eccentric exercise gives greater improvements in strength. For example, lowering from the plank to the push-up gives a greater training effect than coming up from push-up to plank.

12.3.3 Training for Increased Recruitment of Motor Units

A person with relatively small muscles may be physically stronger than someone with larger muscles if they are able to recruit (activate or turn on) a greater number of motor units. (A motor unit is an individual motor nerve and all the muscle fibres it innervates).

Training to increase recruitment of motor units may include the following strategies:
i) Training with the opposite limb
ii) Mental practice (visualisation)
iii) Feedback (auditory, visual, tactile and biofeedback)
iv) Practice.

12.3.4 Cardiopulmonary Training

To improve <u>aerobic capacity</u> you need to exercise at 60% of your maximum <u>heart rate</u> for a period of 15-60 minutes, 3-5 days per week. Your maximum <u>heart rate</u> (HR_{max}) can be approximated with the equation: HR_{max}= 220 minus your age.

Aerobic capacity is a measure of a person's maximal <u>oxygen</u> (O_2) uptake, ie the maximal amount of <u>oxygen</u> capable of being transported to and being utilised by the working muscles, per unit time and per unit body weight.

<u>Maximal oxygen uptake</u> is referred to as VO_{2max}. A trained cross country skier may have a VO_{2max} of 80-90 ml O_2/min/ kg, while a sedentary middle-aged man in poor fitness may have a VO_{2max} of 20-30 ml O_2/min/kg.

<u>Maximal oxygen uptake</u> (VO_{2max}), and hence physical work capacity, is dependent upon the following factors:
- <u>Stroke volume</u> of the <u>heart</u>
- Maximal <u>heart rate</u>
- Amount of blood available to the active muscles
- Maximal <u>oxygen</u> extraction at the tissue level
- <u>Oxygen</u> carrying capacity of the blood (<u>haemoglobin</u> concentration)

12.4. EFFECTS OF IMMOBILISATION OR MINIMAL ACTIVITY

A muscle that is not used for a length of time will begin to weaken and atrophy. Similarly a joint that is not moved for a length of time will begin to stiffen and, if the time is long enough, begin to calcify. The amount of muscle weakness or joint stiffness depends on the following factors:
- **Duration** of immobilisation
- **Extent** of the immobilisation
- **Position/angle** of immobilisation
- **Nature of the specific muscles and joints** immobilised
- **Degree of the injury**: whether the immobilised body part had been injured and to what extent
- **Pain**: presence or absence of pain
- **Age** of the person.

<u>Immobilisation</u> of a muscle in a shortened position will cause muscle shortening due to loss of <u>sarcomeres</u>; while immobilisation of a muscle in the lengthened position causes muscle lengthening by the addition of new sarcomeres.

<u>Selective atrophy</u> may occur between <u>agonists</u> and <u>antagonists</u>. Joint damage generally results in greater weakness of its <u>extensors</u> than its <u>flexors</u>. For example, after an injury to the <u>knee joint complex</u> <u>quadriceps</u> weakness is often greater than hamstring weakness. This may be due to <u>reflex</u> activity causing <u>extensor inhibition</u> and <u>flexor facilitation</u>. <u>Reflex inhibition</u> of <u>muscle activation</u> may be due to pain, joint effusion, intra-articular pressure, and joint position.

Selective wasting may also occur in the <u>quadriceps</u>. <u>Vastus medialis</u> tends to be more prone to atrophy than the other muscles of the <u>quadriceps</u> group. This is thought to be a major cause of <u>patellofemoral maltracking</u> [Section 5.5.4].

12.5. FITNESS TESTING

Assessment of an individual's physical fitness is essential for the safe prescription of any exercise programme. Factors to be considered include:
i) Lifestyle
ii) Blood pressure
iii) Resting heart rate
iv) Amount of body fat
v) Aerobic capacity
vi) Flexibility
vii) Muscle strength

12.6. FUNCTIONAL ANALYSIS OF THE GAIT (WALKING) CYCLE

A functional analysis of gait (walking) serves as a practical example of how to apply the information from the anatomy component of this book with the applied anatomy component.

Gait analysis involves breaking down walking into its essential components and then examining gait-defective individuals for absence of these components. This analysis facilitates the correct prescription of exercises for stretching and strengthening muscles and mobilisation of joints.

Walking consists of a stance phase where the foot is in contact with the floor and a swing phase where the foot is not in contact with the floor. Stance phase normally takes up 60% of the gait cycle while swing takes up 40%.

12.6.1 Essential Components of the Gait (Walking) Cycle
Many of the musculoskeletal problems faced in everyday life are brought to light in a person's gait (walking) cycle. The two main parts of the gait cycle stance phase and swing phase, are described in the text below and the table following.

Stance Phase is that part of the gait cycle where the foot is on the floor. The essential components of stance phase are:
1. Hip extension throughout (angular displacement taking place at ankle as well as hip)
2. Lateral horizontal shift of the pelvis and trunk (normally 4-5 cm in total)
3. Knee flexion (~15°) initiated on heel contact
   Followed by knee extension, then knee flexion prior to toe-off
4. Ankle dorsiflexion
   Followed by ankle plantarflexion at heel-off.

Swing-Phase is that part of the gait cycle where the foot is in the air. The essential components of swing phase are:
1. Knee flexion, with the initial hip extension
2. Lateral pelvic tilt downwards (~5°) in the horizontal plane at toe-off
3. Hip flexion
4. Rotation of the pelvis forward on the swinging leg
   (3-4° on either side of the central axis).
5. Knee extension plus ankle dorsiflexion immediately prior to heel contact.

By examining the essential components of the stance phase and swing phase in normal people, and then comparing the individual components of each phase to *yoga* postures, you can begin to devise exercises that can improve people's walking ability. In the table below the essential components or stages of walking are listed and after each stage photographs of postures that may enhance that stage are shown.

STAGES OF STANCE PHASE OF GAIT WALKING	POSTURES THAT MAY ASSIST IN IMPROVING STANCE PHASE OF GAIT WALKING (*= optional harder versions of postures)
1. Hip extension	
2. Lateral horizontal shift of the pelvis and trunk	
3. Knee flexion (~15°) initiated on heel contact	
Followed by knee extension,	
then knee flexion prior to toe-off	
4. Ankle dorsiflexion	
Followed by ankle plantarflexion at heel-off	

STAGES OF SWING PHASE OF WALKING	POSTURES THAT MAY ASSIST IN IMPROVING SWING PHASE OF WALKING (*= optional harder versions of postures)
1 Knee flexion, with the initial hip extension	
2 Lateral pelvic tilt downwards (~5°) in the horizontal plane at toe-off	
3 Hip flexion	
4 Forward pelvic rotation on the swinging leg	

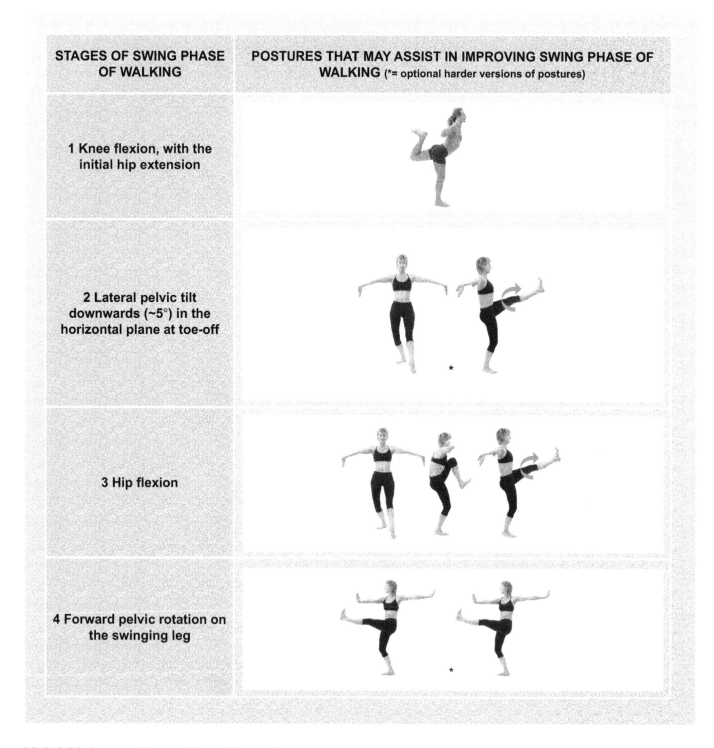

12.6.2 Major problems found in walking

The major problems seen in walking are listed below. For each of these there are possible causes which should be checked. One quick way of helping to establish the possible cause is to recognise the compensatory behaviour (<u>compensations</u>) that it can cause. Next to each possible cause is a picture of a posture, variations of which may be used to assist in strengthening the weakened muscles involved or helping to lengthen (stretch) shortened muscles. Probably the most important problem in walking that is not mentioned below is over-tension in the trunk muscles often caused by excessive 'drawing the navel to the spine' that prevents natural spinal movement during walking and the inability for the pelvis to move freely. This can be usually remedied by allowing the <u>abdomen</u> to feel relaxed while walking and allowing the hips and spine to freely move. Relaxed walking with natural pelvic motion and natural <u>diaphragmatic</u> (<u>abdominal</u>) breathing gives trunk firmness and helps promote circulation while helping to reduce excess muscular and nervous tension.

MAJOR PROBLEMS FOUND IN STANCE PHASE OF GAIT IN THE AFFECTED LEG

PROBLEMS IN STANCE PHASE OF GAIT and COMPENSATIONS	POSSIBLE CAUSES OF A PROBLEM	POSTURES THAT MAY HELP CORRECT THE PROBLEM
1. Decreased peak hip extension in late stance phase COMPENSATIONS: • Lumbar spine extension • Rotation of trunk and pelvis over swing leg	Weak hip extensors	
	Tight or overactive hip flexors	
	Tight or overactive plantarflexors	
	Weak hip flexors	
2. Excessive lateral horizontal pelvic shift in stance phase COMPENSATIONS: • Trunk contralateral lateral flexion • Decreased lateral pelvic shift by decreased stance time	Weak abductors	
	Tight or overactive adductors	
3. Decreased lateral horizontal pelvic shift in stance phase	Weak adductors	
4. Excessive downwards pelvic shift on the intact side associated with excessive lateral pelvic shift to the affected side	Weak hip abductors	

359

5. **Knee hyperextension or decreased knee flexion** COMPENSATIONS: • Increased trunk flexion • Increased knee flexion • Limping, short time spent on bad leg	Weak knee extensors	
	Tight or overactive plantarflexors	
	Weak knee flexors	
	Overactive knee extensors	
6. **Increased knee flexion/ decreased knee extension** RESULTS: • Sometimes keeping the knee flexed • Sometimes keeping the knee extended	Tight or overactive knee flexors	
	Weak knee extensors	
7. **Decreased ankle plantarflexion activity at toe-off and activity to control ankle dorsiflexion in stance phase** RESULTS: • Less effective swing phase • Less hip extension in stance phase • Less propulsion	Weak ankle plantarflexors	
	Tight or overactive ankle dorsiflexors	

MAJOR PROBLEMS FOUND IN SWING PHASE OF GAIT IN THE AFFECTED LEG

PROBLEMS IN SWING PHASE OF GAIT and COMPENSATIONS	POSSIBLE CAUSES OF A PROBLEM	POSTURES THAT MAY HELP CORRECT THE PROBLEM
1. Decreased hip flexion in early swing phase. COMPENSATIONS: • Rotation of trunk and pelvis • Increased lumbar spine extension and posterior pelvic tilt	Decreased peak hip extension in late stance phase	
	Weak hip flexors	
2. Lack of knee flexion at toe-off. COMPENSATIONS: • Circumduction • Hip hitching	Decreased hip extension in late stance	
	Weak knee flexors	
	Overactive knee extensors (especially rectus femoris)	
3. Decreased knee extension prior to heel strike COMPENSATIONS: • Excessive contralateral hip extension and knee flexion • Increased speed of gait cycle	Weak knee extensors	
	Tight or overactive knee flexors	

361

4. **Decreased ankle dorsiflexion in swing phase**	Weak dorsiflexors
COMPENSATIONS: • Circumduction	Tight or overactive plantarflexors
• Hip hitching	

12.7 APPLIED *YOGIC* ANATOMY & PHYSIOLOGY

To examine *yoga* practically, the *astanga yoga* system of Patanjali can be used to divide it into two parts, physical *yoga* and non-physical *yoga*. The two main activities of physical *yoga* are (i) physical exercises (*Asana*) and (ii) breath-control (*Pranayama*). The two main activities of non-physical *yoga* are (i) ethical disciplines (*Yama* and *Niyama*) and (ii) meditative practices (*Pratayahara, Dharana, Dhyana* and *Samadhi*). A *yogin* (experienced *yoga* practitioner) can practice any combination or all of these *yogic* activities at the same time. Ancient *yogic* texts advise that it is safest and most effective for the new *yoga* practitioner to have some practical understanding of the ethical disciplines before learning first physical exercises, then breath-control. Once these are mastered, the *yogin* can then progress to the seated meditative practices. However, in their simplest forms, breath-control and physical exercises can be practised in conjunction with ethical disciplines and meditative practices by anyone. In fact, it is a natural process for most people to achieve some sort of meditative state doing any sort of physical exercise including running, swimming or weight-training; and, at these times, a person's breath is often consciously or unconsciously regulated.

12.7.1 The Anatomy and Physiology of Physical *Yoga*: Physical Exercises (*Asana*) and Breath-control (*Pranayama*)

In most conventional exercise training for strength, flexibility and cardiovascular fitness are practised separately. In physical *yoga*, physical exercises and breath-control can be used to simultaneously develop strength, flexibility, and relaxation in conjunction with joint stabilisation, improved circulation and increased levels of energy. By working holistically, physical *yoga* can improve performance of functional tasks, while decreasing the effort involved.

12.7.1.1 Physical exercises (*Asana*)

Yogic physical exercises (*Asana*) include *asanas* (static postures), *vinyasas* (dynamic exercises), *sat kriyas* (purification processes) and *mudras* (energy-control practices). *Sat kriyas* and *mudras* are thought to be the best *yogic* physical exercises and the best preparation for the meditative practices. They involve a combination of complicated breath-control and physical exercise and will be described after the section on breath-control, for clarity.

Yogic physical exercises can increase the range of joint motion (ROM), increase muscle length and tension (stretch) *nadis* (nerves and other channels) while maintaining joint stability. Nerve reflexes can be utilised to develop muscular strength throughout ROM and to train muscles to be voluntarily active or relaxed at any length. Synergistic muscle activations can be used to maximise the distance between proximal and distal attachments of a muscle and to increase flexibility. Muscle co-activations around the major joints (*bandha*s) can help stabilise these joints, assist in generation of energy, and promote circulation.

Yogic physical exercises can be weight-bearing on any part of the legs, arms, trunk, head or any combination of these parts. Weight-bearing exercises may minimise the risk of osteoporosis by maintaining bone mineral density in the area that is weight-bearing [OBrien, 2001].

12.7.1.1.1 Static postures (*asanas*)

According to *yogic* texts such as the *Siva-Samhita*, there are 8,400,000 *asanas* [Vishnu-Devananda, 1987, Bernard, 1950]. It is a testament to the anatomical knowledge of the ancient sages that you can use simple mathematics to verify this number almost exactly.

If you consider only the major joint-complexes (2 ankles, 2 knees, 2 hips, 1 spine, 2 shoulders, 2 elbows and 2 wrists), and only the main positions possible (flexion/extension in each ankle, knee, elbow and wrist; flexion/extension, abduction/adduction, and internal/external rotations in each hip and flexion/extension, left/ right lateral flexion, and left/right axial rotation in the spine), then the number of postures possible is then calculated to be almost exactly 8.4 million (number of possible postures = 2^2(ankle positions) x 2^2(knee positions) x $(2^3)^2$ (hip positions) x $(2^3)^1$ (spinal positions) x $(2^3)^2$ (shoulder positions) x 2^2(elbow positions) x 2^2 (wrist positions) = $2^2 \times 2^2 \times 2^6 \times 2^3 \times 2^6 \times 2^2 \times 2^2 = 2^{23}$ = 8,388,608) [Borg-Olivier & Machliss, 2003]. Although it is possible to perform any of these postures, a few classical postures offer the greatest benefit with a minimum of effort. Some *asanas* can be performed with completely relaxed muscles, while others impose obligatory isometric muscle activations. Within the full range of *asanas* it is possible to voluntarily activate any muscle in the body isometrically. Each *asana* may be held for any length of time from a few seconds to several hours, depending on the level of difficulty.

12.7.1.1.2 Dynamic exercises (*vinyasas*)

Vinyasa is the term for a linked series of postures and the linking movements between postures. *Vinyasas* can vary in speed: from those so slow that the movement is almost imperceptible to the eye, to those that are too fast for the eye to follow. One example of very fast *yoga* is B.K.S. Iyengar practising 108 gymnastic-like back-flips (*viparita cakrasana*) in four and a half minutes [Iyengar, 1990].

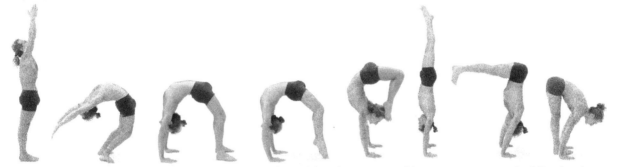

Concentric and eccentric muscle control is developed in *vinyasa*, and because one part of the body can resist against another, isokinetic muscle control can also be developed.

12.7.1.2 Breath-control (*Pranayama*)

Breath-control (*Pranayama*) is considered the link between the body and the mind, as it can be practised during both the physical exercises and the meditative practices. *Pranayama*, which literally means expansion and regulation (*ayama*) of the life force in the breath (*prana*) [Iyengar, 1993], develops internal energy and very efficient breathing which can reduce the amount of oxygen required to do a specific amount of work [Bernardi et al., 2001a]. Breath-control can be used to increase strength [Raghuraj et al., 1997], flexibility and cardiovascular fitness; to reduce blood pressure [Bhargava et al., 1988; Telles et al., 1996] and to regulate blood chemistry, hormone levels and the nervous system.

Yogic breathing is usually performed through both nostrils but can, at times, be through the mouth or through individual and alternating nostrils. *Pranayama* can affect breathing by modifying the length of inhalation, inhalation retention (holding the breath in), exhalation and exhalation retention (holding the breath out). The sound of the breath, the position of the tongue and regulation of the diet all affect *Pranayama*. Control of the muscles used for breathing and control of minute ventilation (the amount of air breathed per minute) are the most important factors determining the outcome of breath-control.

The adverse effects of incorrect yogic breathing, especially excessive breathing, can be extreme and dangerous [Teramoto et al., 1997]. *Yogic* texts stress that physical exercises (*Asana*) should be mastered before advanced breath-control (*Pranayama*) is attempted [Iyengar, 1993]. New practitioners of *yoga* who practise physical exercises (*Asana*) while breathing naturally prepare their bodies and mind for the eventual practise of breath-control (*Pranayama*).

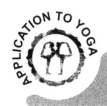

No 12.2 *Bhramari pranayama* (the humming breath) causes nitric oxide formation in the sinuses

Bhramari, also known as the humming breath or the bumble bee breath, is a type of *pranayama* that involves audible humming on the exhalation through the mouth. Humming has been shown to cause fifteen times the normal production of nitric oxide (NO) gas in the sinuses of the skull [Weitzberg & Lundberg; 2002]. NO has been shown to have several beneficial effects on the body. It is an important signalling molecule that acts in many tissues to regulate a diverse range of physiological processes including vasodilation (expansion of the blood vessel width), neuronal function, inflammation, immune function and in programmed cell death (apoptosis). NO has also been implicated in smooth muscle relaxation, pregnancy and blood vessel formation (angiogenesis). NO functions as a neurotransmitter in both the central and peripheral nervous systems [Snyder; 1992]. Endogenous and exogenous NO possesses anti-parasitic effects on both protozoa and metazoa [Ascenzi et al., 2003]. NO has a central anti-stress effect, apparently mediated by limiting the release of catecholamines [Bondarenko et al., 2001]. This may explain why yogic texts have always regarded *bhramari pranayama* with high esteem.

12.7.1.2.1 Yogic regulation of ventilation

A *yogin* (experienced *yoga* practitioner) can regulate blood chemistry by modifying minute ventilation (i.e. the average volume of air breathed per minute). Short periods of hyperventilation (increased minute ventilation) assist in internal cleansing; helps to increase strength, flexibility, and fitness; and prepare the *yogin* for meditation, which mainly involves hypoventilation (reduced minute ventilation).

12.7.1.2.1.1 Yogic use of hyperventilation

Hyperventilation can benefit the *yogin* in several ways. Breathing deeper and faster than normal can strengthen chest and abdominal musculature and reduce physiological dead space in the lungs. Hyperventilation alkalises the body by expelling carbon dioxide and increases sensitivity of the nervous system [Guyton, 1991]. The resultant mild alkalosis increases mobility (flexibility) of joints, muscles and nerves because fluid surrounding these structures becomes less viscous in alkaline conditions. Hyperventilation increases colonic tone [Bharucha et al., 1996] and can therefore be helpful in promoting bowel movements. Breath-holding or breath retention (*kumbhaka*) can be performed for an extended period if preceded by hyperventilation [Marks et al., 1997].

Hyperventilation is used in the *kriya* (yogic cleansing process) known as *kapala-bhati*, which involves rapid breathing through one or two nostrils. *Kapala-bhati-kriya* is an advanced practice that exercises chest and abdominal muscles, eliminates acid residues via the kidneys [Bhole, 1977], decreases urea in the blood [Desai & Gharote, 1990], generates specific brain wave patterns [Stancak et al., 1991a], modifies the status of the autonomic nervous system (ANS) [Raghuraj et al., 1998], exerts changes on blood pressure [Stancak et al., 1991b], increases breath retention times [Joshi, 1981] and prepares the *yogin* for periods of hypoventilation.

12.7.1.2.1.2 Dangers of hyperventilation

Prolonged or excessive hyperventilation and the associated alkalosis can cause adverse effects including provocation of an asthma attack [Helenius et al., 1997] due to bronchoconstriction; dizziness, fainting and headaches due to vasoconstriction and unsteadiness, paraesthesia, skin rashes, excessive appetite and emotional instability due to increased nervous sensitivity [Guyton, 1991]. Therefore, periods of hyperventilation in a *yoga* practice need to be balanced with periods of hypoventilation.

New practitioners of Patabhi Jois' *astanga vinyasa yoga* tend to hyperventilate during the entire physical part of their practice with deep relatively fast breathing. Although this type of hyperventilation confers several benefits – trunk strength, flexibility, cardiovascular fitness and mental focus – it can elicit many adverse reactions including emotional instability, excessive hunger and others listed above. These can usually be countered by a subsequent period of supine relaxation (*savasana*) of ten to thirty minutes in which natural hypoventilation (minimal breathing) is performed. Experienced practitioners of Patabhi Jois' *astanga vinyasa yoga* and other *yogins* (experienced *yoga* practitioners) tend to hypoventilate during their practice because they can maintain *tha-uddiyana bandha* (an expanded chest) and *ha-mula bandha* (a firm lower abdomen) throughout each breath cycle during their entire practice. This effectively reduces <u>minute ventilation</u> (i.e. becomes <u>hypoventilation</u>) while still conferring most of the benefits of normally attributed <u>hyperventilation</u> such as increased joint mobility (through heating the joints with the *bandhas* rather than alkalising them with <u>hyperventilation</u>) and accessing the most difficult-to-access parts of the lungs (by specifically directing the air to those parts of the lungs rather than by taking in excessive air).

12.7.1.2.1.3 Yogic use of hypoventilation

The *yogin* (experienced *yoga* practitioner) can achieve *yoga* (union) by using <u>hypoventilation</u> in the form of (i) respiratory suspension (breath-holding), (ii) long slow deep breathing or (iii) minimal breathing [Section 9.8.2.1] to 'still the fluctuations in the breath' [*Hatha Yoga Pradipika*] in order to 'still the fluctuations in the mind' [*Patanjali Yoga Sutras*]. <u>Hypoventilation</u> causes physiological <u>acidosis</u> (acidic blood), <u>hypoxia</u> (reduced <u>oxygen</u> in blood) and <u>hypercapnia</u> (increased <u>carbon dioxide</u> in blood). <u>Acidosis</u> desensitises the <u>nervous system</u> [Guyton, 1991] thus allowing the *yogin* to withdraw from the body senses and calm the emotions. <u>Hypoxia</u> and <u>hypercapnia</u> also promote <u>vasodilation</u> of the <u>blood vessels</u> to the <u>brain</u>, and <u>bronchodilatation</u> of the air passages to the <u>lungs</u>. <u>Hypercapnia</u> appears to have an active role in recovery after organ injury, as raised concentrations of <u>carbon dioxide</u> are protective, and low concentrations are injurious [Laffey & Kavanagh, 1999]. Mild physiological <u>acidosis</u>, <u>hypoxia</u>, and <u>hypercapnia</u> resulting from <u>hypoventilation</u>, are associated with the generation of <u>coherent synchronous brain wave patterns</u> that are characteristic of the <u>meditative state</u> [Badawi et al, 1984].

12.7.1.2.1.4 Dangers of hypoventilation

Extreme <u>hypoventilation</u> is not suited to the inexperienced practitioner. <u>Hypercapnia</u> (increased <u>carbon dioxide</u>) associated with <u>hypoventilation</u> causes <u>vasodilation</u> which can increase <u>intra-cranial pressure</u> (ICP; pressure in the head). This is especially so when the <u>intra-abdominal pressure</u> (IAP) is increased [Rosenthal et al., 1998] using chest and <u>abdominal muscles</u> (*bandhas*) during respiratory suspension (*kumbhaka*) in many advanced <u>breath-control</u> (*Pranayama*) exercises.

<u>Hypoventilation</u> can only be maintained for long periods without adverse effects if the practitioner adopts an <u>alkaline</u> lifestyle and diet. A low-protein vegetarian diet is the traditional *yogic* diet [Satyananda, 1996], and esoteric *yogi* masters of the Indian forest live solely on a diet of fruit and roots [Yogeshwarananda, 1959]. In the *Yoga-yajnavalkya-samhita* (verses 160-64) it states that those who practise *kevala-kumbhaka*, which has breath so minimal it is not noticeable, will have mastery over hunger [Desikachar, 2001].

12.7.1.3 *Yogic* purification and energy control (*bandhas*, *mudras* and *kriyas*)

<u>Breath-control</u> is also used in most of the unique exercises known as *sat kriyas* (purificatory processes), and *mudras* (energy-control practices). *Sat kriyas* (or simply *kriyas*) *are* cleansing processes that literally purify the body inside and out. *Mudras* are special gestures, postures and muscle-control exercises that regulate the flow of energy in the body. Most *sat kriyas* and *mudras* require the use of *bandhas* (muscle locks). *Bandhas*, *kriyas* and *mudras* are very powerful therapeutic agents, but few teachers are qualified to teach them.

12.7.1.3.1 *Bandhas* – muscle locks and energy guides

Bandhas can be thought of as muscle locks and energy guides. *Bandhas* are actually a special category of *mudra*, which are used in many *kriyas* and in *mudras* that are more complex. On a physical level, a *bandha* is essentially the <u>co-activation</u>, or simultaneous tensing, of opposing (<u>antagonistic</u>) muscles across a <u>joint complex</u>. *Bandhas* help to stabilise <u>joint-complexes</u> by balancing joint flexibility with muscular strength, and also generate and move energy through the body. Studies have shown that <u>co-activation</u> of pairs of one-joint <u>antagonistic</u> (opposing) muscles is not possible, whereas <u>co-activation</u> of pairs of multi-joint <u>antagonistic</u> (opposing) muscles is possible [Herzog & Binding, 1993]. *Bandhas* are explained in detail in the *bandha* sections of previous chapters.

12.7.1.3.2 *Kriyas* – yogic internal cleansing processes

Using the *bandhas* as a base, *hatha yoga* uses *kriyas* to cleanse and purify the inside of the body, and *mudras* to develop energy in the body and then channel it wherever it is needed. Probably the most powerful *kriyas* and *mudras* are those that apply all the main *bandhas* at the same time. This includes the series of *kriyas* related to *nauli* and the series of *mudras* related to *maha mudra*.

Nauli-kriya [Figure 12.1b] clearly defines (shows) the <u>rectus abdominis</u> muscle. *Nauli* generates a negative (sub-atmospheric) pressure in the colon, even greater than that of *tha-uddiyana bandha* alone [Kuvalayananda, 1956]. This moves every part of the intestines and redistributes their contents [Kuvalayananda, 1925]. *Nauli* facilitates the absorption of nutrients and the elimination of wastes [Rosemarynowski, 1981]. *Lauliki kriya* [Figure 12.1a-e] or churning, is a rolling version of *nauli* that activates the longitudinal components of the <u>rectus abdominis</u> sequentially and gives the appearance of the abdomen moving sideways. Advanced *yogins* can use *nauli-kriya* and *lauliki-kriya* to draw liquids into their colons while sitting in water, effectively giving themselves a colonic irrigation (*basti-kriya*), and to also draw liquids into their urethra to cleanse their bladder [Rosemarynowski, 1979, 1981].

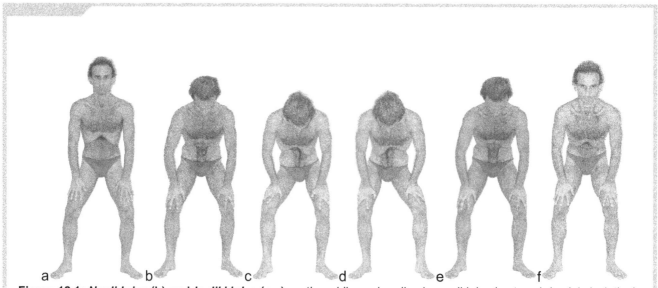

Figure 12.1: ***Nauli kriya* (b) and *lauliki kriya* (a-e):** *a. tha-uddiyana bandha*; b. *nauli kriya* (rectus abdominis isolation); c. left aspect of *nauli kriya*; d. right aspect of *nauli kriya*; e. *nauli kriya*; f. *tha-uddiyana bandha* with *ha-mula bandha* (obliquus externus abdominis isolation)

Other *kriyas* described in ancient *yogic* texts include *neti*, *dhauti*, and *trataka*. *Neti-kriya*, which uses air (*prana neti*), water (*pani neti*) or a long string (*sutra neti*) to clean the channels from the mouth to the nose [Rosemarynowski, 1981], has the ability to relieve headaches and throat problems [Yogeshwarananda, 1975]. *Dhauti-kriya*, which involves swallowing a cloth that is used to clean the stomach [Rosemarynowski, 1981], has been shown to help asthmatics [Gore & Bhole, 1982]. *Trataka*, which involves gazing continually at one point without blinking until the eyes begin to water, helps to clean the eyes. Throughout a *yoga* practice a *yogin* (experienced *yoga* practitioner) practices *dristi sadhana*, which involves gazing on specific points called *dristhis*. *Trataka* and *dristi sadhana* help focus the mind and assist in <u>meditative practices</u> by reducing the input to the <u>optic nerve</u>, the largest nerve entering the <u>brain</u>.

It should be noted that the *kriyas* are not for everyone. Experienced teachers such as B.K.S. Iyengar have cautioned against their use in most cases [Iyengar, 1988]. The more difficult *kriyas,* especially *basti, dhauti* and *sutra neti* are potentially dangerous and should only be practised under the supervision of an experienced teacher.

12.7.1.3.3 *Mudras – yogic* energy-control

12.7.1.3.3.1 *Maha mudra* (great energy-control)

Maha mudra [Figure 12.2] involves the *ha-* and *tha-* forms of *mula bandha, uddiyana bandha* and *jalandhara bandha*. In the many variations of *maha mudra*, the *bandhas* are applied while the breath is held in, while the breath is held out, and during breathing. The tongue is stretched into various positions such as *khecari mudra* (tongue towards the back of the throat) and *simha mudra* (tongue towards the chin) [Figure 12.2 d, e, h] throughout *maha mudra*. This assists in lengthening the <u>spine</u>, <u>tensioning</u> nerves, and stimulating glands. The effect of *maha mudra* is so powerful that *yogic* texts say that if practised enough, *maha mudra* can cure all disease [Ghosh, 1999].

Figure 12.2: *Maha mudra* **and some of its variations: (NB There are many types of** *maha mudra.* **Full sequences of this** *mudra* **are however not shown here as they should only be practised with the guidance of an experienced teacher).**

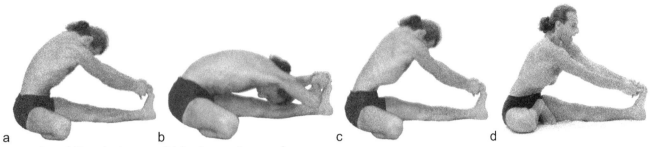

a   b   c   d

a.b.c.d Fourt stages of *bhadra maha mudra* **sequence:**
a. Upward phase with *antara kumbhaka* (inhalation retention) and *ha-jalandhara ha-uddiyana ha-mula bandha*
b. Downward phase with *antara kumbhaka* and *ha-jalandhara ha-uddiyana ha-mula bandha*
c. Upward phase with *bahya kumbhaka* (exhalation retention) and *ha-jalandhara tha-uddiyana ha-mula bandha*
d. *Bhaga maha mudra* with *bahya kumbhaka*, *simha mudra* and *ha-jalandhara tha-uddiyana ha-mula bandha*

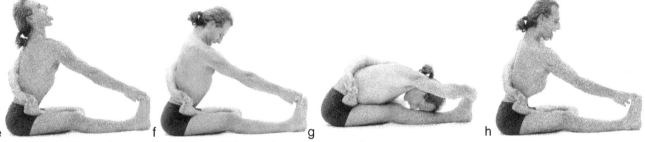

e   f   g   h

e.f.g.h. Four stages of *ardha baddha padma maha mudra* **sequence:**
e. Upward phase with *antara kumbhaka*, *simha mudra*, and *tha-jalandhara tha-uddiyana ha-mula bandha*
f. Upward phase with *antara kumbhaka* and *ha-jalandhara ha-uddiyana ha-mula bandha*
g. Downward phase with *antara kumbhaka* and *ha-jalandhara ha-uddiyana ha-mula bandha*
h. Upward phase with *bahya kumbhaka*, *simha mudra*, and *ha-jalandhara tha-uddiyana ha-mula bandha*

12.7.1.3.3.2 *Viparita karani mudra* (inverted practice)

Viparita karani mudra regulates the gravitational forces and represents inverted postures, such as headstand and shoulderstand, and the many partially inverted postures. The headstand (*sirsasana*) is held in high regard in *yoga* because it reverses the normal flow of gravity and bears the body weight directly on the head, neck and spine. Inverting the body is uncommon in most exercise forms, and with some minor exceptions, prolonged inversion exercises such as the headstand and shoulderstand (*sarvangasana*) are unique to *hatha yoga*.

The *yoga* texts say that *viparita karani mudra* has many health benefits, and scientific studies of head down tilt agree [Bonde-Petersen et al., 1983; Boocock et al., 1990]. Head down tilt is the expression used in scientific papers to describe inverted or semi-inverted postures usually studied on a tilted board. Within the first few minutes of inversion there are marked changes in both the cardiovascular and respiratory systems. Cardiac output and stroke volume increase but heart rate tends to fall [Soubiran et al., 1996]. Body inversion promotes hypoventilation, as shown by decreased minute ventilation, mild acidosis and hypoxia [Soubiran et al., 1996], which are all factors associated with meditative states [Farrow & Herbert, 1982; Kesterson & Clinch, 1989; Sudsuang et al., 1991]. Other immediate effects of even partial inversion include increase in heart volume [Knitelius & Stegemann, 1987], increase in diameter of the right internal jugular vein [Schreiber et al., 2002], changes in volume of body segments [Watenpaugh et al., 1997]; increase of thoracic fluid and changes in fluid regulating hormones [Grundy et al., 1991].

Prolonged effects of inversion include improved kidney function [Merzon & Zeligman, 1978], increased concentrations of energy-carrying molecules such as adenosine triphosphate (ATP) in arterial blood and blood flowing from the brain [Katkov et al., 1979], decreased respiration rate, lung ventilation, and oxygen consumption, and increased exhalation time and levels of blood acidity [Golikov et al., 1980].

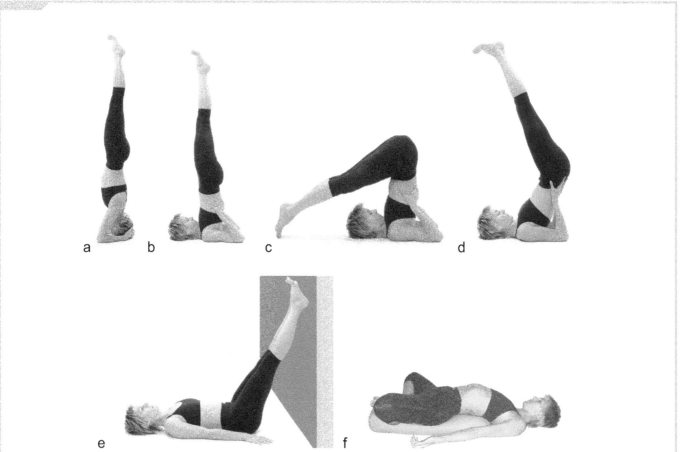

Figure 12.3: *Viparita karani mudra*: a. *sirsasana* (headstand); b. *sarvangasana* (shoulderstand); c. *halasana* (plough pose); d. *ardha sarvangasana* (half shoulderstand); e. *urdhva prasarita padasana* (legs resting up a wall); f. *supta baddha konasana* (with raised support for buttocks)

Viparita karani mudra is an excellent preparation for the meditative practices. A simple version of *viparita karani mudra* that is attainable to most people is simply resting the legs up a wall [Figure 12.3e] for a few minutes or resting the buttocks on a bolster with the shoulders on the floor [Figure 12.3f]. These semi-inverted practices, like the more advanced practice of headstand, impose a type of breath-control (*Pranayama*) that naturally increases the length and depth of thoracic breathing while promoting hypoventilation and mild acidosis.

12.7.1.3.3.3 San mukhi mudra (energy-control and sense-control)

San mukhi mudra [Figure 12.4] is another important *mudra* that is highly regarded in all the ancient texts because it immediately brings about a meditative state. In *san mukhi mudra*, the eyes are pressed closed with the fingers and the ears are pressed closed with the thumbs. The pressure of the thumbs against the ears causes an increased loudness of the breath. The *yogin* (experienced *yoga* practitioner) thus becomes immediately aware of their breath and meditative sense-control (*Pratayahara*) is initiated. As in *viparita karani mudra,* a natural breath-control begins with awareness of the breath. To maintain continual and even pressure of the fingers and thumb over the eyes and ears requires tremendous meditative concentration (*Dharana*). Pressure on the eyes also stimulates powerful images that can be gazed at as in *trataka kriya*. The optic nerve is one of the largest inputs to the brain. Focusing on an image with the eyes open, or visualising an image (meditative contemplation or *Dhyana*) with the eyes open or closed, helps to reduce unnecessary thoughts (described as 'fluctuations of the mind' in the *Patanjali-yoga-sutra*) and create a meditative state with coherent synchronous brain wave patterns as found in scientific studies on mental imagery.

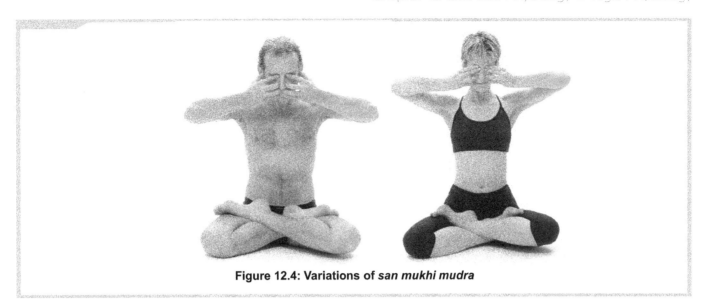

Figure 12.4: Variations of *san mukhi mudra*

12.7.2 Effects of Physical *Yoga*

Many positive and some negative effects of *yoga* are reported in the literature. The effects of *yoga* can be considered both in the long term and also in the short term.

12.7.2.1 Long-term effects of physical *yoga*

Reported long-term positive effects of *yoga* include increases in strength [Madanmohan et al., 1992; Raghuraj & Telles, 1997; Garfinkle *et al.*, 1998; Dash & Telles, 2001], flexibility [Moorthy, 1982; Ray et al., 2001], cardiovascular fitness [Raju et al., 1986; 1994], anaerobic threshold, mental function [Ray et al., 2001], and sense of well-being [Schell et al., 1994], decrease in reaction times [Madanmohan et al., 1992] and improved blood pressure [Patel & North, 1975; Selvamurthy et al., 1998].

Many of the well-documented benefits of the seated meditative practices [Section 9.8.1] can be obtained by practising purely physical *yoga*. This is because meditative states can be generated in any posture (*asana*) and even during movement (*vinyasa*). Physiological phenomena typical of those observed in seated meditative states, such as coherent synchronous brain wave patterns [Aftanas & Golocheikine, 2001] and hypoventilation [Travis & Pearson, 2000], have been demonstrated in people practising physical *yoga* [Junker & Dworkis, 1986; Kamei et al., 2001; Arambula et al., 2001; Vempati & Telles, 2002].

Physical *yoga* can have a simultaneous effect on the brain and the immune system. Kamei *et al* [2001] have demonstrated that during *yoga* exercises alpha brain waves increased while serum cortisol decreased. *Yogic* physical exercises can be thought of as a type of moderate exercise, the long-term effects of which, have been repeatedly shown to enhance the function of the immune system [Pedersen & Toft, 2000; Fairey et al., 2002]. Similarly, stress reduction and relaxation techniques, probably derived from *yoga,* have been shown to enhance immune function [Rood et al., 1993; Lowe et al., 2001].

12.7.2.2 Immediate effects of physical *yoga*

An integral aspect of *yoga* is living in the present moment. Therefore, it is important to note the immediate effects of an intelligent and correctly performed practice of *yogic* physical exercises (*Asana*) and breath-control (*Pranayama*). These effects include increased circulation [Gardner et al., 2001], facilitation of neuro-muscular control [Kocher, 1976; Telles et al, 1993; 1994a], regulation of blood chemistry [Raju et al., 1986; 1994; Miyamura et al., 2002], and control over the nervous system [Vempati & Telles, 2002] and the brain [Kamei et al., 2000].

12.7.2.2.1 Increased circulation through *yoga*

A primary goal of *yoga* is to integrate the body and mind as a whole. This communication is achieved and managed by the four circulatory systems (cardiovascular, lymphatic, nervous and acupuncture meridian sytems) that each form part of our *nadi* (subtle channel) system. Together these systems effectively transport information energy and matter throughout the body, defining the union of body and mind. Circulation is enhanced during a *yoga* practice by generating forces (*hatha*), in the form of high pressures (*ha*) and low pressures (*tha*), which act as circulatory pumps (Pressure = Force per unit of area). *Yoga* utilises six circulatory pumps to assist in the regulatory function of the heart. These pumps exist as a result of muscle activation and relaxation (*vinyasa*), breath-control (*Pranayama*), orientation to gravity (*viparita-karani*), posture (*asana*), co-activation of opposing muscles across joints (*bandha*) and movement (*vinyasa*).

Yoga utilises the musculoskeletal pump of circulation [Orsted et al., 2001] by moving in and out of each posture (*vinyasa*). When muscles tense, they increase local pressure in the veins and push blood and intracellular fluid in the direction of the heart. One-way back-flow valves in the veins prevent movement of venous blood away from the heart. When a muscle relaxes, it decreases local venous pressure and pulls blood to that region from regions more distal to the heart.

The respiratory pump of circulation is also employed in *yoga* [Hillman & Finucane, 1987] with breath-control (*Pranayama*). Breath-control (*Pranayama*) can affect the pre-load of the blood into the heart, which can alter heart rate. Inhalation directed to the thorax increases heart rate, while inhalation directed to the abdominal region decreases heart rate.

A gravitational pump of circulation also exists by virtue of *viparita-karani* [Section 12.7.1.3.3.2], the inverted or

semi-inverted postures. Simple postures such as resting the legs vertically up a wall, and more

advanced poses like *sirsasana* (headstand), reverse the natural flow of gravity in the body and can offer the same benefits as the technique referred to in physiotherapy as postural drainage [Fink, 2002].

The postural pump of circulation uses *asanas,* which are static postures. Relative to normal postures (such

as the anatomical position or *savasana*) *asanas* can physically compress (increase the pressure) on one region of the body while expanding or stretching (decreasing the pressure) in another region of the body.

The muscle co-activation pump of circulation employs *bandhas* (muscle co-activation around joints) to create regions of high pressure (*ha-bandhas*) or regions of low pressure (*tha-bandhas*). Energy in the form of blood and heat (amongst other things) tries to move from the regions of high pressure to the regions of low pressure. Intelligent control of the formation of these *bandha*s during a *yoga* practice can regulate the circulation in any part of the body.

Finally, the centripetal pump of circulation uses the movement between the postures (*vinyasa*) to create centripetal, centrifugal and inertial forces in the body [Resnick & Halliday, 1977]. When the body moves, it tends to move in circular movements. For example, when the upper limb moves from shoulder flexion to shoulder extension there is a circular path traced by the hand. The faster the hand moves, the more the centrifugal forces will pull blood to the hand and centripetal forces will be created to balance these centrifugal forces. The blood and intracellular fluids in the body will move with the body or with a body part until the body changes its velocity, changing its direction or speed. When the body changes its velocity, the blood and intracellular fluids keep trying to move in the same direction they were initially going due to the inertia they have attained. Moving intelligently and effectively can stimulate blood flow to any part of the body via the use of the centripetal pump of circulation.

The six circulatory pumps also assist in the movement of food through the intestines, the absorption of nutrients and the elimination of wastes. The six circulatory pumps can effectively massage internal organs and endocrine glands, assisting in their function.

12.7.2.2.2 *Yogic* facilitation of neuromuscular control
Another important way that *yoga* can effectively achieve union between body and mind is through integrated control and regulation of skeletal muscles and the nervous system. This requires a basic understanding and application of the principles of motor nerve reflexes and nerve tensioning (stretching).

12.7.2.2.2.1 *Yogic* use of nerve reflexes [Sections 1.7.2.2.1, 9.4.2 & 9.7.4]

A reflex is an automatic nerve response to some type of stimulus. Three important reflexes, which should be taken into account and which can be taken advantage of in any physical posture, are the stretch (myotatic) reflex, the reciprocal relaxation reflex and the inverse myotatic reflex.

The myotatic (stretch) reflex is the reflex activation of a muscle whenever a muscle is suddenly tensioned or stretched [Alter, 1996]. If the myotatic (stretch) reflex is activated during a stretching exercise then it will reduce the ability to stretch very far. If forced, the muscle may be damaged. The *yogin* (experienced *yoga* practitioner) tries to inhibit the myotatic (stretch) reflex by:

- Moving slowly into a stretch
- Exhaling (from the thorax) while moving into a stretch (which slows the heart)
- Concentrating on the muscle being stretched
- Activating antagonistic (opposing) muscles (reciprocal relaxation reflex)

The myotatic (stretch) reflex can be taken advantage of by its ability to cause the recruitment (activation) of adjoining and distant muscles and muscle groups by virtue of the fascial connections (connective tissue) between muscles. In order to activate a muscle which is difficult to isolate, the *yogin* can activate any of the muscles in the region of that muscle. They will exert a gentle pull or stretch on neighbouring muscles that are joined by fascial connections and may then become activated via the myotatic (stretch) reflex.

The reciprocal relaxation reflex is the reflex inhibition of a muscle following the activation of its antagonist or opposing muscle [Alter, 1996]. The *yogin* can go deeper into a stretch by consciously activating the muscles opposing the muscles being stretched. An understanding of the reciprocal relaxation reflex gives the *yogin* the means to deeply relax a muscle, stretch it further and also help to strengthen the opposing muscle. In the hamstring stretch, the *yogin* activates and helps strengthen the knee extensors (eg. quadriceps) in order to reciprocally relax and further stretch the knee flexors (eg. hamstrings). Similarly, tensing the muscles under the armpits (shoulder depressors) by pulling the shoulders towards the hips, causes a reflex relaxation of the muscles between the shoulders and the neck (shoulder elevators).

The inverse myotatic reflex is the reflex relaxation of a muscle after it has been subjected to a prolonged intense stretch [Alter, 1996]. This phenomenon, known as a lengthening reaction, is believed to take at least 12-15 seconds to occur if the stretched muscle is initially in a relaxed state. The lengthening reaction is most noticeable if a muscle is activated while being stretched. The *yogin* takes advantage of the inverse myotatic reflex by activating and helping to strengthen the muscle being stretched in order to inversely relax that muscle and subsequently help it stretch further. After the active tension is released, the muscle usually stretches even further.

Antagonistic muscle co-activation (*bandha*) has a variable effect on the nervous system depending on the individual. In some cases, it may result in the activation of all three nerve reflexes mentioned above, leading to an overall stimulation of the nervous system. However, since co-activation is sometimes under voluntary control, all the nerve reflexes may be inhibited, leading to an overall calming effect on the nervous system. Research has shown that during co-activation there is a significant interaction with the nervous system [Proske *et al.*, 2000; Aagaard *et al.*, 2000; Barbeau *et al.* 2000]. However, further research is needed to establish exactly what is taking place in the nervous system, both in the co-activations that are generated by the activities of everyday life and with awareness of the voluntary co-activations generated as *bandhas*.

12.7.2.2.2.2 *Yogic* use of nerve tensioning (stretching)

When *yogic* physical exercises create differential regions of pressure within the body, *prana* (life-force or vital energy) is made to move along the *nadis*. *Nadis* are subtle channels found within the body along which move *prana* and *citta* (consciousness) [Goswami, 1980]. When the body is stretched in a *yoga* practice, it is not just muscles but also *nadis* that are stretched. Blood vessels and nerves are examples of gross manifestations of the *nadis* but are not actually the *nadis* themselves. More subtle *nadis* include the acupuncture meridians of eastern medicine [Motoyama, 1993].

When the *nadis* are stretched, a significant proportion of the physical sensation that may be experienced results from nerves and acupuncture meridians being tensioned (stretched). An increased sense of well-being can result if nerves are carefully tensioned. Tensioning (stretching) nerves mobilises and allows them to function more effectively as instigators of muscle activation. However, over-tensioning (over-stretching) may result in nerve damage, pain, or loss of muscle strength or control.

The practice of *hatha yoga* takes into account the presence of *nadis* and in particular on the gross level, the presence of the nerves because:
- Nerves are an important method of communication in the body.
- Nerve impingement can have a debilitating effect on the body.
- Nerves can have a profound effect on the body if they are tensioned (stretched). Such tensioning can be very relieving and energising when given at an appropriate intensity, or it can be extremely damaging if given in excess.
- Nerve reflexes can affect the activation or inhibition of muscle groups.

Certain postures require care in order not to over-tension (over-stretch) the spinal cord or various nerves. All poses which include flexion of the neck, spine and hip with extension at the knees and ankles, strongly tension (stretch) the spinal cord and the sciatic nerves and can be damaging. In this category are all the straight-legged forward-bending hamstring stretches such as *pascimottanasana*

which may cause an over-stretch of the sciatic nerve and possibly the spinal cord, if the head and neck are in a flexed position (i.e. chin brought towards the chest). Also in this category

is the *yoga* plough pose (*halasana*), which is weight-bearing on the neck and upper back, and can over-stretch and perhaps damage the spinal cord and the nerves around the lower back.

Similarly, all lunging poses, including the front splits movement (*hanumanasana*) and other similar hip flexor stretches, may cause an over-stretch and perhaps possible damage to the femoral nerves. In addition, all postures in which the arms are outstretched and the neck is being moved, may cause an over-stretch and perhaps possible damage to the brachial plexus, median nerve, radial nerve and/or ulnar nerve.

12.7.2.2.3 *Yogic* control over blood chemistry

The *yogin* (experienced *yoga* practitioner) can significantly alter blood chemistry with breath-control. Hyperventilation (increased breathing) decreases carbon dioxide in the blood (hypocapnia) and causes an increase in pH or alkalinity, while hypoventilation (reduced breathing) leads to an increase of carbon dioxide in the blood (hypercapnia), and a decrease in pH or (increased acidity). Various studies of *yoga* exercises have demonstrated changes in levels of noradrenaline [Bharucha et al., 1996], cortisol [Kamei et al., 2000] and lactate [Solberg et al., 2000] and changes in blood-clotting ability [Chohan et al., 1984]. *Yoga* training has been shown to be comparable to sub-maximal endurance training in increasing levels of LDH (lactate dehydrogenase), which is a glycolytic enzyme utilised during exercise to provide energy to contracting muscles [Pansare et al., 1989].

12.7.2.2.4 Yogic regulation of the autonomic nervous system (ANS)

Experienced *yogin*s can regulate the autonomic nervous system (ANS) using physical exercises, or breath-control. Expansion of the chest while emphasising thoracic inhalations, or while practising *tha-uddiyana bandha* with the breath held out, stimulates the sympathetic nervous system and increases heart rate. This is due to the effects of the respiratory pump, which draws blood to the heart as the intra-thoracic pressure (ITP) reduces with chest expansion. Lengthening exhalations stimulates the parasympathetic nervous system and reduces heart rate. [Zeier, 1984].

Another effect on the <u>nervous system</u> through <u>breath-control</u> is via *mudra*. For example in *maha mudra* [Section 12.7.1.3.3.1], trunk muscles are <u>activated</u> in order to increase <u>intra-abdominal pressure</u> (IAP) and <u>intra-thoracic pressure</u> (ITP) while the breath is held in (*ha-bandha antara kumbhaka*). This leads to an increase in <u>blood pressure</u> that is detected by <u>baroreceptors</u> of the circulatory system. These <u>baroreceptors</u> then signal the PNS to slow the <u>heart rate</u> in order to reduce <u>blood pressure</u>.

*Yogin*s can effectively regulate the ANS by selectively breathing through one nostril at a time, through manipulation of the nasal passages with the fingers or tongue. Studies have shown that breathing through the right nostril stimulates the <u>sympathetic nervous system</u> [Mohan, 1996]; increases body heat, <u>oxygen</u> consumption, <u>blood pressure</u> [Telles et al., 1996], and <u>heart rate</u> [Shannahoff-Khalsa & Kennedy, 1993]; stimulates the left cerebral hemisphere [Schiff & Rump, 1995]; and may stimulate verbal task performance [Jella & Shannahoff-Khalsa, 1993]. Breathing through the left nostril stimulates the <u>parasympathetic nervous system</u> [Backon et al., 1990], decreases body heat, <u>heart rate</u> and <u>blood pressure</u> [Telles et al., 1994b]; stimulates the <u>right cerebral hemisphere</u> [Werntz et al., 1987]; and increases spatial task performance [Jella & Shannahoff-Khalsa, 1993]. Alternate nostril breathing (*nadi sodhana pranayama*) balances the ANS and the right and left cerebral hemispheres [Backon et al., 1990], increases alpha and beta <u>brain waves</u> [Stancak & Kuna, 1994], and increases handgrip strength [Rajuraj et al., 1997]. *Yogic* science has had this type of knowledge for millennia [Ghosh, 1999]. However, most of the *yogic* information about this subject has either been lost, or is not being taught by those who know about it, because the ancient texts say that this information should be kept secret [Desikachar, 1998].

Asymmetrical postures can affect the <u>nasal cycle</u> [Haight & Cole, 1986; 1989], the ANS [Backon & Kullok, 1990], and emotional states [Schiff & Lamon, 1994]. When one side of the body is compressed the contralateral nostril becomes more open [Mohan, 1991], which stimulates the corresponding hemisphere of the <u>brain</u> [Schiff & Truchon, 1993]. The *yogin* (experienced *yoga* practitioner) influences the ANS by performing only one side of certain asymmetrical postures. Similarly, by doing the right side of posture first, or by rolling to the right side from a supine resting

posture (*savasana*) as is a common practice amongst *yogins*, the left side nostril becomes less congested, the <u>sympathetic nervous system</u> relaxes and the <u>parasympathetic nervous system</u> is stimulated, thus reducing stress and increasing calmness.

12.7.2.2.5 Use of meditative practices to regulate the nervous system
*Yogin*s can significantly influence the ANS with <u>physical exercises</u> (*Asana*), <u>breath-control</u> (*Pranayama*) and <u>meditative practices</u>. Magnetic resonance imaging (MRI) studies of the <u>brain</u> [Lazar et al., 2000] indicate that <u>meditative practices</u> activate neural structures that are involved in attention and control of the ANS.

12.7.3 The Relationship between Western Physiology and *Yogic* Physiology
Conventional Western science and the science of *hatha yoga* have some features in common and in some areas they have come to exactly the same conclusions. However, the basic premise in Western science and in the Western approach to physiology, until recently, comes from a reductionist philosophy that says that we are but the sum of our individual parts.

On the other hand, the word *yoga* literally means union, a binding together or a oneness. *Yoga* is the ultimate holistic science. In *yogic* physiology (along with its sister science of *ayurveda*), everything is seen to affect and interrelate with everything else. The whole body is greater than the sum of its parts and the whole body is reflected and can be seen in every part of the body.

Due to the difference in the basic premises of *yogic* and Western physiologies, the *yogic* physiology allows for more possibilities of the body and the mind than Western physiology currently allows or can prove to be true. This is only possible because *yogic* physiology has been developed from personal and practical experience, whereas Western physiology is meant to be objective and not subjective or personal. This means that much of what is stated in *yogic* physiology has not yet been proven by Western science, and might not ever be able to be proven.

However, in the last three decades much work has been done to promote a more holistic approach to Western science that has allowed a greater scientific acceptance of holistic concepts such as acupuncture and meridian theory. In addition, whole new fields of Western physiology that reflect the holistic nature of the body have recently evolved. One such holistic science is the emerging field of psychoneuroimmunology [Section 11.1.4.1], which essentially says that the body can think in many ways like the brain. Another developing field of Western physiology is exploring the holistic relationships between cerebral hemispheric contra-laterality, the autonomic nervous system (ANS), the nasal cycle and their effects on physiology and emotional states [Section 9.7.5]. The relatively new holistic ideas in Western physiology are not new to *yoga*. The notion that the nervous system is linked with the endocrine system, as described in the relatively new science of psychoneuroimmunology, is integral to the *yogic* concept of *cakras* as shown in Table 12.2. The effect of regulating the nasal cycle on the ANS is integral to *yoga* practices such as *nadi sodhana pranayama* (the alternate nostril breath). Table 12.2 compares various aspects of Western physiology with *yogic* physiology.

Hopefully it can be seen that both *yogic* and Western physiologies are valid and useful within their realms, but it is some sort of synthesis or synergy between the two which may be the most fruitful way of rediscovering information about the body which was probably once known but now is lost, or confused.

12.7.4 *Ayurveda* and *Yogic* Physiology

Ayurveda is a *Sanskrit* word, derived from two roots: *ayur*, which means life, and *veda*, knowledge. *Ayurveda*, which literally means 'the science of life', is a 6000-year-old healing tradition of India. The same great sages who introduced *yoga* and meditation established *ayurveda*. *Ayurveda* is more than just a medical system, it's a way of life that co-operates with nature and lives in harmony with her. A comprehensive review of *ayurveda* is beyond the scope of this book. What follows is a brief overview.

According to *ayurveda* the union of *purusa* (soul) and *prakruti* (nature) forms the entire universe and the animal kingdom. From the *trigunas* (three qualities of nature), *sattva* (luminosity), *rajas* (vibrancy), and *tamas* (dormancy or inertia), the five main elements (*tatwas*): ether (*akasha*), fire (*tejas*), air (*vayu*), water (*apa*) and earth (*prithvi*) and are formed. In terms of Western physiology ether implies space, fire implies energy, air implies the gaseous state of matter, water implies the liquid state of matter and earth implies the solid state of matter. *Ayurveda* defines three fundamental energies or principles called *dosas* (also called *tri-dosas*) that govern our constitution and the function of our bodies on the physical and emotional level. The *tridosas* (three energies) *vata*, *pitta* and *kapha*, are formed from the five elements with a relationship as described by Lele *et al.* [1999] [Table 12.3].

* These concepts are relatively new to Western or conventional science.

Table 12.2 Relationship between Western physiology & *yogic* physiology

	WESTERN PHYSIOLOGY (WP)	YOGIC PHYSIOLOGY (YP)
PREMISE	• REDUCTIONISTIC	• HOLISTIC
CIRCULATORY CHANNELS	• NERVOUS SYSTEM (**NS**) • CARDIOVASCULAR SYSTEM (**CVS**), • LYMPHATIC SYSTEM (**LS**) Circulatory channels of WP flow with energy in the form of heat, electrochemical energy, and energy carrying molecules (eg. sugars and ATP); & information in the form of electrochemical energy neurotransmitters, immunotransmitters & hormones.	*Nadis* (energy channels of the *yoga* system) *Nadis* include the nerves, blood and lymph vessels, and the acupuncture meridians The *nadis* flow with **prana** (Life Force or energy in one of its many forms including matter) & **citta** (consciousness, which is considered to be a subtle form of energy).

CIRCULATORY MECHANISMS	(1) CARDIOVASCULAR PUMP (**CVP**) (2) MUSCULOSKELETAL PUMP (**MSP**) (3) RESPIRATORY PUMP (**RP**) (4) GRAVITATIONAL PUMP (**GP**) [Chapter 8]	• Use of *hatha* (= force) implies differential forces or pressures represented by *ha* (= Sun, representing heat or high pressure force) & *tha* (= Moon representing cooling or low pressure force), which generate and move energy throughout the body. • Includes **CVP**, **MSP**, **RP**, **GP** & POSTURAL PUMP (**PP**). • **PP**: POSTURES (*asanas*) used to improve circulation in **CVS**, **LS**, & **AMS**. • **POSTURES** used to tension (stretch) nerves and influence **autonomic nervous system.** • **RESPIRATORY PUMP** maximizes use when the central *bandhas* are applied.
BREATHING	WP has good theoretical understanding of normal and unhealthy CardioPulmonary System (CPS), with little practical application to discover the true potential of the CPS [Chapter 8].	• Practical application of principles of hatha *yoga* allows true potential of the cardio-pulmonary system (cps), to be realised. • Use of *bandhas* & *mudras* to guide *prana* through the body. • *Yogis* reduce & regulate the number of breaths taken, in order to extend life.
MAJOR CENTRES OF CIRCULATION	**(1) NERVE PLEXUSES** [Chapter 9] **(2) ENDOCRINE GLANDS** [Chapter 11] (3) *TRIGGER (**ACUPUNCTURE**) POINTS INTERSECTING NERVES & BLOOD VESSELS	*Cakras* are subtle energy centres, or whirling vortexes of energy that can be in charged or uncharged states at various key points (*marmas*) in the body. These can be compared with windmills that can catch wind energy and transform it to electrical energy. 1) **Major *Cakras*** are found at intersecting points of the two major *nadis* (*ida & pingala*) which spiral down from the nostrils and intersect along the spinal cord. 2) **Minor *cakras*** are found at intersecting points of blood vessels and nerves between opposite acupuncture meridians throughout the body [Bhan, 1996].
MUSCLE LOCKS	The *Valsalva manoeuvre* is known to affect pressure in the body [Chapter 8]. Co-activations of certain muscle groups can stabilise joints, eg transversus abdominis role in relief of lower back pain [Chapter 7]; Perineum muscles known to assist in organ function [Chapter 11].	*Bandhas* (internal subtle muscular locks that centre on key points on the spine and on all the major joints in the body) • Stimulate the activation of *cakras* (subtle energy centres); • Influence pressure & hence the movement of energy in the body; • Promote stability of major joints; • Assist in slowing & regulating breathing.
FOOD INTAKE	Food pyramid, reductionist view with individual components of diet, high protein diet prevalent leading to **acid** pH in blood and body systems leading to calcium leaching from bones, blockage of joints and vessels, and inability to retain carbon dioxide [Chapter 10].	Idea of *gunas* (food types & person types). Yogic *sattvic* or *phalari* diet (cooked vegetables, salads, & fruits). Low protein diet leading to **alkaline** residues in blood reduces risk of bone leaching or vessel blockage & increased ability to deal with carbon dioxide.
***CEREBRAL HEMISPHERIC CONTRA-LATERALITY**	The ***nasal cycle** (the alternating nature of breathing through different nostrils throughout the day to automatically regulate temperature and metabolism) has been shown to be linked to the sidedness of the cerebral hemispheres, and also affect the autonomic nervous system (ANS) (heat in body, emotional states, stress levels, digestive function etc.) [Chapter 9].	*Hatha yoga* uses breathing techniques such as *nadi sodhana pranayama* (alternate nostril breathing), postural symmetry & nerve tensioning (stretching), to balance the autonomic nervous system (ANS), to improve physiological function, lung function, and emotional well being.

Table 12.3: Relationship between *Ayurvedic Gunas*, Elements and *Dosas*
[After Lele *et al.*, 1999]

Guna	Ayurvedic Element	Dosa	Contains the Gunas
Sattva	Ether		
Rajas	Air	Vata	Sattva Rajas
Sattva + Rajas	Fire	Pitta	Sattva Rajas Tamas
Tamas + Sattva	Water	Kapha	Tamas Sattva
Tamas	Earth		

Ayurveda defines disease as the natural result of living out of harmony with your constitution. Our constitution is the inherent balance of the *tridosas* (three energies) within our bodies and our minds. Because we all have a different balance of energy, *ayurveda* shows that the path to optimal health is different for each person depending upon his or her constitution. The effects of an imbalance in one of the three energies (*tridosas*) are shown in Table 12.4 which is derived from information obtained from Halpern [1998] and Lele *et al.* [1999].

Ayurveda also says that the three *dosas* – *vata, pitta,* and *kapha* – are closely related to three energies: *prana* (vital energy), *tejas* or *agni* (internal fire) and *ojas* or *soma* (subtle energy). The *dosas* function primarily on the *anna maya kosha* or physical body. The energetic counterparts of the *dosas* (*prana, tejas* and *ojas*) function primarily on the *mano maya kosha* or subtle body [Halpern, 1998]. Mind (*manas*), intellect (*buddhi*) and ego (*ahamkara*) are all superficial aspects of, and operate within, the broader field of consciousness (*citta*) [Iyengar, 1993].

We are all a combination of all three *dosic* energies. On a fundamental level, *pitta* represents our metabolism, *kapha* our structure and *vata* the mobility that brings action and life into creation. Without all three energies we simply could not exist.

12.7.5 *Marmas, Bandhas* and *Cakras*

In *ayurveda,* a *marma* point is defined as an anatomical site where important nerves (*dhamani*) meet together with muscles, veins, ligaments and/or joints [Lele *et al.*, 1999]. *Marma* points are also where the *tridosas* – *vata, pitta,* and *kapha* – are present with their subtle forms *prana, ojas* (*soma*) and *tejas* (*agni*), together with the three *gunas* (qualities of nature), *sattva, rajas,* and *tamas*. These areas are related through the *nadis* (subtle channels) to the internal organs. *Marma* points are also vital points in the body known in various martial arts as secret places which, if injured, can cause disease or death. They are also thought to be places where there is union between body and mind [Lele *et al.*, 1999].

The co-activation of opposing muscles in *bandhas* [Section 1.7.3] can protect vital *marma* points. *Bandhas* also serve to energise the *marmas* by generating energy and moving energy through the *nadis*. According to Dr Bhan [1996], who has compared *yoga* and *ayurveda* throughout India, *marma* points lie between two acupuncture points of opposing meridians. *Marma* points, when activated by *prana* flowing through the *nadis,* are the places that *cakras* (whirling energy vortexes) are activated [Bhan, 1996]. When the *cakra* is activated then the *marma* point is no longer a point of susceptibility but a point of strength [Bhan, 1996].

12.7.6 *Hatha Yoga Vidya* (Science) and Western Physiology

The basic concepts of *Hatha Yoga Vidya* (the science or physiology of *hatha yoga*) and its relation to conventional Western physiology are outlined in Table 12.2 and are discussed throughout the text. Some key points are summarised below:

- o **Prana** (vital energy) is taken into the body in its gross form through the food we eat and in a more subtle form from the air.
- o **Pranayama** (breath-control) means the extension (**ayama**) of the breath, the life force (**prana**) and life itself.

[Based on information derived from Halpern, 1998; & Lele *et al.*, 1999].

Table 12.4: Effects of imbalances in the *dosas* and the relationship to a *yoga* practice

DOSA	IMBALANCES IN THE FOLLOWING *DOSAS*		
	VATA	**PITTA**	**KAPHA**
CHARACTERISTIC OF *DOSAS* (EFFECTS OF ELEMENTS & *GUNAS*)	**Elements**: Air & Ether **Gunas**: Sattva & Rajas **Characteristics**: Light (air) Diffuse (ether)	**Elements**: Fire & Water **Gunas**: Sattva, Rajas, Tamas **Characteristics**: Hot, sharp penetrating (fire) Volatile & oily (water)	**Elements**: Water & Earth **Gunas**: Tamas & Sattva **Characteristics**: Cool & moist like water Stable & heavy like earth
BODY TYPE	Light Thin bones Dry skin Dry hair	Feel warm, Oily skin Penetrating eyes Sharp features Moderate weight Good musculature	Dense Heavy bones Lustrous Supple skin Low metabolism Large, stocky frame
PERSONALITY TYPE	Talkative Enthusiastic Creative Flexible Energetic Speak quickly	Focused & Intense Capable & Competitive Courageous & Energetic Clear communicators Get right to the point Like to solve problems Speak with sharp tongue Great as friends Feared as enemies	Stable personality Not prone to quick fluctuations Handle stress well Dislike change Conservative Enjoy comfort
CHARACTERISTICS OF BODY	Lightness Coldness Mobility Cold hands and feet	Hot	Heavy Sluggish Cold Damp
PHYSICAL PROBLEMS (THAT MAY OCCUR WHEN OUT OF BALANCE)	Weight loss Constipation Weak immune system Weak nervous system	Diarrhoea Infections Burning eyes Skin rashes Acne psoriasis Weak liver Weak spleen & blood	Congestion Mucous accumulation Weight gain Lethargy Weakness in lungs and sinuses Diabetes
MENTAL &/OR EMOTIONAL PROBLEMS (THAT MAY OCCUR WHEN OUT OF BALANCE)	Confusion & Anxiety Nervousness & Fearful Become overwhelmed Difficulty focusing Difficulty making decisions Insomnia	Anger Resentment Jealousy	Lack of motivation Depression Lethargy
BEST TYPE OF *YOGA* PRACTICE (THAT HELPS TO RE-BALANCE AN IMBALANCE OF *DOSAS*)	Need a calming & grounding practice Avoid postures and practice which overstimulates nerves	Need calming & cooling practice to cool the body down Avoid overheating with *Yoga* practice	Need to have a practice that reduces congestion, and creates lightness, dryness and warmth. Avoid passive meditation unless balanced with activity

- o *Pranayama* is facilitated by the *bandhas* (internal locks), which generate force (*hatha*) in the form of pressures, drawing *prana* into the <u>lungs</u> and moves it into the *nadis*.
- o *Nadis* (energy channels) carry *prana* (vital energy) and *citta* (consciousness), which move together through the body.
- o The *asanas* (static postures), *vinyasas* (dynamic exercises), *bandhas* (internal locks) and *pranayamas*, create differential regions of high pressure (*ha*) and low pressure (*tha*) within the body. These forces (*hatha*) pump *prana* through the *nadis*, with guidance from the *mudras* (seals), to key places (*marma* **points**) where the *prana* charges the *cakras* (energy centres).
- o Also the *bandhas*, <u>co-activations</u> of opposing muscles, act on the <u>nervous system</u> by stimulating spinal <u>reflexes</u>. Stimulation of nerve <u>plexuses</u> assists in charging the *cakras*.
- o The charged *cakras* actively regulate the flow of *prana* through the *nadis* and into the rest of the body.
- o *Nadi sodhana pranayama* (alternate nostril breathing) helps assist in the conscious regulation of the flow of *prana* through the various *nadis* and *cakras* (energy centres).

<u>Conclusion</u>

Although the *yogic* physiology cannot be proven by the reductionist and objective Western physiology, the *yoga* practitioner is able to examine and consider the ideas of *yogic* physiology. Because *hatha yoga* is a practical, holistic and subjective science, such an assessment is personally valid.

Until the existence of subtle energy can be demonstrated by conventional physiology (then perhaps) the only advice to offer is to keep practising *hatha yoga* and find the subtle energy for yourself.

Finally, keep practising *hatha yoga* in order to better understand the functioning of the body and life force, and keep studying anatomy and physiology in order to discover new ways of practising *hatha yoga* and playing with the life force.

12.7.7 Non-physical *Yoga*: Meditative Practices (*Pratayahara, Dharana, Dhyana, and Samadhi)* and Ethical Disciplines (*Yama* and *Niyama)*

<u>Non-physical *yoga*</u> includes the <u>meditative practices</u> (*Pratayahara, Dharana, Dhyana, and Samadhi)* and the <u>ethical disciplines</u> (*Yama* and *Niyama)*. <u>Non-physical *yoga*</u> is as important to a *yoga* practice as <u>physical *yoga*</u> (*Asana* and *Pranayama)*.

12.7.7.1 Meditative practices (*Pratayahara, Dharana, Dhyana,* and *Samadhi)*

In the Western world today, meditation is usually perceived to be some sort of mental and/or spiritual practice, which may involve some sort of relaxation or concentration component. In fact, meditation is a state of mind, characterised by the presence of <u>coherent synchronous brain wave patterns</u> that can remove the meditator from sensory awareness taking them into deep concentration and contemplation, until finally a state of blissful super-consciousness or total absorption is attained. The <u>meditative state</u> is often synonymous with the art of mental visualisation. Similar <u>brain wave patterns</u> are generated during both visualisation and meditation [von Stein & Sarnthein, 2000]. Meditation can also be dynamic or even physically exerting [Iyengar, 1966]. It can be said that either meditation is a path to creating a clear or empty mind, or that meditation itself is that state of empty or clear mind into which fresh energy, inspiration and ideas can be attracted.

According to ancient *yogic* texts, *yoga* and meditation are the same thing. The main text on *raja yoga* (often thought of as meditation), the *Patanjali-yoga-sutra,* says *yoga* is *citta-vrtti-nirodha*, which means *yoga* is that state in which the fluctuations in the mind cease [Iyengar, 1993]. In scientific terms, this can be interpreted and seen as <u>coherent synchronous brain wave patterns</u>. The main text on *hatha yoga* (often thought of as <u>physical yoga</u>), the *Hatha yoga-pradipika,* says *yoga* is *prana-vrtti-nirodha*, which means *yoga* is that state when the fluctuations in the breath cease [Iyengar, 1988]. In scientific terms, this can be interpreted as <u>hypoventilation</u> (long slow breathing, minimal breathing or breath-suspension). Clinical studies on *raja yoga* and *hatha yoga* have confirmed that these two statements are correct. It is found that raja yogis who 'still their mind' (as evidenced by coherent synchronous brain wave patterns), also simultaneously spontaneously demonstrate hypoventilation (reduced breathing) with periods of breath-suspension [Farrow & Herbert, 1982; Gallois, 1984; Travis & Wallace, 1997]. Similarly, hatha yogis and others who 'still their breath' using different types of hypoventilation, also simultaneously spontaneously demonstrate coherent synchronous brain wave patterns, i.e. when they 'still their breath' they also 'still their mind'. The physiology of meditation is described in Chapter 9. The positive and negative effects of the meditative practices are described in Section 9.8.3.

12.7.7.2 Ethical disciplines (*Yama* and *Niyama*)

The ethical disciplines involved with the practice of *yoga* are termed *Yama* and *Niyama*. According to Iyengar [1988] *Yama* and *Niyama* form the roots and trunk of the *astanga yoga* tree.

Yama reflects our attitudes to our environment (including the people around us) [Desikachar, 1998]. *Yama* includes the principles of *ahimsa* (non-violence), *satya* (truthfulness), *asteya* (freedom from avarice), *brahmacarya* (control of sensual pleasure) and *aparigraha* (freedom from covetousness and possessions beyond need).

Niyama reflects our attitudes to ourselves [Desikachar, 1998]. *Niyama* includes the principles of *sauca* (cleanliness), *santosa* (contentment), *tapas* (ardour or a burning desire), *svadhyaya* (self-study) and *Ishvara-pranidhana* (self-surrender, devotion or love).

Both teachers and students of *yoga* require the correct attitude. *Yama* and *niyama* demand the correct attitudes both to our individual selves and to our environment, which includes the people in our lives. *Yoga* is as much about union with our higher selves as it is the union or relationships with the people in our lives. For a student of *yoga* to receive safe and engaging *yoga* they must have correct attitude to the way they approach their practice and to the way they deal with their teacher. Similarly, for a *yoga* teacher to transmit their knowledge to students they also must have the correct attitudes to themselves and to their students.

Compliance of students and patients of *yoga* is further discussed in Section 12.7.7.2.1. The appropriateness of *yoga* in different situations is discussed in Section 12.7.7.2.2. Contraindications in *yoga are* discussed in Section 12.7.7.2.3. The relationship of *yoga* to the rest of the medical community is discussed in Section 12.7.7.2.4.

12.7.7.2.1 Compliance of students and patients of *yoga*

Student (or patient) compliance, or to put it more in *yoga* terms, the student's ability to attend class or maintain a regular practice, depends on the nature of the *yoga* teacher (*guru*), the student (*sisya*) and the relationship between *guru* and *sisya*. To be of use as a teacher, the *guru* must be able to offer more information to the *sisya* than they already know. It is ideal if the *guru* has a better understanding of *yoga*, anatomy, physiology and psychology than the *sisya*. The *guru* must be able to encourage the *sisya* to strive to work to their personal maximum. The *guru* must be able to advise the *sisya* when it is time to back off in order to avoid physical or psychological injury. If a student does not make an effort in their practice that is close to their personal maximum, which will vary from one day to another, then they will not get the full benefits of their practice and they may become bored and discontinue the practice. If a student over-does physical exercises, breath-control or meditative practices, then physical, physiological or psychological injury may occur. Excessive discomfort on any of these levels, either during or after practise, because of over-doing it, may cause a student to abandon their pursuit of *yoga*.

A student's personality will significantly affect the way they approach *yoga*, and consequently how they should be taught. A student of the typical A-type personality (the over-achiever, competitive type) can easily over-do *yoga* and induce physical, physiological or psychological injury, or over exercise to the point of extreme soreness on the next day. A student with the typical B-type personality (the under-achiever, lazier or disinterested type) may not try hard enough and may not obtain any of the benefits of *yoga*.

12.7.7.2.2 Appropriateness of *yoga* in different situations

Anyone can practise some type of *yoga* in every situation provided there is appropriate adaptation and modifications. Only three conditions apply. First, the teacher must have sufficient understanding and experience in *yoga*, anatomy, physiology and psychology. Second, the student must be willing to learn. Third, it is important that a good relationship exist between *yoga* teacher (*guru*) and student (*sisya*).

Yoga is primarily about relationships and communication. Ultimately, *yoga* is the realisation of the fundamental relationship and identity between the individual self (*jivatma*) and the universal self (*Paramatman*). However, at the commencement of a *yogic* path, the relationships which are most important to develop are those of the self (eg. the connections between body and mind) and the relationship between *guru* and *sisya*. Without a functional relationship between *guru* and *sisya*, the *yoga* may be of limited value [Desikachar, 1998]. This may be the case if the student perceives that the teacher has not enough understanding and experience either in *yoga*, or in human anatomy, physiology and psychology to adequately deal with a student's problem. In addition, if the student is either unwilling to learn, or if the student is over-competitive, then *yoga* can become dangerous.

12.7.7.2.3 Contraindications in *yoga*

A good *yoga* teacher can tailor an individual *yoga* practice to suit anybody. However, few people can safely practise all aspects of *yoga*, as described in this book, without years of training. To learn *yoga*, a student has a choice of a mixed-level open group class, a beginner or higher-level closed course or individual tuition. Traditionally, *yoga* instruction was a one-to-one interaction between teacher and student, but very few good *yoga* teachers now work this way. A good *yoga* teacher can safely guide a student through an individually modified *yoga* practice in a group class, provided they are aware of that student's injuries or medical conditions. Attendance at group *yoga* classes is not recommended unless the teacher is able to adapt and modify the *yoga* to accommodate each student's special needs. Students who should be particularly aware and who need to have special instructions and individual guidance, include those with:

- cancer and other diseases
- cardiovascular problems
- nervous system disorders
- endocrine system disorders
- pregnancy
- spinal abnormalities
- intervertebral disc bulging
- spondylolisthesis
- spinal nerve entrapment
- sciatica
- musculoskeletal problems
- joint instability
- respiratory problems

Finally, although *yoga* can affect all the body systems and may have the potential to help people with specific musculoskeletal problems and medical conditions, very few teachers in the world currently have the necessary combination of theoretical understanding of the body and practical application of *yoga* to help everyone with *yoga*. Most *yoga* teachers are still advised to refer patients to medical practitioners and physiotherapists unless their problems are very straightforward.

12.7.7.2.4 Relationship of *yoga* to the rest of the medical community

Over the years, many people have been injured during *yoga* practice or in classes. *Yoga*-based injuries have especially increased over the last decade as more people have been drawn to the more dynamic and demanding styles of *yoga* such as *astanga vinyasa* [Dembner, 2003]. Injuries are due in part to the limitations of the Western body. Physical *yoga* was initially designed for traditional Indian bodies that have developed strength and flexibility from sitting cross-legged on the floor, squatting to go to the toilet and often carrying large weights on their heads. Lack of understanding of *yoga* and anatomy, physiology and psychology by *yoga* teachers and students is also a prime cause of *yoga*-based injuries. Currently, *yoga* teachers do not require a teaching certificate or medical qualifications to teach. Often injuries can result from students becoming overzealous and trying too hard to achieve certain postures, or by becoming competitive in their practice. In addition, most people are not aware that *yoga* has the potential to be very difficult and can be dangerous if done in its full form by an untrained practitioner. For example, many of the breath-control exercises described in this chapter are very advanced and would not be taught in a standard *yoga* class, but they have been described here to demonstrate the potential that *yoga* can have. Similarly postures shown in the advanced sequence shown in Figure 12.5 are potentially very damaging if they are not done with a balance of strength and flexibility.

The number of *yoga*-based injuries has lead some members of the medical community to doubt the safety and efficacy of *yoga*. When patients come to physiotherapists, doctors, chiropractors, and osteopaths for treatment following *yoga*-based injuries, some of these therapists discourage the practice of *yoga*.

The credibility of *yoga* in the medical world has improved in the last decade with *yoga* teachers required to have more certification and being more qualified in their understanding of anatomy and physiology. In addition, a number of *yoga* teachers are also physiotherapists and have presented papers on the applied anatomy and physiology of *hatha yoga* [Borg-Olivier & Machliss, 1997], while others are doctors who have published papers demonstrating the efficacy of *yoga* [Garfinkle, 1998; Ornish et al., 1990]. *Yoga* teachers now have improved relationships with physiotherapists, doctors, chiropractors, osteopaths and naturopaths.

12.7.7.3 Conclusion

The effects of *yoga* can vary according to the way you practise and the attitude you have when practising. Our attitudes are trained by the *yogic* ethical disciplines, *Yama* and *Niyama*, which form the most fundamental differences between *yoga* and conventional exercise.

Yama and *Niyama*, the first two stages of *astanga yoga*, hold the key to *yoga* and the fulfilment of one's life. *Yama* includes the principles of non-violence (*ahimsa*), truthfulness (*satya*), non-stealing (*asteya*), continence (*brahmacarya*), and non-covetousness (*aparigraha*). On the simplest level, these principles are learnt during a *yoga* practice. For example, to prevent physical or psychological injury during *yoga*, practise without aggression (*ahimsa*), with an honest recognition of any limitations and without a competitive nature. *Niyama* includes the principles of purity (*sauca*), contentment (*santosa*), fervour (*tapas*), self-study (*svadhyaya*), and devotion (*isvara pranidhana*) or love. On the simplest level, to rid oneself of things that are not needed, to be ultimately content with any limitations, but to nevertheless strive to keep improving body and mind through self-study and devotion (*Ishvara pranidhana*).

To achieve complete success in *yoga* one must embrace at least part of the philosophy behind it. *Yoga* is such that its ongoing practice can teach the ethical disciplines. Success in *yoga* may be seen when the ethical disciplines enter into one's daily life.

The practice of *yoga* is a means to enhance all aspects of life, but ideally *yoga* can also become a way of life. Correct application of physical *yoga*, namely physical exercises (*Asana*) and breath-control (*Pranayama*) has been shown to improve physical health and fitness. Mindfulness of the non-physical *yoga*, namely ethical disciplines (*Yama* and *Niyama*) and meditative practices (*Pratyahara*, *Dharana*, *Dhyana* and *Samadhi*), has been shown to augment mental and emotional well-being.

When one practices physical *yoga*, even basic stretching exercises, the best effects on the body are achieved when ethical disciplines such as the principle of non-aggression (*ahimsa*), and meditative practices, such as meditative concentration (*Dharana*), are applied simultaneously. Conversely, when one practices non-physical *yoga*, in particular meditative contemplation (*Dhyana*), the most easily achieved benefits for the mind and emotions and perhaps the best meditations can be achieved while engaged in a physical *yoga* (*Asana* and *Pranayama*) practice involving breath-control exercise (*pranayama*), posture (*asana*) and even movement (*vinyasa*).

The ongoing practice of physical *yoga* (*Asana* and *Pranayama*), in particular correct posture (*asana*), movement (*vinyasa*) and breathing (*pranayama*), can translate to one's everyday life. Some *yogins* can eventually obtain the physical benefits of physical *yoga* through the activities of daily life alone (*karma yoga*). In similar fashion ethical disciplines such as truthfulness (*satya*), self-study (*svadhyaya*) and devotion or love (*isvara pranidhana*), and meditative practices such as meditative sense-control (*Pratyahara*) and meditative concentration (*Dharana*) of non-physical *yoga* can also translate to every day life. The mental and emotional benefits of non-physical *yoga* may also be eventually replaced by the activities of everyday life.

Therefore, even though the paths of *yoga* are many, there is really only one type of *yoga*. *Yoga* is the integration of your actions and deeds, via the interplay between posture, movement and breathing, with thoughts, attitudes and feelings and the effects you have on people and the environment.

****

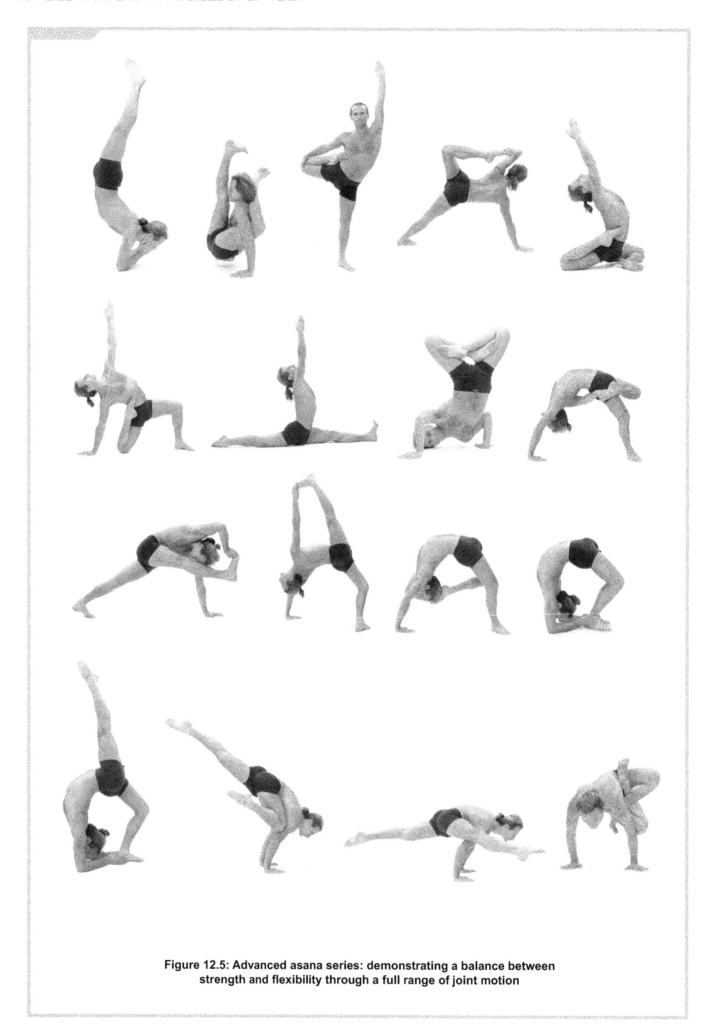

Figure 12.5: Advanced asana series: demonstrating a balance between
strength and flexibility through a full range of joint motion

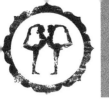

Almost any muscle or muscle group can be activated (ie made to generate tension) during any posture, but the most useful postures for eliciting a muscle activation are those that oblige a muscle group to become activated. This means that the posture can not even be attempted without some basic activation of that muscle group. This is especially helpful for those people who have no body awareness in a particular part of the body.

Column 1 of Table A1 lists each pair of muscle groups that represent the primary movements of the main non-spinal joint complexes [Chapters 2-6].

Column 2 of Table A1 lists some of the postures that each muscle group must be activated to attempt the pose.

Column 3 of Table A1 lists some of the postures that each muscle group will be lengthened or stretched relative to the anatomical position (savasana).

To make a posture work more deeply than what the basic form offers additional muscle groups should be activated correctly.

Abbreviations: ST = scapulothoracic joint of the shoulder; GH = glenohumeral joint of the shoulder; WB= weight-bearing; NWB = non weight-bearing; OC = open-chain; CC = closed chain; R= right side; L = left side;

Table A1 Obligatory activations and lengthening (stretching) of muscle groups in hatha yoga postures

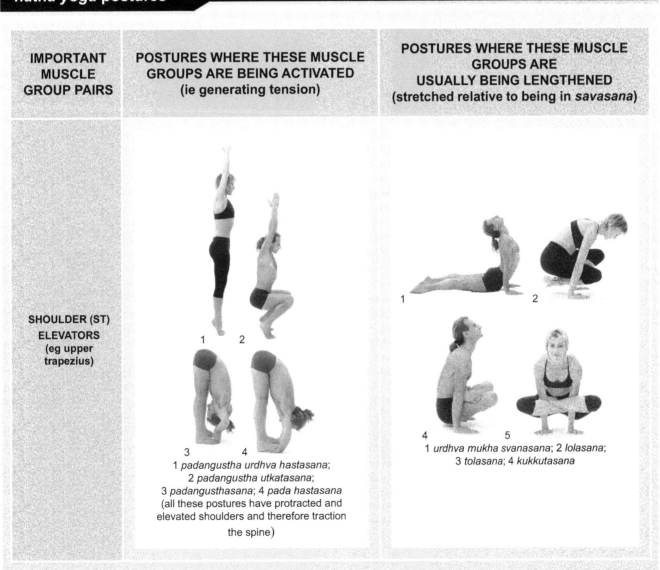

IMPORTANT MUSCLE GROUP PAIRS	POSTURES WHERE THESE MUSCLE GROUPS ARE BEING ACTIVATED (ie generating tension)	POSTURES WHERE THESE MUSCLE GROUPS ARE USUALLY BEING LENGTHENED (stretched relative to being in savasana)
SHOULDER (ST) ELEVATORS (eg upper trapezius)	1 padangustha urdhva hastasana; 2 padangustha utkatasana; 3 padangusthasana; 4 pada hastasana (all these postures have protracted and elevated shoulders and therefore traction the spine)	1 urdhva mukha svanasana; 2 lolasana; 3 tolasana; 4 kukkutasana

IMPORTANT MUSCLE GROUP PAIRS	POSTURES WHERE THESE MUSCLE GROUPS ARE BEING ACTIVATED (ie generating tension)	POSTURES WHERE THESE MUSCLE GROUPS ARE USUALLY BEING LENGTHENED (stretched relative to being in *savasana*)
SHOULDER (ST) DEPRESSORS (eg latissimus dorsi, pectoralis major)	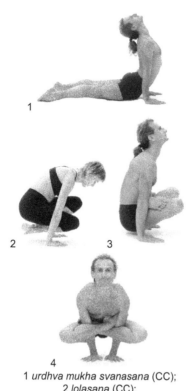 1 *urdhva mukha svanasana* (CC); 2 *lolasana* (CC); 3 *tolasana* (CC); 4 *kukkutasana*	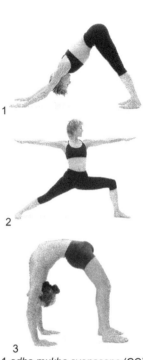 1 *adho mukha svanasana* (CC); 2 *parsvakonasana* (OC); 3 *urdhva dhanurasana* (CC);
SHOULDER (ST) PROTRACTORS (eg serratius anterior, pectoralis minor)	1 *san tolanasana* (plank pose)(CC, WB); 2 *niralamba setu bandhasana* (OC, NWB); 3 *garudasana*; 4 *tittibhasana*	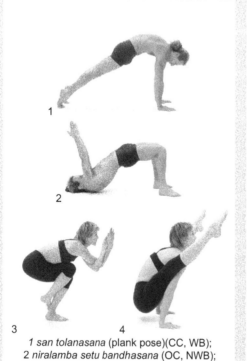 1 *baddha hasta setu bandhasana* (OC, NWB); 2 *baddha kulpha setu bandhasana* (OC, NWB); 3 *purvottanasana*; 4 *baddha prasarita padottanasana*; 5 *raja simhasana*; 6 *dhanurasana*

IMPORTANT MUSCLE GROUP PAIRS	POSTURES WHERE THESE MUSCLE GROUPS ARE BEING ACTIVATED (ie generating tension)	POSTURES WHERE THESE MUSCLE GROUPS ARE USUALLY BEING LENGTHENED (stretched relative to being in *savasana*)
SHOULDER (ST) RETRACTORS (eg rhomboids, middle trapezius)	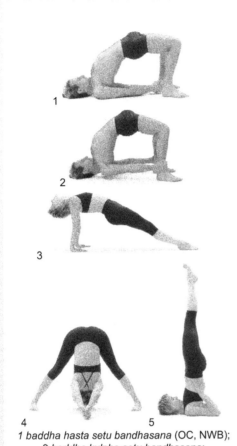 1 *baddha hasta setu bandhasana* (OC, NWB); 2 *baddha kulpha setu bandhasana*; 3 *purvottanasana*; 4 *baddha prasarita padottanasana*; 5 *salamba sarvangasana*	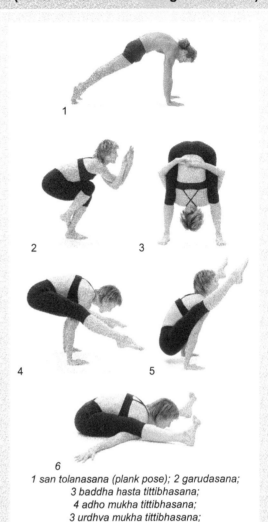 1 *san tolanasana (plank pose)*; 2 *garudasana*; 3 *baddha hasta tittibhasana*; 4 *adho mukha tittibhasana*; 3 *urdhva mukha tittibhasana*; 6 *kurmasana*;
SHOULDER (GH) FLEXORS (eg anterior deltoid)	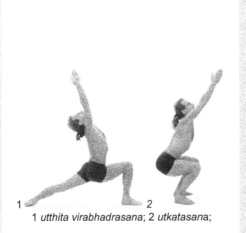 1 *utthita virabhadrasana*; 2 *utkatasana*;	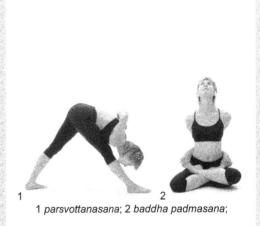 1 *parsvottanasana*; 2 *baddha padmasana*;

385

IMPORTANT MUSCLE GROUP PAIRS	POSTURES WHERE THESE MUSCLE GROUPS ARE BEING ACTIVATED (ie generating tension)	POSTURES WHERE THESE MUSCLE GROUPS ARE USUALLY BEING LENGTHENED (stretched relative to being in *savasana*)
SHOULDER (GH) EXTENSORS (eg posterior deltoid	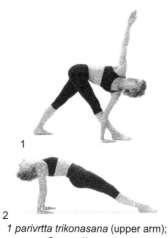 *1 parivrtta trikonasana* (upper arm); *2 purvottanasana*	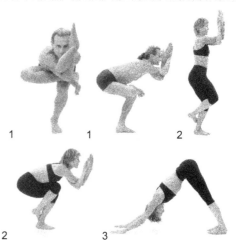 *1 utthita swastikasana; 2 garudasana* (OC, NWB); *3 adho mukha svanasana* (CC, WB);
SHOULDER (GH) ABDUCTORS (eg deltoid)	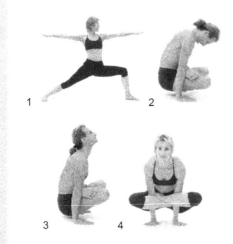 *1 parsva virabhadrasana; 2 adho mukha tolasana; 3 urdhva mukha tolasana; 4 kukkutasana*	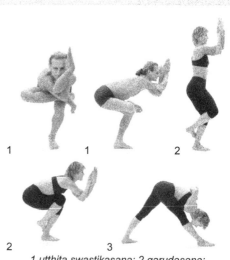 *1 utthita swastikasana; 2 garudasana; 3 parsvottanasana*
SHOULDER (GH) ADDUCTORS (eg latissimus dorsi, pectoralis major)	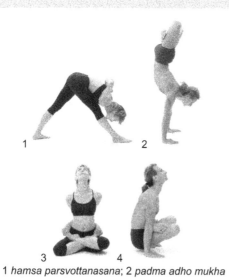 *1 hamsa parsvottanasana; 2 padma adho mukha vrksasana; 3 baddha padmasana; 4 tolasana*	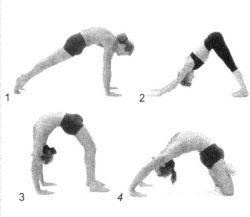 *1 san tolanasana* (plank pose) (CC, W*B*); *2 adho mukha svanasana; 3 urdhva dhanurasana; 4 padma urdhva dhanurasana;*

IMPORTANT MUSCLE GROUP PAIRS	POSTURES WHERE THESE MUSCLE GROUPS ARE BEING ACTIVATED (ie generating tension)	POSTURES WHERE THESE MUSCLE GROUPS ARE USUALLY BEING LENGTHENED (stretched relative to being in *savasana*)
SHOULDER (GH) INTERNAL ROTATORS (eg latissimus dorsi, pectoralis major)	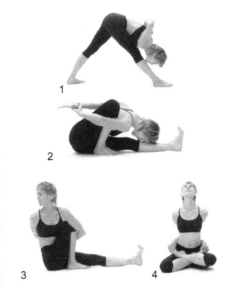 1 *hamsa parsvottanasana*; 2 *maricyasana*; 3 *parivrtta maricyasana*; 4 *baddha padmasana*	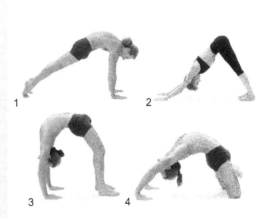 1 *san tolanasana (plank pose)* (CC, WB); 2 *adho mukha svanasana*; 3 *urdhva dhanurasana*; 4 *padma urdhva dhanurasana*
SHOULDER (GH) EXTERNAL ROTATORS (eg posterior deltoid)	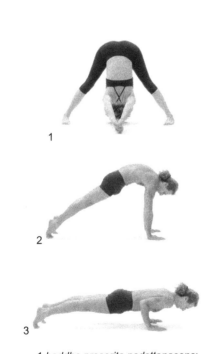 1 *baddha prasarita padottanasana*; 2 *san tolanasana*; 3 *cataranga dandasana*;	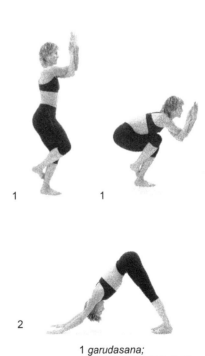 1 *garudasana*; 2 *adho mukha svanasana* (CC, WB);

IMPORTANT MUSCLE GROUP PAIRS	POSTURES WHERE THESE MUSCLE GROUPS ARE BEING ACTIVATED (ie generating tension)	POSTURES WHERE THESE MUSCLE GROUPS ARE USUALLY BEING LENGTHENED (stretched relative to being in *savasana*)
ELBOW FLEXORS (eg biceps brachii)	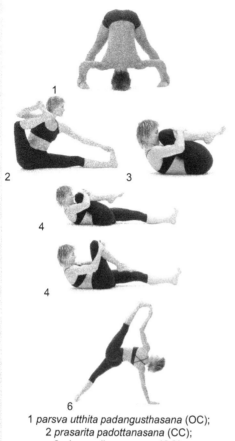 1 *parsva utthita padangusthasana* (OC); 2 *prasarita padottanasana* (CC); 3 *akarna dhanurasana* (OC); 4 *supta pavanmuktasana* (CC, *NWB)*; 5 *vasisthasana*	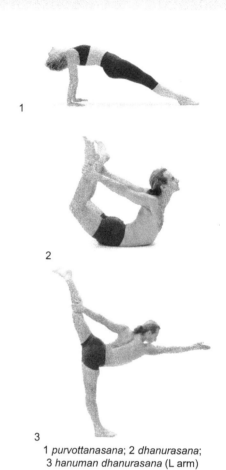 1 *purvottanasana*; 2 *dhanurasana*; 3 *hanuman dhanurasana* (L arm)
ELBOW EXTENSORS (eg triceps brachii)	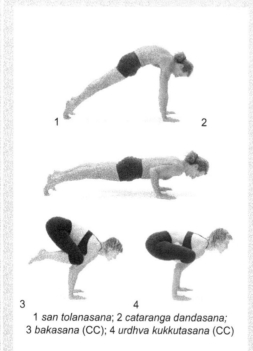 1 *san tolanasana*; 2 *cataranga dandasana*; 3 *bakasana* (CC); 4 *urdhva kukkutasana* (CC)	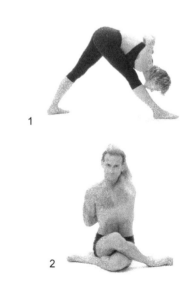 1 *parsvottanasana*; 2 *gomukhasana* (upper arm gets a greater triceps stretch than the lower arm)

IMPORTANT MUSCLE GROUP PAIRS	POSTURES WHERE THESE MUSCLE GROUPS ARE BEING ACTIVATED (ie generating tension)	POSTURES WHERE THESE MUSCLE GROUPS ARE USUALLY BEING LENGTHENED (stretched relative to being in *savasana*)
WRIST FLEXORS	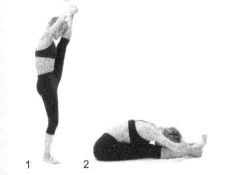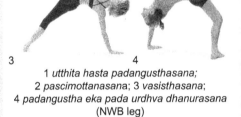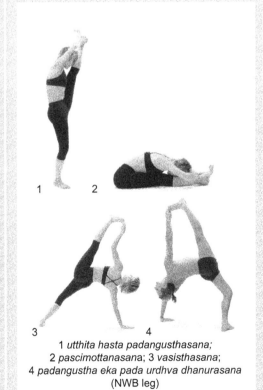1 *utthita hasta padangusthasana*; 2 *pascimottanasana*; 3 *vasisthasana*; 4 *padangustha eka pada urdhva dhanurasana* (NWB leg)	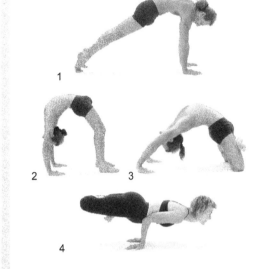1 *san tolanasana (plank pose)* 2 *urdhva dhanurasana*; 3 *padma urdhva dhanurasana*; 4 *padma mayurasana*
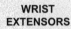**WRIST EXTENSORS**	1 *utthita hasta padangusthasana*; 2 *pascimottanasana*; 3 *vasisthasana*; 4 *padangustha eka pada urdhva dhanurasana* (NWB leg)	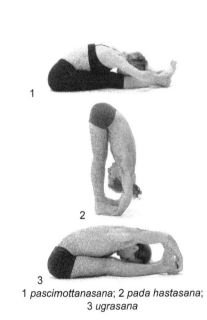1 *pascimottanasana*; 2 *pada hastasana*; 3 *ugrasana*

IMPORTANT MUSCLE GROUP PAIRS	POSTURES WHERE THESE MUSCLE GROUPS ARE BEING ACTIVATED (ie generating tension)	POSTURES WHERE THESE MUSCLE GROUPS ARE USUALLY BEING LENGTHENED (stretched relative to being in *savasana*)
HIP FLEXORS (eg iliopsoas, sartorius)	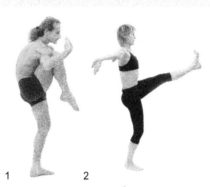 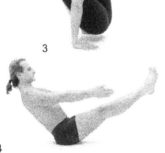 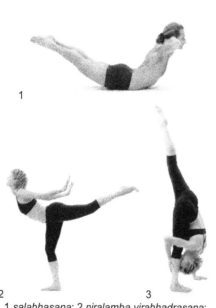 1 *niralamba utthita pavanmuktasana;* 2 *niralamba utthita padangusthasana;* 3 *cakorasana* (L leg) 4 *navasana*	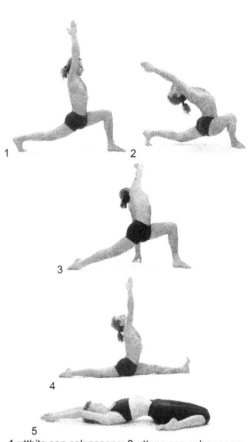 1 *utthita san calanasana;* 2 *uttana san calanasana;* 3 *parsva san calanasana;* 4 *hanumanasana;* 5 *supta virasana*
HIP EXTENSORS (eg gluteus maximus, hamstrings)	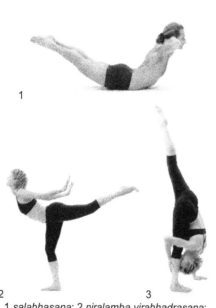 1 *salabhasana;* 2 *niralamba virabhadrasana;* 3 *urdhva prasarita ekapadasana* (L, OC, NWB)	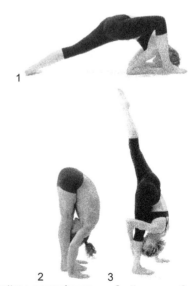 1 *uttana parsvakonasana;* 2 *uttanasana;* 3 *urdhva prasarita ekapadasana* (R, CC, WB)

IMPORTANT MUSCLE GROUP PAIRS	POSTURES WHERE THESE MUSCLE GROUPS ARE BEING ACTIVATED (ie generating tension)	POSTURES WHERE THESE MUSCLE GROUPS ARE USUALLY BEING LENGTHENED (stretched relative to being in *savasana*)
HIP ABDUCTORS (eg gluteus medius, tensor facia latae)	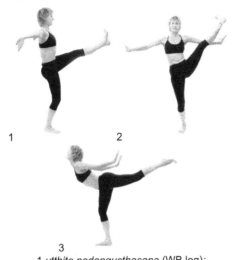 1 *utthita padangusthasana* (WB leg); 2 *parsva utthita padangusthasana* (NWB leg); 3 *niralamba virabhadrasana* (WB leg)	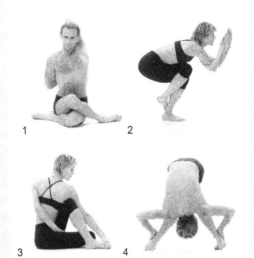 1 *gomukhasana*; 2 *garudasana*; 3 *ardha matsyendrasana*; 4 *meru danda vakrasana*
HIP ADDUCTORS (eg adductor longus, adductor magnus)	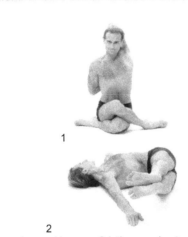 1 *gomukhasana*; 2 *jathara parivartanasana*;	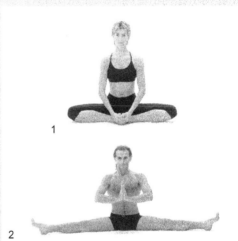 1 *baddha konasana*; 2 *samakonasana*;
HIP INTERNAL ROTATORS (eg hip adductors)	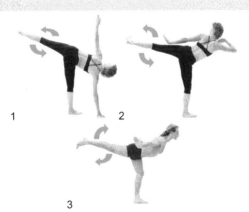 1 *ardha candrasana*; 2 *niralamba ardha candrasana*; 3 *sukha niralamba virabhadrasana* (all these postures with WB leg in hip internal rotation)	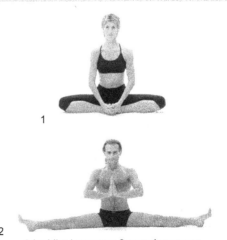 1 *baddha konasana*; 2 *samakonasana*;

391

IMPORTANT MUSCLE GROUP PAIRS	POSTURES WHERE THESE MUSCLE GROUPS ARE BEING ACTIVATED (ie generating tension)	POSTURES WHERE THESE MUSCLE GROUPS ARE USUALLY BEING LENGTHENED (stretched relative to being in *savasana*)
HIP EXTERNAL ROTATORS eg gluteus maximus)	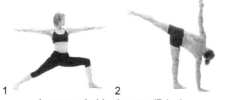 1 *parsva virabhadrasana* (R leg); 2 *ardha candrasana* (floor leg)	1 *adho mukha swastikasana*; 2 *garbha pindasana*
KNEE FLEXORS (eg hamstrings, gastrocnemius)	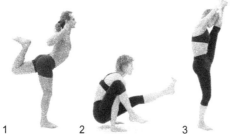 1 *utthita niralamba natarajasasana* (bent leg); 2 *eka hasta bhujasana* (bent leg); 3 *utthita hasta padangusthasana*	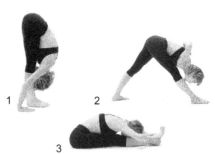 1 *uttanasana*; 2 *parsvottanasana*; 3 *pascimottanasana*
KNEE EXTENSORS (quadriceps)	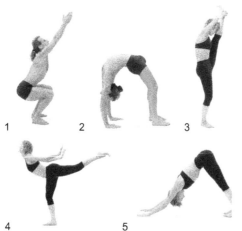 1 *utkatasana*; 2 *urdhva dhanurasana*; 3 *utthita hasta padangusthasana* (WB leg); 4 *niralamba virabhadrasana* (WB leg); 5 *eka pada galavasana* (bent leg)	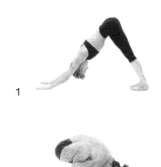 1 *adho mukha virasana*; 2 *bhekasana*; 3 *supta bhekasana*
ANKLE PLANTAR-FLEXORS (eg gastrocnemius, soleus)	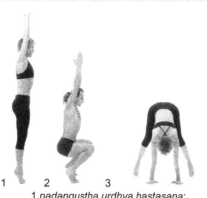 1 *padangustha urdhva hastasana*; 2 *padangustha utkatasana*; 3 *padangustha prasarita padottonasana*	1 *adho mukha svanasana*; 2 *malasana*

392

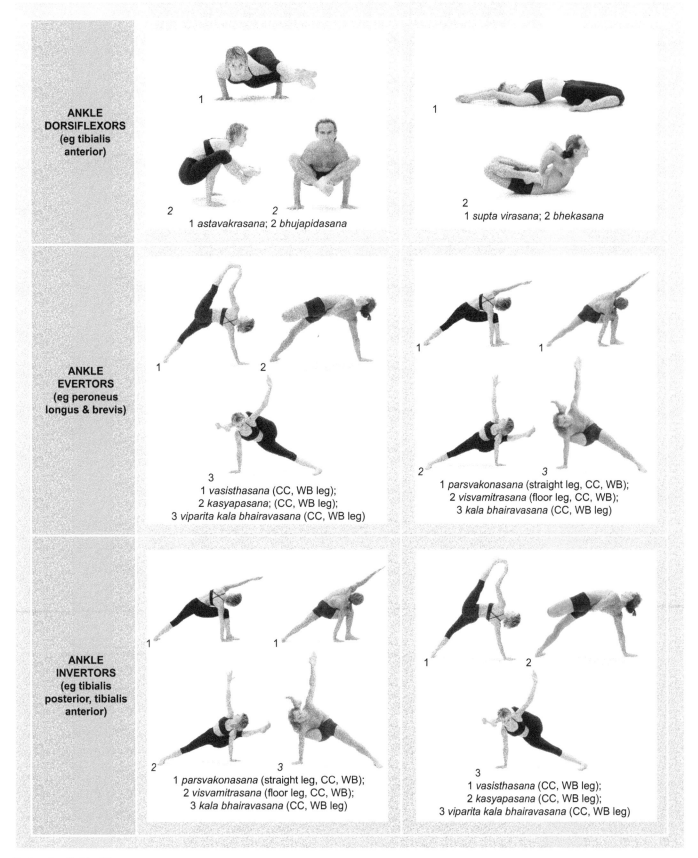

ANKLE DORSIFLEXORS (eg tibialis anterior)

1 *astavakrasana*; 2 *bhujapidasana*

1 *supta virasana*; 2 *bhekasana*

ANKLE EVERTORS (eg peroneus longus & brevis)

1 *vasisthasana* (CC, WB leg);
2 *kasyapasana*; (CC, WB leg);
3 *viparita kala bhairavasana* (CC, WB leg)

1 *parsvakonasana* (straight leg, CC, WB);
2 *visvamitrasana* (floor leg, CC, WB);
3 *kala bhairavasana* (CC, WB leg)

ANKLE INVERTORS (eg tibialis posterior, tibialis anterior)

1 *parsvakonasana* (straight leg, CC, WB);
2 *visvamitrasana* (floor leg, CC, WB);
3 *kala bhairavasana* (CC, WB leg)

1 *vasisthasana* (CC, WB leg);
2 *kasyapasana* (CC, WB leg);
3 *viparita kala bhairavasana* (CC, WB leg)

Notes for Table A1:

- Many postures that cause an obligatory activation of shoulder (scapulothoracic) (ST) protractors also stretch the shoulder (ST) retractors.
- Many postures that cause an obligatory activation of shoulder (ST) retractors also stretch the shoulder (ST) protractors.
- Hip adductors and hip internal rotators include many of the same muscles and, as a general rule, they can be stretched in the same way.
- Ankle evertors can be activated with the same type of postures that ankle invertors are stretched in.
- Ankle invertors can be activated with the same type of postures that ankle evertors are stretched in.

Observation of the body in various postures can give a lot of information about that body that may then be utilised to help correct and improve any deviations from normal body alignment. Observation is best practiced with a partner but may also be done with mirrors, photographs or video.

Initially, study a body in the anatomical position. Use either *savasana* 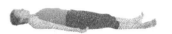 or

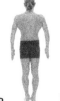

tadasana . Following are a few points to look for in a simple observation.

General observation: examine the following:
- Bony & soft tissue contours, limb positions, skin colour and texture, deformities.

Observation from anterior view: examine general symmetry of trunk and limbs:
- Head position: look for unwanted side flexion (tilting) or rotation
- Shoulders: look for contours and height
- Trunk: check ribs, clavicle, sternum and hips
- Hips: check for genu varum (bow-legged) or genu valgus (knock-knees)
- Knees: compare positions of patellas (knee caps)
- Feet: check for excessive and asymmetrical inversion or eversion.

Observation from posterior view: examine general symmetry of trunk and limbs:
- Head position: look for unwanted side flexion (tilting) or rotation
- Shoulders: look at scapulas and examine for height, muscle mass etc
- Trunk: check spine for curvature (scoliosis).
- Hips: compare positions of iliac crests (top of hips) and gluteal folds (buttocks crease)
- Knees: check for line of posterior knee crease
- Feet: check achilles tendon and feet for excessive pronation or eversion.

Observation from lateral view: examine plumb line between shoulders, hips ankles:
- Head position: look for unwanted flexion, or extension or rotation
- Shoulders: check to see whether the shoulders are more anterior or posterior.
- Trunk: check for thoracic kyphosis, lumbar lordosis and any trunk rotation.
- Hips: check for excessive anterior or posterior pelvic tilt
- Knees: check for genu recurvatum (hyper-extended knees)
- Feet: check for excessive and asymmetrical inversion or eversion

Later, practise on other symmetrical postures which weight-bear on other parts of the body, eg *uttanasana*, *adho mukha svanasana* (down-dog pose), *swastikasana* (crossed-leg) *baddha konasana*, *adho mukha vrksasana* (handstand), *sirsasana* (headstand) etc.

Compare the two sides of the body in each posture and see if there really is symmetry. If there is no symmetry, check what muscle actions it takes to change the posture so that it becomes more symmetrical.

Then progress your observations to the asymmetrical postures such as *trikonasana, parsvakonasana, janu sirsasana, ardha matsyendrasana* and other forward bends and twists. Compare one side of each pose with the other.

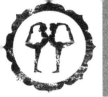

The generation of each of the nine (9) major joint *bandhas* is possible in every *yoga* posture. However when the *bandhas* are initially being learnt it difficult to know exactly how to create them. Table C1 shows postures that can be used to generate the *bandhas* in their *ha-* (hot and compressive) and *tha-* (cool and expansive) forms relatively easily with a few simple instructions.

Abbreviations: ST = Scapulothoracic Joint; GH = Glenohumeral Joint; WB= Weight-bearing; NWB = Non-weight-bearing;
OC = Open-chain; CC = Closed-chain; R= Right side; L = Left side;

Table C1 Generating *bandhas* in *hatha yoga* postures

BANDHA & RELATED JOINT COMPLEX	POSTURES WHERE SPECIFIC *BANDHAS* ARE AUTOMATICALLY CREATED OR ARE RELATIVELY EASY TO CREATE	NOTES AND VERBAL INSTRUCTIONS THAT MAY HELP FACILITATE CREATION OF *BANDHAS*
HA-KULPHA BANDHA A compressive and heating co-activation of opposing muscles of the ANKLE JOINT COMPLEX	1 *tadasana*; 2 *trikonasana*; 3 *parsvottanasana*; 4 *utthita padangusthasana* (wb leg); 5 *niralamba virabhadrasana* (wb leg); 6 *janu sirsasana* (left ankle extended and toes flexed to achieve *ha-kulpha bandha*)	*Ha-kulpha bandha* *Ha-kulpha bandha* is a compressive and heating *bandha* that pushes energy away from the ankle joint complex. It is engaged when there is toe flexor activity and ankle extensor (dorsiflexor) activity. This is achieved by making a clenched fist with the feet or by attempting to make a clenched fist even though the feet may remain flat to the floor. Some ankle evertor activity (ie pulling the outer feet towards you) is also useful to stabilise the ankle and render this *bandha* more effective in stabilising the joint. For WB feet of all standing postures, where the feet are on the floor, verbal instructions for creating *ha-kulpha bandha* may include: • Grip the floor with the feet like you are trying to grab the floor • Try to make a closed fist with the feet as you can with the hands • Lift the arches of the feet, especially the outer arch For the NWB feet of all postures, where the feet are not pressing on the floor, such as *janu sirsasana*, verbal instructions for creating *ha-kulpha bandha* may include: • Bend the ankle joint towards you and pull the foot towards you but curl the toes away from you • Try to make a closed fist with the feet as you can with the hands

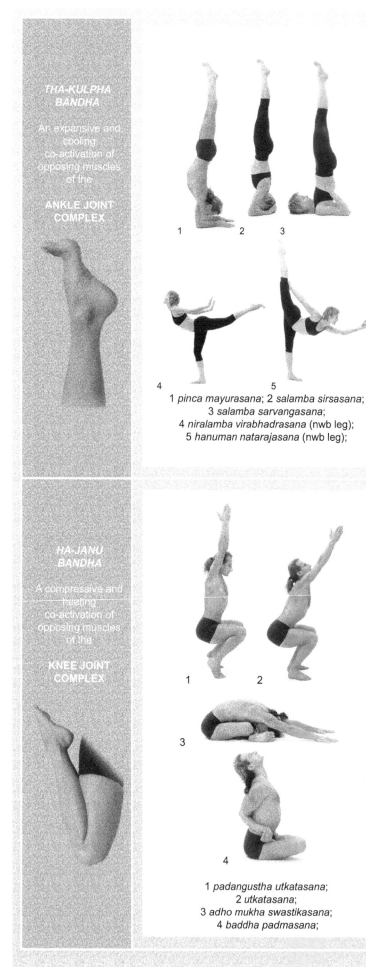

THA-KULPHA
BANDHA

An expansive and
cooling
co-activation of
opposing muscles
of the

ANKLE JOINT
COMPLEX

1 *pinca mayurasana*; 2 *salamba sirsasana*;
3 *salamba sarvangasana*;
4 *niralamba virabhadrasana* (nwb leg);
5 *hanuman natarajasana* (nwb leg);

HA-JANU
BANDHA

A compressive and
heating
co-activation of
opposing muscles
of the

KNEE JOINT
COMPLEX

1 *padangustha utkatasana*;
2 *utkatasana*;
3 *adho mukha swastikasana*;
4 *baddha padmasana*;

Tha-kulpha bandha

Tha-kulpha bandha is an expansive and cooling *bandha* that pulls energy towards the ankle joint complex. It is engaged when there is toe extensor activity and ankle flexor (plantarflexor) activity ie like trying to pull the toes towards you while trying to press the base of the big toe and the front of the foot away from you. Some ankle evertor activity (ie pulling the outer feet towards you) is also useful to stabilise the ankle and render this *bandha* more effective in stabilising the joint.

For WB feet of all standing postures, where the feet are on the floor, verbal instructions for creating *tha-kulpha bandha* may include:

- Try and raise the heels of the floor (without actually having to lift them) ie bring body weight towards the front of the foot
- Keep the ankle bones moving inwards
- Try to lift the arches of the feet, especially the outer arch of the foot (even if does not actually lift) ie activate the evertors

For NWB feet of all standing postures, where the feet are off the floor, verbal instructions for creating *tha-kulpha bandha* may include:

- Spread and stretch the toes
- Push the base of the big toe furthest away from you while pulling the tips of the toes closer to you
- Pull the outer edges of the feet closer towards you than the inner edges of the feet

Ha-janu bandha

Ha-janu bandha is a compressive and heating *bandha* that pushes energy away from the knee joint complex. It is engaged when there is a co-activation of knee flexors and knee extensors that may cause an impingement of the blood flow through the knee joint complex. This happens most effectively when the knee is flexed and internally rotated.

For all activations of *janu bandha*:
- Press into the base of the big toe
- Pull the outer arch of the foot towards you

For postures where the knee is semi-flexed, such as *utkatasana*, verbal instructions for creating *ha-janu bandha* may include:

- Pull up the knee caps by tightening the front of the thighs (to activate knee extensors), then try and bend the knee (without actually bending it) while keeping the front of the thighs firm (in order to co-activate knee flexors with knee extensors)
- Press onto the front of the foot as if you are about to raise the heel

For postures where the knee is fully flexed, like cross-legged (*swastikasana*) or *baddha padmasana*, verbal instructions for creating *ha-janu bandha* may include:

- Tighten the calf and hamstring muscles at the same time as trying to straighten the leg at the knee (similar to making a bulging biceps around the elbow joint complex)

Generating Bandhas: Ways to Co-activate Opposing Muscles Around The Nine (9) Major Joint Complexes Using Various Yoga Postures

APPENDIX C

THA-JANU BANDHA

An expansive and cooling co-activation of opposing muscles of the

KNEE JOINT COMPLEX

1 *hanuman natarajasana*;
2 *utthita trivikramasana*;
3 *niralamba virabhadrasana*;
4 *parsvottanasana*;
5 *(a-f) utthita mandala vinyasa*

Tha-janu bandha

Tha-janu bandha is an expansive and cooling *bandha* that pulls energy towards the knee joint complex. It is engaged when there is a co-activation of knee flexors (including hamstrings and calf muscles) and knee extensors that enhances the flow of blood through the knee joint complex. This is best achieved when the knee is fully extended.

For WB limbs of postures, where the feet are on the floor, such as *tadasana*, verbal instructions for creating *tha-janu bandha* may include:

- Straighten the knee and gently pull up the knee cap tightening the front of the thighs.

- At the same time try to bend the knee (without actually bending it) in order to tighten the hamstrings and the back of the thigh

For NWB limbs in postures where the feet are off the floor and the hip is extended, like *niralamba virabhadrasana*, verbal instructions for creating *tha-janu bandha* may include:

- Straighten the knee and gently pull up the knee cap tightening the front of the thighs

- Rotate the thigh inwards in order to activate the hamstrings and the inner thigh muscles

- Press into the base of the big toe in order to activate ankle plantarflexors

- Pull the outer arch of the foot towards you in order to activate ankle evertors

For NWB limbs in postures where the feet are off the floor and the hip is flexed, like *niralamba padangusthasana*, verbal instructions for creating *tha-janu bandha* may include:

- Straighten the knee and tighten the front of the thigh while turning the thigh outwards

- Pull up the knee caps and tighten the front of the thigh, and then try to bend the knee without letting the thighs soften

- Press into the base of the big toe in order to activate ankle plantarflexors

- Pull the outer arch of the foot towards you in order to activate ankle evertors

HA-KATI
BANDHA

A compressive and
heating
co-activation of
opposing muscles
of the

HIP JOINT
COMPLEX

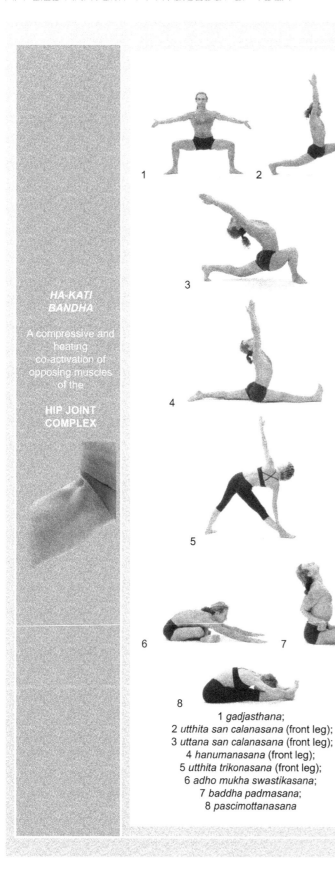

1 *gadjasthana*;
2 *utthita san calanasana* (front leg);
3 *uttana san calanasana* (front leg);
4 *hanumanasana* (front leg);
5 *utthita trikonasana* (front leg);
6 *adho mukha swastikasana*;
7 *baddha padmasana*;
8 *pascimottanasana*

Ha-kati bandha

Ha-kati bandha is a compressive and heating *bandha* that pushes energy away from the hip joint complex. It is effectively engaged when there is a co-activation of hip flexors and extensors, abductors and adductors, and/or internal rotators and external rotators, which can cause an impingement of the blood flow through the hip joint complex.

For all lunge-like standing postures verbal instructions for creating *ha-kati bandha* may include:

- Try and squash the floor with your feet, as if your legs are scissors trying to cut the floor

- At the same time gently squeeze the buttocks

For all postures, such as *prasarita padottonasana* or *gadjasthana*, verbal instructions for creating *ha-kati bandha* may include:

- Squeeze your heels inwards

- At the same time push the feet outwards

For the leading (front) leg of all other standing postures, verbal instructions for creating *ha-kati bandha* may include:

- Try and stretch the floor with you feet

- At the same time, turn the thighs out and squeeze the heel inwards

For floor postures, like *swastikasana*, *padmasana* and *pascimottanasana*, verbal instructions for creating *ha-kati bandha* may include:

- Press down with your feet

- At the same time try to lift the inner thighs

and/or

- Squeeze your thighs together

- At the same time squeeze the buttock muscles

PLEASE NOTE: Do not overstretch the hips especially when bending forward. If you are bending forward with your body then the hips are part of the movement but approximately 24/25ths of the movement could come from the spine. Excessive hip flexion and constant ha-kati bandha activation with spinal extension tends to cut the blood supply to the lower limbs and can predispose the practitioner to physiological problems.

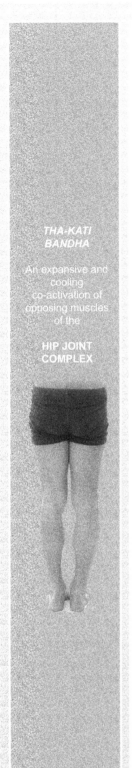

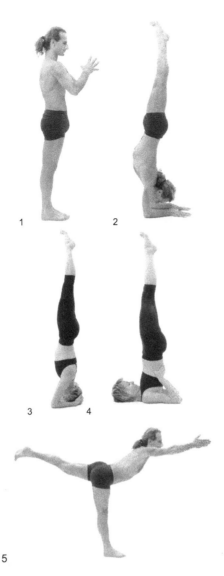

1 *tadasana* (with big toes touching and heels
slightly apart);
2 *pinca mayurasana*;
3 *sirsasana*;
4 *sarvangasana*;
5 *niralamba virabhadrasana* (with the NWB left leg
turning inwards and the gluteus maximus gently
activated in a lengthened state)

Tha-kati bandha

Tha-kati bandha [Section 4.5.1] is an expansive and cooling *bandha* that pulls energy towards the hip joint complex. It is engaged when there is a co-activation of hip flexors and extensors, hip abductors and adductors, or hip internal rotators and external rotators, which enhances the flow of blood through the hip joint complex. This is best achieved when the hip is slightly extended and internallly rotated.

Tha-kati bandha is formed when the blood and energy flowing through the hip joint complex is the least impinged. The best positions to generate *tha-kati bandha* are those where the hip joint is kept in a neutral or slightly extended position as in *Tadasana*. Co-activation of opposing muscles of the hip joint complex is generated either by directing the focus to the feet for weight-bearing (WB) postures such as *tadasana* or to the hips themselves in non weight-bearing (NWB). Co-activation of the internal and external rotators of the hip can be achieved in this fashion while still maintaining a relatively open space in the hip (coxafemoral) and sacroiliac joints.

For the WB hip of all standing poses, where the feet are on the floor, verbal instructions for creating *the-kati bandha* may include:

- Start with feet slightly turned inwards

- Gently squeeze the heels inwards, while pushing the front of the feet outwards

For the NWB feet of all poses, where the feet are off the floor, verbal instructions for creating *tha-kati bandha* may include:

- Turn your NWB thigh(s) inwards & move the legs behind you (extend at the hip joint), using your hamstring muscles

- Gently activate the buttocks muscles (gluteus maximus) when they are stretched at the maximum point of hip internal rotation and hip extension

HA-MULA BANDHA
A compressive and heating co-activation of opposing muscles of the **LUMBAR SPINE JOINT COMPLEX** (a circumferential compressional co-activation around the lumbar joint complex)

1

2   3

4   5

6

1 *uddiyana* with *mula bandha* (defining the obliquus externus abdominis); 2 relaxed breathing; 3 diaphragmatic inhale; 4 thoracic inhale (complete inhale); 5 passive thoracic exhale; 6 active abdominal exhale to gently draw the navel towards the spine with using the muscles of forced abdominal exhalation and thus generating a gentle *ha-mula bandha*.

Ha-mula bandha

Ha-mula bandha is a compressive and heating *bandha* that pushes energy away from the lumbar spine joint complex. *Ha-mula bandha* is the *mula bandha* that is spoken of in many *yoga* texts. It is effectively engaged when there is a circumferential co-activation around the trunk using the perineum, the transverse and oblique abdominal muscles and the diaphragm.

Ha-mula bandha can also be effectively engaged by increasing intra-abdominal pressure (IAP) using the transverse and oblique abdominal muscles through use of the breath or without the breath

Verbal instructions for creating ha-mula bandha with the exhaled breath may include:
- Gently contract the muscles of the perineum just before each exhale in order to activate transversus abdominis
- Then exhale fully

Verbal instructions for creating ha-mula bandha with a breath retention after the exhalation (defining the obliquus externus abdominis) may include:
- Gently contract the perineum and exhale completely
- Close the glottis (opening to the channel to the lungs) and make a false inspiratory effort with the chest (*tha-uddiyana bandha*) then tighten the lower abdomen *(ha-mula bandha)* as if you are about to exhale fully from the abdomen

Verbal instructions for creating ha-mula bandha with a breath retention after the inhalation may include:
Breathe with full exhalations but only inhale between one third to two thirds of the entire lungs, then hold the breath in briefly and then gently and carefully tense the lower abdomen as if about to exhale fully from the abdomen

Ha-mula bandha can also be effectively engaged by increasing intra-abdominal pressure (IAP) using the diaphragm through use of the breath or without the breath

Verbal instructions for creating ha-mula bandha using abdominal breathing or using the diaphragm with or without breathing may include:
- Practice breathing from the abdomen so that the abdomen expands with each gentle inhalation
- Learn to recognise this type of breathing as coming from the movement of the diaphragm towards the abdomen with the inhale
- Use the abdominal muscles (transverse and oblique muscles) for making full (gently forced) exhalation
- Keep the abdomen firm with the muscles of gentle forced exhalation and once again try and breathe using the diaphragm, i.e. breathe into the abdomen without letting it puff out
- Eventually learn to activate the diaphragm without breathing

The practice of *asvini mudra*, which is an alternating contraction and expansion (or relaxation) of the anal constrictor muscles can also assist in developing the control of *ha- mula bandha*.

APPENDIX C

Generating Bandhas: Ways to Co-activate Opposing Muscles Around The Nine (9) Major Joint Complexes Using Various Yoga Postures

THA-MULA BANDHA
An expansive and cooling co-activation of opposing muscles of the lower trunk or **LUMBAR SPINE JOINT COMPLEX**

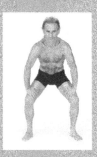

Nauli (Tha Uddiyana Bandha with tha-mula bandha) (defining the rectus abdominis on an exhalation retention) (nauli is a type of tha-mula bandha)

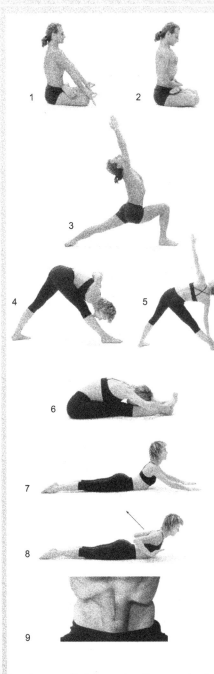

1 *padmasana* with *jnana mudra* with more natural spinal curvature (reduced tha-mula bandha effect);
2 *padmasana* with *dharana mudra* with more straightened spine (more effective *tha-mula bandha* effect) 3 *utthita virabhadrasana*; 4 *parsvottanasana*; 5 *trikonasana*; 6 *pascimottanasana* 7 *bhujanasana* 8 *salabhasana* 9 *tha-mula bandha* with *tha-uddiyana* to create nauli (defining the rectus abdominis) (Also photo on left)

Tha-mula bandha

Tha-mula bandha is an expansive and cooling co-activation of opposing muscles around the lumbar spine that gives stability to the lumbar spine joint complex and enhances the blood flow through this region. Simple positions for *tha-mula bandha* are those where the spine is made to be as lengthened as possible in seated or standing. Other means to create include 'stretching the mat with one's feet', pushing the hips down and forward and bringing the middle back, and creating nauli.

Tha-mula bandha is used to maintain an erect spinal posture such as (figures 1 and 2) *padmasana* (lotus posture) or cross-legged posture for prolonged periods. *Tha-mula bandha* maximises the length (height) of the spine equally anteriorly and posteriorly by lifting the thoracic spine upwards while keeping the sitting bones (ischial tuberosities) on the floor. In addition simultaneously lifting the sternum upwards while keeping the anterior perineum on the floor. This leads to reduction or loss in the natural spinal curvature to the point where the spine can become almost straight. This is done with a minimum of muscle activity. A completely relaxed or flaccid spine will initially adopt its natural curvature and then slump forward. Initial attempts to lengthen a collapsed or totally relaxed (flaccid) spine using spinal muscle activity will result in a reduction in the forward slump of the spine, followed by a return to the natural curvature of the spine. Further lengthening of the spine leads to reduction or loss in the natural spinal curvature to the point where the spine can become almost straight. The distances between each vertebrae will have increased anteriorly and posteriorly. This process is analogous to the co-activation of the wrist and finger extensors and flexors that cause the fingers to straighten and stretch in *tha-mani* (wrist) *bandha*.

Verbal instructions for creating *tha-mula* bandha as a co-activation of opposing muscles of the spine in standing poses such as (3) *utthita virabhadrasana*, (4) *parsvottanasana* and (5) *trikonasana* may include:
- Either stretch the floor with your feet or squeeze the floor with your feet or do both at the same time using the front and the back of the feet separately
- Use your abdominal muscles to press from each sitting bone towards each respective foot

Verbal instructions for creating tha-mula bandha as a co-activation of opposing muscles of the spine in seated forward bends such as (6) *pascimottanasana* and prone extended postures such as (7) *bhujanasana* (cobra pose) and (8) *salabhasana* (lifting chest and hands) may include:
- Press the sitting bones down and forward (to activate the spinal flexors) and
- Try to pull the middle back inwards (to activate the spinal extensors)

Verbal instructions for creating (9) nauli (tha-mula bandha with tha-uddiyana bandha) with a breath retention after the exhalation may include:
- Stand with your knees bent and have hands on thighs with shoulders turned inwards
- Gently contract the perineum and exhale completely
- Close the glottis (opening to the channel to the lungs) and make a false inspiratory effort with the chest *(tha-uddiyana bandha)*. This is like expanding the chest and upper back as if you are trying to inhale but not actually inhaling
- Push the hips and thighs into the shoulders and hands (to activate the spinal flexors)

For other poses verbal instructions may include:
- First pick the part of your back that can move inwards (extends) most easily, and consciously move it outwards (flex it) as much as you can in order to activate spinal flexor muscles
- Then pick the part of your back that moves outwards (flexes) most easily, and consciously move it inwards (extend it) as much as you can in order to activate spinal extensor muscles

HA-UDDIYANA BANDHA
A compressive and heating co-activation of opposing muscles of the **THORACIC SPINE JOINT COMPLEX**

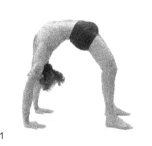

1

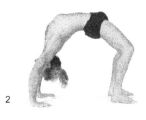

2

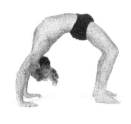

3

A

B

C

1 *urdhva dhanurasana* with *ha-uddiyana bandha*
2 *ardha urdhva dhanurasana* without *ha-uddiyana bandha* (ribs flaring out between the chest and the abdomen resulting in greater impingement (squashing) in the lower back and less extension in the middle back at the lumbothoracic junction)
3 *ardha urdhva dhanurasana* with *ha-uddiyana bandha* (ribs held in between the chest and the abdomen resulting in lesser impingement (squashing) in the lower back and greater extension in the middle back at the lumbothoracic junction) 4 *tadagi kriya* ABC (see details on right and photos on left)

Ha-uddiyana bandha

Ha-uddiyana bandha [Section 7.4.1.1] is a compressive and heating *bandha* that pushes energy away from the chest and thoracic spine joint complex. It is effectively engaged when there is a co-activation of internal and external intercostal muscles and other muscles that can compress the chest and upper back. *Ha-uddiyana bandha* can cause an impingement of the blood flow through the thoracic spine joint complex (as demonstrated by its ability to slow the heart). *Ha-uddiyana bandha* is essentially the same type of muscular compression of the thorax that would be used in a forced expiration.

Ha-uddiyana bandha gives a very effective protective effect to the lower back. If the front ribs are held in firmly, then the lower back, especially the commonly weak region around L4-L5, is less likely to over-stretch (over-extend or over-flex) and is more likely to encourage mobility of the region around the lumbothoracic junction (middle back), which is usually very stiff. The lumbothoracic junction is where the kidneys are and thererfore *ha-uddiyana bandha* can massage, compress and stimulate the kidneys and improve their function, as well help to mobilise this usually very stiff region of the back in both spinal flexion and extension as well as side flexion.

Ha-uddiyana bandha is very important to use in backward bending (spinal extension) postures like *urdhva dhanurasana* (back arch).

Ha-uddiyana bandha is often described (especially in Ashtanga Vinyasa yoga) as being a toning or tightening of the upper abdomen, because that is what it can feel like and that is what it can cause. However, you do not need to tighten the abdomen at all to effectively tense the thoracic cage. This is the case in *Tadagi mudra* described below.

Ha-uddiyana bandha can be used in *tadagi kriya*. *Tadagi kriya* is powerful exercise for the muscles of the chest and abdomen in which the abdomen can be rolled up and down in a manner similar in appearance to *lauliki* [Figure 12.1], which is an alternating isolation of the rectus abdominis. *Ha-uddiyana bandha* is the compressive form of *uddiyana bandha* that is rarely used by the beginner in *yoga* except during the process of a forced expiration. However the experienced practitioner can use this *ha-uddiyana bandha* in exercises such as *tadagi kriya* (photos on left) to enhance blood flow through all the body systems, to bring strength and energy to any part of the body, and even to suspend the pulse and sometimes the heart beat itself.

An introductory form of *tadagi mudra* is described by Saraswati [1996] in *Asana Pranayama Mudra bandha* in which the above process is alluded to by the suggestion to do forced exhalations with a soft abdomen, forcing the muscles of the chest (e.g. Intercostals) to compress the chest wall and cause an increase in intra abdominal pressure (IAP)

Tadagi kriya (photos on left): This is a *yogic* internal cleansing process done here with an inhalation retention and *ha-jalandhara bandha* in ABC. These three positions can be practiced repeatedly in this sequence like a vertical lauliki kriya [Figure 12.1].
A: *maha bandha = tha-uddiyana bandha* (expanded chest) plus *ha-mula bandha* (contracted lower abdomen);
B: *ha-tadagi mudra = ha-uddiyana bandha* plus *ha-mula bandha* with a relaxed upper abdomen;
C: *tha-tadagi mudra = ha-uddiyana bandha* plus *tha-mula bandha* ie a completely relaxed upper & lower abdomen)

APPENDIX C

Generating Bandhas. Ways to Co-activate Opposing Muscles Around The Nine (9) Major Joint Complexes Using Various Yoga Postures

THA-UDDIYANA BANDHA
An expansive and cooling co-activation of opposing muscles of the **THORACIC SPINE JOINT COMPLEX**

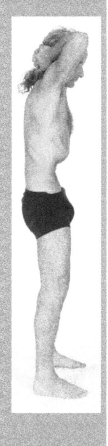

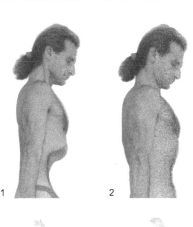

1   2

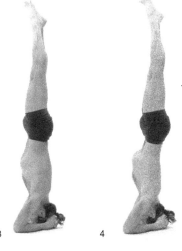

3   4

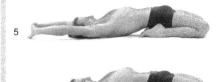

5

6

1 *tha-uddiyana bandha* with exhalation retention
2 *tha-uddiyana bandha* with inhalation retention (Note that when *tha-uddiyana bandha* is effectively engaged the chest looks almost the same size and shape regardless of whether the tha- uddiyana bandha has been activated either on exhalation retention (Figure 1 above) or inhalation retention (Figure 2 above).
3 *sirsasana* without *tha-uddiyana bandha* 4 *sirsasana* with *tha-uddiyana bandha* 5 *supta virasana* without *tha-uddiyana bandha* 6 *supta virasana* with *tha-uddiyana bandha*

Tha-uddiyana bandha

Tha-uddiyana bandha is essentially an expansion of the thorax (chest and upper back) equally from the front of the body and from the back of the body. *Tha-uddiyana bandha* is an internal process but postures such as san tolanasana (plank pose) and *urdhva dhanurasana* (back arch) can assist to get the idea of what stretching the chest (*urdhva dhanurasana*) and upper back (*san tolanasana*) feels like.

The best time to practice *tha-uddiyana bandha* is on the exhalation retention (i.e. when there is no air in the lungs. However, it can also be performed while holding the breath in and even while breathing in and out.

If the body is 'bending' in a position that is no different from a movement in that person's every day life then there is no need to grip ha-uddiyana bandha (i.e. to compress the chest) and so it is possible to do tha-uddiyana bandha to advantage. While this is theoretically possible to do in any pose it is safest in postures where the spine is relatively safe such as in (3,4) sirsasana (headstand) and (5,6) supta virasana

Verbal instructions for creating tha-uddiyana bandha during inhalation and exhalation may include:
- Make the chest expand (tha-uddiyana bandha) with each inspiration and contract the lower abdomen (ha-mula bandha) with each expiration
- Maintain the firmness of the lower abdomen (ha- mula bandha) as you inhale to assist in the expansion of the chest (tha-uddiyana bandha)
- Maintain the expansion of the chest (tha-uddiyana bandha) as you exhale

Verbal instructions for creating tha-uddiyana bandha with a breath retention after the exhalation may include:
- Gently contract the perineum and exhale completely
- Close the glottis (opening to the channel to the lungs) and make a false inspiratory effort with the chest (tha-uddiyana bandha). This is like expanding the chest and upper back as if you are trying to inhale but not actually inhaling

Verbal instructions for creating tha-uddiyana bandha with a breath retention after the inhalation may include:
- Inhale between two thirds to three quarters of your lungs
- Close the glottis (opening to the channel to the lungs) and make a false inspiratory effort with the chest (tha-uddiyana bandha). This is like expanding the chest and upper back as if you are trying to inhale more but not actually inhaling.

403

HA-JALANDHARA
BANDHA
A compressive and
heating
co-activation of
opposing muscles
of the

CERVICAL SPINE
JOINT COMPLEX

Ha-jalandhara bandha

Ha-jalandhara bandha [Section 7.4.1.2.1] is a compressive and heating *bandha* that pushes energy away from the cervical spine joint complex. It is effectively engaged when there is a co-activation of neck flexors and extensors, which can cause an impingement of the blood flow through the cervical spine joint complex.

Ha-jalandhara bandha is engaged when there is head flexor activity and neck extensor activity. This is achieved when one tries to bring the chin to the chest as in the shoulderstand.

Ha-jalandhara bandha is best learnt in postures such as *niralamba setu bandhasana* but once learnt it is a useful practice in many postures which involve abdominal strength such as the push up called *cataranga dandasana* and sit up style postures. This is because *ha-jalandhara* causes a reflex activation of *ha-mula bandha*.

Ha-jalandhara bandha pushes blood and energy away from the neck and head. *Pranayama* is best done using *ha-jalandhara bandha* unless under the supervision of an experienced teacher.

Verbal instructions for creating *ha-jalandhara bandha* in postures may include:

- Move the head down (towards to sternum) and the neck back (away from the sternum)

- Bring the chin down and in towards the throat

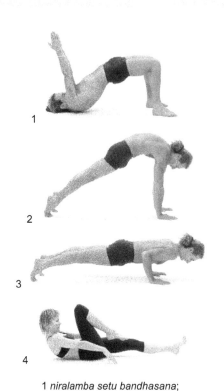

1 *niralamba setu bandhasana*;
2 *san tolanasana*;
3 *cataranga dandasana*;
4 *niralamba eka pada supta pavan muktasana*

THA-
JALANDHARA
BANDHA
An expansive and
cooling
co-activation of
opposing muscles
of the

CERVICAL SPINE
JOINT COMPLEX

Tha-jalandhara bandha

Tha-jalandhara bandha [Section 7.4.1.2.2] is an expansive and cooling *bandha* that pulls energy towards cervical spine joint complex. It is effectively engaged when there is a co-activation of neck flexors and extensors, which enhances the flow of blood through the cervical spine joint complex. This is best achieved when the cervical spine is slightly extended and internally rotated.

Tha-jalandhara bandha is engaged when there is head extensor activity and neck flexor activity. This is achieved by raising the chin and stretching the front of the neck.

Tha-jalandhara bandha is best learnt in postures such as *utthita virabhadrasana* (warrior pose), *urdhva mukha svanasana* (upwards facing dog pose) *and tolasana*.

Tha-jalandhara bandha pulls blood and energy towards the neck and head. It is sometimes nice to practice meditation with this *bandha* as it can keep the blood flowing to the head.

Verbal instructions for creating *tha-jalandhara bandha* in postures may include:

- Take the head up and the neck forward

- Take the chin up and the throat forward

1 *urdhva mukha svanasana*; 2 *utthita virabhadrasana*;
3 *tolasana*; 4 *bakasana*;
5 *kukkutasana*; 6 *urdhva kukkutasana*;
7 *purvottanasana*; 8 *dhanurasana*

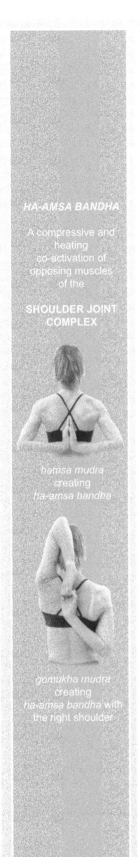

HA-AMSA BANDHA

A compressive and heating co-activation of opposing muscles of the

SHOULDER JOINT COMPLEX

hamsa mudra creating *ha-amsa bandha*

gomukha mudra creating *ha-amsa bandha* with the right shoulder

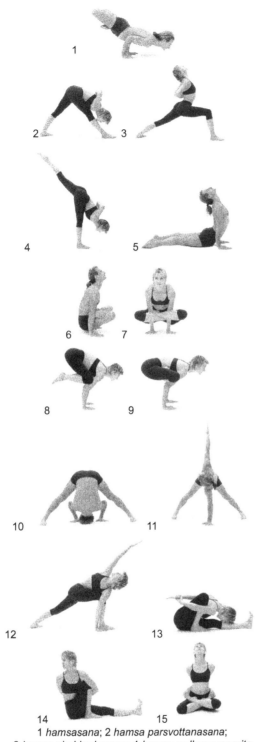

1 *hamsasana*; 2 *hamsa parsvottanasana*; 3 *hamsa virabhadrasana*; 4 *hamsa urdhva prasarita padasana*; 5 *urdhva mukha svanasana*; 6 *tolasana*; 7 *kukkutasana*; 8 *bakasana*; 9 *urdhva kukkutasana*; 10 *prasarita padottanasana*; 11 *parivrtta prasarita padottanasana*; 12 *parivrrta parsvakonasana*; 13 *maricyasana*; 14 *parivrtta maricyasana*; 15 *baddha padmasana*

Ha-amsa bandha

Ha-amsa bandha is a compressive and heating *bandha* that pushes energy away from the shoulder joint complex. *Ha-amsa bandha* is engaged when there is a co-activation of shoulder flexors and extensors, abductors and adducers, or internal rotators and external rotators, which can cause an impingement of the blood flow through the shoulder joint complex.

Ha-amsa bandha is effectively generated when the scapula is depressed and the underarm muscles pectoralis major and latissimus dorsi are active in a shortened state. That a blood flow impingement can occur with strong shoulder depression is evidenced by a loss or reduction of the radial pulse when shoulder depressors, such as the underarm muscles pectoralis major and latissimus dorsi, are actively moving the shoulder joint complex away from the neck and towards the hip.

Ha-amsa bandha is most effective when the underarm muscles pectoralis major and latissimus dorsi are actively shortening and moving the shoulder joint complex away from the neck and towards the hip and at the same time internally rotating the shoulder and adducting it.

The combined main actions of the underarm muscles pectoralis major and latissimus dorsi, which are the strongest and most important muscles in *ha-amsa bandha*, bring the shoulder into the perfect position to perform the *namaskar* (prayer) position behind the back. This position is actually referred to in many texts as *hamsa mudra* (meaning the swan gesture), presumably because it resembles the wings of the swan but also perhaps because of the *ha-amsa* (*hamsa*) *bandha* required to create it. Coincidentally, five fingers of each hand are brought together in the *hamsa mudra* with the help of *ha-amsa bandha*, and in many old languages in the world spoken today the word *hamsa* means the number five.

Additionally the sounds *ham* and *sa* are used for meditation on the breath in the *soham mantra* which is also known as the *hamsa mantra*. The sound *soooo* sounds like the sound of inhalation and the sound *ham* sounds like the sound of exhalation. *Hamsa mudra* is a very good posture to open the chest and practice *pranayama*. When *ha-amsa bandha* is engaged fascial connections between latissimus dorsi and the transverse abdominus and the activity of the myotatic (stretch) reflex make it much easier to activate *ha-mula bandha* which is essential for a complete exhalation. Similarly, fascial connections between pectoralis major and the chest musculature and the activity of the myotatic reflex enable *ha-amsa bandha* to enhance the activity of *tha-uddiyana bandha* which is essential for a complete inhalation.

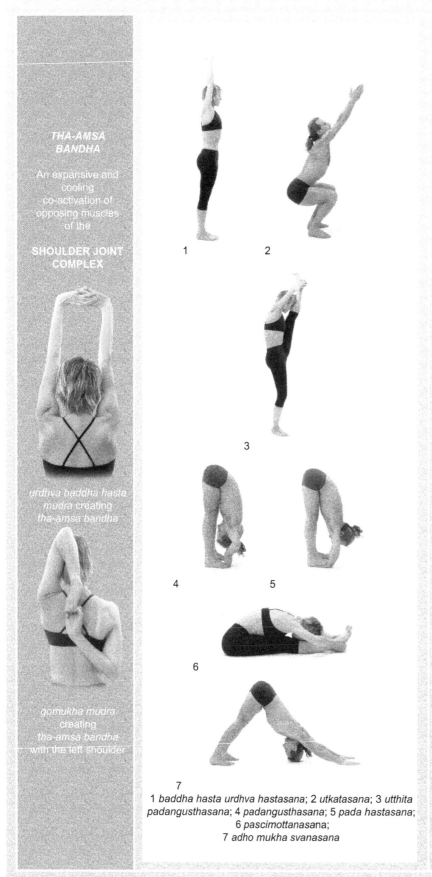

*THA-AMSA
BANDHA*

An expansive and
cooling
co-activation of
opposing muscles
of the

**SHOULDER JOINT
COMPLEX**

*urdhva baddha hasta
mudra creating
tha-amsa bandha*

*gomukha mudra
creating
tha-amsa bandha
with the left shoulder*

1 *baddha hasta urdhva hastasana*; 2 *utkatasana*; 3 *utthita
padangusthasana*; 4 *padangusthasana*; 5 *pada hastasana*;
6 *pascimottanasana*;
7 *adho mukha svanasana*

Tha-amsa bandha

Tha-amsa bandha is an expansive and cooling *bandha* that pulls energy towards the shoulder joint complex. It is engaged when there is a co-activation (simultaneous tensing) of antagonistic muscles around the shoulder joint complex that enhances the flow of blood through the shoulder joint complex.

The best positions for *tha-amsa bandha* are those where the shoulder is flexed, abducted, internally rotated, protracted and elevated, but with the underarm muscles pectoralis major and latissimus dorsi active in a lengthened position to counter the effects of the abductor, flexor and external rotator actions which are primarily from the deltoid group.

The strength of radial pulse is noticably greater in *tha-amsa bandha* than in *ha-amsa bandha*. This can be easily demonstrated if the radial pulse strength is assessed when *ha-amsa bandha* and *tha-amsa bandha* are adopted while the body is in a horizontal position.

HA-KURPARA
BANDHA

A compressive
co-activation of
opposing muscles
of the

ELBOW JOINT
COMPLEX

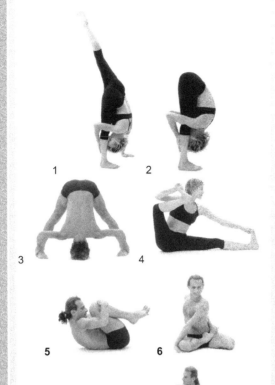

1 *urdhva prasarita ekapadasana* (R *elbow*);
2 *kulpha uttanasana*; 3 *baddha kulpha prasarita
padottanasana*; 4 *akarna dhanurasana* (R *elbow*);
5 *supta pavanmuktasana*; 6 *padma bharadvajasana*;
7 *ardha baddha padma pascimottanasana*;
8 *padma ardha matsyendrasana*

Ha-kurpara bandha

Ha-kurpara bandha is engaged when there is a co-activation of elbow flexors and extensors that causes an impingement of the blood flow through the elbow joint complex. This is effectively when the elbow is flexed about half way through its range of movement.

Ha-kurpara bandha is most obviously achieved when a bulging biceps is made visible. This can only occur in postures such as *niralamba utthita padangusthasana* when making a voluntary co-activation of elbow flexors and extensors.

In postures such as *akarna dhanursana* (R elbow) and *urdhva prasarita ekapadasana* (R elbow) shown opposite, the biceps is usually obliged to be active (Table A1), but in order to activate *ha-kurpara bandha* there should be conscious activation of the triceps brachii to counter the flexor effects of the biceps brachii.

Ha-kurpara bandha is more effective when the bulging biceps is activated while the forearm is being pronated, as this will allow the supination action of the biceps brachii to counter the pronator effects of pronator teres. This can be achieved in postures such as *padma bharadvajasana, ardha baddha padma pascimottanasana* and *padma ardha matsyendrasana* as both arms can be flexed and pronated at the elbow.

THA-KURPARA
BANDHA

An expansive
co-activation of
opposing muscles
of the

ELBOW JOINT
COMPLEX

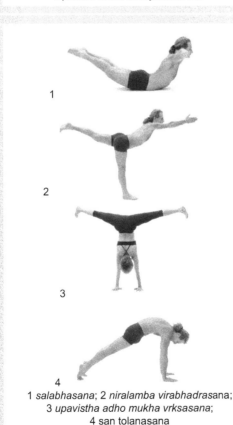

1 *salabhasana*; 2 *niralamba virabhadrasana*;
3 *upavistha adho mukha vrksasana*;
4 san *tolanasana*

Tha-kurpara bandha

Tha-kurpara bandha is engaged when there is a co-activation of elbow flexors and extensors that causes no impingement of the blood flow through the elbow joint complex. This is where the elbow is kept extended as in the handstand or plank postures, but there should be conscious activation of the biceps brachii to counter the effect the extensor effects of the triceps brachii.

Tha-kurpara bandha is most effective when the bulging biceps is activated while the forearm is being pronated, as this will allow the supination action of the biceps brachii to counter the pronator effects of pronator teres.

HA-MANI BANDHA

An compressive and
heating
co-activation of
opposing muscles
of the

**WRIST JOINT
COMPLEX**

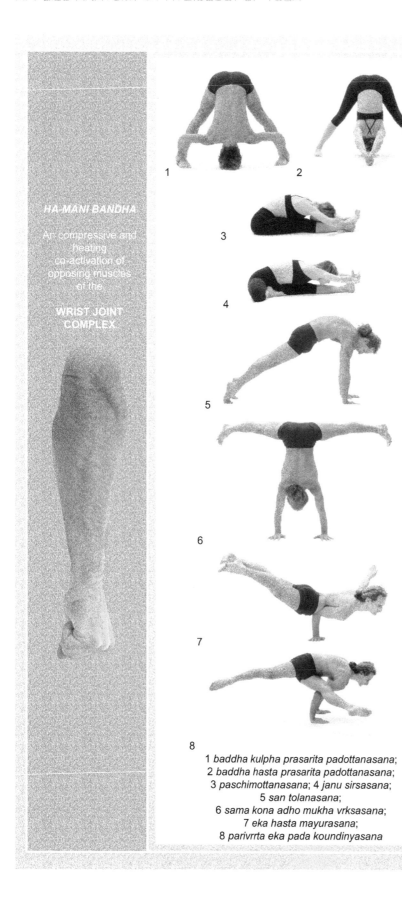

1 *baddha kulpha prasarita padottanasana*;
2 *baddha hasta prasarita padottanasana*;
3 *paschimottanasana*; 4 *janu sirsasana*;
5 *san tolanasana*;
6 *sama kona adho mukha vrksasana*;
7 *eka hasta mayurasana*;
8 *parivrrta eka pada koundinyasana*

Ha-mani bandha

Ha-mani bandha is a compressive and heating *bandha* that pushes energy away from the wrist joint complex. It is engaged when there is finger flexor activity and wrist extensor activity. This is like when one makes a clenched 'fist' or when one tries to make a clenched 'fist' even though the hands are kept flat to the floor as in the handstand or plank postures.

THA-MANI BANDHA

An expansive and
cooling
co-activation of
opposing muscles
of the

**WRIST JOINT
COMPLEX**

1 *parsva virabhadrasana*;
2 *utthita virabhadrasana*;
3 *utthita parsvakonasana*;
4 *parivrtta parsvakonasana*; 5 *urdhva hastasana*;
6 *padangustha urdhva hastasana*;
7 *padangustha utkatasana*; 8 *utkatasana*

Tha-mani bandha

Tha-mani bandha is an expansive and cooling *bandha* that pulls energy towards the wrist joint complex. *Tha-mani bandha* is engaged when there is finger extensor activity and wrist flexor activity. This is like actively stretching into the fingers.

Tha-mani bandha generates a relatively low pressure and can therefore pull blood and energy to the hand. Hence, when the arms are raised above the head it usually feels lighter and easier to stretch into the fingers (*tha-mani bandha*) than it is to make a fist (*ha-mani bandha*) even though activation of the same muscle groups is involved in both cases.

409

Abbreviations:

R	=	Right
L	=	Left
Jt	=	Joint
Fl	=	Flexion
Ex	=	Extension
Ab	=	Abduction
Ad	=	Adduction
IR	=	Internal Rotation
ER	=	External Rotation

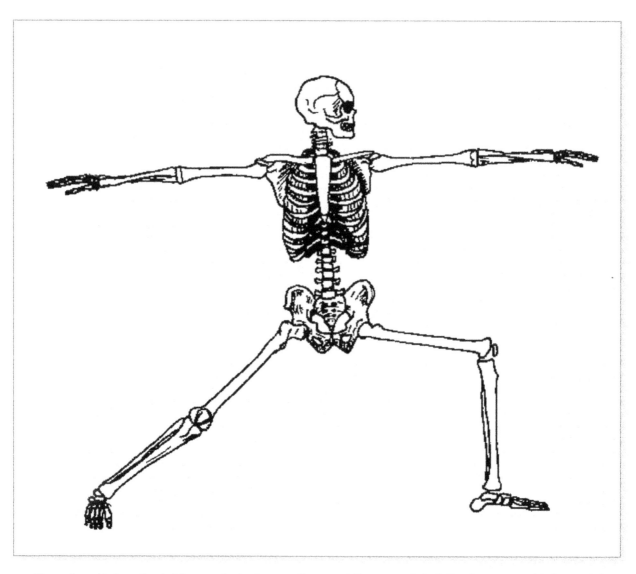

Exercise: Using the tables and photos on the next 2 pages, label the bones and joints of the above skeleton and indicate what position each joint is in as has been done in the table on the next page

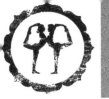

The following descriptions refer to the pictures on the following page:

Abbreviations:

Fl	=	Flexion
Ex	=	Extension
Ab	=	Abduction
Ad	=	Adduction
IR	=	Internal Rotation
ER	=	External Rotation
PF	=	Plantarflexion of ankle
DF	=	Dorsiflexion of ankle
Ev	=	Eversion of ankle
Pr	=	Pronation of forearm
Su	=	Supination of forearm
Pt	=	Protraction of scapula
Rt	=	Retraction of scapula
N	=	Neutral or normal position (i.e. as in *savasana* or corpse posture)

Table D1 Description of joint positions in yoga postures

Body joint or part	Posture → Side of body ↓	1. Padmasana with Jnana Mudra	2. Ustrasana	3. Urdhva Dhanur-asana	4. Utthita Virabhadr-asana	5. Paripurna Matsyendr-asana (to L)	6. Eka Pada Sirsasana (L leg over head)
Ankles	Right	PF, In	PF, Ev	DF, Ev	DF, Ev	PF, Ev	N, Ev
	Left	PF, In	PF, Ev	DF, Ev	N, In	PF, In	N, Ev
Knees	Right	Fl	Fl	Fl	Fl	Fl	Ex
	Left	Fl	Fl	Fl	Ex	Fl	Fl
Hips	Right	Fl, ER	Ex	Ex	Fl	Fl, Ad, ER	Fl
	Left	Fl, ER	Ex	Ex	Ex	Fl, Ad, IR	Fl, ER
Spine		N	Ex	Ex	Ex	Fl	Fl
Wrists	Right	N	Ex	Ex	N	N	Ex
	Left	N	Ex	Ex	N	Ex	Ex
Forearms	Right	Su	Pr	Pr	Pr	Pr	Pr
	Left	Su	Pr	Pr	Pr	Pr	Pr
Elbows	Right	Ex	Ex	Ex	Ex	Ex	Fl
	Left	Ex	Ex	Ex	Ex	Fl	Fl
Shoulders	Right	Ab, Fl, ER	Ex, ER	Fl, ER	Fl, ER	Fl, Ab, ER	N
	Left	Ab, Fl, ER	Ex, ER	Fl, ER	Fl, ER	Ex, Ad, IR	N
Scapulas	Right	N	Rt	Pt	Pt	Pt	N
	Left	N	Rt	Pt	Pt	Rt	N
Neck		N	Ex	Ex	Ex	N	Ex

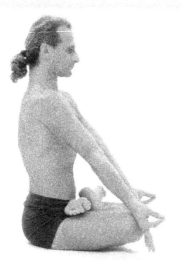

1. *Padmasana with jnana mudra*

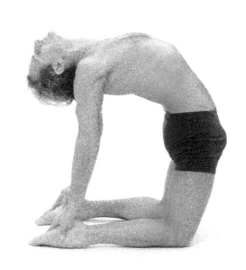

2. *Ustrasana*

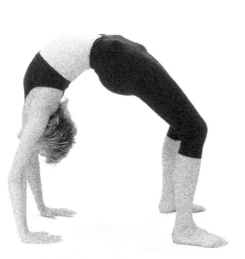

3. *Urdhva dhanurasana*

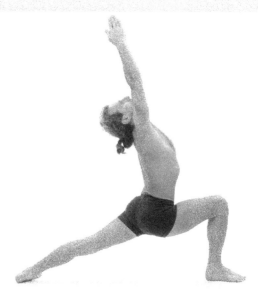

4. *Utthita virabhadrasana*

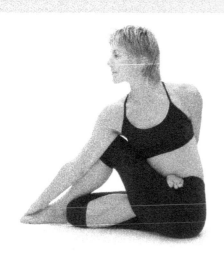

5. *Paripurna matsyendrasana*

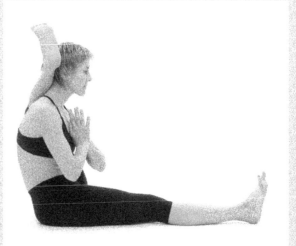

6. *Eka pada sirsasana*

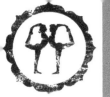

A *yoga* teacher or body worker may be effective without knowing any technical jargon regarding anatomy and physiology. However, an understanding of the terms used in anatomy and physiology can help deepen understanding by being able to read books and articles that are more technical in nature. Understanding technical terms also makes it easier to communicate with medical practitioners and helps in understanding medical reports.

Further information is available in the glossaries of the **Anatomy Colouring Book** [Kapit & Elson, 1993] and the **Principles of Anatomy & Physiology** [Tortora, & Grabowski, 1993].

- **Abduction**: movement away from the midline of the body.
- **Action**: muscle action is defined to be the movement produced (eg flexion, extension) when a muscle activates concentrically (i.e. shortens) in isolation. By definition, it will always be the same for any given muscle.
- **Active insufficiency**: a muscle is said to be actively insufficient if it is either in a too shortened or too lengthened position to actively generate tension.
- **Acute injuries**: are usually recent and have tissue damage with inflammation.
- **Adduction**: movement towards the midline of the body.
- **Afferent**: bringing to or leading towards a central organ or point, (opposed to efferent). An afferent blood vessel or nerve is about to enter a structure.
- **Agonist:** a muscle takes the role of agonist if it is the principle muscle producing a movement.
- **Anatomical position**: the standard position which most anatomical terminology relates to. It is standing erect with the arms placed by the side of the body and with the forearms supinated (i.e. palms facing forward, like a standing version of the corpse posture sometimes called *Savasana*).
- **Antagonist:** a muscle takes the role of antagonist if it must relax to allow the desired movement to occur. The antagonist opposes the agonist.
- **Anterior pelvic tilt**: anterior movement of the superior pelvis (i.e. forward movement of the top of the hips)
- **Anterior**: relatively closer to the front of the body.
- **Appendicular skeleton** consists of the 126 bones contained in the upper (60) and lower (60) limbs and the pectoral (shoulder) (4) and pelvic (hip) (2) girdle.
- **Articular system**: joints, joint capsules and articular discs.
- **Articulation**: see **joint.**
- **Axial skeleton:** consists of 80 bones that lie around the central axis of the body: the skull bones (22), auditory ossicles (6), hyoid bone (1), ribs (24), sternum (breastbone) (1), and the spinal vertebrae (26).
- **Baroreceptor**: nervous system receptor sensing changes in pressure.
- **Bi-articular (two-joint) muscle**: A bi-articular, or two-joint muscle, crosses two joints, for example *Rectus femoris* is a bi-articular muscle as it crosses both the hip and the knee joints.
- **Bi-lateral:** two sided.
- **Blood pressure**: the pressure of the blood; when used alone this term refers to the average arterial blood pressure [Moffett et al., 1993].
- **Bursae**: Closed flattened sacs filled with synovial fluid.
- **Cardio-vascular system**: heart, blood vessels and flow of blood.
- **Chronic injuries**: are those where the inflammation has subsided.
- **Closed-chain (CC) movement or exercises**: are where the distal end of limb, or limb segment is fixed (i.e. attached to the floor or wall etc.). Here the origin of a muscle is the distal attachment and the insertion is the proximal attachment. The limb is said to be acting in a ***closed kinetic chain***. Many of the movements in everyday life and during exercise are closed chain movements or exercises.
- **Co-activation**: Activation of agonist and antagonist muscle groups at the same time is referred to as co-activation or simultaneous tension. A co-activation around a joint has the effect of limiting joint mobility thereby leading to an increased joint stability.
- **Co-contraction**: see **co-activation**. The use of the terms '*contraction*' of muscles and '*co-contraction*' of muscles are avoided in these notes as '*contract*' can also mean to shorten, yet much of the work that muscles do does not always involve shortening. For example, muscles can be generating tension or working while lengthening (eccentric muscle activation) or staying the same length (isometric muscle activation).
- **Concentric muscle activation**: muscle shortens while working or generating tension.
- **Contra-**: opposing (Latin prefix).
- **Contra-lateral**: the opposite side.
- **Depression**: movement of the scapular inferiorly (i.e. movement of the shoulder blade away from the head).
- **Digestive system**: assimilation & breakdown of food.
- **Distal**: relatively further from the attachment of a limb, or the point of origin.

- **Dorsiflexion**: moving the foot towards the body. Dorsiflexion at the ankle joint is analogous to extension at the wrist.
- **Eccentric muscle activation**: muscle lengthens while working/tensing.
- **Efferent**: bringing to or leading away from a central organ or point, (opposed to afferent). An efferent blood vessel or nerve is leaving a structure.
- **Elevation**: movement of scapular superiorly (i.e. movement of the shoulder blade towards the head).
- **Endocrine system**: control & communication by chemical signals.
- **Eversion**: turning the sole of the foot to face outwards (lateral movement).
- **Extension**: straightening or increasing the angle between the bones of a joint. One exception is the shoulder, where taking the arm towards your body from above your head is called extension.
- **External (lateral) Rotation**: rotation away from the midline of the body.
- **Fixator** or **stabiliser**: when it supports a body part so that another muscle may have a firm base to act on to produce the desired movement.
- **Flexion**: bending or reducing the angle between the bones of a joint. One exception is the shoulder where taking the arm towards the head (not the body) is called flexion.
- **Gravitational pump** [Section 1.0.4]: pumps blood around the body by the force of gravity. The part that is closest to the floor usually is where all the blood is going.
- **Hyperventilation**: breathing more than you need in the situation you are in
- **Hypoventilation**: breathing less than you need in the situation you are in
- **Immune system**: body defence mechanisms.
- **Inferior**: relatively further from the head.
- **Inflammation:** is a localised, protective response to tissue injury designed to destroy, dilute, or wall off the infecting agent or injured tissue. Inflammation is characterised by (i) Redness, (ii) Pain, (iii) Heat, (iv) Swelling, and sometimes (v) Loss of function.
- **Infra-**: below (Latin prefix).
- **Internal (Medial) Rotation**: rotation toward the midline of the body.
- **Inversion**: turning the sole of the foot to face inwards (medial movement).
- **Irritable conditions:** musculoskeletal conditions that are easily stirred up and must be treated very carefully or else they can become very sore after exercise or after a treatment.
- **Joint:** is the point of contact or **articulation** between bones, between cartilage and bones, or between teeth and bones.
- **Kyphosis**: posteriorly convex curvature of the spine usually in the thoracic spine and in the sacrococcygeal spine.
- **Lateral rotation**: see external rotation
- **Lateral**: relatively further from the midline of the body.
- **Lengthening reaction**: when a muscle is initially stretched it will tend to tense and resist the movement into the stretch due to the myotatic reflex (stretch reflex) but after a period of time this resistance suddenly collapses and the muscle is able to more easily stretch or lengthen due to autogenic inhibition (the inverse myotatic reflex), in what is termed the 'lengthening reaction' [Section 1.7.2.2.1.3].
- **Lordosis**: anteriorly concave curve of the spine usually in the lumbar spine and in the cervical spine.
- **Lymphatic system**: lymph flow and recovery of tissue fluid.
- **Medial rotation**: see internal rotation.
- **Medial**: relatively closer to midline of the body.
- **Minute ventilation:** the average amount of air inhaled per minute
- **Mole**: a chemical unit of measurement. One mole of a substance is defined to be the weight in grams of the molecular weight of that substance.
- **Multi-articular (many joint) muscle**: a muscle that crosses more than one joint. They are economic since they are able to produce motion at more than one joint.
- **Muscle activation**: increasing local pressure.
- **Muscle attachments**: muscles attach to bones by tendons, which consist of dense regular connective tissue.
- **Muscle co-activation pump** [Section 1.7.3]: pumps blood around the body using the ha-bandhas to compress the body and the tha-bandhas to expand the body.
- **Muscle insertion:** the insertion of a muscle is by definition the muscle attachment that is not fixed during movement. It is usually the distal attachment of a muscle in classical muscle charts, which generally only describe closed chain movements. However, the muscle insertion is the proximal insertion of a muscle in open chain movements.
- **Muscle origin:** the origin of a muscle is by definition the muscle attachment that is stable during movement. Hence, it is usually the proximal attachment of a muscle in classical muscle charts which generally only describe closed chain movements. However, the muscle origin is the distal insertion of a muscle in open chain movements.
- **Muscle relaxation**: decreasing local pressure.
- **Muscular system**: muscles and tendons which join them to bones.
- **Musculoskeletal pump** [Section 8.1.2.3.1]: pumps blood around the body by skeletal muscles activating and pushing blood towards the heart. When muscles relax, valves prevent backflow.

- **Nervous system**: control & communication via electrochemical signals.
- **Neutraliser:** when it cancels out unwanted movements that would otherwise be produced by the agonist.
- **Non-irritable conditions:** musculoskeletal conditions that are able to be treated or exercised quite firmly and while they may have a sense of discomfort while exercising or while being treated, the discomfort settles down after the treatment.
- **Non-weight-bearing (NWB) exercises:** are static or dynamic exercises in which a particular limb or body part is taking little or no body weight and is said to be **unloaded**. Many non-weight-bearing exercises are open chain exercises.
- **Open-chain (CO) movement or exercises** are where the distal end of a limb is not fixed (i.e. free to move). Here the origin of a muscle is the proximal attachment and the insertion is the distal attachment. The limb is said to be acting in an *open kinetic chain*. Muscle actions in the tables in these notes (and in other texts) are described in terms of open chain movements.
- **Pain gate control theory:** says there is neural gate that can be relatively open or closed modulating incoming nociceptive signals before the brain experiences them as pain.
- **Passive insufficiency:** occurs when a muscle is of insufficient length while relaxed and acting passively as a antagonist too short to allow the agonist to complete it's full range of movement (ROM).
- **Perfusion**: how much air is actually getting into the pulmonary blood vessels from the alveoli of the lungs.
- **Plantarflexion**: moving the foot away from the body. Plantarflexion at the ankle joint is analogous to flexion at the wrist.
- **Posterior pelvic tilt**: posterior movement of the superior pelvis (backward movement of the top of the hips).
- **Posterior**: relatively closer to the back of the body.
- **Postural pump** [Section 1.0.4]: pumps blood around the body in each posture by compression of one part of the body and expansion or stretch of another part.
- **Pronation**: turning the palm of the hand downwards (like internal rotation of the forearm).
- **Protraction**: movement of the scapular anteriorly (i.e. movement of the shoulder blade away from the spine).
- **Proximal**: relatively closer to the attachment of a limb, or the point of origin.
- **Receptor**: a receptor is a structure of any size or complexity that collects and usually also edits information about conditions, inside or outside the body e.g. the eye, muscle spindle, and the free ending of the peripheral neural of a sensory neuron. Information about the external and internal environment reaches the central nervous system following the activation of a sensory receptor. Receptors convert one form of energy in the environment in response to changes in membrane permeability (transduction).
- **Reflex arc**: a mono-synaptic reflex arc (which has only one synapse) is the basic unit of integrated neural activity. It has 5 main components: (i) Receptor, (ii) Afferent neuron, (iii) Centre, (iv) Efferent neuron, & (v) Effector organ.
- **Reflex**: a stereotyped reaction of the CNS to a sensory stimulus, can be somatic or visceral.
- **Reproductive system**: sexual organs.
- **Respiratory pump** [Section 8.1.2.3.2]: pumps blood around the body on inspiration. The diaphragm descends towards the abdomen resulting in a decrease in thoracic pressure and an increase in abdominal pressure. Blood flows from high to low pressure, therefore from the abdomen to the thorax. On expiration the reverse would occur, however the valves prevent backflow.
- **Respiratory system**: lungs, windpipe (trachea) and nasal cavity.
- **Retraction**: movement of the scapular posteriorly (i.e. movement of the shoulder blade towards the spine).
- **Role**: the role of any muscle may vary with every movement that is made.
- **Skeletal system**: bones and ligaments that join the bones.
- **Stroke volume**: the amount of blood ejected from the heart ventricle in one beat or contraction.
- **Superior**: relatively closer to the head.
- **Supination**: turning the palm of the hand upwards (external rotation of the forearm).
- **Supra-**: above (Latin prefix).
- **Synergist**: a muscle is said to be a synergist when it works with other muscles to produce a desired effect.
- **Synovial fluid**: fluid inside the joint cavity that lubricates joints, also present between muscles and fascia, and also around nerve sheaths.
- **Synovial Joints**: synovial joints are generally easily moveable joints, which always have a joint cavity, articular cartilage, ligaments, and articular capsule. They also have a synovial membrane, filled with synovial fluid and are susceptible to becoming inflamed.
- **Tone**: the state of excitability of the nervous system controlling or influencing skeletal muscles; also can be an ongoing tension or activation exhibited by a muscle while it is holding a posture or moving from one posture to another.
- **Transduction of energy**: transduction is the conversion of one from of energy to another.
- **Uni-articular (single-joint) muscle**: a muscle that crosses only one joint.
- **Unilateral**: one sided.
- **Urinary system**: the body system that functions in water and acid-base balance, and in the excretion of wastes.
- **Valsalva's manoeuvre**: contraction of the abdominal muscles while the breath has been retained in, i.e. an attempt at forced expiration with a closed glottis [Astrand & Rodahl, 1986]. This is essentially the same as making a *ha-mula bandha*

(contacting the abdomen) and a *ha-uddiyana bandha* (contracting the chest) with the breath held in.

- **Ventilation**: how much air is actually getting into the alveoli of the lungs.
- **Weight-bearing (WB) exercises:** are static or dynamic exercises in which a particular limb or body part is taking part or all of the weight of the body and is said to be **loaded**. Many weight-bearing exercises are closed-chain exercises.
- **Wolff's Law**: states that "*The form of a bone being given, bone elements will place or displace themselves in the direction of the functional stress, and will increase or decrease their mass to reflect the amount of the functional stress.*" This 'law' describes the nature of the effect of the external environment and therefore the choice and will of an individual to affect the growth and development of a bone.

****

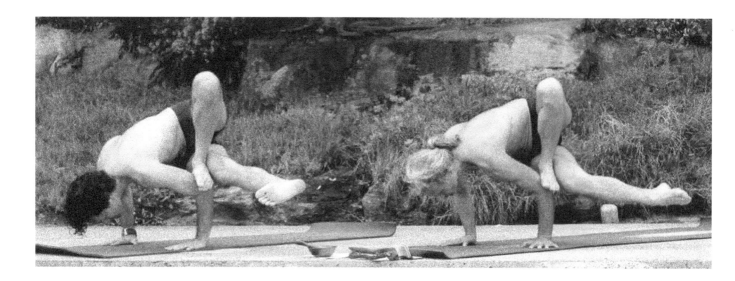

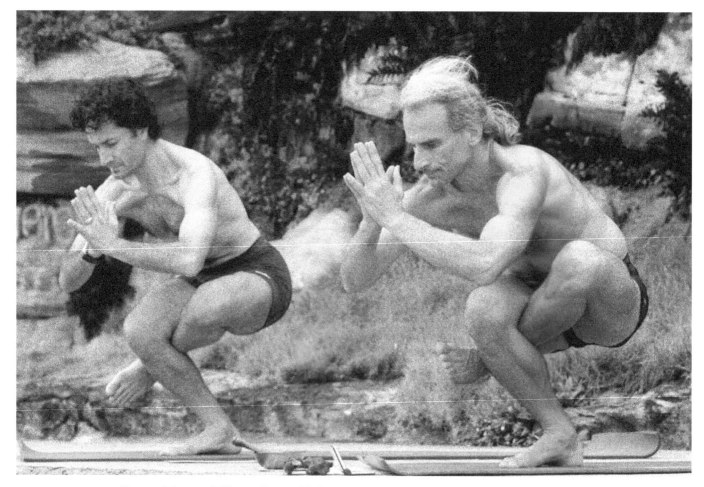

Danny May and Simon Borg-Olivier, photos courtesy of Martin Renwick.

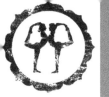

A *yoga* teacher may be effective without knowing any *Sanskrit* terms regarding *yoga* and other Indian systems. However, an understanding of these terms can help deepen one's knowledge of *yoga* by being able to read books and articles using these terms. Further information is available from the glossaries of many *hatha yoga* books [Iyengar, 1966, 1988, 2001; Yogeshwaranandaji, 1977; Goswami, 1980.].

Abbreviation: pr. = pronounced

- **Adho**: downward [Iyengar, 1966]
- **Agni**: metabolism, metabolic fire
- **Amsa bandha**: on a subtle level it is the binding of the energy of the shoulder; on a more anatomical level it is a joint stabilisation or co-activation of opposing muscle groups crossing the shoulder joint complex
- **Amsa**: the shoulder [Capp, 2000]
- **Anumukha**: small mouthed [Capp, 2000]
- **Apana**: a type of prana which functions below the naval [Yogeshwaranandaji, 1977]; an *Upanishad* (ancient Indian text) term for inspiration [Goswami, 1980]
- **Aratni bandha**: more commonly called *Kurpara bandha*. On a subtle level it is the binding of the energy of the elbow; on a more anatomical level it is a joint stabilisation or co-activation of opposing muscle groups crossing the elbow joint complex
- **Aratni**: the elbow [Capp, 2000]
- **Ardha**: half [Iyengar, 1966]
- **Asana**: a pose or posture in which the body is maintained motionless [Goswami, 1980], static posture
- **Asanam**: static postures, poses
- **Atanu**: large [Capp, 2000]
- **Ayur**: life
- **Ayurveda**: ancient Indian science of life [Lele *et al.*, 1999]
- **Baddha**: bound [Iyengar, 1966]
- **Bandha**: a lock an internal locking mechanism. On a subtle level it is the binding of the energy of a region of the body; on a more anatomical level it is a joint stabilisation or co-activation of opposing muscle groups crossing a joint complex.
- **Bheka**: a frog [Iyengar, 1966]
- **Buddhizuddhi**: purification of the heart [Capp, 2000]
- **Bukka**: heart [Capp, 2000]
- **Cakra (pr. Chakra)**: a subtle circular organisation within the body containing *mahabhuta* (meta-matter), *tanmatra* (sense forces) and *prana*, not part of the material world but a supra-material power centre [Goswami, 1980]
- **Catur (pr. Chatur)**: four [Iyengar, 1966]
- **Cikitsa (pr. Chikitsa)**: therapy (as in *Yoga Chikitsa* – Yoga therapy)
- **Citta (pr. Chitta)**: sense-consciousness, perceptive mind [Goswami, 1980]
- **Danda**: a rod
- **Dhamani**: nerves [Lele *et al.*, 1999]
- **Dhanu (ra)**: a bow [Iyengar, 1966]
- **Dharana**: holding concentration, the 6th stage of *ashtanga yoga* [Goswami, 1980]
- **Dhyana**: meditation [Iyengar, 1966]
- **Doshas (tridoshas)**: three fundamental energies or principles, *sattva* (luminosity), *rajas* (vibrancy), and *tamas* (dormancy or inertia), [Lele *et al.*, 1999; Iyengar, 1993]
- **Drishti**: insight, intellective vision [Goswami, 1980]
- **Dwi**: two [Iyengar, 1966]
- **Eka**: one [Iyengar, 1966]
- **Garuda**: an eagle [Iyengar, 1966]
- **Gunas**: the qualities of nature [Iyengar, 1993]
- **Ha**: sun, hot, compressive, or relatively high pressure [Iyengar, 1966; Yogeshwaranandaji, 1977; Goswami, 1980; Iyengar, 2001]
- **Ha-bandha**: a compressive (or relatively high pressure) subtle energy lock (*bandha*), which on the physical level takes the form of a co-activation of opposing muscle groups around a joint complex. A *ha-bandha* generates a lot of heat energy due to muscle activation, but prevents energy from entering that region, and in its extreme form does not allow blood to pass through that region or *prana* (vital energy) to flow through the *nadis* (subtle energy channels) in that region.
- **Hala**: a plough [Iyengar, 1966]
- **Hanuman**: the monkey [Iyengar, 1966]

- **Hasta bandha**: another name for *mani bandha*. On a subtle level it is the binding of the energy of the hand; on a more anatomical level it is a joint stabilisation or co-activation of opposing muscle groups crossing the hand joint complex
- **Hasta**: the hand [Iyengar, 1966]
- **Hatha**: force, forcibly [Kapp, 2001]; with rigorous effort [Pranavanada, 1992]
- **Ida & Pingala**: the two vital force lines or nadis residing on left and right side of vertebral column respectively [Goswami, 1980]
- **Jalandhara bandha**: on a subtle level it is the binding of the energy of the cervical spine and neck region; on a more anatomical level it is a joint stabilisation or co-activation of opposing muscle groups crossing the cervical spine joint complex.
- **Janu bandha**: on a subtle level it is the binding of the energy of the knee; on a more anatomical level it is a joint stabilisation or co-activation of opposing muscle groups crossing the knee joint complex.
- **Janu**: the knee [Capp, 2000]
- **Jathara**: the abdomen, stomach [Capp, 2000]
- **Kanda mula** (or **Kanda**): force concentration centre from which all the *nadis* originate, and which is situated inside the coccyx just below the *muladhara chakra* [Iyengar, 1966; Goswami, 1980].
- **Kati bandha**: on a subtle level it is the binding of the energy of the hip; on a more anatomical level it is a joint stabilisation or co-activation of opposing muscle groups crossing the hip joint complex.
- **Kloman**: lung [Capp, 2000]
- **Kona**: an angle [Iyengar, 1966]
- **Kulpha bandha**: on a subtle level it is the binding of the energy of the ankle; on a more anatomical level it is a joint stabilisation or co-activation of opposing muscle groups crossing the ankle joint complex.
- **Kulpha**: the ankle [Capp, 2000]
- **Kumbhaka**: breath suspension [Goswami, 1980]
- **Kurpara (Aratni) bandha**: on a subtle level it is the binding of the energy of the elbow; on a more anatomical level it is a joint stabilisation or co-activation of opposing muscle groups crossing the elbow joint complex
- **Kurpara**: elbow [Capp, 2000]
- **Mani bandha**: on a subtle level it is the binding of the energy of the wrist; on a more anatomical level it is a joint stabilisation or co-activation of opposing muscle groups crossing the wrist joint complex
- **Mani**: the wrist [Capp, 2000]
- **Marma**: a vital anatomical point which is at the union between an important nerve and also a muscle, vein, ligament and/or bone [Lele et al., 1999]. Marma points lie between 2 acupuncture points of opposing meridians [Bhan, 1996]
- **Mudra**: a seal or sealing posture [Iyengar, 1966] control exercise [Goswami, 1980]
- **Mukha**: the face [Iyengar, 1966]
- **Mula bandha**: on a subtle level it is the binding of the energy of the lumbar spine and lower trunk; on a more anatomical level it is a joint stabilisation or co-activation of opposing muscle groups crossing the joint complex of the lumbar spine
- **Mula**: the root or base [Iyengar, 1966]
- **Nadi**: a subtle channel of energy found within the body [Pranavanada, 1992]; that which is motion or motional; a subtle line of direction along which the prana (and other *vayus* move); a *pranic* force-radiation-line [Goswami, 1980]
- **Namaskar**: a salute, salutation, generally indicated by Namaskara mudra which has the palms placed together resembling the prayer position [Iyengar, 1966]
- **Namaste**: a salute, salutation; generally indicated by Namaskara mudra which has the palms placed together resembling the prayer position [Iyengar, 1966]
- **Nidra**: sleep [Iyengar, 1966]
- **Niralamba**: unsupported [Iyengar, 1966]
- **Pada bandha**: on a subtle level it is the binding of the energy of the foot; on a more anatomical level it is a joint stabilisation or co-activation of opposing muscle groups crossing the foot joint complex
- **Pada**: a foot [Iyengar, 1966]
- **Padangustha**: a big toe [Iyengar, 1966]
- **Padma**: a lotus [Iyengar, 1966]
- **Padottana**: legs spread apart position [Iyengar, 1966]
- **Parivartana**: turning around, revolving [Iyengar, 1966]
- **Parivrtta**: turned around revolved [Iyengar, 1966]
- **Parsva**: the side, lateral [Iyengar, 1966]
- **Pascha**: west, the back of the body [Iyengar, 1966]
- **Pashimotana**: intense stretch of the back of the body [Iyengar, 1966]
- **Prakruti (Prakrti)**: nature, the original source of the material world, consisting of the 3 gunas (= trigunas), sattva, rajas and tamas [Iyengar, 1966]
- **Prana**: the basic life force, present as different forms of bio-energy, also a term for expiration [Goswami, 1980]
- **Pranayama**: a system of bio-energy control through short-quick and long-slow breathing and breath suspension exercises [Goswami, 1980]

- **Prasarita**: spread out, stretched out [Iyengar, 1966]
- **Puraka**: inhalation [Iyengar, 1988]
- **Puritat**: intestine [Capp, 2000]
- **Purusha**: the seer or the soul [Iyengar, 1993]
- **Purva**: east, the front of the body [Iyengar, 1966]
- **Purvottana**: intense stretch of the front of the body [Iyengar, 1966]
- **Rachana**: anatomy [Lele et al., 1999]
- **Rajas**: vibrancy, one of the 3 gunas (qualities of nature) Iyengar, 1993]
- **Rechaka**: exhalation [Iyengar, 1988]
- **Sama**: same, equal, upright [Iyengar, 1966]
- **Sarvanga**: whole body [Iyengar, 1966]
- **Sattva**: luminosity, one of the 3 gunas (qualities of nature) [Iyengar, 1993]
- **Sava**: a dead body, corpse [Iyengar, 1966]
- **Setu**: a bridge [Iyengar, 1966]
- **Sthira**: firm, fixed, steady, steadfast [Iyengar, 1993]
- **Sukha**: happiness, pleasure, comfort [Iyengar, 1966]
- **Sukham**: happiness, delight [Iyengar, 1993]
- **Supta**: lying down, reclining, sleeping [Iyengar, 1966]
- **Surya**: the sun [Iyengar, 1966]
- **Svana**: a dog [Iyengar, 1966]
- **Svastika**: a swastika symbol, usually denoting a cross legged position [Iyengar, 1966]
- **Tada**: a mountain [Iyengar, 1966]
- **Tamas**: dormancy or inertia, one of the 3 gunas (qualities of nature) [Iyengar, 1993]
- **Tha**: moon, cool, expansive, or relatively low pressure [Iyengar, 1966; Yogeshwaranandaji, 1977; Goswami, 1980; Iyengar, 2001]
- **Tha-bandha**: an expansive (or relatively low pressure) subtle energy lock (*bandha*), which on the physical level takes the form of a co-activation of opposing muscle groups around a joint complex. A *tha-bandha* generates some heat energy due to muscle activation, but allows energy to enter that region, and in its extreme form actually 'pulls' blood to that region and 'pulls' *prana* (vital energy) through the *nadis* (subtle energy channels) in that region.
- **Tittibha**: insect [Iyengar, 1966]
- **Tri**: three [Iyengar, 1966]
- **Uddiyana bandha**: on a subtle level it is the binding of the energy of the thoracic spine and upper trunk; on a more anatomical level it is a joint stabilisation by co-activation of opposing muscle groups crossing the thoracic spine and rib joint complex, this especially includes the external and internal intercostal muscles
- **Upavistha**: seated [Iyengar, 1966]
- **Urdhva**: upward [Iyengar, 1966]
- **Utkata**: powerful [Iyengar, 1966]
- **Uttan**: intense [Iyengar, 1966]
- **Utthita**: extended, raised up, stretched [Iyengar, 1966]
- **Vasti**: bladder [Capp, 2000]
- **Veda**: science
- **Vidya**: science; as used in *hatha yoga vidya*, the science of *hatha yoga* [Iyengar, 1966]
- **Vinyasa**: dynamic exercise, movement exercise, linking movement between 2 static poses, linked series of postures
- **Viparita karani**: inverted and semi-inverted postures
- **Vira**: a hero [Iyengar, 1966]
- **Virabhadra**: a warrior [Iyengar, 1966]
- **Vrksa**: a tree [Iyengar, 1966]
- **Yoga**: union [Iyengar, 1966]

Tensioning (stretching) and Stimulation of Acupuncture Meridian stretches in various postures

Meridian name Names of possible yoga poses for meridian tensioning (stretching)	Positions of meridians on each joint complex	Positions of joint for meridian tensioning (stretching)	Postures or joint positions that cause meridian stimulation with muscle activation or joint/muscle compression
Lung meridian (LU): Median nerve stretch (i) and (ii) Purvottanasana Vasisthasana Parsvakonasana	Wrist: anterior radius Elbow: lateral anterior Shoulder: anterior shoulder	Wrist extension, ulnar deviation Elbow extension, pronation/ supination? Shoulder retraction, depression, abduction, extension, external rotation	Direct pressure and activation in all arm balances especially mayurasana Padahastasana stimulates with toe pressure
Pericardium meridian (PC): Median nerve stretch (i) and (ii) Purvottanasana Vasisthasana Parsvakonasana	Wrist: anterior radioulnar joint Elbow: mid anterior Shoulder: anterior shoulder	Wrist extension, Elbow extension, pronation/ supination? Shoulder retraction, depression, abduction, extension, external rotation	Direct pressure and activation in all arm balances especially mayurasana Padahastasana stimulates with toe pressure
Heart meridian (HT): Median nerve stretch (i) and (ii) Ulnar nerve stretch (i) Purvottanasana Vasisthasana Parsvakonasana	Wrist: anterior ulnar Elbow: medial anterior Shoulder: axilla, armpit	Wrist extension, radial deviation Elbow extension/flexion?, pronation/supination? Shoulder protraction/ retraction?, elevation/ depression?, abduction, extension, external rotation	Direct pressure and activation in all arm balances especially mayurasana Padahastasana stimulates with toe pressure
Small intestine meridian (SI): Gomukhasana (flexed/ raised arm) (with wrist flexion) Padahastasana	Wrist: lateral ulnar Elbow: medial posterior] Shoulder: lateral posterior scapula	Wrist flexion, radial deviation Elbow flexion, pronation/ supination? Shoulder protraction, depression, adduction, flexion, internal rotation	Direct pressure and activation in all arm balances Padahastasana stimulates with toe pressure
San jao meridian (SJ): Gomukhasana (raised arm) (with wrist flexion) Padahastasana	Wrist: posterior radius Elbow: posterior (olecronon) Shoulder: posterior deltoid	Wrist flexion, Elbow flexion, pronation/ supination? Shoulder protraction, depression/elevation?, adduction, flexion, internal rotation	Direct pressure in pinca mayurasana and sayanasana Activation and stretching in pinca mayurasana and cataranga dandasana
Large intestine meridian (LI): Radial nerve stretch Gomukhasana (lower arm) (with wrist flexion) Padahastasana	Wrist: posterior radioulnar joint Elbow: lateral Shoulder: superior deltoid	Wrist flexion, ulnar deviation Elbow flexion/extension?, pronation/supination? Shoulder protraction, depression, abduction/ adduction?, extension, internal rotation	Direct pressure in Activation and stretching in pinca mayurasana and cataranga dandasana
Stomach meridian (ST): Supta virasana Bhugangasana Urdhva dhanurasana	Toes: mid anterior, dorsal Ankle: anterior Knee: anterior Hip: anterior Trunk: anterior Neck: anterior	Toe flexion Ankle plantarflexion Knee flexion Hip extension Spinal extension Neck flexion and head extension	Direct pressure activation and stretching in Rajakapotasana

Spleen meridian (LI): Parsva san calanasana	Toes: medial, dorsal Ankle: anterior medial Knee: anterior medial Hip: anterior medial Trunk: anterior lateral	Toe flexion Ankle plantarflexion, eversion Knee extension/flexion? Hip extension Spinal extension, lateral flexion	Direction pressure (stimulation of spleen 6 acupuncture point) with Kulpha simhasana
Liver meridian (LR): Urdhva samakonasana Eka pada upavistha konasana Bhujangasana	Toes: medial, dorsal Ankle: anterior medial Knee: medial Hip: anterior medial Trunk: anterior lateral	Toe flexion Ankle plantarflexion, eversion Knee extension/flexion? Hip abduction, extension Spinal extension, lateral flexion	Direct pressure while squeezing the legs together especially in postures such as astavakrasana and also in eka hasta bhujasana, eka pada sirsasana Activation in all postures with active internal rotation and extension of hip
Kidney meridian (K): Urdhva mukha pascimottanasa (i.e. extended spine floor Pascimottanasana) Urdhva samakonasana Upavistha konasana Simha mudra, sitali mudra, kecari mudra	Ankle: mid sole of foot, lateral ankle Knee: medial posterior Hip: medial posterior Trunk: mid anterior slightly lateral Head: meridian terminates at tip of tongue	Ankle plantarflexion, eversion Knee extension Hip flexion, abduction Spinal extension Tongue lengthening	Direct pressure in pascimottanasana Activation in salabhasana Stimulation with all tongue stretching mudras
Bladder meridian (BL): Janu sirsasana with jalandhara bandha Halasana Pascimottanasana	Toes: lateral little toe Ankle: lateral heel Knee: posterior Hip: posterior Trunk: posterior slightly lateral Neck: posterior slightly lateral to crown of head	Toe flexion Ankle dorsiflexion Knee extension Hip flexion Spinal flexion and lateral flexion Neck extension with head flexion and lateral flexion of head and neck	Direct pressure in pascimottanasana Activation in salabhasana
Gall bladder meridian (GB): Parsva urdhva hastasana Merudanda vakrasana Ardha matyendrasana	Toes: lateral fourth toe Ankle: lateral Knee: lateral Hip: lateral Trunk: lateral Neck: posterior lateral to lateral crown of head	Toe flexion Ankle plantarflexion Knee extension or flexion Hip adduction Spinal lateral flexion Neck extension with head flexion and lateral flexion of head and neck	Direct pressure in all lateral supine postures such as anastasana Closed chain activation in the weight bearing limb on all one legged postures such as niralamba padangusthasana
Governing or Du Vessel (DU): Halasana Pascimottanasana	Trunk: tailbone to first thoracic vertebrae Neck: posterior along the spine to crown of head	Trunk flexion Neck extension with head flexion	Direct pressure, stretch and choice to activate in halasana and supta urdhva mukha pascimottanasana Activation in salabhasana and mayurasana
Conception or Ren Vessel (REN): Bhugangasana Urdhva dhanurasana	Trunk: pubis to the sternum in the midline Neck: anterior along the neck, anterior face to crown of head	Trunk extension Neck flexion and head extension	Direct pressure, stretch and choice to activate in salabhasa and viparita salabhasa Activation in ardha navasana

Following is a list of some of the literature we have used in developing this course, and of the research articles that have been referred to.

1. Aagaard, P., Simonsen, E.B., Andersen, J.L., Magnusson, S.P., Bojsen, Miller, F., Dyhre Poulsen, P. (2000). Antagonist muscle co-activation during isokinetic knee extension. Scandinavian Journal of Medical Science & Sports. 04, 10: 2, 58-67.

2. Ada, L. & Canning, C. (Eds.) (1990). Key Issues in Neurological Physiotherapy, London: Butterworth Heinemann.

3. Aftanas LI, Golocheikine SA, (2001). Human anterior and frontal midline theta and lower alpha reflect emotionally positive state and internalized attention: high-resolution EEG investigation of meditation., Neuroscience letters 310: 1, 57-60

4. Aganoff JA, Boyle GJ (1994), Aerobic exercise, mood states and menstrual cycle symptoms, Journal of psychosomatic research 38: 3, 183-92.

5. Alexander CN, Langer EJ, Newman RI, Chandler HM, Davies JL, (1989). Transcendental meditation, mindfulness, and longevity: an experimental study with the elderly., Journal of Personality and Social Psychology 57: 6, 950-64

6. Allred, C.D., Allred, K.F., Helferich, W.G. (2001). Soy diets containing varying amounts of genistein stimulate growth of estrogen-dependent (MCF-7) tumors in a dose-dependent manner., Cancer Research.61: 13, 5045-50.

7. Alter, M.J. (1996). Science of Flexibility. Human Kinetics. South Australia.

8. Arambula P, Peper E, Kawakami M, Gibney KH, (2001). The physiological correlates of Kundalini Yoga meditation: a study of a yoga master., Applied psychophysiology and biofeedback 26: 2, 147-53

9. Ascenzi P, Bocedi A, Gradoni L, (2003). The anti-parasitic effects of nitric oxide., IUBMB Life 55: 10-11, 573-8.

10. Astin JA, (1997). Stress reduction through mindfulness meditation. Effects on psychological symptomatology, sense of control, and spiritual experiences., Psychotherapy and Psychosomatics 66: 2, 97-106

11. Astrand, P., Rodahl, K. (1986). Textbook of Work Physiology. McGraw Hill, New York.

12. Atanassova, N., McKinnell, C., Turner, K.J., Walker, M., Fisher, J.S., Morley, M., Millar, M.R., Groome, N.P., Sharpe, R.M. (2000). Comparative effects of neonatal exposure of male rats to potent and weak (environmental) estrogens on spermatogenesis at puberty and the relationship to adult testis size and fertility: evidence for stimulatory effects of low oestrogen levels. Endocrinology Oct;141(10):3898-907.

13. Atwood, J.D. & Maltin , L. (1991). Putting eastern philosophies into western psychotherapies, American Journal of Psychotherapy, XLV, pp. 368-82

14. Backon J (1990). Forced unilateral nostril breathing: a technique that affects brain hemisphericity and autonomic activity. Brain Cognition, 12:1, 155-7.

15. Backon J, Kullok S, (1990). Why asthmatic patients should not sleep in the right lateral decubitus position., The British journal of clinical practice 44: 11, 448-9

16. Backon J, Matamoros N, Ramirez M, Sanchez RM, Ferrer J, Brown A, Ticho U, (1990). A functional vagotomy induced by unilateral forced right nostril breathing decreases intraocular pressure in open and closed angle glaucoma., The British journal of ophthalmology 74: 10, 607-9

17. Badawi K, Wallace RK, Orme-Johnson D, Rouzere AM, (1984). Electrophysiologic characteristics of respiratory suspension periods occurring during the practice of the Transcendental Meditation Program., Psychosomatic Medicine 46: 3, 267-76

18. Balasubramanian B, Pansare MS, (1991). Effect of yoga on aerobic and anaerobic power of muscles., Indian journal of physiology and pharmacology 35: 4, 281-2

19. Banquet JP, (1973). Spectral analysis of the EEG in meditation. Electroencephalography and Clinical Neurophysiology 35: 2, 143-51

20. Barbeau, H., Marchand, Pauvert, V., Meunier, S., Nicolas, G., Pierrot, Deseilligny, E. (2000). Posture-related changes in heteronymous recurrent inhibition from quadriceps to ankle muscles in humans. Experimental Brain Research, 02, 130: 3, 345-61.

21. Barnes VA, Treiber FA, Davis H, (2001). Impact of Transcendental Meditation on cardiovascular function at rest and during acute stress in adolescents with high normal blood pressure., Journal of psychosomatic research 51: 4, 597-605

22. Barnes VA, Treiber FA, Turner JR, Davis H, Strong WB, (1999). Acute effects of transcendental meditation on hemodynamic functioning in middle-aged adults., Psychosomatic medicine 61: 4, 525-31

23. Bazak I (1990) Clinical use of the Valsalva manoeuvre. Harefuah 118 (6): 323-325

24. Benca RM, Obermeyer WH, Larson CL, Yun B, Dolski I, Kleist KD, Weber SM, Davidson RJ, (1999). EEG alpha power and alpha power asymmetry in sleep and wakefulness., Psychophysiology 36: 4, 430-6

25. Benson H, Malhotra MS, Goldman RF, Jacobs GD, Hopkins PJ, (1990). Three case reports of the metabolic and electroencephalographic changes during advanced Buddhist meditation techniques., Behavioral Medicine 16: 2, 90-5, Summer,

26. Bera, T.K., Gore, M.M., Oak, J.P. (1998). Recovery from stress in two different postures and in Savasana--a yogic relaxation posture. Indian Journal of Physiology and Pharmacology, 42: 473-478.

27. Bernard, T. (1950). Hatha Yoga. Rider and Company, London.

28. Bernardi L, Passino C, Wilmerding V, Dallam GM, Parker DL, Robergs RA, Appenzeller O, (2001a). Breathing patterns and cardiovascular autonomic modulation during hypoxia induced by simulated altitude., Journal of hypertension 19: 5, 947-58

29. Bernardi L, Sleight P, Bandinelli G, Cencetti S, Fattorini L, Wdowczyc-Szulc J, Lagi A, (2001b). Effect of rosary prayer and yoga mantras on autonomic cardiovascular rhythms: comparative study., BMJ (Clinical research ed.) 323: 7327, 1446-9

30. Bhan, Dr., (1996). The relationship between Marma Points and Cakras in Yoga and Ayurveda. Unpublished manuscript, Goa India

31. Bhargava R, Gogate MG, Mascarenhas JF (1988). Autonomic responses to breath holding and its variations following pranayama. Indian Journal of Physiology and Pharmacology 32 (4): 257-264

32. Bharucha AE, Camilleri M, Ford MJ, O'Connor MK, Hanson RB, Thomforde GM (1996). Hyperventilation alters colonic motor and sensory function: effects and mechanisms in humans. Gastroenterology Aug;111(2):368-377

33. Bhole, M.V. (1977). Immediate effect of pranayama and Kapala-bhati on urinary output. Yoga Mimamsa; quarterly Journal Kaivalyadhama Yoga Research Institution, Lonavala, India, Volume XIX:1: pp38-46

34. Blimkie, C.J., Rice, S., Webber, C.E., Martin, J., Levy, D., & Gordon, C.L. (1996). Effects of resistance training on bone mineral density in adolescent females. Canadian Journal of Physiology & Pharmacology, 74: 1025-1033.

35. Bondarenko ON, Bondarenko NA, Malyshev Ilu, Manukhina EB, (2001) [Anti-stress effect of nitric oxide], Izvestiia Akademii nauk. Seriia biologicheskaia / Rossiiskaia akademiia nauk. 4, 459-66.

36. Bonde-Petersen F, Suzuki Y, Sadamoto T, (1983). Gravitational effects on human cardiovascular responses to isometric muscle contractions., Advanced Space Research 3: 9, 205-8

37. Boocock MG, Garbutt G, Linge K, Reilly T, Troup JD, (1990). Changes in stature following drop jumping and post-exercise gravity inversion., Medicine and science in sports and exercise 22: 3, 385-90

38. Borg-Olivier, S.A. & Machliss, B.E. (1995-2005). Yoga Synergy: Anatomy & Physiology Course for Yoga Teachers and Students. Yoga Synergy Pty. Ltd Sydney.

39. Borg-Olivier, S.A. & Machliss, B.E. (2003). Yoga and Meditation. In An Introduction to Complementary Medicine (Edited by T. Robson) Allen and Unwin, Australia.

40. Borg-Olivier, S.A. & Machliss, B.E. (1997). Hatha yoga stretching & muscle strengthening A Guide for Physiotherapists. The Australian Physiotherapy Association 1997 Conference for Alternative Therapies, Available at http://www.yogasynergy.com

41. Borg-Olivier, S.A. & Machliss, B.E. (1998). Integrating yoga & physiotherapy. Proceedings of the Australian Physiotherapy Association 1998 on 'Physiotherapy: Balancing the Art with the Science Sydney Australia.

42. Braden et al. (1967).The oestrogenic activity and metabolism of certain isoflavones in sheep. Australian Journal of Agricultural Research 18:335-348

43. Brown D, Forte M, Dysart M, (1984). Visual sensitivity and mindfulness meditation. Perceptual and Motor Skills 58: 3, 775-84

44. Bullen BA, Skrinar GS, Beitins IZ, von Mering G, Turnbull BA, McArthur JW (1985) Induction of menstrual disorders by strenuous exercise in untrained women, The New England Journal of Medicine 312: 21, 1349-53.

45. Bushinsky, D.A., Gavrilov, K., Chabala, J.M., Featherstone, J.D., Levi Setti, R. (1997). Effect of metabolic acidosis on the potassium content of bone. Journal of Bone Mineral Research. Oct, 12:10, 1664-71.

46. Butler, D. (1991). Mobilisation of the Nervous System. Churchill Livingstone

47. Cantero JL, Atienza M, Salas RM, Gomez C, (1999). Alpha power modulation during periods with rapid oculomotor activity in human REM sleep., Neuroreport 10: 9, 1817-20

48. Capano G, Guandalini S, Guarino A, Caprioli A, Falbo V, Giraldi V, Ruggeri FM, Vairano P, Vegnente A, Vairo U (1984). Enteric infections, cow's milk intolerance and parenteral infections in 118 consecutive cases of acute diarrhoea in children. European Journal of Pediatrics 142: 4, 281-5.

49. Carr, J.H. & Shepherd, R.B. (1987). A Motor Relearning Programme for Stroke. (2nd Ed.). Oxford: Butterworth-Heinemann.

50. Cassidy, A, Bingham, S, and Setchell, KDR. (1994). Biological effects of soy protein rich in isoflavones on the menstrual cycle of premenopausal women. Am. J. Clin. Nutr. 60, 333-340,.

51. Chohan IS, Nayar HS, Thomas P, Geetha NS, (1984). Influence of yoga on blood coagulation., Thrombosis and Haemostasis 51: 2, 196-7

52. Cholewicki J, Juluru K, McGill SM, (1999). Intra-abdominal pressure mechanism for stabilizing the lumbar spine. 1, 13-7

53. Cholewicki J, Panjabi MM, Khachatryan A, (1997). Stabilizing function of trunk flexor-extensor muscles around a neutral spine posture. 19, 2207-12

54. Chorazy, P.A., Himelhoch, S., Hopwood, N,J., Greger, N.G., and Postellon, D.C. (1995). Persistent hypothyroidism in an infant receiving a soy formula: Case report and review of the literature. Pediatrics 148–150.

55. Clark, H.R. (1999). The Cure for all Advanced Cancers. New Century Press. USA

56. Clark WL, Trumble TE, Swiontkowski MF, Tencer AF (1992) Nerve tension and blood flow in a rat model of immediate and delayed repairs, The Journal of hand surgery 17: 4, 677-87.

57. Cohen, R (2001). The Not Milkman. http://www.notmilk.com

58. Coker, K.H. (1999). Meditation and prostate cancer: integrating a mind/body intervention with traditional therapies. Seminars on Urology & Oncology. May, 17:2, 111-8.

59. Cook, N.E., Rogers, Q.R., Morris, J.G. (1996). Acid-base balance affects dietary choice in cats. Appetite, Apr, 26:2, 175-92.

60. Corby JC, Roth WT, Zarcone VP Jr, Kopell BS, (1978). Psychophysiological correlates of the practice of Tantric Yoga meditation., Archives of General Psychiatry 35: 5, 571-7

61. Cordain, L. (1999). Cereal grains: humanity's double-edged sword. World Review of Nutrition and Dietetics, vol. 84, pp. 19-73.

62. Corliss, R. (2001). The power of Yoga. Time Magazine, April 23 pp44-53

63. Corrigan GE (1969). Fatal air embolism after Yoga breathing exercises JAMA 210 (10): 1923

64. Craven, J.L. (1989). Meditation and psychotherapy, Canadian Journal of Psychiatry, 34, pp. 648-653

65. Crosbie, J. & McConnell, J. (Eds.) (1993). Issues in Musculoskeletal Physiotherapy, London: Butterworth Heinemann.

66. Cumming RG, Klineberg RJ (1994) Case-Control Study of Risk Factors for Hip Fractures in the Elderly, American Journal of Epidemiology, 139: 493-505.

67. Dalton CB, Austin CC, Sobel J, Hayes PS, Bibb WF, Graves LM, Swaminathan B, Proctor ME, Griffin PM (1997). An outbreak of gastroenteritis and fever due to Listeria monocytogenes in milk. New England Journal of Medicine 336: 2, 100-5.

68. Dash M, Telles S, (2001). Improvement in hand grip strength in normal volunteers and rheumatoid arthritis patients following yoga training., Indian journal of physiology and pharmacology 45: 3, 355-60

69. Davies, DF Rees, BW Davies, PT (1980). Cow's milk antibodies and coronary heart disease., Lancet. 1: 8179, 1190-1..

70. De Crée C (1998) Sex steroid metabolism and menstrual irregularities in the exercising female. A review. Sports Medicine, 25:6, 369-406.

71. Delmonte MM, (1989). Meditation, the unconscious, and psychosomatic disorders., International Journal of Psychosomatics 36: 1-4, 45-52

72. Dembner, A. (2003). 'Om…Om…oh my aching back'. Increases in the number of yoga-related injuries. Reprinted from the Boston Globe in the Sydney Morning Herald, January 14, 2003 page 8. Sydney

73. Desai BP, Gharote ML (1990) Effect of Kapalabhati on blood urea, creatinine and tyrosine. Activitas nervosa superior (Praha) 32 (2): 95-98

74. Desikachar, T.K.V. (1995). The Heart of Yoga. Inner Traditions International.

75. Desikachar, T.K.V. (1998). Health Healing and Beyond. Krishnamacharya Yoga Mandiram.

76. Desikachar, T.K.V. (2000). Yoga-yajnavalkya Samhita. Krishnamacharya Yoga Mandiram.

77. Dettori JR, Bullock SH, Sutlive TG, Franklin RJ, Patience T, (1995). The effects of spinal flexion and extension exercises and their associated postures in patients with acute low back pain., Spine 20: 21, 2303-12

78. Devananda, V. (1987). Hatha Yoga Pradipika of Swatmarama: The Classic Guide for the Advanced Practice of Hatha Yoga, with 1897 commentary of Brahmananda, and 1987 commentary of Devandana. OM Lotus Publishing Company, New York.

79. Devi, I. (1953). Forever Young, Forever Healthy, Prentice Hall, Inc.

80. Dillbeck M.C. & Orme-Johnson, D.W (1987). Psychological differences between transcendental meditation and rest, American Psychology, 42, PP. 879-81

81. Dillbeck MC, (1977). The effect of the Transcendental Meditation technique on anxiety level., Journal of Clinical Psychology 33: 4, 1076-8

82. Dillbeck MC, Vesely SA, (1986). Participation in the transcendental meditation program and frontal EEG coherence during concept learning., International Journal of Neuroscience 29: 1-2, 45-55

83. Dillbeck, M.C., Bronson, E.C. (1981).Short-term longitudinal effects of the transcendental meditation technique on EEG power and coherence., International Journal of Neuroscience 14: 3-4, 147-51

84. Dua, J.K & Swinden, M.L (1992). Effectiveness of negative-thoughts-reduction, meditation and placebo training treatment in reducing anger, Scandinavian Journal of Psychology, 33(2), pp. 135-46

85. DuBose, T.D. (1982) Acid-base physiology in uraemia. Artificial Organs, 6:4, 363-9.

86. Dunn BR, Hartigan JA, Mikulas WL, (1999). Concentration and mindfulness meditations: unique forms of consciousness?, Applied psychophysiology and biofeedback 24: 3, 147-65

87. Dwyer J, Foulkes E, Evans M, Ausman L (1985). Acid/alkaline ash diets: time for assessment and change. Journal of the American Dietary Association. 85 (7): 841-845.

88. Ekstrom RA, Holden K (2002) Examination of and intervention for a patient with chronic lateral elbow pain with signs of nerve entrapment, Physical Therapy 82: 11, 1077-86.

89. Elias A.N. & Wilson A.F. (1995). Serum hormonal concentrations following transcendental meditation: potential role of gamma aminobutyric acid, Med. Hypotheses, 44, pp. 287-291

90. Elias AN, Guich S, Wilson AF, (2000). Ketosis with enhanced GABAergic tone promotes physiological changes in transcendental meditation., Medical Hypotheses 54: 4, 660-2

91. Ellis, E. & Alison, J. (Eds.) (1992) Key Issues in Cardiopulmonary Physiotherapy, London: Butterworth Heinemann.

92. Eppley KR, Abrams AI, Shear J, (1989). Differential effects of relaxation techniques on trait anxiety: a meta-analysis., Journal of clinical psychology 45: 6, 957-74.

93. Fairey AS, Courneya KS, Field CJ, Mackey JR, (2002). Physical exercise and immune system function in cancer survivors: a comprehensive review and future directions., Cancer 94: 2, 539-51

94. Farrow JT, Hebert JR, (1982). Breath suspension during the transcendental meditation technique., Psychosomatic Medicine 44: 2, 133-53

95. Feskanich D, Willet, W.C, Stampfer, M.J, et al (1997)Milk, Dietary Calcium, and Bone Fractures in Women: A 12-Year Prospective Study. American Journal of Public Health, 992-997.

96. Feuerstein, G. (1996) The Shambala Guide to Yoga. Shambala Publications: Boston.

97. Fink JB, (2002). Positioning versus postural drainage., Respiratory care 47: 7, 769-77

98. Foley, B. & Gregg, G.W. (1997) BodyWorks 6.0: Medical Library: A 3D Journey Through The Human Anatomy. Interactive CD ROM, Mythos Software Inc, Utah

99. Fong KY, Cheung RT, Yu YL, Lai CW, Chang CM (1993) Basilar artery occlusion following yoga exercise: a case report. Clin Exp Neurol 30: 104-109

100. Fort P, Moses N, Fasano M, Goldberg T, Lifshitz F. (1990). Breast and soy-formula feedings in early infancy and the prevalence of autoimmune thyroid disease in children. Journal of the American College of Nutrition Apr;9(2):164-7

101. Fukutake M, Takahashi M, Ishida K, Kawamura H, Sugimura T, Wakabayashi K, (1996). Quantification of genistein and genistin in soybeans and soybean products. Food & Chemical Toxicology, 34: 5, 457-61.

102. Gallois P, (1984). [Neurophysiologic and respiratory changes during the practice of relaxation technics], (Modifications neurophysiologiques et respiratoires lors de la pratique des techniques de relaxation.), L'Encephale. 10: 3, 139-44

103. Gardner AW, Katzel LI, Sorkin JD, Bradham DD, Hochberg MC, Flinn WR, Goldberg AP, (2001). Exercise rehabilitation improves functional outcomes and peripheral circulation in patients with intermittent claudication: a randomized controlled trial., Journal of the American Geriatrics Society 49: 6, 755-62

104. Garfinkel MS, Schumacher HR Jr, Husain A, Levy M, Reshetar RA, (1994). Evaluation of a yoga based regimen for treatment of osteoarthritis of the hands., The Journal of Rheumatology 21: 12, 2341-3

105. Garfinkel, M.S., Singhal, A., Katz, W.A., Allan, D.A., Reshetar, R., Schumacher, H.R. (1998). Yoga-based intervention for carpal tunnel syndrome: a randomized trial. Journal of the American Medical Association. 280: 18, 1601-1603.

106. Gentile, A.M. (1987). Skill acquisition: action, movement, & neuromotor processes. In Carr, J.H. & Shepherd, R.B. (Eds.). Movement Science: Foundations for Physical Therapy in Rehabilitation. (pp. 93-154). Rockville, Maryland: Aspen.

107. Ghosh, S (1999). The Original Yoga: as expounded in Sivasamhita, Gherandasamhita and Patanjala Yogasutra. Munshiram Manoharlal Publishers Pvt. Ltd. New Delhi.

108. Giannini, S., Nobile, M., Sartori, L., Calò, L., Tasca, A., Dalle Carbonare, L., Ciuffreda, M., Dangelo, A., Pagano, F., Crepaldi, G. (1998). Bone density and skeletal metabolism are altered in idiopathic hypercalciuria. Clinical Nephrology, Aug, 50:2, 94-100.

109. Gillard BK, Simbala JA, Goodglick L (1983) Reference intervals for isoenzymes in serum and plasma of infants and children. Clinical Chemistry 29, 1119–1123.

110. Ginn, K. (1993, 1994). Lecture notes for Anatomy. Faculty of Health Sciences, University of Sydney

111. Gioia G, Lin B, Katz R, DiMarino AJ, Ogilby JD, Cassel D, DePace NL, Heo J, Iskandrian AS, (1995). Use of a tantalum-178 generator and a multiwire gamma camera to study the effect of the Mueller maneuver on left ventricular performance: comparison to hemodynamics and single photon emission computed tomography perfusion patterns., American heart journal 130: 5, 1062-7

112. Glasscock NF, Turville KL, Joines SB, Mirka GA, (1999). The effect of personality type on muscle coactivation during elbow flexion. 1, 51-60.

113. Goldberg, B.A., Nowinski, R.J., & Matsen, F.A. 3rd (2001). Outcome of nonoperative management of full-thickness rotator cuff tears. Clinical Orthopaedics & Related Research. 382, 99-107.

114. Goldish GD, Quast JE, Blow JJ, Kuskowski MA (1994) Postural effects on intra-abdominal pressure during Valsalva manoeuvre. Archives Phys. Med. Rehabilitation 75 (3): 324-327

115. Golikov AP, Vorob'ev VE, Abdrakhmanov VR, Stazhadze LL, Bogomolov VV, (1980). (Human external respiratory function and blood acid-base balance during prolonged antiorthostatic hypokinesia and during the recovery period], Kosm Biol Aviakosm Med 14: 1, 42-6

116. Goswami, S.S. (1980). Layayoga: An Advanced Method of Concentration. Routledge & Kegan Paul, London.

117. Goyeche, J.R., Abo, Y., & Ikemi, Y. (1982). Asthma: the yoga perspective. Part II: Yoga therapy in the treatment of asthma. Journal of Asthma, 19:189-201.

118. Greene JW (1999) Menstrual irregularities associated with athletics and exercise, Comprehensive therapy 25: 4, 209-15.

119. Gregorevic P, Lynch GS, Williams DA, (2000). Hyperbaric oxygen improves contractile function of regenerating rat skeletal muscle after myotoxic injury., Journal of Applied Physiology 89: 4, 1477-82

120. Gribble PL, Ostry DJ, (1998). Independent coactivation of shoulder and elbow muscles. 3, 355-60.

121. Griggs, S.M., Ahn, A., Green, A. (2000). Idiopathic adhesive capsulitis. A prospective functional outcome study of nonoperative treatment. Journal Of Bone And Joint Surgery. American Volume. 82-A: 10, 1398-407.

122. Grigorov, G.U., Sineok, L.L. (1982). Age-specific peculiarities of the acid base balance and the influence of various diets. ZFA, 1982 Jul, 37:4, 241-7.

123. Grosvenor, C. (1992). Hormones and Growth Factors in Milk Endocrine Reviews, 14:6.

124. Grundy D, Reid K, McArdle FJ, Brown BH, Barber DC, Deacon CF, Henderson IW, (1991). Trans-thoracic fluid shifts and endocrine responses to 6 degrees head-down tilt., Aviation, space, and environmental medicine 62: 10, 923-9

125. Gupta YP [1987] "Anti-nutritional and toxic factors in food legumes: a review." Plant Foods for Human Nutrition, vol. 37, pp. 201-228.

126. Guyton, A.C. (1991). A Textbook of Medical Physiology. W.B. Saunders, Co, Philadelphia. USA.

127. Haight JS, Cole P, (1986). Unilateral nasal resistance and asymmetrical body pressure., J Otolaryngol Suppl 16:, 1-31

128. Haight JS; Cole P (1989). Is the nasal cycle an artefact? The role of asymmetrical postures. Laryngoscope, May, 99:5, 538-41

129. Hale RW (1983) Exercise, sports, and menstrual dysfunction, Clinical obstetrics and gynecology 26: 3, 728-35.

130. Hallberg L (1989) Search for nutritional confounding factors in the relationship between iron deficiency and brain function. Am J Clin Nutr Sep 50:3 Suppl 598-604; discussion 604-6

131. Halpern, M. (1998). Tridosha: The Science of Ayurveda. www.ayurvedacollege.com

132. Halpern, M. (2000). Pranayama, Yoga, and Ayurveda. www.ayurvedacollege.com

133. Hancock, (2002). Underworld. Penguin Books. ,England.

134. Hänninen, O., Nenonen, M., Ling, W.H., Li, D.S., Sihvonen, L. (1992). Effects of eating an uncooked vegetable diet for 1 week. Appetite, 19:3, 243-54.

135. Hanus SH, Homer TD, Harter DH (1977). Vertebral artery occlusion complicating yoga exercises. Archives of Neurology 34 (9): 574-5

136. Hart, W. (1987). Vipassana Meditation as taught by Goenka. Harper San Francisco.

137. Harte, J.L., Eifert, G.H. & Smith, R. (1995). The effects of running and meditation on beta-endorphin, corticotrophin-releasing hormone and cortisol in plasma and on mood, Biological Psychology, 40(3), pp. 251-65

138. Helenius IJ, Tikkanen HO, Haahtela T (1997). Association between type of training and risk of asthma in elite athletes. Thorax Feb; 52(2):157-160

139. Herbert RD, Gabriel M, (2002). Effects of stretching before and after exercising on muscle soreness and risk of injury: systematic review., BMJ (Clinical research ed.)325: 7362 - 468

140. Herbert, R. (1993). Human strength adaptations - Implications for therapy. In J. Crosbie & J. McConnell (Eds.) Key Issues in Musculoskeletal Physiotherapy, London: Butterworth Heinemann (pp. 142-171).

141. Herzog H, Lele VR, Kuwert T, Langen KJ, Kops ER, Feinendegen LE, (1990). Changed pattern of regional glucose metabolism during yoga meditative relaxation., Neuropsychobiology 23: 4, 182-7, -91

142. Herzog W, Binding P, (1993). Cocontraction of pairs of antagonistic muscles: analytical solution for planar static nonlinear optimization approaches. 118: 1, 83-95

143. Hewitt J. (1983).The yoga of breathing posture and meditation. London: Random House, 89-91

144. Hightower M (1997) Effects of exercise participation on menstrual pain and symptoms, Women and Health 26: 4, 15-27.

145. Hillman DR, Finucane KE, (1987). A model of the respiratory pump., Journal of Applied Physiology 63: 3, 951-61

146. Hollingsworth, E. (2000). Take control of your health & escape the sickness industry. Empowerment Press International.

147. Horne, R. (1985). The Health Revolution. Happy landings Publishers.

148. Hsieh CY, Santell RC, Haslam SZ, Helferich WG. (1998) Estrogenic effects of genistein on the growth of estrogen receptor-positive human breast cancer (MCF-7) cells in vitro and in vivo. Cancer Res Sep 1 58:17 3833-8.

149. Hubley-Kozey, C. & Earl, E.M. (2000). Co-activation of the ankle musculature during maximal isokinetic dorsiflexion at different angular velocities. European Journal of Applied Physiology. 82: 289-96.

150. Hudetz JA, Hudetz AG, Klayman J, (2000). Relationship between relaxation by guided imagery and performance of working memory., Psychological reports 86: 1, 15-20

151. Hughes LO, Heber ME, Lahiri A, Harries M, Raftery EB (1989) Haemodynamic advantage of the Valsalva manoeuvre during heavy resistance training. European Heart Journal 10 (10): 896-902

152. Il'in VM, (1999). (The circulatory changes as dependent on the type of autonomic homeostasis in divers in dives to a depth of 65 m), Fiziolohichhnyi Zhurnal 45: 5, 38-48

153. Irvine, CHG, Fitzpatrick, MG, and Alexander, SL. (1998). Phytoestrogens in soy-based infant foods: Concentrations, daily intake, and possible biological effects. Proc. Soc. Exp. Biol. Med. 217, 247-253,.

154. Ishizuki, Y., Hirooka, Y., Murata, Y., and Togasho, K (1991). The effects on the thyroid gland of soybeans administered experimentally to healthy subjects. Nippon Naibunpi gakkai Zasshi 67, 622-629,. Kimura, S, Suwa, J, Ito, B and Sato, H. (1976). Development of malignant goiter by defatted soybean with iodine-free diet in rats. Gann 67, 763-765.

155. Iyengar, B.K.S. (1966). Light on Yoga. Schocken Books, New York.

156. Iyengar, B.K.S. (1988). The Tree of Yoga. Fine Line Books, Oxford.

157. Iyengar, B.K.S. (1990). Interview of Guruji by Teenagers. In 70 Glorious Years of Yogacharya B.K.S. Iyengar (Commemoration Volume). Light on Yoga Research Trust, pp 48-61

158. Iyengar, B.K.S. (1993). Light on the Yoga Sutras of Patanjali. Aquarian Press, London.

159. Iyengar, B.K.S. (2001). Yoga: the Path to Holistic Health. Dorling Kindersley Limited, London.

160. Iyengar, G.S. (1983). Yoga a Gem for Women. Allied Publishers.

161. Jain S.C., & Talukdar B. (1993). Evaluation of yoga therapy programme for patients of bronchial asthma. Singapore Medical Journal, 34:306-308.

162. Jain, S.C., Rai, L., Valecha, A., Jha, U.K., Bhatnagar, S.O., & Ram, K. (1991). Effect of yoga training on exercise tolerance in adolescents with childhood asthma. Journal of Asthma, 28:437-442.

163. Janse de Jonge XA (2003) Effects of the menstrual cycle on exercise performance, Sports Medicine 33: 11, 833-51.

164. Jella SA, Shannahoff-Khalsa DS, (1993). The effects of unilateral forced nostril breathing on cognitive performance The International journal of neuroscience 73: 1-2, 61-8

165. Jenson, B (1981). Tissue cleansing through bowel management. Published by Bernard Jenson, California.

166. Jevning R, Anand R, Biedebach M, (1996). Fernando G, Effects on regional cerebral blood flow of transcendental meditation., Physiology and Behavior 59: 3, 399-402.

167. Jevning R, Wallace RK, Beidebach M, (1992). The physiology of meditation: a review. A wakeful hypometabolic integrated response, Neuroscience and Biobehavioral Reviews 16: 3, 415-24

168. Jin P, (1992). Efficacy of Tai Chi, brisk walking, meditation, and reading in reducing mental and emotional stress., Journal Of Psychosomatic Research 36: 4, 361-70

169. Jong Weon Choi, Moon Whan Im and Soo Hwan Pai (2002) Nitric oxide Production Increases during Normal Pregnancy and Decreases in Preeclampsia Annals of Clinical and Laboratory Science 32:257-263

170. Joshi, K.S. (1981). Effect of kapala-bhati on retention of breath. Yoga Mimamsa; quarterly Journal Kaivalyadhama Yoga Research Institution, Lonavala, India, Volume XX:1-2: pp29-35

171. Junker, A., Dworkis, S. (1986). Investigation of brain wave activity during yoga postures and meditation. Dayton, Ohio: Results of a research project at Wright Patterson Air Force Base also incorporated into Andrew Junker's PhD thesis. For more information, see http://www.extensi-

onyoga.com/7Principles.htm

172. Kalkman CJ, Boezeman EH, Ribberink AA, Oosting J, Deen L, Bovill JG, (1991). Influence of changes in arterial carbon dioxide tension on the electroencephalogram and posterior tibial nerve somatosensory cortical evoked potentials during alfentanil/nitrous oxide anesthesia., Anesthesiology 75: 1, 68-74

173. Kamei T, Toriumi Y, Kimura H, Ohno S, Kumano H, Kimura K, (2000). Decrease in serum cortisol during yoga exercise is correlated with alpha wave activation., Perceptual and motor skills 90: 3 Pt 1, 1027-32

174. Kannus, P., Alosa, D., Cook, L., Johnson, R.J., Renstrom, P., Pope, M., Beynnon, B., Yasuda, K., Nichols, C., & Kaplan, M. (1992) Effect of one-legged exercise on the strength, power & endurance of the contralateral leg. A randomized, controlled study using isometric & concentric isokinetic training. European Journal of Applied Physiology. 64: 117-126.

175. Kapit, W. & Elson, L.M. (1993) The Anatomy Coloring Book. (2nd Ed.) by New York: Harper Collins (ACB).

176. Karambelkar, P.V., Deshpande, R.R., Bhole, M.V. (1982). Oxygen consumption during Ujjayi pranayama. Yoga Mimamsa, Volume XXI: 3 & 4.

177. Katkov VE, Chestukhin VV, Lapteva RI, Yakovleva VA, Mikhailov VM, Zybin OK, Utkin VN, (1979). Central and cerebral hemodynamics and metabolism of the healthy man during head-down tilting., Aviation, space, and environmental medicine 50: 2, 147-53

178. Kesterson J, Clinch NF, (1989). Metabolic rate, respiratory exchange ratio, and apneas during meditation., American Journal of Physiology 256: 3 Pt 2, R632-8

179. Key, T.J., Roe, L., Thorogood, M., Moore, J.W., Clark, G.M., Wang, D.Y. (1990) Testosterone, sex hormone-binding globulin, calculated free testosterone, and oestradiol in male vegans and omnivores. British Journal of Nutrition 64 (1): 111-119.

180. Kjeldsen-Kragh, J., Haugen, M., Borchgrevink, C.F., Laerum, E., Eek, M., Mowinkel, P., Hovi, K., Forre, O. (1991) Controlled trial of fasting and one-year vegetarian diet in rheumatoid arthritis. Lancet 338 (8772): 899-902.

181. Klimesch W, Doppelmayr M, Schimke H, Ripper B, (1997). Theta synchronization and alpha desynchronization in a memory task., Psychophysiology 34: 2, 169-76

182. Klimesch W, Doppelmayr M, Schwaiger J, Auinger P, Winkler T, (1999). ,Paradoxical' alpha synchronization in a memory task., Brain research. Cognitive brain research 7: 4, 493-501

183. Klimesch W, Schimke H, Pfurtscheller G, (1993). Alpha frequency, cognitive load and memory performance., Brain topography 5: 3, 241-51

184. Klimesch, W. (1999). EEG alpha and theta oscillations reflect cognitive and memory performance: a review and analysis. Brain research reviews 29: 2-3, 169-95

185. Knitelius H, Stegemann J, (1987). Heart volume during short-term head-down tilt (-6 degrees) in comparison with horizontal body position., Aviation, space, and environmental medicine 58: 9 Pt 2, A61-3

186. Kocher, H.C. (1976). Effects of savasana on the extent of knee-jerk. Yoga Mimamsa; quarterly Journal Kaivalyadhama Yoga Research Institution, Lonavala, India, Volume XVIII:3-4: pp40-47

187. Kominars KD, (1997). A study of visualization and addiction treatment., Journal of substance abuse treatment 14: 3, 213-23

188. Kroner-Herwig B, Hebing G, van Rijn-Kalkmann U, Frenzel A, Schilkowsky G, Esser G, (1995). The management of chronic tinnitus--comparison of a cognitive-behavioural group training with yoga., Journal of psychosomatic research 39: 2, 153-65

189. Kubota Y, Sato W, Toichi M, Murai T, Okada T, Hayashi A, Sengoku A, (2001). Frontal midline theta rhythm is correlated with cardiac autonomic activities during the performance of an attention demanding meditation procedure., Brain research. Cognitive brain research 11: 2, 281-7

190. Kutz, I., Borysenko, J.K. & Benson, H. (1985a). Meditation and psychotherapy: a rationale for the integration of dynamic psychotherapy, the relaxation response and mindfulness meditation, American Journal of Psychiatry, 142, pp. 1-8.

191. Kutz, I., Leserman, J., Dorrington, C., Morrison, C.H., Borysenko, J. & Benson, H. (1985b). Meditation as an adjunct to psychotherapy, an outcome study, Psychotherapy Psychosomatics, 43, pp. 209-18

192. Kuvalayananda, S. (1924). Barometric experiments on nauli: 'Madhavdas vacuum'. Yoga Mimamsa; quarterly Journal Kaivalyadhama Yoga Research Institution, Lonavala, India, Volume I:1-2: pp27-100

193. Kuvalayananda, S. (1925). X ray experiments on uddiyana and nauli in relation to the colon contents. Yoga Mimamsa; quarterly Journal Kaivalyadhama Yoga Research Institution, Lonavala, India, Volume I:1-4: pp15-254

194. Kuvalayananda, S. (1928). Experiments on intra-gastric pressures. Yoga Mimamsa; quarterly Journal Kaivalyadhama Yoga Research Institution, Lonavala, India, Volume III:1: pp10-17

195. Kuvalayananda, S. (1957). Comparative study of radiographic and manometric experiments on uddiyana and nauli. Yoga Mimamsa; quarterly Journal Kaivalyadhama Yoga Research Institution, Lonavala, India, Volume VI:4 287-94

196. Kuvalayananda, S. (1982). Comparison between uddiyana bandha and uddiyanaka with Mueller's and Valsalva maneuvers respectively. Yoga Mimamsa; quarterly Journal Kaivalyadhama Yoga Research Institution, Lonavala, India, Volume XXI:1-2: pp35-46

197. La Perriere, A., Ironson, G., Antoni, M.H., Schneiderman, N., Klimas, N., & Fletcher, M.A. (1994) Exercise & psychoneuroimmunology. Medicine & Science in Sports & Exercise. 26: 182-190.

198. Laffey, J G Kavanagh B P (1999). Carbon dioxide and the critically ill--too little of a good thing? Lancet; 354: 1283-86

199. Lazar SW, Bush G, Gollub RL, Fricchione GL, Khalsa G, Benson H, (2000). Functional brain mapping of the relaxation response and meditation. Neuroreport 11: 7, 1581-5

200. Lee, M. (1993). Dynamics of the Human Body (3rd Ed.). Sydney: Zygal.

201. Lele, A., Ranade, S., & Frawley, D. (1999). Secrets of Marma. International Academy of Ayurveda. Pune, India. Website: www.ayurved-int.com

202. Leopold AS. (1976). Phytoestrogens: Adverse effects on reproduction in California Quail. Science 191: 98-100

203. Lepicovska V, Dostalek C, Kovarova M, 1990. Hathayogic exercise jalandharabandha in its effect on cardiovascular response to apnoea., Activitas nervosa superior (Praha) 32: 2, 99-114

204. Lewis, N.M., Marcus, M.S., Behling, A.R.; Greger, J.L. (1989). Calcium supplements and milk: effects on acid-base balance and on retention of calcium, magnesium, and phosphorus American Journal of Clinical Nutrition Mar, 49:3, 527-33.

205. Liener IE [1994] "Implications of anti-nutritional components in soybean foods." Crit Rev Food Sci Nutr., vol. 34, pp. 31-67.

206. Lindahl, O., Lindwall, L., Spangberg, A., Stenram, A., Ockerman, P.A. (1984) A vegan regimen with reduced medication in the treatment of hypertension. British Journal of Nutrition 52 (1): 11-20.

207. Liu GL, Cui RQ, Li GZ, Huang CM, (1990). Changes in brainstem and cortical auditory potentials during Qi-Gong meditation., The American Journal of Chinese Medicine 18: 3-4, 95-103

208. Liu, D. (1991). Taoist Health Exercise Book. Paragon House New York.

209. Lowe G, Bland R, Greenman J, Kirkpatrick N, Lowe G, (2001). Progressive muscle relaxation and secretory immunoglobulin A., Psychological reports 88: 3 Pt 1, 912-4

210. Lunven, P. [1990] 'Roots, tubers, plantains and bananas in human nutrition' FOOD AND AGRICULTURE ORGANIZATION OF THE UNITED NATIONS Rome http://www.fao.org/inpho/vlibrary/t0207e/T0207E00.htm

211. MacDougall JD, McKelvie RS, Moroz DE, Sale DG, McCartney N, Buick F, (1992). Factors affecting blood pressure during heavy weight lifting

and static contractions., Journal of applied physiology 73: 4, 1590-7

212. Mackinnon SE, Novak CB (2002) Thoracic Outlet Syndrome. Current Problems in Surgery; 39:1070-145.

213. MacLean CR, Walton KG, Wenneberg SR, Levitsky DK, Mandarino JP, Waziri R, Hillis SL, Schneider RH, (1997). Effects of the Transcendental Meditation program on adaptive mechanisms: changes in hormone levels and responses to stress after 4 months of practice., Psychoneuro-endocrinology 22: 4, 277-95

214. Madanmohan, Thombre DP, Balakumar B, Nambinarayanan TK, Thakur S, Krishnamurthy N, Chandrabose A (1992) A Effect of yoga training on reaction time, respiratory endurance and muscle strength Indian Journal of Physiology and Pharmacology 36(4):229-33

215. Maestroni GJ, (2001). The immunotherapeutic potential of melatonin. Expert Opinion On Investigational Drugs 10: 3, 467-76

216. Magee, D.J. (1992). Orthopaedic Physical Assessment (2nd Ed.). USA: W.B. Saunders Company.

217. Maheshwarananda, PS (2004) The hidden power in humans: chakras and kundalini. European University Press. Vienna, Austria.

218. Maier, S.F., Watkins, L.R., & Fleshner, M. (1994). Psychoneuroimmunology. The interface between behaviour, brain, & immunity. American Psychologist. 49: 1004-1017.

219. Maier, S.F., Watkins, L.R., & Fleshner, M. (1994). Psychoneuroimmunology. The interface between behaviour, brain, & immunity. American Psychologist. 49: 1004-17

220. Malathi A, Damodaran A, (1999). Stress due to exams in medical students--role of yoga., Indian journal of physiology and pharmacology 43: 2, 218-24

221. Manchanda SC, Narang R, Reddy KS, Sachdeva U, Prabhakaran D, Dharmanand S, Rajani M, Bijlani R, (2000). Retardation of coronary atherosclerosis with yoga lifestyle intervention., The Journal of the Association of Physicians of India 48: 7, 687-94

222. Manjunath NK, Telles S, (2001). Improved performance in the Tower of London test following yoga., Indian journal of physiology and pharmacology 45: 3, 351-4

223. Marks B, Mitchell DG, Simelaro JP (1997) Breath-holding in healthy and pulmonary-comprised populations: effects of hyperventilation and oxygen inspiration.Journal of Magnetic Resonance Imaging May;7(3):595-97

224. Marsh, A.G., Sanchez, T.V., Michelsen, O., Chaffee, F.L., Fagal, S.M. (1988). Vegetarian lifestyle and bone mineral density. American Journal of Clinical Nutrition. 48:3 Supplement, 837-41.

225. Martin, P. (2003). Milk: Is The White Stuff The Right Stuff? London Times. Available at http://www.vnv.org.au/Milk.htm

226. Masion, A.O., Teas, J., Herbert, J.R., Werheimer, M.D. & Kabat-Zinn, J. (1995). Meditation, melatonin and breast/prostate cancer: hypothesis and preliminary data, Medical Hypotheses, 44, pp. 39-46

227. McArdle , W.D., Katch, F.L., Katch, V.L. (1991). Exercise Physiology: Energy, Nutrition & Human Performance, (3rd Ed). Lea and Febiger, Philadelphia.

228. McCarty, M.F. (1999) Vegan proteins may reduce risk of cancer, obesity, and cardiovascular disease by promoting increased glucagon activity. Medical Hypotheses, Dec, 53:6, 459-85.

229. McMichael-Phillips DF, Harding C, Morton M, Roberts SA, Howell A, Potten CS, Bundred NJ (1998). Effects of soy-protein supplementation on epithelial proliferation in the histologically normal human breast. Am J Clin Nutr Dec 68:6 Suppl 1431S-1435S

230. Mehta, S., Mehta, M. & Mehta, S. (1990). Yoga The Iyengar Way. Simon & Schuster: Australia.

231. Merzon AK, Zeligman VS, (1978) [Change in human kidney activity in passive orthostatism and head-down tilting], Kosm. Biol. Aviakosm. Med. 12: 6, 25-8

232. Metcalfe, A. (1996). Stretch Your Mind & Body with Yoga. A Manual for Yoga Teachers published by Amoona Metcalfe, Australia, tel: 61 2 9524 9481.

233. Metzger BL, Therrien B, (1990). Effect of position on cardiovascular response during the Valsalva maneuver. Nursing Research. 39: 4, 198-202

234. Miksicek, RJ. (1995). Estrogenic flavonoids: Structural requirements for biological activity. Proc. Soc. Exp. Biol. Med. 208, 44-50,

235. Miyamura M, Nishimura K, Ishida K, Katayama K, Shimaoka M, Hiruta S, (2002). Is man able to breathe once a minute for an hour?: the effect of yoga respiration on blood gases., Japanese journal of physiology 52: 3, 313-6

236. Moffett, D., Moffett, S., Stauf, C. (1993). Human Physiology: Foundations and Frontiers. Mosby, Missouri.

237. Mohamed AI, Ponnamperuma AJP, Hafez YS 1986 New Chromophore for Phytic Acid Determination. Cereal Chem 63:6 475-8

238. Mohan SM, (1991). Reversal of nostril dominance by posture., Journal of the Indian Medical Association 89: 4, 88-91

239. Mohan SM, (1996). Svara (nostril dominance) and bilateral volar GSR Indian journal of physiology and pharmacology 40: 1, 58-64

240. Mohan SM; Eccles R (1989). Effect of inspiratory and expiratory airflow on congestion and decongestion in the nasal cycle. Indian Journal Physiology Pharmacology, Jul, 33:3, 191-3.

241. Mohan, A.G. (2000). Yoga-yajnavalkya. Ganesh & Co Madras.

242. Monteiro Pedro, V., Vitti, M., Bérzin, F., Bevilaqua Grosso, D. (1999). The effect of free isotonic and maximal isometric contraction exercises of the hip adduction on vastus medialis oblique muscle: an electromyographic study. Electromyographic Clinical Neurophysiology 39:7, 435-40.

243. Moore, K.L., (1992). Clinically Oriented Anatomy. Wiliams & Wilkins.

244. Moorthy, A.M. (1982). Effect of selected yoga asanas and physical exercises on flexibility. Yoga Review. Vol. II:3: pp161-66

245. Motoyama H. (1993). 'A study of Yoga from Eastern a& Western Medical Viewpoints – Control of Body & Mind through the Activation of Prana (Ki)'. Human Science Press, Japan.

246. Nagarathna, R., & Nagendra, H.R (1985). Yoga for bronchial asthma: a controlled study. British Medical Journal, 291:1077-1079.

247. Nagata C, Takatsuka N, Kurisu Y, Shimizu H, (1998). Decreased serum total cholesterol concentration is associated with high intake of soy products in Japanese men and women. Journal of Nutrition128: 2, 209-13,

248. Nagendra, H.R., & Nagarathna, R. (1986). An integrated approach of yoga therapy for bronchial asthma: a 3-54-month prospective study. Journal of Asthma, 23:123-137.

249. Nagendra, H.R., & Nagarathna, R. (1986). An integrated approach of yoga therapy for bronchial asthma: a 3-54-month prospective study. Journal of Asthma, 23:123-37.

250. Narayan R, Kamat A, Khanolkar M, Kamat S, Desai SR, Dhume RA (1990). Quantitative evaluation of muscle relaxation induced by kundalini yoga with the help of E.M.G. integrator, Indian Journal Physiological Pharmacology, 34(4), pp. 279-81

251. Narloch JA, Brandstater ME, (1995). Influence of breathing technique on arterial blood pressure during heavy weight lifting., Archives of physical medicine and rehabilitation 76: 5, 457-62

252. Naveen KV, Nagarathna R, Nagendra HR, Telles S, (1997). Yoga breathing through a particular nostril increases spatial memory scores without lateralized effects., Psychological reports 81: 2, 555-61

253. New, S.A., Bolton Smith, C., Grubb, D.A., Reid, D.M. (1997). Nutritional influences on bone mineral density: a cross-Sectional study in pre-menopausal women. American Journal of Clinical Nutrition. 65:6, 1831-9.

254. Nishimura RA, Tajik AJ (1986).The Valsalva maneuver and response revisited., Mayo Clinic Proceedings 61: 3, 211-7

255. Noah ND, Bender AE, Reaidi GB, Gilbert RJ, [1980]. Food poisoning from raw red kidney beans. British Medical Journal, vol. 2, pp. 236-237.

256. Nobrega AC, Williamson JW, Araujo CG, Friedman DB (1994) Heart rate and blood pressure responses at the onset of dynamic exercise: effect of Valsalva manoeuvre. European Journal of Applied Physiology 68 (4): 336-340.

257. Norkin, C.C. & Levangie, P.K. (1992). Joint Structure & Function: A Comprehensive Analysis (2nd Ed.). Philadelphia: F.A. Davis Company.

258. O'Brien M, (2001). Exercise and osteoporosis., Irish journal of medical science 170: 1, 58-62

259. O'Connor, P., Sforzo, G.A., & Frye, P. (1989). Effect of breathing instruction on blood pressure responses during isometric exercise. Physical Therapy, 69: 757-761.

260. Ogilvie, D. (2001). Dietary Omega-3 Fatty Acids: Are They "Essential"? Vegetarian Network Victoria. Available at http://www.vnv.org.au/Nutrition/Omega3.htm

261. Ornish D, Brown SE, Scherwitz LW, Billings JH, Armstrong WT, Ports TA, McLanahan SM, Kirkeeide RL, Brand RJ, Gould KL, (1990). Can lifestyle changes reverse coronary heart disease? The Lifestyle Heart Trial., The Lancet 336: 8708, 129-33.

262. Orsted HL, Radke L, Gorst R, (2001). The impact of musculoskeletal changes on the dynamics of the calf muscle pump., Ostomy Wound Management 47: 10, 18-24

263. Pan W, Zhang L, Xia Y, (1994). The difference in EEG theta waves between concentrative and non-concentrative qigong states--a power spectrum and topographic mapping study. Journal of traditional Chinese medicine 14: 3, 212-8

264. Panjwani U, Gupta HL, Singh SH, Selvamurthy W, Rai UC, (1995). Effect of Sahaja yoga practice on stress management in patients of epilepsy., Indian journal of physiology and pharmacology 39: 2, 111-6

265. Pansare MS, Kulkarni AN, Pendse UB, (1989). Effect of yogic training on serum LDH levels., The Journal of sports medicine and physical fitness 29: 2, 177-8

266. Parfitt, A.M. (1987). Bone and plasma calcium homeostasis. Bone, 8 Supplement 1: S1-8.

267. Parrino L, Smerieri A, Terzano MG, (2001). Combined influence of cyclic arousability and EEG synchrony on generalized interictal discharges within the sleep cycle., Epilepsy research 44: 1, 7-18

268. Patel C, North WR (1975) Randomised controlled trial of yoga and bio-feedback in management of hypertension. Lancet 2 (7925): 93-95

269. Pattabhi Jois K., & Miele, L. (1994). Ashtanga Yoga. Ashtanga Yoga Research Institute, Mysore.

270. Pedersen BK, Toft AD, (2000). Effects of exercise on lymphocytes and cytokines., British journal of sports medicine 34: 4, 246-51

271. Peltonen, R., Nenonen, M., Helve, T., Hanninen, O., Toivanen, P., Eerola, E. (1997) Faecal microbial flora and disease activity in rheumatoid arthritis during a vegan diet. British Journal of Rheumatology 36 (1): 64-68.

272. Peng CK, Mietus JE, Liu Y, Khalsa G, Douglas PS, Benson H, Goldberger AL, (1999). Exaggerated heart rate oscillations during two meditation techniques., International Journal of Cardiology 70: 2, 101-7

273. Perez-De-Albeniz, A., Holmes, J. (2000). Meditation: concepts, effects and uses in therapy International Journal of Psychotherapy, 5:1, p49-59

274. Piha SJ (1995). Autonomic responses to the Valsalva manoeuvre in healthy subjects. Clinical Physiology 15 (4): 339-347.

275. Pranavananda, Y. (1992). Pure Yoga. Motilal Banarsidass Publishers Pvt Ltd, Delhi, India

276. Proske, U., Wise, A.K., Gregory, J.E. (2000). The role of muscle receptors in the detection of movements. Progress in Neurobiology. 01, 60: 1, 85-96.

277. Puente AE, Beiman I, (1980). The effects of behavior therapy, self-relaxation, and transcendental meditation on cardiovascular stress response., Journal of Clinical Psychology 36: 1, 291-5

278. Pusztai A, Clarke EM, Grant G, King TP. [1981]. The toxicity of Phaseolus vulgaris lectins: Nitrogen balance and immunochemical studies. Journal of the Science of Food & Agriculture, vol. 32, pp. 1037-1046.

279. Raghuraj P, Nagarathna R, Nagendra HR, Telles S, (1997). Pranayama increases grip strength without lateralized effects. Indian journal of physiology and pharmacology 41: 2, 129-33

280. Raghuraj P, Ramakrishnan AG, Nagendra HR, Telles S, (1998). Effect of two selected yogic breathing techniques of heart rate variability., Indian journal of physiology and pharmacology 42: 4, 467-72

281. Raghuraj P, Telles S, (1997). Muscle power, dexterity skill and visual perception in community home girls trained in yoga or sports and in regular school girls., Indian journal of physiology and pharmacology 41: 4, 409-15

282. Raju PS, Kumar KA, Reddy SS, Madhavi S, Gnanakumari K, Bhaskaracharyulu C, Reddy MV, Annapurna N, Reddy ME, Girijakumari D, et al (1986). Effect of yoga on exercise tolerance in normal healthy volunteers. Indian Journal of Physiology and Pharmacology 30 (2): 121-32

283. Raju PS, Madhavi S, Prasad KV, Reddy MV, Reddy ME, Sahay BK, Murthy KJ (1994). Comparison of effects of yoga & physical exercise in athletes. Indian Journal of Medical Research 100: 81-6

284. Raman, K. (1998). A Matter of Health: Integration of Yoga Western Medicine for Prevention and Cure. Eastwest Books, Madras

285. Rauma, A.L., Torronen, R., Hanninen, O., Verhagen, H., Mykkanen, H. (1995) Antioxidant status in long-term adherents to a strict uncooked vegan diet. American Journal of Clinical Nutrition 62 (6): 1221-1227.

286. Ray US, Mukhopadhyaya S, Purkayastha SS, Asnani V, Tomer OS, Prashad R, Thakur L, Selvamurthy W, (2001). Effect of yogic exercises on physical and mental health of young fellowship course trainees., Indian journal of physiology and pharmacology 45: 1, 37-53

287. Ray WJ, (1997). EEG concomitants of hypnotic susceptibility., The International journal of clinical and experimental hypnosis 45: 3, 301-13

288. Reid, D.C. (1992). Sports Injury Assessment & Rehabilitation. Churchill Livingstone, New York.

289. Resnick, R., & Halliday, D. (1977). Physics. John Wiley and Sons Inc, Canada.

290. Richardson, C.A. & Jull, G.A. (1995). Muscle Control - Pain Control what exercises should you prescribe. Manual Therapy Journal 1: 2 -10

291. Roberts, J.M., Wilson, K. (1999). Effect of stretching duration on active and passive range of motion in the lower extremity. British Journal of Sports Medicine, 33:4, 259-63.

292. Ron S. Miller (2005) Spine health http://www.spine-health.com/topics/conserv/sciaex/sciaex08.html

293. Rood YR, Bogaards M, Goulmy E, Houwelingen HC, (1993). The effects of stress and relaxation on the in vitro immune response in man: a meta-analytic study., Journal of behavioral medicine 16: 2, 163-81

294. Rosemarynowski, M. (1979}. Experiments with Vajroli. Yoga Mimamsa; quarterly Journal Kaivalyadhama Yoga Research Institution, Lonavala, India, Volume XIX:4: pp36-45

295. Rosemarynowski, M. (1981}. Sat-karma-sadana. In Life in the 21st Century. Ed Kulvinskas, V., & Tasca, R. Omangod Press, Connecticut. pp273-97

296. Rosenthal RJ, Friedman RL, Chidambaram A, Khan AM, Martz J, Shi Q, Nussbaum M, (1998). Effects of hyperventilation and hypoventilation on PaCO2 and intracranial pressure during acute elevations of intra-abdominal pressure with CO2 pneumoperitoneum: large animal observations., Journal of the American College of Surgeons 187: 1, 32-8

297. Ruiz, F.P. (2001). Krishnamacharya's Legacy: You may never have heard of him, but Tirumalai Krishnamacharya influenced or perhaps even invented your yoga. Yoga Journal May/June 2001. This article can be found online at http://www.yogajournal.com/wisdom/465_1.cfm

298. Sanders, T.A., and Purves, R, (1981). An anthropometric and dietary assessment of the nutritional status of vegan preschool children. Journal of Human Nutrition. 35 (5): 349-357.

299. Sanders, T.A., Ellis, F.R., Dickerson, J.W. (1978). Studies of vegans: the fatty acid composition of plasma choline phosphoglycerides, erythrocytes, adipose tissue, and breast milk, and some indicators of susceptibility to ischemic heart disease in vegans and omnivore controls. American Journal of Clinical Nutrition. 31 (5): 805-813.

300. Santti R, Makela S, Strauss L, Korkman J, Kostian ML, (1998). Phytoestrogens: potential endocrine disruptors in males., Toxicolology & Industrial Health 14: 1-2, 223-37.

301. Saraswati, Swami Satyananda (1985). 'Kundalini Tantra'. Bihar School of Yoga, India.

302. Sat Chuen Hon (2003) Taoist Qigong for Health and Vitality: A Complete Program of Movement, Meditation, and Healing Sounds. Shambhala. Also available at http://users.erols.com/dantao/breath.html

303. Satyananda, S. (1984) Kundalini Tantra. Bihar Yoga Bharati. Munger, Bihar, India.

304. Satyananda, S. (1996) Asana, Pranayama, Mudra, Bandha. Bihar Yoga Bharati. Munger, Bihar, India.

305. Schecter, A., Cramer, P., Boggess, K., Stanley, J., Olson, J.R. (1997) Levels of dioxins, dibenzofurans, PCB and DDE congeners in pooled food samples collected in 1995 at supermarkets across the United States. Chemosphere 34 (5-7): 1437-1447

306. Scheler, M.F. (1992). Effects of optimism on psychological and physical wellbeing: theoretical and empirical update, Cognitive Therapy and Research, 16, pp. 201-228

307. Schell FJ, Allolio B, Schonecke OW (1994). Physiological and psychological effects of Hatha-Yoga exercise in healthy women. Int J Psychosom 41 (1-4): 46-52

308. Schiff B.B., Rump S.A. (1995). Asymmetrical hemispheric activation and emotion: the effects of unilateral forced nostril breathing. Brain Cognition, 29:3, 217-31

309. Schiff BB, Lamon M, (1994). Inducing emotion by unilateral contraction of hand muscles., Cortex; a journal devoted to the study of the nervous system and behavior 30: 2, 247-54

310. Schiff BB, Truchon C, (1993). Effect of unilateral contraction of hand muscles on perceiver biases in the perception of chimeric and neutral faces., Neuropsychologia 31: 12, 1351-65

311. Schiff BB; Rump SA (1995). Asymmetrical hemispheric activation and emotion: the effects of unilateral forced nostril breathing. Brain Cognition, 29:3, 217-31.

312. Schreiber SJ, Lambert UK, Doepp F, Valdueza JM, (2002). Effects of prolonged head-down tilt on internal jugular vein cross-sectional area., British Journal of Aanaesthesia 89: 5, 769-71

313. Seer P, Raeburn JM, (1980). Meditation training and essential hypertension: a methodological study. Journal of Behavioral Medicine 3: 1, 59-71

314. Sei H, Morita Y, (1996). Acceleration of EEG theta wave precedes the phasic surge of arterial pressure during REM sleep in the rat., Neuroreport 7: 18, 3059-62

315. Selvamurthy W, Sridharan K, Ray US, Tiwary RS, Hegde KS, Radhakrishan U, Sinha KC, A new physiological approach to control essential hypertension., Indian journal of physiology and pharmacology 42: 2, 205-13

316. Setchell KDR et al. (1987). Dietary estrogens - a probable cause of infertility and liver disease in captive cheetahs. Gastroenterology 93: 225-23

317. Setchell, K.D.R., (1997). "Naturally occurring non-steroidal estrogens of dietary origin," in "Estrogens in the Environment", John A. McLachlan, Editor, Elsevier Science Publishing Co. Inc., pp 79/80 and p 70

318. Setchell, KDR, Zimmer-Nechemias, L, Cai, J, and Heubi, JE. (1997). Exposure of infants to phyto-estrogens from soy-based infant formula. Lancet, 350, 23-27,

319. Shaffer HJ, LaSalvia TA, Stein JP, (1997). Comparing Hatha yoga with dynamic group psychotherapy for enhancing methadone maintenance treatment: a randomized clinical trial., Alternative therapies in health and medicine 3: 4, 57-66

320. Shah, C.S. (2001). The Tantras and the Concept of Kundalini Shakti http://www.boloji.com/hinduism/kundalini.htm

321. Shannahoff-Khalsa D. (1993). The ultradian rhythm of alternating cerebral hemispheric activity. International Journal of Neuroscience 70: 3-4, 285-98.

322. Shannahoff-Khalsa DS, Kennedy B, (1993). The effects of unilateral forced nostril breathing on the heart., The International journal of neuroscience 73: 1-2, 47-60

323. Shapiro DH, (1992). Adverse effects of meditation: a preliminary investigation of long-term meditators. International Journal of Psychosomatics 39: 1-4, 62-7

324. Sharpe RM, Skakkebaek NE (1993) Are oestrogens involved in falling sperm counts and disorders of the male reproductive tract? Lancet May 29 341:8857 1392-5

325. Sheehan, D.M. (1997). Isoflavone content of breast milk and soy formulas: Benefits and risks. Clin. Chem., 43:850,.

326. Sheehan, D.M. (1998a). Literature analysis of no-threshold dose-response curves for endocrine disruptors. Teratology, 57, 219,

327. Sheehan, D.M. (1998b). Herbal medicines and phytoestrogens: risk/benefit considerations. Proc. Soc. Exp. Biol. Med., 217, 379-385,.

328. Shepherd, R.B. (1994, 1995,1996). Lecture notes for Physiotherapy in Neurology. Faculty of Health Sciences, University of Sydney.

329. Shiba, Y., Obuchi, S., Saitou, C., Habata T., Maeda M. (2001), Effects of Bilateral Upper-Limb Exercise on Trunk Muscles. Journal of Physical Therapy Science, Vol.13 No.1, 65-67

330. Sim, M.K. & Tsoi, W.F. (1992). The effects of centrally acting drugs on the EEG correlates of meditation, Biofeedback Self-Regulation, 17(3), pp. 215-20

331. Singh, V., Wisniewski, A., Britton, J., & Tattersfield, A. (1990). Effect of yoga breathing exercises (pranayama) on airway reactivity in subjects with asthma. Lancet, 335:1381-1383.

332. Sivananda, S. (1994). Kundalini Yoga (10th Ed). The Divine Life Trust Society, India.

333. Smith AM, (1981). The coactivation of antagonist muscles. 7, 733-47.

334. Smith ML, Beightol LA, Fritsch-Yelle JM, Ellenbogen KA, Porter TR, Eckberg DL (1996) Valsalva's manoeuvre revisited: a quantitative method yielding insights into human autonomic control. American Journal of Physiology 271 (3 Pt 2): H1240-H1249

335. Snyder SH, (1992). Nitric oxide and neurons., Current opinion in neurobiology 2: 3, 323-7.

336. Solberg EE, Halvorsen R, Sundgot-Borgen J, Ingjer F, Holen A, (1995). Meditation: a modulator of the immune response to physical stress? A brief report., British Journal of Sports Medicine 29: 4, 255-7

337. Solberg EE, Ingjer F, Holen A, Sundgot-Borgen J, Nilsson S, Holme I, (2000). Stress reactivity to and recovery from a standardised exercise bout: a study of 31 runners practising relaxation techniques., British Journal of Sports Medicine 34: 4, 268-72

338. Soubiran C, Harant I, de Glisezinski I, Beauville M, Crampes F, Riviere D, Garrigues M, (1996). Cardio-respiratory changes during the onset of head-down tilt., Aviation, Space, and Environmental Medicine 67: 7, 648-53

339. Sperry K (1994) Achalasia, the Valsalva manoeuvre, and sudden death: a case report. Journal of Forensic Science 39 (2): 547-551

340. Spindler, S.R. (2001). Reversing the genomic effects of aging with short-term calorie restriction. The Scientific World 1, 544–546.

341. St George, F., (1999). Bodyworks. ABC Books, Sydney

429

342. Stancak A Jr, Kuna M, Srinivasan, Dostalek C, Vishnudevananda S, (1991b). Kapalabhati--yogic cleansing exercise. II. EEG topography analysis., Homeostasis in health and disease 33: 4, 182-9

343. Stancak A Jr, Kuna M, Srinivasan, Vishnudevananda S, Dostalek C, (1991a). Kapalabhati--yogic cleansing exercise. I. Cardiovascular and respiratory changes., Homeostasis in health and disease : international journal devoted to integrative brain functions and homeostatic systems 33: 3, 126-34

344. Stancak A Jr, Pfeffer D, Hrudova L, Sovka P, Dostalek C, (1993). Electroencephalographic correlates of paced breathing., Neuroreport 4: 6, 723-6

345. Stancak A Jr; Kuna M (1994). EEG changes during forced alternate nostril breathing. International Journal of Psychophysiology. 18:1, 75-9

346. Stanescu DC, Nemery B, Veriter C, Marechal C (1981). Pattern of breathing and ventilatory response to C02 in subjects practising hatha-yoga. Journal of Applied Physiology. 51: 1625-9

347. Stigsby B, Rodenberg JC, Moth HB, (1981). Electroencephalographic findings during mantra meditation (transcendental meditation). A controlled, quantitative study of experienced meditators., Electroencephalography and Clinical Neurophysiology 51: 4, 434-42

348. Sudsuang R, Chentanez V, Veluvan K. (1991).Effect of Buddhist meditation on serum cortisol and total protein levels, blood pressure, pulse rate, lung volume and reaction time. Physiology and Behavior 50: 3, 543-8

349. Sun TF, Kuo CC, Chiu NM, (2002). Mindfulness meditation in the control of severe headache., Chang Gung Medical Journal 25: 8, 538-41

350. Suzuki, H. (1995) Serum vitamin B12 levels in young vegans who eat brown rice. Journal of Nutritional Science & Vitaminology (Tokyo) 41 (6): 587-594

351. Tabrizi P, McIntyre WM, Quesnel MB, Howard AW, (2000). Limited dorsiflexion predisposes to injuries of the ankle in children. Journal of Bone and Joint Surgery. 82: 8, 1103-6

352. Tal-Akabi A, Rushton A (2000) An investigation to compare the effectiveness of carpal bone mobilisation and neurodynamic mobilisation as methods of treatment for carpal tunnel syndrome. Manual Therapy, 5(4):214-22.

353. Telles S, Hanumanthaiah B, Nagarathna R, Nagendra HR, (1993). Improvement in static motor performance following yogic training of school children., Perceptual and motor skills 76: 3 Pt 2, 1264-6

354. Telles S, Hanumanthaiah BH, Nagarathna R, Nagendra HR, (1994a). Plasticity of motor control systems demonstrated by yoga training., Indian journal of physiology and pharmacology 38: 2, 143-4

355. Telles S, Nagarathna R, Nagendra HR, (1994b) Breathing through a particular nostril can alter metabolism and autonomic activities., Indian journal of physiology and pharmacology 38: 2, 133-7

356. Telles S, Nagarathna R, Nagendra HR, (1995). Autonomic changes during "OM" meditation, Indian Journal of Physiology and Pharmacology 39: 4, 418-20

357. Telles S, Nagarathna R, Nagendra HR, (1996). Physiological measures of right nostril breathing., Journal of alternative and complementary medicine (New York, N.Y.)2: 4, 479-84

358. Telles S. & Desraju, T. (1993). Autonomic changes in Brahmakumaris Raja yoga meditation, International Journal of Psychophysiology, 15(2), pp. 147-152

359. Teramoto S, Sugai M, Saito E, Matsuse T, Eto M, Toba K, Ouchi Y (1997). Hyperventilation syndrome in a very old woman. Nippon Ronen Igakkai Zasshi Mar;34(3):226-29

360. Tooley GA, Armstrong SM, Norman TR, Sali A, (2000). Acute increases in night-time plasma melatonin levels following a period of meditation., Biological psychology 53: 1, 69-78

361. Tortora, G.J. & Grabowski, S.R. (1993). Principles of Anatomy & Physiology (7th Ed.). New York: Harper Collins College Publishers.

362. Travis F, (2001). Autonomic and EEG patterns distinguish transcending from other experiences during Transcendental Meditation practice. International Journal of Psychophysiology. 42: 1, 1-9

363. Travis F, Wallace RK, (1997). Autonomic patterns during respiratory suspensions: possible markers of Transcendental Consciousness., Psychophysiology 34: 1, 39-46

364. Travis F.T & Orme-Johnson, D.W (1989). Field model of consciousness: EEG coherence changes as indicators of field effects, International Journal of Neuroscience, 49, pp. 203-11

365. Underwood MR, Morgan J, (1998). The use of a back class teaching extension exercises in the treatment of acute low back pain in primary care., Family practice 15: 1, 9-15

366. Vasconcelos IM, Trentim A, Guimarães JA, Carlini CR Arch (1994). Purification and physicochemical characterization of soyatoxin, a novel toxic protein isolated from soybeans (Glycine max). Biochem Biophys 1 312:2 357-66

367. Vempati RP, Telles S, (2002). Yoga-based guided relaxation reduces sympathetic activity judged from baseline levels., Psychological reports 90: 2, 487-94

368. Vishnu-Devananda, S. (1987). Hatha Yoga Pradipika of Swatmarama: The Classic Guide for the Advanced Practice of Hatha Yoga, with 1897 commentary of Brahmananda, and 1987 commentary of Vishnu-Devandana. OM Lotus Publishing Company, New York.

369. Vogiatzis I, Spurway NC, Jennett S, Wilson J, Sinclair J. (1996). Changes in ventilation related to changes in electromyograph activity during repetitive bouts of isometric exercise in simulated sailing. European Journal of Applied Physiology;72(3):195-203

370. Vogt F, Klimesch W, Doppelmayr M, (1998). High-frequency components in the alpha band and memory performance., Journal of clinical neurophysiology 15: 2, 167-72, Mar,.

371. von Stein A, Sarnthein J, (2000). Different frequencies for different scales of cortical integration: from local gamma to long range alpha/theta synchronization., International journal of psychophysiology 38: 3, 301-13

372. Walford, R.L., Harris, S.B., Gunion, M.W. (1992). The calorically restricted low-fat nutrient-dense diet in Biosphere 2 significantly lowers blood glucose, total leukocyte count, cholesterol, and blood pressure in humans. Proceedings of the National Academy of Science U S A, 89:23, 11533-7.

373. Wallace RK, Dillbeck M, Jacobe E, Harrington B, (1982). The effects of the transcendental meditation and TM-Sidhi program on the aging process., International Journal of Neuroscience 16: 1, 53-8

374. Wall EJ, Massie JB, Kwan MK, Rydevik BL, Myers RR, Garfin SR (1992) Experimental stretch neuropathy. Changes in nerve conduction under tension, The Journal of bone and joint surgery. British volume 74: 1, 126-9.

375. Ward, B. (1995). Holistic medicine. Australian Family Physician, 24: 761-762.

376. Watenpaugh DE, Breit GA, Ballard RE, Hargens AR, (1997). Monitoring acute whole-body fluid redistribution by changes in leg and neck volumes., Aviation, space, and environmental medicine 68: 9 Pt 1, 858-62

377. Waxman MB, Wald RW, Finley JP, Bonet JF, Downar E, Sharma AD (Oct 1980) Valsalva termination of ventricular tachycardia. Circulation 62 (4): 843-851

378. Weber, S. (1996). The effects of relaxation exercises on anxiety levels in psychiatric inpatients. Journal of Holistic Nursing, Sep, 14:3, 196-205.

379. Weinstein M, Smith JC, (1992). Isometric squeeze relaxation (progressive relaxation) vs meditation: absorption and focusing as predictors of state effects., Perceptual and Motor Skills 75: 3 Pt 2, 1263-71

380. Weitzberg E, Lundberg JO, (2002). Humming greatly increases nasal nitric oxide., American journal of respiratory and critical care medicine 166: 2, 144-5.

381. Wenneberg SR, Schneider RH, Walton KG, Maclean CR, Levitsky DK, Salerno JW, Wallace RK, Mandarino JV, Rainforth MV, Waziri R, (1997). A controlled study of the effects of the Transcendental Meditation program on cardiovascular reactivity and ambulatory blood pressure., The International journal of neuroscience 89: 1-2, 15-28

382. Werntz DA, Bickford RG, Shannahoff-Khalsa D, (1987). Selective hemispheric stimulation by unilateral forced nostril breathing., Human Neurobiology 6: 3, 165-71

383. White, L, Petrovich, H, Ross, GW, Masaki, KH, Abbot, RD, Teng, EL, Rodriguez, BL, Blanchette, PL, Havlik, RJ, Wergowske, G, Chiu, D, Foley, DJ, Murdaugh, C, and Curb, JD. (1996b). Prevalence of dementia in older Japanese-American men in Hawaii, JAMA 276, 955-960,

384. White, L, Petrovitch, H, Ross, GW, and Masaki. Association of mid-life consumption of tofu with late life cognitive impairment and dementia: The Honolulu-Asia Aging Study. (1996a) The Neurobiology of Aging, 17 (suppl 4), S121,.

385. Wiley, R.L., Dunn, C.L., Cox, R.H., Hueppehen, N.A., & Scott, M.S. (1992). Isometric exercise training lowers resting blood pressure. Medicine & Science in Sports & Exercise. 24: 749-754.

386. Wilson, A.F., Jevning, R. & Gulch, S. (1987). Marked reduction of forearm carbon dioxide production during states of decreased metabolism, Physiology and Behavior, 41, pp. 347-352

387. Witoonchart C, Bartlet L, (2002). The use of a meditation programme for institutionalized juvenile delinquents., Journal of the Medical Association of Thailand 85 Suppl 2:, S790-3

388. Witvrouw, E., Lysens, R., Bellemans, J., Peers, K,, Vanderstraeten, G., (2000). Open versus closed kinetic chain exercises for patellofemoral pain. A prospective, randomized study, American Journal Of Sports Medicine 28: 687-94.

389. Wolkove N, Kreisman H, Darragh D, Cohen C, Frank H, (1984). Effect of transcendental meditation on breathing and respiratory control., Journal of Applied Physiology: Respiratory, Environmental and Exercise Physiology 56: 3, 607-12

390. Wood C, (1993). Mood change and perceptions of vitality: a comparison of the effects of relaxation, visualization and yoga., Journal of the Royal Society of Medicine 86: 5, 254-8

391. Wood CJ, (1986). Evaluation of meditation and relaxation on physiological response during the performance of fine motor and gross motor tasks., Percept Mot Skills 62: 1, 91-8

392. Woodhams, D.J. (1995) Soy Information Newsletter.Soy Information Network C/- Dr DJ Woodhams, Whatarangi Road, R D 2, Featherston 5952, New Zealand.

393. Woodroffe, J. (1986). The Serpent Power. 13th Ed. Ganesh & Co., Madras.

394. Yamazaki Y, Itoh H, Ohkuwa T, (1995). Muscle activation in the elbow-forearm complex during rapid elbow extension. 3, 285-95,.

395. Yan, Q., Sun, Y. (1996). Quantitative research for improving respiratory muscle contraction by breathing exercise. Chinese Medical Journal (Engl), Oct, 109:10, 771-5.

396. Yeshe, L. (1999). Make your mind an ocean: Aspects of Buddhist Psychology. Lama Yeshe Wisdom Archive, Boston.

397. Yogananda, P. (1946). Autobiography of a Yogi. Republished (1991) Self Realisation Fellowship. Or original 1946 edition Available Online at http://www.crystalclarity.com/yogananda/

398. Yogeshwarananda, S. (1959). 'Atma Vijnana - Science of Soul'. Yoga Niketan Trust, Bharat India.

399. Yogeshwarananda, S. (1970). 'Bahiranga Yoga - First Steps to Higher Yoga'. Yoga Niketan Trust, Bharat India

400. Zamarra JW, Schneider RH, Besseghini I, Robinson DK, Salerno JW, (1996). Usefulness of the transcendental meditation program in the treatment of patients with coronary artery disease. American Journal of Cardiology 77: 10, 867-70

401. Zehr EP, Sale DG, Dowling JJ, (1997). Ballistic movement performance in karate athletes. 10, Oct 1366-73.

402. Zeier H, (1984). Arousal reduction with biofeedback-supported respiratory meditation. Biofeedback Self Regulation 9: 4, 497-508

403. Zuroff DC, Schwarz JC, (1980). Transcendental meditation verus muscle relaxation: two-year follow-up of a controlled experiment., American Journal of Psychiatry 137: 10, 1229-21

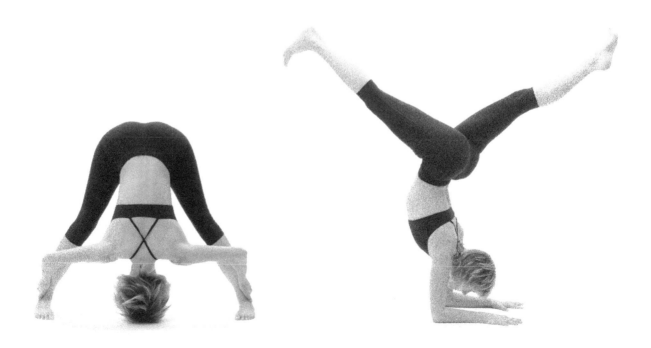

Bianca Machliss in *Baddha Prasarita Padottanasana* and *Pinca Mayurasana*.
Photos courtesy of Alejandro Rolandi.

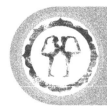

Yoga Synergy

Yoga Synergy Pty. Ltd. ACN: 082 087 634; ABN: 94 082 087 634
Postal Address: P.O. Box 9, Waverley, 2024;
School Addresses: Bondi: 115 Bronte Rd, Bondi Junction 2026;
                     Newtown 196 Australia St., Newtown 2042;
Telephone: (61 2) 9389 7399
Email: yoga@yogasynergy.com
Website: http://www.yogasynergy.com
Directors: Bianca Machliss BSc BAppSc (Physiotherapy) ;
                     Simon Borg-Olivier MSc BAppSc (Physiotherapy)

Yoga Synergy was established in Newtown in 1984, in Bondi Junction in 1997. This dynamic style of *hatha yoga*, devised by the directors, who are both qualified physiotherapists, Simon Borg-Olivier MSc BAppSc (Physiotherapy) & Bianca Machliss BSc BAppSc (Physiotherapy) , represents a synthesis between *astanga vinyasa yoga*, *Iyengar yoga*, *Tibetan yoga* and modern medical science. The *hatha yoga* taught at *Yoga Synergy* is derived from the work of Professor T. Krishnamacharya. Sri Krishnamacharya, who died in 1989 at the age of 101, was the teacher of three of the most influential yoga masters alive today. These *yoga* masters are Sri B.K.S. Iyengar (author of "Light on *Yoga*"); Sri K. Pattabhi Jois, who teaches *astanga vinyasa yoga* and, Sri T.K.V. Desikachar (author of "The Heart of *Yoga*").

Synergy-style yoga is an *astanga* based *vinyasa* flow-style meditative practice, linking postures with the breath while maintaining an awareness of anatomical and physiological alignment, and allowing students to progress with guidance at their own pace. *Yoga Synergy-style* is a dynamic moving meditation, that improves cardiovascular fitness, strength and flexibility.

There are five (5) key *Synergy-style* sequences that can each be approached from the beginner to the advanced level. At the *Yoga Synergy* schools each sequence is taught for a period of 9 weeks. At the Yoga Synergy schools, each sequence is taught for a period of 9 weeks in 'open classes' and 'pre-booked courses. Each of the five *Synergy-style* sequences is taught at seven (7) different levels: Open, Beginner Level 1 and 2, Intermediate Level 1 and 2, and Advanced Level 1 and 2. Each *asana* (static posture), *vinyasa* (dynamic exercise) and *pranayama* ('breath-control' exercise) has a range of variations from the simplest least complicated version through to the full or hard version. Design of these sequences takes into consideration that each exercise must have an easy or safe version for beginners and for students with musculoskeletal problems or with medical conditions, and a full or challenging version for experienced students, athletes, dancers, martial artists etc. The practitioner is guided to choose the level of intensity for each pose that is appropriate for them at the time of practice. A sequence sheet of the postures in each sequence and DVD's of each sequence are available to assist students in their own practice.

By regularly attending *Synergy-style yoga* classes, the student is able to learn a *yoga* sequence enough to do self-practice and yet still be stimulated every 9 weeks by a new set of postures and exercises. *Yoga Synergy* is a team of professional teachers, trained personally by Bianca and Simon, with years of experience teaching the *Synergy-style* of *yoga*.

The pre-booked courses and casual attendance classes (Open classes) at *Yoga Synergy* are suitable for people with non-severe musculoskeletal problems such as back and neck pain, knee pain or instability, and for those who need to increase strength, stability, range of motion in any of the major joints, flexibility and cardiovascular fitness.

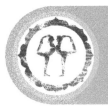

Yoga Synergy

Applied Anatomy & Physiology of Yoga

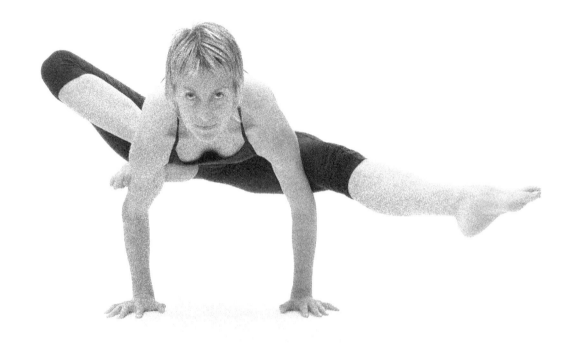

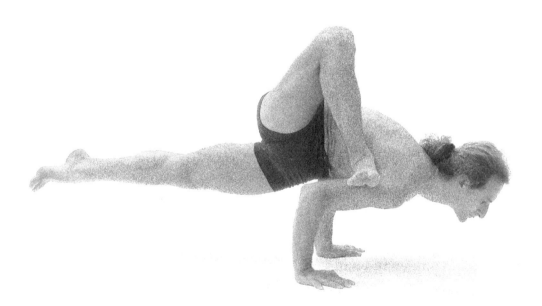

Simon Borg-Olivier
MSc BAppSc (Physiotherapy)

&

Bianca Machliss
BSc BAppSc (Physiotherapy)

About the Authors:

Simon Borg-Olivier

Simon Borg-Olivier MSc BAppSc (Physiotherapy) is a director of YogaSynergy, one of Australia's oldest and most respected yoga schools with a style based on a deep understanding of yoga anatomy, yoga physiology and traditional hatha yoga. Simon has been teaching since 1982. He is a registered physiotherapist, a research scientist and a University lecturer. Simon has been regularly invited to teach at special workshops and conferences interstate and overseas since 1990.

Simon was introduced to yoga at age six, learning breath retentions from his father and the main bandhas (internal locks) by Basil Brown, (an Olympic athletic). At age 17, Simon studied for one year with a Tibetan Lama who introduced Simon to the philosophy and practice of tantric yoga. In 1980, Simon started the postures and movements of hatha yoga, eventually learning with BKS Iyengar, K. Pattabhi Jois and TKV Desikachar.

Simon met his main teacher Natanaga Zhander (Shandor Remete) in 1985 and had the privilege of studying intensively with him for almost two decades. Simon credits Zhander as being the most important person in his pursuit, passion and understanding of hatha yoga. To this day, Zhander remains as Simon's foremost yoga inspiration and mentor.

Simon studied and taught at Sydney University over a period of 20 years. In that time he completed a Bachelor of Science in human biology, a research based Master of Science in molecular biology and a Bachelor of Applied Science in Physiotherapy. In 1988, Simon met physiotherapist and yoga teacher Bianca Machliss. Together, over the last 20 years, Simon and Bianca have developed the unique YogaSynergy system.

Simon has regularly taught yoga to dance companies (Sydney Dance Company, Darc Swan, Bangarra Dance Company) and lectured at the University of NSW and the University of Western Sydney Dance Departments. In addition, he has performed with several dance productions and numerous yogic dance performances. Simon regularly gives artistic demonstrations of advanced yoga vinyasa (linked sequences of postures) to music.

Author and journalist Alix Johnson featured Simon's personal history and philosophy of yoga in her book 'Yoga: The Essence of Life: Eight Yogis Share Their Journeys' (2004). Simon has contributed chapters on yoga to several technical books including 'An Introduction to Complementary Medicine' (2005) Edited by Terry Robson and 'Integrative Medicine Perspectives' (2007) Edited by Professor Marc Cohen. He regularly contributes articles to 'Australian Yoga Life Magazine', 'Well Being Magazine', 'Australian Natural Health Magazine', Art of Healing Magazine' and several Russian Yoga Journals. Simon's postures have also been featured in many yoga books, including Christina Brown's bestselling book 'The Yoga Bible' (2003), Jesse Chapman's books 'Yoga Postures for Your Body, Mind and Soul' (2000) and 'Yoga for Inner Strength' (2004) and James Houston's book 'One' (2005).

Simon is regularly invited to speak on radio and has had numerous television appearances. He is featured in the recently released film 'Yoga and Me' (2009) produced by Robbie Baldwin. He has also been invited to be a guest lecturer/ presenter at many conventions and annual conferences, including the Australian Physiotherapy Association (APA) (1997, 1998), Pilates Australia (2004, 2007) Sydney Yoga Expo (2004, 2005, 2006, 2007, 2008), Byron Bay Yoga Festival (2006), the 'Yoga and Science' Conventions (1996, 2005, 2006), the Asia Yoga Conference (Kuala Lumpur, 2007), the 13th International Holistic Health Conference (2007) the FILEX Convention (Australian Fitness Leaders Network) (2007, 2008, 2009) and the International Ayurveda and Yoga Conference (2006, 2009).

Since 1995 Simon has been teaching courses in the Applied Anatomy and Physiology of Yoga internationally. Apart from training many teachers in YogaSynergy System with Bianca Machliss, Simon has also been an invited guest lecturer at many major yoga teacher training courses throughout the world, including the International Yoga Teachers Association (IYTA) (1990, 1997, 2001, 2002, 2005, 2006), 'Sydney Yoga Centre Teacher Training' (1995, 1996), 'Yoga Arts Teacher Training' (Byron Bay, 2000, 2001), 'InspyaYoga Teacher Training' (Byron Bay, 2006, 2007, 2008), the Yoga Teachers Association of Australia (YTAA) (2007, 2008, 2009), 'Yoga Zone Teacher Training (Kuala Lumpur, 2007), Ysynergy Teacher Training (Kuala Lumpur, 2008), 'Vibrant Living Yoga Teacher Training' (Bali, 2008, 2009) and 'Yoga Jaya Teacher Training' (Tokyo and Osaka, 2009).

In 2007 Simon was approached by Professor Marc Cohen of RMIT University (Melbourne) to create a course called 'Integrative Applied Eastern Anatomy and Physiology'. Simon is now the main lecturer and course co-ordinator of this course which he developed and wrote with Bianca Machliss. The course has been running since 2008. It uses this book (Applied Anatomy and Physiology of Yoga) as its main text book and forms part of two new internationally recognised degrees, Bachelor of Wellness and Master of Wellness.

Simon regularly teaches about 10 classes during the week and undertakes a number of private consultations. He travels interstate or overseas to teach at special workshops and conferences between 20 to 30 weekends every year. He lives in Sydney with his wife Vitoria and their two children Amaliah and Eric.

Bianca Machliss

Bianca Machliss BSc BAppSc (Physiotherapy) is a director of Yoga Synergy, one of Australia's largest and oldest yoga schools. Bianca has taught yoga since 1989. She is a registered physiotherapist, research scientist and ACHPER graduate. Bianca has organised and taught workshops on yoga, applied anatomy and physiology of yoga and yogic nutrition throughout the world since 1990.

Bianca initially learnt yoga from Andrew Nethery and Simon Borg-Olivier. She studied intensively in Australia with Natanaga Zhander (Shandor Remete). She also studied with Sri BKS Iyengar, Sri K Pattabhi Jois and Clive Sheridan.

Bianca first began yoga in the 1980's, while studying for a Bachelor of Science at the University of Sydney. Before beginning yoga, Bianca had been a passionate athlete since her youth. Her interest in yoga was stimulated by her university studies in human psychology and biology and her trips to India. Bianca taught yoga to school children in India and she was subsequently invited to perform yoga dance in an Indian circus. She later performed on many occasions with Simon Borg-Olivier at festivals and conferences throughout the world.

After completing her BSc, Bianca worked at the University of Sydney as a research scientist in biology, while co-directing Yoga Synergy. After many trips to India to study Yoga, Bianca was inspired to return to Sydney University from 1994 to 1997 to attend a full-time Physiotherapy degree. Bianca became a physiotherapist to further her knowledge of the human body and western medical science in order to enhance her yoga teaching.

As a physiotherapist and yoga therapy teacher Bianca has helped thousands of individuals to heal from musculoskeletal problems such as knee and shoulder dislocations, chronic lower back pain, sprained wrists and ankles, broken bones and neck injuries. Bianca has also successfully used her understanding of traditional hatha yoga and exercise-based physiotherapy to help many people with medical conditions such as asthma, diabetes, arthritis, cancer, heart attack, stroke, infertility and epilepsy.

Bianca has become an expert in prenatal and postnatal yoga. She was recently featured as the main teacher and lecturer in the recently released and very popular Prenatal YogaSynergy DVD, which was filmed before the birth of her first child Lorenzo.

Bianca has personally trained more than 50 yoga teachers in individual intensive three year apprenticeship programmes at Yoga Synergy over the last 12 years. Bianca is highly acknowledged for her ability to teach the essence of physical adjustments and verbal instruction to yoga teachers. Many of the teachers Bianca trained now run successful Yoga Schools around the world.

Bianca has produced five three-hour DVDs in which she teaches the finer points of yoga and instructs beginner to advanced YogaSynergy sequences. She has also contributed chapters on yoga to several technical books including 'An Introduction to Complementary Medicine' (2005) Edited by Terry Robson and 'Integrative Medicine Perspectives' (2007) Edited by Professor Marc Cohen. Bianca has a regular column for questions on yoga anatomy and physiology in 'Australian Yoga Life Magazine' and regularly contributes articles to magazines such 'Well Being', 'Australian Natural Health' and 'The Art of Healing'. Bianca's postures have also been featured in Christina Brown's bestselling book 'The Yoga Bible' (2004) and James Houston's book 'One' (2005).

Bianca is also guest lecturer in the course 'Integrative Applied Eastern Anatomy and Physiology'. This course, which she helped develop with Simon Borg-Olivier, uses this book (Applied Anatomy and Physiology of Yoga) as its main text book, and is part of two degrees in the School of Health Sciences at RMIT University (Melbourne).

Bianca regularly teaches about 10 classes per week, as well as participating in special workshops. She is responsible for the administration and organization of the two main YogaSynergy school's daily running as well as the YogaSynergy Teacher Training Program. She lives in Sydney with her partner Juliano and their young son Lorenzo.

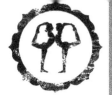

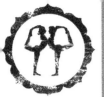

The purpose of *yoga* **is to** realise that jivatma (individual consciousness) is one with Paramataman (universal consciousness).

The purpose of *hatha yoga* **is:**

* To help your body to live long enough and be healthy enough for your mind to realise yoga.
* To physically realise (on a more mundane level) that your brain and your body are connected and are in fact one.
* To improve communication within the body by enhancing the circulation of prana (energy) and citta (consciousness/ information) through the nadis (subtle channels), thus helping us to educate, energise, nourish and heal the various parts of our body.

Yoga Synergy is traditional hatha yoga for the modern/western body with an understanding from exercise-based physiotherapy – based on the principles of practically applied anatomy and physiology of yoga. Yoga Synergy is generally taught as five specific sequences, but the method can be applied to any hatha yoga sequence. It can be either very hard or very easy. You should modify and adapt each pose and the way you enter and exit each pose according to your physical limitations and how you feel at the time – this has to be re-assessed from one day to the next from one pose to the next and eventually with every breath and every movement.

Modify your practice to make your yoga harder or easier in 3 main ways:

1. **Don't overstrain your brain** by trying to comprehend too much information or trying to do too much in each exercise.
1. **Don't overstrain your physiology** by breathing too much or forcing the breath – less breath is best.
1. **Don't overstrain your body** by over-tensing or over-stretching the muscles, or by moving too quickly.

General rule for safety in *hatha yoga*: **Balance, strength and flexibility with relaxation**

* The more you are bending a part of your body beyond what you would in everyday life, then the more you should tense that part of the body to keep its structure stable.
* However, if tensioning that part of the body causes discomfort or prevents you from feeling relaxed, especially in the face or neck, then you need to tense that part of the body less which means you should also bend that part of the body less.

YOGA SYNERGY'S MAIN PRINCIPLES OF PRACTICE

Yoga Synergy sequences are designed to control the flow of energy and information (consciousness) in the body, to nourish and cleanse the body's systems, and to create a dynamic balance between strength, flexibility and cardiovascular fitness. Therefore:

* Keep your body safe where necessary by doing more simple forms of each posture and more simple forms of the sequence.
* Bring your mind to a more meditative state of concentration or inner peace by the end of the practice.
* Work towards gathering energy with your practice rather than expending it.

Yoga Synergy is traditional hatha yoga for the modern/western body with an understanding from exercise-based physiotherapy and the main principles of applied anatomy and physiology of yoga. These principles include:

* **Sequencing for the western body** – Do not assume that a western body has the flexibility and strength of the traditional Indian body. Most traditional sequences assume flexibility of the spine and hip, as *well* as adequate strength in the knees shoulders and spine. Therefore, if you are practicing a traditional sequence take this into account.
* **Gradation of exercises** – Use a range of easy (simple) versions to hard (complex) versions of each posture where you 'bend' less at each joint for a simple version of a pose.
* **Active movements** – Move actively into each posture going initially only as far into the pose as the body will take you, without helping with another part of your body. Balance, strength, flexibility and the ability to relax by stimulating the reciprocal reflex. Activate (tense) muscles (strengthening them) in their shortened state.
* **Resisted movements** – Once having stabilised the spine with a full exhalation, you can deepen the posture by trying to escape out of each pose once you have got there. Balance, strength, flexibility and the ability to relax with the nervous system by stimulating the relaxation reflex. Activate (tense) muscles (strengthening them) in their lengthened state.

- *Mudras* - Many traditional *yoga* poses are also *mudras* and hence they can stimulate the flow of blood, the nervous system and the acupuncture meridian system. *Mudra* has many meanings. In *yoga*, *mudra* can also mean a 'seal', a 'current' or 'a control exercise'. *Mudras* are used to generate energy, regulate and control the circulation of energy and information in the body, and regulate and control the nervous system. *Mudras* can stimulate or tension (stretch) *nadis*. The *nadis*, or subtle channels, include blood vessels, nerves and acupuncture meridians.
- *Bandhas* – Learn ways to generate *bandhas* at each joint in each pose. A *bandha* is the co-activation (simultaneous tensing) of opposing muscle groups around a joint complex. *Bandhas* are a specific subset of *mudras*.
- *Pranayama* – learning how to breathe less for better cleansing, nourishment, communication and meditation.
- 'The yogi measures life by the number of breaths they take not the years'.
- *Pranayama* is the opposite of what many people think. It is learning how to breathe less air - not more.
- Provided you occasionally exhale fully, breathing less than normal builds up carbon dioxide, which causes more blood to flow to the brain and heart, more air to the lungs and more oxygen to the cells. Carbon dioxide is dissolved as carbonic acid which calms the mind and nervous system in general and to a certain extent suppresses hunger.
- Sustained exhalation retention with *bandhas* (including *tha-mula bandha* with *tha-uddiyana bandha* in the form of nauli) allows superior control and manipulation of the spine, increased circulation of energy and information, as well as an increased absorption of nutrients and elimination of wastes.
- Sustained inhalation retention with *bandhas* (including *ha-mula bandha* with *ha-uddiyana bandha* which both increase internal pressure and compress the *prana* within the body) helps to increase the flow of oxygen to the cells via a type of mild autogenous hyperbaric oxygen therapy (Borg-Olivier and Machliss, 2007, in 'Integrative Medical Perspectives' edited by Professor Marc Cohen, AIMA) and increase internal strength and musculoskeletal stability.
- Once diet is regulated and the bandhas are understood then less breath is best for musculoskeletal stability, strength, internal cleansing, nourishment, communication and meditation.

CREATING THE BANDHAS AROUND EACH JOINT-COMPLEX (APCh 1, 2,4, 7 Appendix C)

- *Bandha* is defined as co-activation (simultaneous tensing) of antagonistic (opposing) muscle groups around a joint complex; *Bandhas* require multi-joint muscles and multi-joint complexes; *Bandhas* strengthen and stabilise joint-complexes; *Bandhas* help to move *prana* (energy) and *citta* (consciousness) through the *nadis* (subtle channels including nerves, blood vessels, lymph vessels and acupuncture meridians).
- **Ha-bandhas are compressive**, create heat and increase local pressure. They push energy and blood away from their region and reduce local blood flow.
- **Tha-bandhas are expansive**, decrease temperature and local pressure. They pull energy and blood away from their region and increase local blood flow.
- **There are many ways to generate bandhas at each of the nine main joint complexes**. The main ways are listed below with simple instructions to guide you in the posture.

Kulpha (ankle) *bandha* (APpp 178-186, 395-396)

Ha-kulpha bandha (This pushes the blood away from the feet and should mainly be used when the foot is on the floor).
- Grip (flex) the toes (like trying to make a closed fist).
- Lift the arches of the feet – mostly lift the outer feet.

Tha-kulpha bandha (This pulls the blood towards the feet and should mainly be used when the foot is off the floor).
- Spread (extend) the toes and push away with the ball of the foot (the base of the big toe).
- Pull the outer feet towards the knee.

Janu (knee) *bandha* (APpp 158-163, 396-397)

Ha-janu bandha (This restricts blood flow through the knee and should mainly be used when the knee is flexed in a squat-like posture e.g. the leg is weight-bearing onto the floor).
- Press into the front of the foot as if you are trying to straighten the knee (to tense in front of the knee).
- Press into the front of the foot as if you are trying to raise up the heel (to tense the back of the knee).

Ha-janu bandha (This restricts blood flow through the knee and should mainly be used with the knee flexed with a non weight-bearing leg).
- Tighten the back of the knee (like trying to the make a 'bulging biceps' at the elbow).
- If the foot or shin is touching something then try and straighten the knee against resistance.

Tha-janu bandha (This enhances blood flow through the knee and should mainly be used with the knee extended in a weight-bearing posture).
- Pull up the knee caps (in order to activate knee extensors).

- Try to bend the knee with knee caps still pulled up and/or press into the front of the foot (activate knee flexors).

Tha-janu bandha (This enhances blood flow through the knee and should mainly be used with the knee extended in a non-weight-bearing hip extended posture).

- Pull up the knee caps (in order to activate knee extensors).
- Turn the thigh inwards (in order to activate inner thigh muscles as hip internal rotators and hamstrings as hip extensors and knee flexors).

Kati (hip) *bandha* (mainly in standing or with the leg in the air) (APpp 134-142, 398-399)

Ha-kati bandha (This restricts blood flow through the hip and should mainly be used with the hip flexed, i.e. in thigh moving towards the front of the body, in standing or in the air).

- Stretch the mat with the feet from the hips (if the foot is on the floor) and try to turn the thigh outwards.
- OR press/move the heel inwards and press/move the front of the foot outwards (this is like trying to turn the thigh outwards, but effectively co-activates hip abductors and adductors).

Tha-kati bandha (This enhances blood flow through the hip and should mainly be used with hip extended, i.e. in thigh moving towards the back of the body, in standing or in the air).

- Stretch the mat with the feet from the hips (if the foot is on the floor) and try to turn the thigh inwards OR press/ move the heel outward and press/move the front of the foot inwards (this is like trying to turn the thigh inwards, but effectively co-activates hip abductors and adductors).

Kati (hip) *bandha* (for mainly on the floor). (APpp 134-142, 398-399)

Ha-kati bandha (This restricts blood flow through the hip and should mainly be used with hip flexed sitting on the floor).

- Try to press down with the feet and lift the inner thighs.
- Turn the thigh out (can be done by pressing/moving the heel inwards and pressing/moving the front of the foot outwards).

Tha-kati bandha (This enhances blood flow through the hip and should mainly be used with hip extended).

- Try to press thighs towards each other and press the buttocks cheeks together.
- Turn the thigh in (can be done by pressing/moving the heel outward and pressing/moving the front of the foot inwards).

Mula (lower trunk) bandha (APpp 207-209, 400-401)

Ha-mula bandha (This restricts blood flow through the lower trunk).

- Narrow and compress the waist (using the abdominal muscles).
- Grip the perineum then exhale fully and tighten the anus, abdominal and armpit muscles.
- Contract the diaphragm with or without an inhalation.
- Learn how to inhale using the diaphragm (abdominal breathing) while not letting the abdomen puff out and this will increase intra-abdominal pressure and add to the stability of the lumbar spine.

Tha-mula bandha (This enhances blood flow through the lower trunk).

- For straight spine postures, lunges and all simple forward bends and backward bending postures, activate the muscles at the front and back of the trunk and relax the sides of the trunk. This can be done by:
- Lifting or lengthening the spine
- Pushing the sitting bones down and forward and pull the middle back in and up (co-activate the rectus abdominis and the spinal extensors)
- Stretching the mat with the feet if standing with one leg in front of the other
- Pulling with the heels and pushing from the sitting bones if sitting
- Performing *Nauli* in any of these types of postures (co-activation the rectus abdominis and the spinal extensors while generating *tha-uddiyana bandha* on exhalation retention) (Figures 6a and 6b)
- For side bending postures, activate the left and right side of the trunk while remaining relaxed at the front and back of the trunk. This can be done by trying to stretch or squash your mat with your feet.
- For spinal twisting postures to the right side push forward from the right hip and left shoulder before, during and while releasing from a twist (conversely push from left hip and right shoulder for twists to the left side).
- These ways of activating tha-mula bandha are all enhanced by inhaling using the diaphragm (abdominal breathing).

Uddiyana (chest and upper back) bandha (APpp 208, 211, 402-403)

Ha-uddiyana bandha (This restricts blood flow through the upper trunk and is good to use during spinal bending

postures, i.e. use when bending forward, backward, sideways or twisting in order to stabilise the spine).
- Contract the lower rib cage and the rear kidney region inwards towards each other.
- Exhale fully (*ha-uddiyana bandha* is easiest to feel on safely performed forced exhalation).
- Equally round out the upper back then lift the collar bones so the front and the back of the chest are equally stretched.

Tha-uddiyana bandha (This enhances blood flow through the upper trunk and is safest to use in neutral spine postures).
- Expand the lower rib cage.
- Inhale to the chest or expand the chest as if you are inhaling (this can be done at any time of the breath cycle).
- Equally round out the upper back then lift the collar bones so the front and the back of the chest are equally expanded.

Jalandhara (neck & head) bandha (APpp 209-211, 404)

Ha-jalandhara bandha (This restricts blood flow through the neck).
- Move the head down and move the neck back.
- If you rotate the head to the right then move the right ear away from the right shoulder.

Tha-jalandhara bandha (This enhances blood flow through the neck).
- Move the head up and move the throat forwards.
- If you rotate the head to the right then move the right ear away from the right shoulder.

Amsa (shoulder) bandha (APpp 87-92, 405-406)

Generally to create *amsa* (shoulder) *bandha*, move or push the armpits in the direction they are facing and move the elbows in the opposite direction.

Ha-amsa bandha (This restricts blood flow through the shoulders and is best used when the shoulders are extended by the side of the body or abducted out to the sides).
- Push the shoulders down towards the hips and push the elbows away from the hips.

Ha-amsa bandha (This restricts blood flow through the shoulders and is best used when the shoulders are extended behind the body).
- Push the armpits towards each other and towards the spine, and push the elbows away from each other and away from the spine

Tha-amsa bandha (This enhances blood flow through the shoulders and is best used when the shoulders are flexed, i.e. arms above the head).
- Push the shoulders forward towards the chest and push the elbows backwards away from the chest.

Kurpara (elbow) bandha (APpp 112-113, 407)

Ha-kurpara bandha (This restricts blood flow through the elbows and is best used when the elbows are flexed).
- If the arm is not pulling or pushing then try and simultaneously tighten (bulge) the biceps and triceps brachii.
- If the arm is pushing to try and straighten (extend) the elbow then try to rotate the forearm outwards (elbow supination).
- If the arm is pulling to try and bend (flex) the elbow then try to rotate the forearm inwards (elbow pronation).

Tha-kurpara bandha (This enhances blood flow through the elbows and is best used when the elbows are extended).
- If the arm is not pulling or pushing then try and simultaneously tighten (bulge) the biceps and triceps brachii.
- If the arm is pushing to try and straighten (extend) the elbow then try to rotate the forearm outwards (elbow supination).
- If the arm is pulling to try and bend (flex) the elbow then try to rotate the forearm inwards (elbow pronation).

Mani (wrist) bandha (APpp 113-120, 408-409)

Ha-mani bandha (This pushes the blood away from the hand and should mainly be used when the hand is weight-bearing or grabbing something).
- Grip (flex) with the fingers and pull the back of the hand towards the wrist (extend the wrist), make a closed fist with the hand.
- In an open handed position try to make a tight closed fist with the hand.

Tha-mani bandha (This pulls the blood towards the feet and should mainly be used when the hand is not weight-bearing or grabbing something).
- Stretch (extend) the fingers and slightly pull the front of the hand towards the wrist (i.e. slightly extend the wrist) OR in a closed hand position try and stretch (extend) the fingers and slightly pull the front of the hand towards the wrist (i.e. slightly extend the wrist).

MEDITATIVE PRACTICE (APpp 277-284)

The benefits of a meditative practice including reduced needs for sleep and food and a greater ability to remain relaxed, pain-free and generally content are more accessible when you establish the following six things in each pose:

1. **Stillness:** Keep still when in a posture, move gracefully and smoothly while in motion.

2. **Length:** Use gentle versions of the 9 bandhas to keep length in the subtle channels (nadis) of energy (prana) and consciousness (citta) and stability in the joints.

3. **Softness**: Stay as soft as you can while not losing length and stability.

4. **Quietness:** Have quiet minimal breathing that is less through the lungs and more through the skin.

5. **Visualisation:** Maintain stillness in the eyes (dristhi). Maintain a visualisation of your body in the pose (a useful visualisation). In each static posture visualise each bandha and its related joint complex and mentally chant the associated words TOES, KNEE, HIPS, WAIST, CHEST, NECK, SHOULDERS, ELBOWS, FINGERS. VISUALISE each part to be STILL, LONG, and as SOFT as possible with QUIET breathing through the skin.

6. **Contentment:** Manifest or rediscover the natural state of inner bliss and contentment; i.e. having done your best (tapas) in a non violent and non-aggressive way (ahimsa), be happy for now with what you have done (santosa) in your practice and your life, and be happy with how you are now, where you are now and who you are.

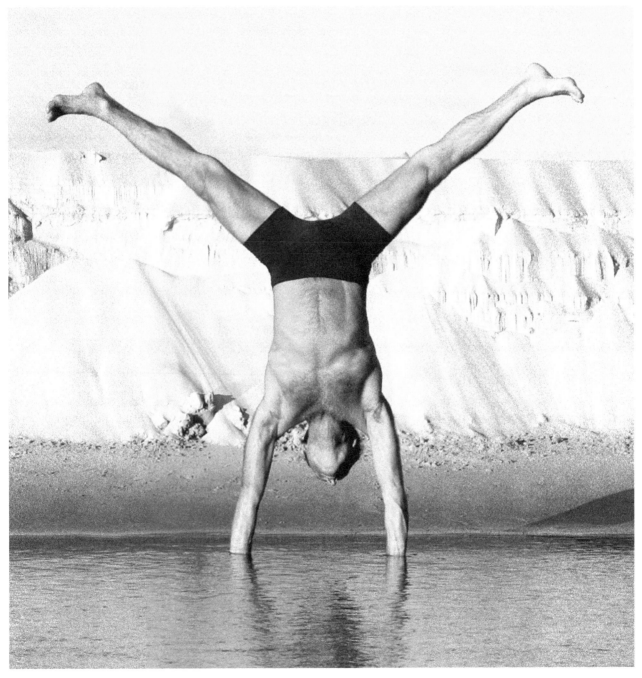

Simon Borg-Olivier in *Upavistha Kona Adho Mukha Vrksasana*. Photo courtesy Donatella Parisini.

TRADITIONAL *HATHA YOGA* WITH AN UNDERSTANDING FROM EXERCISE BASED PHYSIOTHERAPY

By Simon Borg-Olivier **MSc BAppSc (Physiotherapy)** and Bianca Machliss **BSc BAppSc (Physiotherapy)**, (adapted from a previously published magazine article)

YogaSynergy is traditional *hatha yoga* with an understanding from exercise based physiotherapy. This unique style of *yoga* is very fluid and dynamic and has been developed in Sydney since 1989 by Simon Borg-Olivier and Bianca Machliss. It incorporates all the postures seen in other popular *yoga*'s but also includes many novel postures and exercises that do not appear elsewhere. Although strength, flexibility and cardiovascular fitness can be by-products of practicing the **Yoga**Synergy style, they are not the main aim. The main aim of *yoga* is communication and the realisation that we are all connected. The main physical aim of **Yoga**Synergy is the enhancement of the flow of energy and information through the various channels of the body. When this is understood then a **Yoga**Synergy style practice can leave you energised yet calm, with a reduced need for food and sleep. In addition, because this system enhances the flow of information though the body it can be used to heal many injuries and illnesses, and can prevent many of the common *yoga*-based injuries from occurring.

The **Yoga**Synergy system has been developed over a 20 year period based on the teaching we have been lucky enough to receive from our *yoga* teachers, and our understanding of the theory and practice of the applied anatomy and physiology of *yoga* as research based scientists and physiotherapists. The **Yoga**Synergy system can be adapted to any system of physical exercise, but it is most easily applied in the five specific sequences designed and refined by **Yoga**Synergy over a 10 year period from 1989 to 1999. These specifically designed sequences are named after the elements earth, water, fire, air and ether. Each sequence is taught at seven levels ranging from beginner to advanced. Studies have shown that repetition is important for learning therefore, learning a set sequence is important, but because training is specific it is also important to vary the approach to learning something like a sequence of exercises. Each sequence is taught progressively over a nine week period and in each class, group level and circumstances such as weather, time of day and general energy at the time of the class is taken into account. **Yoga**Synergy encourages practitioners to approach their practice intelligently and use it as a tool to enhance their lives. One of the main methods of doing this is to have variations for each of the postures, ranging from a simple version to a more complex version. All practitioners are taught the simple versions and are encouraged to use those when they are not feeling 100% and thus are still able to practice. As a result many different versions of the basic form of any of the sequences are available and we have classes for people with many different types of bodies and levels of experience, enjoying their practice together.

It was never our intention to create a particular style of *yoga*. Initially we practiced the *yoga* we were taught by our main teachers Natanaga Zhander, Sri B.K.S Iyengar, Sri K. Pattabhi Jois and Sri T.V.K. Desikarchar. These great masters helped us greatly in our own path of *yoga*. However, after many years of practice and teaching we realised that we had missed something in our understanding of the body. So we both went back to university and studied to become physiotherapists. This dramatically changed the way we approached our *yoga* practice and teaching, and over the next few years a unique **Yoga**Synergy style began to emerge almost by itself.

The main features of this style of *yoga* are:

- Modification of traditional *yoga* postures and sequences to take account of the modern body and variations between practitioners.
- Gradation of postures with a personal choice ranging from simple (easy) to complex (hard) versions of each posture or sequence.
- Use of active movements to enter each pose.
- Use of resistance work during each pose.
- Use of co-activation (simultaneous tensing) of the muscles around the nine main joint complexes of the body in order to stabilise these joints.
- Use of seven circulatory pumps to aid in the movement of energy and information through the body.
- Use of special *mudras* (energy control gestures) that can tension (stretch) nerves and acupuncture meridians.
- Use of specific breath control to gradually reduce the amount of air required per minute in order to lessen the need for sleep and food, bring more oxygen to the brain and calm the nervous system.

1. Modification of traditional yoga postures and sequences to take account of the modern body and variations between practitioners

Traditional *hatha yoga* is taught with the assumption that those practicing it have traditional Indian bodies and/or are beginning *yoga* practice at a young age. Generally, in the modern world, where *yoga* has become very popular, this is not the case. In general, people living in India may very easily come to the squatting position, something they have been doing since they were children. Similarly, they can readily do the lotus position because of a lifetime of sitting cross-legged on the floor as opposed to sitting on chairs.

Many traditional *yoga* sequences place deep squats and full-lotus or half-lotus postures relatively early on in the sequence without allowing much time to warm up the hips, knees or ankles. These postures are not considered to be deep or difficult stretches for the traditional Indian body. Yet they are often the cause of injury and found quite difficult by most people, especially when starting *yoga* practice over the age of 20.

The **Yoga**Synergy system does not assume that the practitioner has natural flexibility. Postures are sequenced in such a way that one posture prepares the body for the postures to come after it. Each posture can also be modified to take into account the stiffness that tends to be prevalent in typical modern bodies.

2. Gradation of postures with a personal choice ranging from simple (easy) to complex (hard) versions of each posture or sequence

In the **Yoga**Synergy system each pose can be modified by each individual so that they can balance the needs of their body and their mind at that time. Flexibility in this system is to do with the mental flexibility to do each posture or exercise in such a way that it supports your current needs. Some examples include the following:
*   If the back of the legs are stiff when bending forward (Figure 1a), then simply bend the knees (Figure 1b). When a one legged balance is not possible simply come to the toe-tips of one leg.
*   If balancing on the hands is not possible then simply lean on the hands.

Figure 1a: *Hasta Uttanasana*

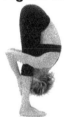

Figure 1b: *Sukha Hasta Uttanasana* (modified forward bend with bent knees)

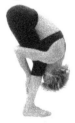

3. Use of active movements to enter each pose

One misconception of *yoga* is that it is all about stretching or relaxation. In fact, learning how to activate (tense) muscles and strengthen the body is as important as learning how to stretch and relax muscles. The **Yoga**Synergy system appreciates that to achieve the healthiest physical body as well as the best physical *yoga*, you need to have a controlled balance between strength and flexibility as well as the ability to relax. This brings consciousness and awareness throughout the whole body, which is an important aim in physical *yoga*.

Many problems can manifest in the body if it is forced to 'bend' too far or if you over-stretch ligaments. The **Yoga**Synergy system uses the 'active movement' approach in which you only take the body as far into a pose as it can go by itself without the aid of gravity. For example, instead of letting the body bend with gravity into a potentially damaging soft spined 'upward facing dog pose' (Figure 2a), one can simply lie on the abdomen and lift the chest and hands (Figure 2b). This forces the body to bend only as far as it is actively capable to bend while building strength at the same time. Using this approach in all the poses helps to simultaneously develop strength, flexibility, fitness and the ability to relax. Active movements are a necessary prerequisite of doing many advanced postures safely (e.g. Figures 3b, 4b and 5b).

Figure 2a: *Urdhva Mukha Svanasana* (upward facing dog pose)

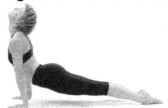

Figure 2a: *Sukha Urdhva Mukha Svanasana* (modified upward facing dog pose)

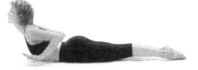

4. Use of resistance work during each pose

In **Yoga**Synergy, resistance can be applied in each position at each joint. If a muscle is tensed for a few seconds or more while it is being stretched, it not only strengthens the muscles involved, but also stretches them further and allows them to subsequently relax more easily.

For example, if you are doing a forward bending postures such as the simple cross-legged forward bend (Figure 3a) or the advanced lotus arm balance (Figure 3b), it is mainly the buttocks muscles that are being stretched. You can tense the buttocks by trying to press the feet towards the floor. This not only rapidly stretches, strengthens and subsequently relaxes the buttocks but can also help the health of the lower back.

Another example of how resistance can be used is the simple lunge posture (Figure 4a) which stretches the front of the groin. In the lunge you can tense the front of the groin while it is being stretched by trying to press the two feet together or by trying to 'squash the mat with your feet'. This action not only quickly stretches, strengthens and subsequently relaxes the front groin but can also help the health of the spine. Similar but more complicated processes can be applied in the 'advanced balancing lunge' shown in Figure 4b.

The use of active movements and resistance work in the **Yoga**Synergy style allow muscles to be trained through the full range of joint movement.

5. Use of co-activation (simultaneous tensing) of the muscles around the nine main joint complexes of the body in order to stabilise these joints

n recent times there has been a lot written about core stabilisation and its benefits for health of the lower back. Core stabilisation is essentially the same as the co-activation or simultaneous tensing of the muscles around the lower trunk. In *yoga* this is called *bandha* (internal lock). Most *yoga* only refers to three main *bandha*s but **Yoga**Synergy incorporates nine *bandha*s that are very effective at stabilising and strengthening the entire body. These *bandha*s are sometimes referred to as the 'yogi's suit of armour'. Understanding and applying the nine *bandha*s not only helps to fix spinal problems but also helps to fix problems of the ankles, knees, hips, shoulders, elbows and wrists.

6. Use of seven circulatory pumps to aid in the movement of energy and information through the body

The heart is thought of as the main circulatory pump of energy and information in the body, but in fact it is only effective in pumping the blood about a metre from the heart. There are six other pumps that are taken advantage of by the **Yoga**Synergy system to enhance circulation.

(1) The gravitational pump functions to improve circulation when posture is changed in the field of gravity.
(2) The musculoskeletal pump works to pump blood in the veins to the heart when muscles contract then

relax. This can be done either voluntarily or as you move in and out of postures.

(3) The respiratory pump works to enhance the flow of blood to the heart as the chest expands and then retards the flow of blood as the chest contracts.

(4) The postural pump works by physically compressing one part of the body and 'pushing' the blood further from that part, and by stretching another part of the body, which 'pulls' the blood towards that region.

(5) The co-activation (*bandha*) pump works to effectively move energy and information through the body at will because each of the *bandha*s have two opposing forms. There are positive or high pressure *bandha*s that push the energy away from a joint, and negative or low pressure *bandha*s that pull energy and information toward that joint. For example, a high pressure *bandha* can be made around the wrist by making a closed fist, which pushes energy away from the wrist, while a low pressure *bandha* can be made around the wrist by stretching the fingers, which pulls energy towards the wrist.

(6) The centripetal pump uses the circular motions of the bones around their joints to move blood (and energy and information) mainly to the extremities. The centripetal pump becomes more effective the faster the body moves.

7. Use of special *mudras* (energy control gestures) that can tension (stretch) nerves and acupuncture meridians

The **Yoga**Synergy system uses knowledge of the pathways of nerves and acupuncture meridians to tension (stretch) some nerves where appropriate, and lessen the tension (stretch) of other nerves that have been unintentionally and dangerously stretched. For example, opening the palms with the shoulders pushing towards the hips and rotating outwards (Figure 5a) tensions (stretches) the median nerve and the lung acupuncture meridian. Bending the elbow and taking the fingers to the shoulders tensions (stretches) the ulna nerve and the heart acupuncture meridian (Figure 5b).

Figure 5a: *Gadjasthana* (tensioning (stretching) the median nerve and the lung acupuncture meridian)

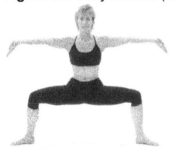

Figure 5b: *Niralamba Ardha Candrasana* (with the right hand tensioning (stretching) the ulnar nerve and the heart acupuncture meridian and the left hand tensioning the median nerve and pericardium meridian)

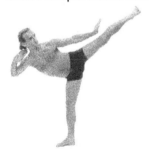

8. Use of specific breath control to gradually reduce the amount of air required per minute in order to lessen the need for sleep and food, bring more oxygen to the brain and calm the nervous system

While most exercise and *yoga* encourages hyperventilation (breathing more than you actually need) which stimulates the nervous system and encourages you to eat heavy food after practice, traditional *hatha yoga* as well as the **Yoga**Synergy system, encourages hypoventilation (breathing less than you think you need). **Yoga**Synergy generally encourages complete exhalations, which clears the lungs of stale air and helps to stabilise the spine, but inhalations are generally only small in order to retain the firmness of the spine and its internal pressure. While all movements of the chest and abdomen are important to practice, it is the ventilation (amount of air coming in and out of the lungs per minute) that has the most important physiological effects on the body. Reduced ventilation builds up carbon dioxide in the body. Carbon dioxide is not a poison as many people think, but is in fact a substance that helps to calm the nerves, expand the blood vessels, and reduce the need for sleep and food.

A flexible approach to your *yoga* practice

One of the most important features of **Yoga**Synergy is the flexible approach it adopts for each practice. The main guiding principles of **Yoga**Synergy come from the *Bhagavad Gita*, the ancient Indian poem contained in the classic Indian text the *Mahabharata*, and the *Patanjali Yoga Sutras*. Loosely translated these say 'Don't be attached to the fruits of your actions but rather be engaged in the actions themselves. Don't be attached to either success or failure, but don't be attached to laziness either. *Yoga* is this balance between doing your best (*tapas*) without being aggressive or violent in body or mind (*ahimsa*) and then being content with the outcome (*santosa*).' This means that each **Yoga**Synergy practice can be appropriate for your body here and now. Strong when you need strong practice. Soft when you need soft practice. Energising or calming as you need. The secret of flexibility has nothing to with the body. Flexibility is all about your mind!

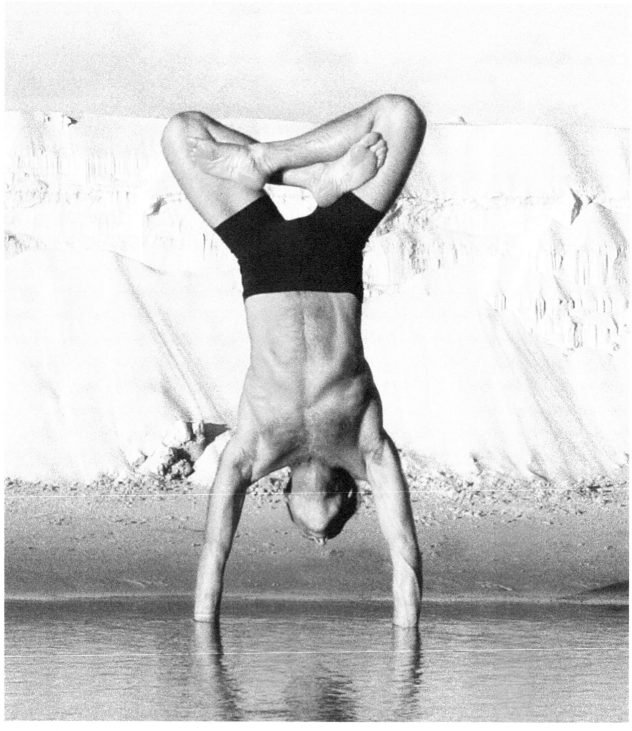

Simon Borg-Olivier *Padma Adho Mukha Vrksasana*. **Photo courtesy Donatella Parisini.**

DYNAMIC RELAXATION AND REJUVENATION

By Simon Borg-Olivier MSc BAppSc **(Physiotherapy)** and Bianca Machliss BSc BAppSc (Physiotherapy) (adapted from a previously published magazine article)

When practised correctly, physical *yoga* can simultaneously relax and rejuvenate you. A main aim of physical *yoga* is to develop the ability to effortlessly deal with life and its challenges so that life can always be experienced in a joyful manner. In this way you can achieve more quality and quantity in your life. The effects of this can then be shared with those around you. You can leave a more positive effect in your community and on the environment.

Relaxation is the opposite of stress or tension. Dictionaries define it as the aim of recreation and leisure activities. It is also when things that are perceived as difficult seem easier and even fun. To be fully effective relaxation addresses your muscles, nerves, brain and your emotions. *Yoga* can address relaxation by using simple techniques that regulate your muscles and nerves and help to direct the way you choose to think and feel.

Rejuvenation is defined as the process of feeling young again or creating beneficial changes. Young people and especially children are renowned for their high energy and vitality, and for having a positive approach to things in their life. *Yoga* uses simple techniques to generate energy and move it through the body. *Yoga* can increase circulation and improve health and vitality without needing to make the heart beat faster.

Tension uses excess energy
If your muscles are constantly tense rather than relaxed this takes energy and can make you feel very tired. A simple practical exercise can demonstrate this. The region between the shoulders and the neck is often hard and tense. Use your hands you to feel the tension in the muscles between your shoulder and your neck that usually comes from lifestyle patterns that include driving and sitting at computers all day. Then, use your hands to feel between your inside thighs, which are usually quite relaxed. Try and squeeze your thighs together and feel how much effort it takes to make your inner thighs as hard and tense as the region around your neck. Now imagine for a moment if you had to do that all day long. It would be exhausting! If you can become aware of releasing any unnecessary tension in the body you can save a lot of energy and not feel so tired.

Tension can block the flow of energy inside you
Often you do not feel energetic simply because excess tension in your muscles physically compresses your blood vessels and other channels preventing blood and energy from moving inside you. In other words, you may have plenty of energy in your chest but if your abdominal muscles are too tense then your legs will feel tired because the flow of your energy was blocked in your abdomen. Therefore, simply learning how to relax can make a big difference to the way you feel on an energetic level.

Yoga teaches you a way of doing stressful things while being relaxed
While there is definite benefit in lying down and being totally relaxed for a period most people do something like that every night in bed. In addition, lying down is not what you can just do any time of the day or night while you are supposed to be working. What you really need is the ability to do stressful things and be relaxed and effortless in doing them. So you can think of a physical *yoga* practice as learning to be relaxed while putting yourself into a set of artificially induced semi-stressful situations in a controlled environment. This can then become a model for your everyday life. For example, if your family or work life is getting really stressful because there so many things to be done and so many things happening at the same time you can't just lie down and relax for a while. That usually is not received well with the people around you that you are supposed to be helping. It is much better to learn how to be relaxed while doing stressful things. At its simplest level *yoga* can teach you this.

Correct *yoga* is active relaxation that rejuvenates you
In *yoga* the synergy between relaxation and the flow of energy within you (your sense of rejuvenation) is enhanced if you can consciously choose where and when to tense and relax. Specific voluntary muscle

activation can result in precise relaxation. Energy naturally flows from tension to relaxation, from hot to cold and from high pressure to low pressure. By selectively tensing only certain parts of your body, you can create regions of high and low pressure. In this way, *yoga* can help in both relaxation and the flow of energy (rejuvenation) at the same time. Practically, this is done in the following five main ways which are elaborated below:

(1) Breathing into the abdomen (diaphragmatic breathing) in order to stimulate that part of the autonomic or automatic nervous system that keeps you calm.

(2) Tensing shortened muscles on one side of a joint in order to automatically relax the lengthened (stretched) muscles on the opposing side of the joint.

(3) Tensing lengthened (stretched) muscles in order to subsequently relax them.

(4) Activating all the muscles around one particular part of the body in order to subsequently reduce blood pressure and make you more relaxed.

(5) Focusing and concentrating the mind, which can quieten the brain and calm the whole body.

1. Abdominal (diaphragmatic) breathing stimulates relaxation and rejuvenation

Breathing into your abdomen, which is actually breathing using your diaphragm, is the most natural way to breathe. Your diaphragm is arguably the most used and most important muscle in the body. Your diaphragm is a large dome shaped muscle that sits across the width of the body at the base of your ribs. Diaphragmatic breathing is also called abdominal breathing because when you in inhale with your diaphragm you can feel the pressure in your abdomen increasing and the abdomen trying to push outwards. Increased use of your diaphragm stimulates the parasympathetic nervous system (PNS), which is that part of your automatic (autonomic) nervous system that keeps you calm. The PNS slows your heart and helps to relax you. This also helps with rejuvenation because it enhances your ability to digest food, absorb food and eliminate waste. This means you can eat less and still be satisfied and nourished. Using your diaphragm as the main muscle of breathing also stimulates the reproductive system and helps to improve your sexual organ function. At times of stress the diaphragm is used less and breathing tends to take place more from the expansion and contraction of the rib cage. This tends to increase heart rate and the amount of air you breathe. It also stimulates the sympathetic nervous system, which is that part of your nervous system which makes you prepared for 'flight or fight'. In other words it makes your body think there is danger around you that you may have to quickly run away from ('flight') or an enemy who is about to attack you and you may have to fight. In such situations your body is not resting or gathering energy (i.e. it is not rejuvenating), instead it is running on 'nervous energy' and using stored energy. Many people are so stressed that they are always like this. Breathing with your diaphragm keeps you calm and relaxed, and allows your body to absorb food, gather energy and rejuvenate.

If your abdominal wall is held firm with some of the abdominal muscles then the diaphragmatic breathing can actually make your spine more stable and allow you greater strength. When the abdomen is toned (kept gently firm with everyday movements and other activities) the increase in abdominal pressure induced by diaphragmatic breathing magnifies the energy stored in your lower trunk. In many eastern exercises, including Indian *hatha yoga* and Chinese Taoist *yoga* (Chi Kung), the lower abdomen and its enhancement intra-abdominal pressure due to diaphragmatic breathing is considered to be your most important source of strength, energy, relaxation and rejuvenation.

2. Tensing one muscle can relax its opposite partner

This process takes advantage of a spinal reflex and can be effectively applied in any part of the body. For example, if you consciously tense the muscles under your armpit by pushing the shoulders towards the hips, then the opposing muscles above the shoulder, that also connect to the neck, can be automatically relaxed. When you do this it instantly frees the circulation of energy and information between the head and the rest of the body, thus helping you to feel rejuvenated. A similar effect can be seen in the lunge like exercise designed to lengthen (stretch) the front of your hip (the front groin) (Figure 4a) and in the Upward facing dog pose (Figure 2a), which can be thought of as a double legged lunge. By making a voluntary activation of the buttocks muscles behind the hip joint, the muscles at the front of the hip around the groin will automatically relax. This not only relieves a lot of back pain, but it also enhances the flow of energy and information through the important channels at the front of the hip such as the femoral artery, the femoral nerve and the stomach acupuncture meridian.

454

This principal of reciprocal relaxation can also be used in the spine. If you can tense only the muscles on the left side of the spine then the right side of spine can automatically relax (Figure 5b). This can be especially useful when bending the spine sideways. Similarly, in certain situations voluntary tension of the muscles at the front of the spine can cause the muscles at the back of the spine to relax. In other situations, voluntary tension at the rear of the spine can cause the muscles at the front of the spine to relax. However, the only way that this process can work in the region of the trunk and the spine, is when the deep abdominal muscles used in complete exhalation are not functioning. The three deepest layers of abdominal muscles are circumferential in nature. That is, they go all around the lower trunk like a belt. Therefore, if they are active then the front, back and sides of the spine will be always active. These muscles can be inhibited to a certain extent with diaphragmatic (abdominal) breathing. Then it is possible to tense one part of the spine in order to relax the opposite part of spine. Energy and information will move from the region of the active (tense) compressed part of the spine to the relaxed lengthened part of the spine. In this way a dynamic periodic relaxation and ongoing rejuvenation then becomes possible within the spine.

3. Tensing a stretched muscle can later relax it

If you lengthen or stretch any muscle for long enough, say at least 30 seconds in most cases, then it will subsequently automatically relax. This is one reason why stretching exercises are generally felt to be relaxing. This reflex relaxation can be made more rapid if you tense a muscle while it is stretched or in a lengthened state. This also has the effect of changing the local pressure, which causes increased blood flow and helps you to feel more rejuvenated.

4. Tensing muscles around one part of the body can later reduce blood pressure and calm you

High blood pressure is often associated with stress. A significant reduction in blood pressure and an overall feeling of relaxation can be obtained by carefully tensing part or all of the body in a controlled way, and ideally with a specific breathing pattern. Voluntary tension, especially in conjunction with appropriate breathing, artificially 'tricks' your body into thinking that blood pressure has increased even more. Your body will then respond with a reflex that reduces your blood pressure. This can leave you feeling more relaxed and rejuvenated.

5. Concentration can help to rest and relax the mind

Often we can feel stressed due to too many thoughts going on in our minds. Exercises that involve concentration such as physical *yoga* and meditation have been shown to relieve stress and bring about relaxation presumably because they help you to focus your mind on one thing at once, rather than having many things going on at the same time. Studies have also shown that when you concentrate on a particular part of the body the flow of blood increases to that area and that region becomes rejuvenated. Therefore, concentration can enhance relaxation and rejuvenation.

All of the exercises described above involve various levels of concentration. The act of concentration can be applied to all of the principles that help in relaxation and rejuvenation. *Yoga* can help you to actively relax by breathing with your diaphragm, or by tensing one or more muscles around a joint. This process of active relaxation gives tremendous assistance to the process of moving energy and information through your body. Circulation is enhanced yet the heart and lungs can stay relatively rested. In this way you can be left with an exhilarating feeling of rest and rejuvenation.

THE RELATIONSHIP BETWEEN BREATH-CONTROL *(PRANAYAMA)* AND THE CONCEPT OF CORE STABILISATION FOR THE WHOLE BODY *(BANDHA)* IN *YOGA* AND EXERCISE

By Simon Borg-Olivier MSc BAppSc(Physiotherapy) and Bianca Machliss BSc BAppSc(Physiotherapy) (adapted from a chapter in 'Integrative Medical Perspectives' (2007) edited by Professor Marc Cohen)

Introduction

The ultimate goal of *yoga* (which means union) is the realisation that the individual's consciousness is one with the universe's consciousness. This is a very lofty goal for most of us. A more achievable and practical goal in the short term is to maximise the effectiveness of the connections between the brain and the body. *Hatha yoga* is the physical form of the ancient Indian science of *yoga* that helps to achieve the union of brain and body by augmenting the circulation of energy (*prana*) and information (*citta*) through the circulatory channels (*nadis*) of the body thus enhancing health, vitality and recovery from injury.

The word *hatha* literally means force. *Hatha yoga* uses physical exercises and breath-control (*pranayama*) to generate pressure forces within the body that aid in circulation. To achieve this it helps to have control of the muscles and joints of the body, as well as a practical understanding of the physiology of breathing. In this paper we describe the use of spinal reflexes in creating four states of muscle activation/ relaxation around the major joint complexes. We present a practical application of musculoskeletal anatomy and cardiopulmonary physiology that can enhance a *hatha yoga* practice and any physical exercise by improving joint stability, strength, flexibility, fitness, energy, relaxation, meditation and ability to heal injuries. We also describe how musculoskeletal control in the form of muscular co-activation around the major joint complexes, referred to as *bandha* in *hatha yoga,* can be used in traditional *yogic* breathing (*pranayama*) to increase the life-force (*prana*) of the cells with hypoventilation and autogenous hyperbaric oxygenation.

Musculoskeletal control

One misconception of *yoga* is that it is all about stretching or relaxation however activating and strengthening the body is just as important. To achieve the healthiest physical body as well as perform *hatha yoga* you need to have a controlled balance between strength and flexibility as well as the ability to relax.

There are more than 200 joints and more than 600 named muscles in the body. To get a simplified but functional understanding of the body it helps to think of the body in terms of nine main joint complexes that work together in the body and behave as one joint and about 20 pairs of opposing muscle groups. The nine major joint-complexes in the body are the ankles, knees, hips, lower back, upper back, neck, shoulders, elbows and wrists.

This simplified yet practical approach to musculoskeletal anatomy is often used by physiotherapists. For example, the knee is a complicated structure made up of 2 main joints and 16 muscles but it can be practically thought of as one knee joint-complex with one pair of opposing muscle groups, the knee flexors and the knee extensors.

To practise *hatha yoga* with a balance between strength and flexibility it is useful to consider three spinal reflexes. These are the myotatic (stretch) reflex, the reciprocal relaxation reflex and the inverse myotatic (relaxation) reflex.

The stretch (myotatic) reflex

This reflex causes activation of the antagonist (the lengthened muscle group) if it is suddenly stretched. Therefore, it is beneficial to try and inhibit this reflex while trying to stretch a muscle. The stretch reflex can be inhibited by:
- mentally focusing on the muscle group being stretched
- exhaling as you stretch
- moving slowly into a stretch
- using the agonist (the shortened muscle group) to actively move the joint complex into the stretched position (which causes reflex reciprocal relaxation - see below).

The stretch reflex can be useful when trying to activate muscles that are otherwise hard to activate. If you activate a muscle that is joined to or is physically close to a second muscle, the second muscle can become activated because of fascial connections which pull on and lightly stretch the second muscle. This is a process that helps in the co-activation of opposing muscle groups (*bandha*) for enhancing joint stability.

For example, it is sometimes difficult for people to activate the abdominal muscles. If you first activate the Latissimus dorsi by trying to pull the shoulders towards the hips, this tensions connective tissue attachments to abdominal muscles such as transversus abdominis and obliquus externus and makes the abdominal muscles much easier to activate (Figure 6c).

The reciprocal relaxation reflex

The reciprocal relaxation reflex causes the antagonist muscle group to relax when the agonist is activated. This reflex can be employed to help you to relax and/or stretch any part of your body. It is most easily utilised by entering a posture in an active manner, i.e. by activating the agonist to enter the pose.

Stiffness in the knee flexors (e.g. hamstring muscles) is usually eased by activating knee extensors (quadriceps). This can be done in a straight-legged forward bending position by simply 'pulling up the knee caps' or 'tensing the front of the thighs' (Figure 1a). This principle is also very useful to apply if there is tension or pain in any part of the body. A tense or painful part of the body can often be relieved by tensing the opposite part of that joint complex – for example, pain or stiffness in the inner thigh or hip can often be relieved by tensing the outer thigh or hip. Similarly, pain in the muscles that normally pull the shoulders up towards the ears (muscles on the side of the neck) can often be relieved by actively trying to pull the shoulders towards the hips (Figures 2a, 6a,6b and 6c).

The inverse myotatic (relaxation) reflex

The inverse myotatic reflex causes the antagonist to relax if it is stretched a sufficient amount. This is termed the 'relaxation reflex' or the 'lengthening reaction' and usually takes place after a minimum of 12 – 15 seconds. However, if the muscle is activated for a few seconds or more while it is being stretched, the relaxation reflex can take place within a few seconds. So if you activate the antagonist (the lengthened muscle group) it not only strengthens the muscles involved, but also stretches them further and allows them to subsequently relax more easily.

For example, if you are doing a forward bending posture such as cross-legged forward bend (Figures 3a and 3b); it is mainly the hip extensors (buttocks muscles) that are being stretched. To rapidly get the effects of the inverse myotatic (relaxation) reflex in this posture, you can choose to either tense the buttocks muscles (Gluteus maximus) or activate the hip extensor group by trying to extend the hip from a flexed hip position. In the cross-legged forward bend this is practically achieved by trying to press the feet into the floor.

Another example of a position where the relaxation reflex can be used is the lunge or hip flexor stretch (Figure 4a). In the lunge you can activate the hip flexors while they are being stretched by trying to press the two feet together or by trying to 'squash the mat with your feet'. This action stimulates the relaxation reflex by helping to stretch the hip flexors quickly and effectively, whilst also strengthening them. Later, it also allows them to relax more easily. Similar processes can be applied in the 'advanced balancing lunge' shown in Figure 4b.

Balancing force provides stability

The techniques of *hatha yoga* eventually allow you to control each muscle enough to be able to activate or relax it at will throughout the range of motion of the joint or joints which each muscle crosses. As we age it is common that some parts of our body become more flexible and less stable while other parts are rarely moved and become relatively stiff. *Yoga* (which can mean 'balance') aims to equalise the forces around each of the main joint complexes in the body by getting opposing muscle groups into a state of balance. These forces can result from either passive or active muscle tension. Passive muscle tension (stiffness) is especially noticeable when a muscle is lengthened. Active muscle tension can be voluntary or involuntary and can happen with a muscle in either a shortened or lengthened state.

Depending on the situation at each joint complex, a *yoga* practitioner can choose to either tense or relax either agonist or antagonist muscle groups. There are four possible states for opposing muscle groups around a joint and at the simplest level the adept *yoga* practitioner can balance the forces around a joint by adopting any one of four states of activation or relaxation. Each of these four states has advantages and disadvantages that make them more or less appropriate.

State 1: Relaxed agonist and antagonist muscle groups: The agonist and the antagonist can both be relaxed. This requires minimal physical effort but usually causes resistance from the stretched muscle due to the stretch-reflex causing muscle tension in the antagonist muscle and does not offer any additional stabilisation to the joint complex.

In certain situations, such as when there is a muscle spasm, it is appropriate to let both opposing muscle groups be completely relaxed and to safely hold each stretch long enough, for the stretch reflex to be over-ridden by the relaxation reflex. This state takes minimal effort and allows the mind to relax as well as the body.

State 2: Agonist muscle group activation: The agonist can be activated and the antagonist can remain relaxed. This helps to strengthen the agonist and stimulates reciprocal reflex relaxation and lengthening of the antagonist whilst the agonist is being strengthened in a shortened state. Pain in the region of the antagonist may also be relieved by agonist activation.

State 3: Antagonist muscle group activation: The antagonist can be activated and the agonist can remain relaxed. This helps to strengthen the antagonist in a lengthened position and stimulates the inverse myotatic (relaxation) reflex, leading to an increase in the stretch and subsequent increase in the ability of the antagonist to relax. This can also stimulate the reciprocal relaxation reflex in the agonist muscle group, helping it to relax and alleviate any unwanted and sometimes pain-producing tension.

Tense or very stiff muscles, which may elicit joint pain, can often be relaxed by actively tensing them when they are in a lengthened state. This can be enhanced if the muscle is further stretched by physically pressing on various parts of the muscle which can be done with various acupressure or massage techniques or using other parts of the body such as in certain *yoga* postures.

State 4: Co-activation of agonist and antagonist muscle groups: Co-activation of the agonist and the antagonist gives stability to the joint, helps to regulate circulation and helps to improve strength, flexibility and the subsequent ability to relax all the muscles involved. Co-activation has been shown to only be possible around joint complexes as opposed to individual joints, and only with multi-joint muscles as opposed to single joint muscles [1].

Bandha – muscular co-activation around a joint complex

In *hatha yoga* co-activation around a joint complex is referred to as a *bandha*. Studies on spinal stability have demonstrated that a joint-stabilising effect from the co-activation of opposing muscles around the lumbar spine [2] can reduce the risk of lumbar spinal injury and help to minimise lower back pain. In *hatha yoga* co-activation around the lumbar spine is called *mula bandha*.

Recent studies have demonstrated that co-activation happens spontaneously around most of the major joint complexes of a healthy person in everyday life. The joint-stabilising effect of co-activation is discussed in studies on the ankle [3], knee [4], shoulder [5], elbow [6], and wrist [7]. The concept of a *bandha* as muscular co-activation around a joint complex can be generalised throughout the body. *Hatha yoga* can generate *bandhas* around the nine major joint complexes that serve to improve stability, strength, flexibility and circulation [8]. If a weak region of a joint complex is not supported by some muscular co-activation when moved to an extreme ('stretched') position, its weakest part will be at risk of damage.

Further research has shown that during co-activation there is a significant interaction with the nervous system [9; 4;10]; but the details of this interaction are yet to be fully elucidated. In some cases a *bandha* may result in the activation of all three nerve reflexes mentioned above. However, since co-activation is sometimes under voluntary control, all the nerve reflexes may be inhibited. The concept of *yoga* as union can also be seen to be reflected in the spinal reflex system uniting the body (muscles) with the brain (central nervous system).

Bandhas pressure and circulation

Bandhas around each of the nine major joint complexes can be generated in many ways. Most bandhas in the body are formed as co-activations of opposing muscles around joint complexes, but some of the spinal bandhas are formed by circumferential co-activation of muscles that go all the way around the spinal joint complexes. These include the diaphragm, transversus abdominis, abdominal oblique muscles and the intercostals muscles. Each bandha can be used to generate high pressure (referred to as a ha-bandha) that 'pushes' blood and energy away from that region, or low pressure (referred to as a tha-bandha), that 'pulls' blood and energy towards that region.

For example, the co-activation of opposing muscle groups around the wrist can generate high pressure (ha-mani bandha) by activating the multi-joint muscle groups, wrist extensors and finger flexors (which include wrist flexors) to try and make a closed fist; or low pressure (tha-mani bandha) by activating wrist flexors and finger extensors (which include wrist extensors) to try and make a stretched open palm. Similarly, circumferential muscular co-activation around the thorax can generate high pressure (ha-uddiyana bandha) by activating muscles of forced thoracic exhalation, which compresses the thorax and 'pushes' blood and energy away from that region and air out the lungs, thus increasing intra-thoracic pressure (ITP); or low pressure (tha-uddiyana bandha) by activating muscles of forced thoracic inhalation, which expands the thorax and 'pulls' blood and energy away from that region and air into the lungs, thus decreasing ITP.

In hatha yoga when tha-uddiyana bandha is performed without any air in the lungs it can create a powerful negative pressure effect, similar to that produced in a Mueller manoeuvre that can be used to manipulate internal organs and the spine. It also forms the basis of many advanced yoga processes (kriyas) such as nauli which incorporates a flexor-extensor co-activation of the lumbar spine (tha-mula bandha) (Figures 6a, 6b). When ha-uddiyana bandha is carefully performed with air in the lungs it increases pressure within the body in the same way as a Valsalva manoeuvre. This can cause changes in blood pressure, circulation, an increase in oxygen saturation [11] and decrease in levels of pain [12].

The hatha yoga texts say that when this is performed with pranayama in conjunction with other bandhas there is a very powerful pressure increasing effect on the body that can compress the air and the prana (life force) contained within it, and force it into the cells in a manner similar to hyperbaric oxygenation therapy [13].

Bandhas, breathing and cardiopulmonary physiology

Spinal bandhas are very important for breathing, especially deep or forced breathing and for changing pressure inside the trunk. Three special types of muscles, the diaphragm, transversus abdominis and the intercostals, can by their nature individually cause a type of circumferential co-activation around the spine during diaphragmatic inhalation, forced abdominal exhalation and forced thoracic breathing respectively. Both thoracic inhalation and forced thoracic exhalation require circumferential co-activation around the thorax, which is referred to in yoga as uddiyana bandha (Figures 6a, 6b and 6c).

Mula bandha via co-activation of opposing muscles

Muscular co-activation around the lumbar spine (referred to in yoga as mula bandha) can be expressed in two distinct ways and can work separately or together. The first type of mula bandha is generated via co-activation of opposing muscles, and the second type is generated via increasing intra-abdominal pressure (IAP) due to circumferential muscular co-activation.

The first type of mula bandha involves co-activation of antagonistic flexor–extensor pairs around the lumbar spine and has been shown to have a stabilising effect on the lumbar spine [2; 14]. Co-activation of trunk flexor and extensor muscles is present around a neutral spine posture in healthy individuals. It is enhanced when a person sits up straight. It is very pronounced if someone leans forward onto the front of their feet with shoulders forward and their arms up into the air. This is a type of expansive co-activation which can be referred to as *tha-mula bandha*. It gives the spine stability with mobility, and allows the spine to lengthen with energy (heat, blood etc.) to freely flow through the trunk. This co-activation is seen to increase as weight is added to the body, and is believed to be part of a neuromuscular system that provides mechanical stability to the lumbar spine [14].

Voluntary generation of *tha-mula bandha* by co-activation of antagonistic (opposing) muscle groups can be achieved in three main ways. Each of these involves making resisted attempts at trying to move two separate parts of the spine in opposite directions at the same time, in any of the three primary movement planes of the spine i.e. flexion–extension, right axial rotation–left axial rotation and right lateral flexion–left lateral flexion.

Mula bandha to increase intra-abdominal and intra-thoracic pressure

A second method that allows a *mula bandha* to give stability and strength to the lower trunk in *yoga* is via the use of intra-abdominal pressure (IAP), which is primarily generated by the transverses abdominis [15] but also by obliquus externus abdominis and obliquus internus abdominis. IAP is supplemented by the effects of other muscles including the diaphragm which exerts a positive pressure on the abdomen when it is active [16]. IAP can be further enhanced by compressing the chest with a circumferential muscular co-activation, like that used for forced expiration (*ha-uddiyana bandha*) [17].

This mechanism can increase spinal stability without the additional co-activation of specific spinal extensors and spinal flexors. Voluntary generation of *mula bandha* via the use of IAP and ITP can be achieved in three main ways:

1. **By making a forced expiration** that compresses the waist and the chest.
2. **By the Valsalva manoeuvre.** This is done by breathing in about half to three quarters of the lungs, holding the breath in, and then carefully tensing the abdomen as if you are exhaling, but not exhaling. It is not appropriate for many people with blood pressure problems, and for many others, and should not be attempted unless under supervision.
3. **By co-activating the diaphragm with some or all of the abdominal muscles.** This is the most powerful, effective and relaxing way to make *mula bandha*. When mastered, it is relatively easy to lift up to a handstand while inhaling with your diaphragm. The diaphragm serves to increase intra-abdominal pressure as well as calm the nervous system. However, it can be difficult to achieve because it is also a type of co-activation of opposing muscles on another level. It is the co-activation of the main muscle of inhalation, the diaphragm, with the main muscles of forced exhalation, the abdominal muscles. For most people, this is very difficult to achieve because activation of the diaphragm generally causes reciprocal relaxation of the abdominal muscles and vice versa.

Increasing IAP and ITP can be performed during *pranayama* [18] which can also be incorporated in the physical exercises of *hatha yoga*. This method of generating circumferential co-activation can be extremely effective in stabilising the spine. It is also able to manifest tremendous amounts of energy, which can be used to heat the body, and to generate the sort of strength required to do many of the arm balancing postures and other exercises where much physical power is required. However, if the body is not adequately prepared, and/or if this *pranayama* is not properly performed, this *pranayama* can be extremely dangerous.

This method should not be attempted with fully inflated lungs unless instructed by an experienced teacher, and only after the body has been strengthened by years of regular practice of *hatha yoga* with *bandhas* and *pranayama*. When IAP and ITP are increased while maintaining an internal breath retention (i.e. holding the breath in), the increase in pressure is able to move energy through the body with great force. *Hatha yoga* masters and others (such as the *Shaolin* monks) have used this method in many public demonstrations over the years to demonstrate great feats of strength, imperviousness to being pierced by sharp objects such as spears, and the ability to stop the heart. A lot of power can be generated when this technique is mastered, but must be contained in a safe way. You have to have a good practical understanding of all the other *bandhas* of the body. If the pressure generated inside the body is not adequately contained there is a risk of rupturing blood vessels that can lead to paralysis, heart attack or stroke, depending on where the rupture takes place. Medical literature contains several references to *yoga* practitioners being injured after practising *hatha yoga* with *bandhas* and *pranayama* [19, 20, 21].

A mild, gentle form of this method of increasing IAP with breath retention can be safely practised if one only inhales one quarter to one third of the full volume of the lungs and then makes only a gentle compression of the abdomen. This can be attempted by people with some experience of *hatha yoga* with *pranayama,* but the effects should be constantly monitored and the practice temporarily or permanently discontinued if headache or other symptoms of high blood pressure are observed.

The effects of *pranayama* on cardiopulmonary physiology

Much debate exists as to what is the most appropriate type of breathing to encourage in *hatha yoga*. Initially *hatha yoga* and *pranayama* were not designed to be given as a therapy for sick people, but rather were a means of achieving extreme psycho-physiological states for the purpose of meditation and to access higher levels of consciousness. However, in modern times, *yoga* in the west is used by a large number of people who have significant physical, physiological and emotional problems that have to be addressed before they can begin to practice the higher levels of *hatha yoga* and especially the breath-control involved in *pranayama*.

Every type of breathing will have some physiological effect and so every type of breathing may be appropriate to use in certain circumstances for certain people. For example, there are pros and cons of hyperventilation versus hypoventilation, deep breathing versus shallow breathing, abdominal breathing versus thoracic breathing, and slow breathing versus fast breathing (See Tables 8.1 and 8.2 in chapter 8). In some situations, such as lying supine, when one is feeling stressed, it may be suitable to do slow relaxed abdominal breathing, but relaxed abdominal breathing is generally not safe if someone is doing exercises that put tensile or compressive forces on the spine. For most people the best and safest type of breathing to do while practising *hatha yoga* or other exercise (especially when there are tensile or compressive forces on the spine) is their own natural breathing while maintaining a muscular co-activation around the spine in the form of the spinal *bandhas*. Once the exercises become easy enough to not pose a threat to musculoskeletal stability then it may be appropriate to begin to regulate the breath with *pranayama*.

Adequate oxygenation of the cells is important to optimum health. Therefore, many people think that *yoga* is concerned with how to breathe more, but actually it is the art of learning how to breathe less while still getting better oxygenation of the cells. The *yogic* science of breathing is termed *pranayama*. *Prana* has been described as the life-force or subtle energy in the air that we breathe. *Prana* is not actually the breath, but it has something to do with the way we breathe and what happens to the air that we take in. *Ayama* means to control, to regulate, to cease or to extend [22]. Therefore, the art and science of *pranayama* is ultimately not about breathing more air, but actually learning to breathe less air over a longer space of time and learning how to make the most effective use of every bit of air that we breathe in and the *prana* we absorb. Like a car that is considered to be more efficient when it runs just as far on less fuel, the human body eventually works better on less fuel (air).

*Bandha*s and breathing during exercising

In *hatha yoga* texts it is frequently stated that the spinal *bandhas* should be maintained throughout the *yoga* practice. The spinal *bandhas* are physically the muscular co-activation around the lumbar, thoracic and cervical spine, and are referred to as *mula, uddiyana* and *jalandhara bandha* respectively. All of the *bandhas* have the possibility of either being compressive or expansive in nature.

In order to protect the spine and maintain a safe and effective practice of *yoga* and other physical exercises that place compressive or tensile forces on the spine, *mula bandha* and *uddiyana bandha* should both be compressive co-activations. If these *bandhas* are maintained throughout the breath cycle then each exhalation is a full exhalation, which doesn't allow the chest to reduce its volume while each inhalation maintains its narrow girth but doesn't allow the chest to expand any further. Hence, the amount of air that is taken in to fill the lungs during each inhalation is no more than the tidal volume of a few hundred millilitres. This in precisely in line with the definition of *pranayama*, which is defined to be a state of reduced breathing (hypoventilation), but contradicts the way that many people practice and teach *yoga* and other exercise. In this type of breathing the diaphragm is active and contracts on inhalation but abdominal muscle activation prevents the usual outward movement of the abdomen and instead causes a further increase in IAP.

Hatha yoga with *pranayama* and *bandhas* uses long slow breathing with or without internal and external breath retentions to induce hypoventilation. By retaining less air for a longer period of time, carbon dioxide concentrations in the blood are increased. Carbon dioxide acts as a vasodilator of the blood vessels going to the brain. An increase in carbon dioxide in the blood causes an increase in the amount of blood and *prana* (life force or energy) flowing to the brain. Similarly, carbon dioxide is a bronchodilator. Therefore, an increase in carbon dioxide will also cause an increase in the amount of air and *prana* going to the lungs. Also, because of the Bohr Effect there is an increased transfer of oxygen from haemoglobin to tissue cells. The Bohr Effect states that an increase in acidity decreases the affinity of haemoglobin for oxygen. Hence, in the presence of carbon dioxide, which dissolves to become carbonic acid, haemoglobin will release its bound oxygen to the surrounding tissues, but in the absence of carbon dioxide and carbonic acid (as in situations such as hyperventilation) haemoglobin binds its oxygen tightly and does not release it to the surrounding tissues.

Pranayama as it is taught in the west today so often involves hyperventilation that many people are unaware that in fact the aim is to progressively learn to hypoventilate. To illustrate this it is interesting to note that *yoga* was introduced to China about 500 CE and developed into *Taoist yoga*. *Taoist yoga* is used by Shaolin monks to tone and flex their bodies, to gather *qi* energy (qi or *chi* in *Taoist yoga* is the equivalent of *prana* in *hatha yoga*), and to prepare for meditation. In *Taoist* training, the breath has four levels:
1. Windy-breath is noisy and usually present upon physical exertion.
2. Raspy-breath can be heard by others and is usually due to disturbed emotions or sickness.
3. *Qi*-breath is so quiet that one cannot even hear one's own breath.
4. Resting-breath is the ultimate *Qi-gong* state of breathing when one cannot tell whether one is breathing or not [23].

The contemporary *Taoist yoga* master Sat Chuen Hon [24] writes of breathing in *Taoist yoga* in exactly the same terms that breathing is described in the ancient Indian texts.
"It is only when one achieves the level of breathing of total smoothness of resting-breath that one can consider to have really attained the beginning level of Qi-gong practice … very few practitioners can practice with Qi-breath and only a few great masters have demonstrated the ability to maintain a flowing state of resting-breath while practising Tai-ji or Qi-gong forms. One experiences resting-breath more readily when doing seated meditation. Once one has reached the level of deep theta brain-waves or the deep Samadhi state, the sound of one's own breathing disappears and one no longer notices whether one is breathing or not." [24]

As the practitioner becomes healthier and more comfortable with breathing less, and in a controlled manner, the body actually begins to become more oxygenated. More blood and oxygen goes to the brain, more air to the lungs, and more oxygen to the cells. With controlled reduced breathing the body adopts a slightly more acidic state that calms the nervous system, reduces your desire for acidic foods and reduces your level of hunger in general.

Pranayama (*yogic* breath control) uses two main methods to help increase oxygenation and the flow of *prana* to the cells of the body.

(1) Hypoventilation: Reducing minute ventilation causes increased levels of carbon dioxide and carbonic acid that leads to increased blood flow to the brain, increased oxygenation of the alveoli, greater oxygenation of the cells via the Bohr Effect and desensitisation of the nervous system.

(2) Autogenous hyperbaric oxygenation: Muscular co-activation around the nine major joint complexes can temporarily increase blood pressure, which can increase the partial pressure and saturation of oxygen in the body. This can lead to oxygenation of the cells and can subsequently calm the nervous system by lowering blood pressure.

Pranayama for hypoventilation
Studies in India [25] have demonstrated that beginner *pranayama* practitioners often tend to hyperventilate while experienced *pranayama* practitioners tend to hypoventilate.

The normal person at rest takes about 12 –16 breaths per minute with a tidal volume of about 500 ml therefore breathing around 6 – 8 litres per minute. The average lung capacity is about five litres, so a beginner *yoga* practitioner who chooses to breathe deeply while maintaining a normal breath rate will be breathing up to 60 litres per minute (ten times as much air as normal). Such excess levels of fuel in a car engine would almost certainly 'flood the engine' or, at best, render it less efficient than it should otherwise be. The body responds in a similar way to excess breathing. Such high levels of breathing 'blows off' carbon dioxide before it can reach levels that signal vasodilation (widening of blood vessels) or bronchodilatation (widening of tubes bringing air to the lungs). Also, because of the Bohr Effect there is an inhibition of transfer of oxygen from haemoglobin to tissue cells. The Bohr Effect states that an increase in alkalinity (a decrease in carbonic acid) increases the affinity of haemoglobin to oxygen. So the paradox of *pranayama* and breath-control is that one actually gets more oxygen and *prana* to the brain, lungs and into tissue cells by taking in less, rather than more, air. However, when the effort required to maintain difficult postures dramatically increases, more fuel (greater amounts of air) obviously needs to be taken in.

Hypoventilation causes a mild increase in the acidity of body fluids such as blood due to the build up of carbon dioxide and carbonic acid. Acidity has the effect of decreasing the sensitivity of the nervous system. Hence hypoventilation leads to decreased emotional sensitivity, decreased levels of pain, decreased skin sensitivity and skin problems and a decreased desire for acid-producing foods and food in general. Reducing the need for acid-producing foods (which include meat, fish, eggs, cooked grains and nuts) reduces leaching of calcium from the bones to neutralise food derived acids by combining with them to form insoluble calcium salts [17]. Reducing the levels of insoluble calcium salts in the blood reduces the risk of arteriosclerosis, renal problems and arthritis.

A mild respiratory acidosis can be generated with hypoventilation by using *bandhas* to assist in making slow complete exhalations, small inhalations and by holding the breath both in and out. Holding the breath (apnoea) is referred to as *kumbhaka* in *hatha yoga*. The highest form of *kumbhaka* is *kevala kumbhaka*. This is when, with sufficient preparation, the breath spontaneously and naturally stops, and is without inhalation and exhalation for long periods and the practitioner enters a meditative state. According to *hatha yoga* texts it is through *kevala kumbhaka* that the experiential knowledge of *kundalini* (energy inside the spine) arises. To enable this to take place physically it is the practitioner's skin not the lungs that breathe the most. Also the practitioner must have sufficient alkaline reserves to tolerate increased amounts of carbonic acid from retaining carbon dioxide. In some ancient *yoga* texts *kevala kumbhaka* is described as when breathing becomes about 30 very small breaths per minute. The phenomenon may be explained in terms of the anatomical dead space for if the tidal volume is less than 150 ml (the volume of the anatomical dead space) then it is essentially like not breathing and may be precisely what the *yogic* texts describe as *kevala kumbhaka*.

A person regularly practicing *hatha yoga* with *pranayama* and *bandhas* who can generate a mild respiratory acidosis can easily derive the benefits of living on the traditional *hatha yoga phalahari* diet of fruit, salad and vegetables. In one of the oldest texts on *hatha yoga* (*Yogayajnavalkya Samhita* Verses VI.60-VI.64), it says that those who can do *kevala kumbhaka pranayama* will have mastery over hunger [25].

Hypoventilation during meditation
If *hatha yoga*, practiced with *pranayama* and *bandhas*, is followed by a period of observation of breath the meditative state can easily ensue. The most consistent findings in the many studies of meditation was the presence of some sort of hypoventilation [27, 28, 29], and coherent synchronous brain wave patterns [30, 31, 32, 33] distinct from that of ordinary waking, hypnosis or sleep [34]. With continued observance of natural breathing when sitting or lying quietly, the practitioner can approach *kevala kumbhaka*. The inhalations and exhalations in *kevala kumbhaka* are so silent, small in volume and so infrequent that a state of non-breathing is approached and the mind is very calm and rested.

Yoga is synonymous with meditation. *Hatha yoga* is said to be the pathway to *raja yoga* (the ultimate *yoga* of the mind and meditation). The main text on *raja yoga* says *yoga* is "*citta vrtti nirodha*", which is when the fluctuations (*vrtti*) of the mind (*citta*) are stilled (*nirodha*) [35]. In scientific terms, this can be interpreted and seen as coherent synchronous brain wave patterns. The main text on *hatha yoga* says *yoga* is "*prana vrtti nirodha*", which is when the fluctuations (*vrtti*) of the breath (*prana*) are stilled (*nirodha*) [36]. In scientific terms, this can be interpreted as hypoventilation.

The ancient *yoga* texts are clear in stating that *citta* (mind/consciousness/information) and *prana* (essential life force in the breath) move as one, and are always together in the body [35]. If '*yoga* is stillness in mind' (*raja yoga*) and '*yoga* is stillness in breath' (*hatha yoga*), then when there is stillness in mind there should be stillness in breath and vice versa. There are therefore essentially two approaches to achieve *yoga* and reach a meditative state, the *raja yoga* approach and the *hatha yoga* approach. These two approaches lead to a meditative state that is physiologically similar in terms of brain wave patterns and type of ventilation. In the *raja yoga* approach, which uses non physical methods such as observation of the natural breathing pattern, the *yoga* practitioner stills the mind, generating coherent synchronous brain wave patterns [37, 38]. The body then responds with *kevala kumbhaka*, a state of hypoventilation in which the breath is almost imperceptible or spontaneously absent [39, 30, 40, 41]. In the *hatha yoga* approach, physical *yoga* (including *pranayama* with *bandhas*) is used to bring stillness to the breath which is seen as some form of hypoventilation [42, 43]. The mind then responds with a calmness that is associated with the presence of coherent synchronous brain wave patterns [44, 45, 31].

The effects of hyperventilation on cardiopulmonary physiology
Although the ultimate aim of *pranayama* (*yogic* breath-control) is controlled hypoventilation there are times when it is useful to hyperventilate. Many of the breathing exercises taught in *yoga* classes unknowingly lead to hyperventilation. Even those exercises which do involve holding the breath tend to cause hyperventilation as many teachers encourage deep breathing, but few practitioners can safely hold full lungs long enough, or breathe deeply slow enough, to breathe less than the normal minute ventilation.

Hyperventilation has some temporary benefits such as training the muscles of the chest and abdomen to increase the rate and depth of the breath. This causes an increase in body heat, which can facilitate joint mobility. The increased chest expansion during inhalation and the rapid compression of chest and abdomen during exhalation in hyperventilation teaches *uddiyana bandha* in its compressive and expansive forms and *mula bandha* in its compressive form. In addition, hyperventilation causes the depletion of carbon dioxide, which results in the body becoming more alkaline because of respiratory alkalosis. The major positive effect of an alkaline system is that it also makes the synovial fluid more liquid and thus increases flexibility in the same way that heat does.

The major clinical effect of alkalosis (an over-alkaline system) is over-excitability of the nervous system, which affects both the central nervous system (CNS) and peripheral nervous system [46]. High levels of alkalinity in the bloodstream and body fluids can make the nervous system hypersensitive, which can manifest as joint pain, allergies, skin rashes and emotional disturbances. The major negative effect of respiratory alkalosis is that chemoreceptors in the carotid arteries and also those in the bronchial tubes detect the reduction in carbon dioxide levels and cause vasoconstriction (narrowing of blood vessels) or bronchoconstriction (narrowing of the tubes bringing air to the lungs). This reduces the flow of blood and air to the brain and lungs respectively. Hyperventilation also tends to speed up the heartbeat and therefore increases sympathetic nervous system stimulation, and decreases parasympathetic nervous system stimulation.

As the practitioner becomes more adapt, the minimal benefits of hyperventilation can be achieved by other means and so they are then free to pursue breathing patterns that lead to hypoventilation. For example the control of the chest and abdominal muscle achieved through rapid breathing can eventually be obtained without breathing at all. Also, the increased fluidity of the synovial fluid obtained through hyperventilation can be obtained by heating the body with *bandhas* and other muscle activations, or by adopting an alkaline diet which is the most supportive of a breathing pattern that is predominantly hypoventilation, thus generating greater levels of carbonic acid.

Mild hyperbaric oxygenation using *bandha* and *pranayama* on cardiopulmonary physiology
Although a main aim of *pranayama* is to hypoventilate, the aim nevertheless is to bring more oxygen to the cells, which is the eventual outcome of hypoventilation. *Hatha yoga* may bring more oxygen to the cells via a type of autogenous mild hyperbaric oxygenation (HBO) and may have effects similar effects as mild HBO therapy [47]. The word *hatha* means force and implies pressure [48, 49]. *Hatha yoga* may increase cellular oxygenation by generating pressures using *bandhas* and other techniques inside the body that increase oxygen saturation and partial pressure of oxygen. *Bandhas* can generate increases in IAP and ITP within the body and can have the same effect as the Valsalva manoeuvre. This has been shown to be significantly

modified when other *bandhas* are applied such as the hand grip [50], which is essentially a co-activation around the wrist referred to as *ha-mani bandha*. Carter *et al* [11] have confirmed that there is an increase in systemic arterial oxygen saturation during the period of increased ITP induced by a Valsalva manoeuvre. Many of the effects seen by practitioners of *hatha yoga* incorporating *bandha* and *pranayama* are the same as those of mild hyperbaric oxygen therapy [13, 51, 52].

SUMMARY AND CONCLUSION

We have presented a simple yet practical division of the body's anatomy using a set of basic principles. The *yoga* body can be thought of in terms of nine joint complexes, about 20 pairs of opposing muscle groups, three spinal nerve reflexes and four states of muscle activation/relaxation for antagonistic muscle groups around a joint complex. One of these states is co-activation, which happens spontaneously in many cases but can also be trained in *hatha yoga* where it is referred to as *bandha*. *Bandhas* interact with the nervous system and can help to promote joint stability, strength, flexibility and the ability to relax. *Bandhas* can be made to either generate high or low pressure and can therefore move energy (*prana*) and information (*citta*) through the body. *Bandhas* are important elements of *pranayama* (the breath-control system of *hatha yoga*) and have a significant effect on respiration and cardiopulmonary physiology. One of the main physical aims of *hatha yoga* and of *pranayama* is to maximise oxygenation of the cells. When the *bandhas* are properly maintained during the respiratory cycle in *pranayama* the natural outcome is hypoventilation. Hypoventilation leads to a build up of carbon dioxide which results in more air to the alveoli (due to bronchodilatation), more blood to the brain and heart (due to vasodilation), and more blood to each cell (due to the Bohr Effect). Hypoventilation also increases levels of carbonic acid, which calms the nervous system, hence enabling easier meditation, and reduces the need and desire for high protein or acidic foods and food in general. When the *bandhas* are applied throughout the body with *pranayama* according to the *hatha yoga* system, they cause pressure changes within the body that can have an effect similar to that of mild hyperbaric oxygen therapy which has been shown to increase oxygenation of the cells.

A *yoga* practice based on the principles of applied anatomy and physiology of *hatha yoga* can be a very effective therapy for many musculoskeletal problems and medical conditions in addition to being a very effective means of improving strength, flexibility, cardiovascular fitness, and the ability to relax and meditate. However, to know how and when it is appropriate to apply these principles as a therapy in a safe and effective manner requires a practical understanding and regular personal practice of *hatha yoga* as learned from an experienced teacher.

References

1. Herzog W, Binding P, (1993). Cocontraction of pairs of antagonistic muscles: analytical solution for planar static nonlinear optimization approaches. Mathematical biosciences.118: 1, 83-95.
2. Richardson, C.A., Jull, G.A. (1995). Muscle Control - Pain Control what exercises should you prescribe. Manual Therapy Journal 1: 2 -10.
3. Hubley-Kozey, C. & Earl, E.M. (2000). Co-activation of the ankle musculature during maximal isokinetic dorsiflexion at different angular velocities. European Journal of Applied Physiology. 82: 289-96.
4. Aagaard, P, Simonsen, EB, Andersen, JL, Magnusson, SP, Bojsen, Miller, F, Dyhre Poulsen, P (2000). Antagonist muscle co-activation during isokinetic knee extension. Scandinavian Journal of Medical Science and Sports. 04, 10: 2, 58-67.
5. Gribble PL, Ostry DJ, (1998). Independent coactivation of shoulder and elbow muscles. 3, 355-60.
6. Yamazaki Y, Itoh H, Ohkuwa T, (1995). Muscle activation in the elbow-forearm complex during rapid elbow extension. 3, 285-95.
7. Smith AM, (1981). The coactivation of antagonist muscles. Canadian journal of physiology and pharmacology. 7, 733-47.
8. Borg-Olivier, S.A. Machliss, B.E. (2003). *Yoga* and Meditation. In An Introduction to Complementary Medicine (Edited by T. Robson) Allen and Unwin, Australia.
9. Proske, U., Wise, A.K., Gregory, J.E. (2000). The role of muscle receptors in the detection of movements. Progress in Neurobiology. 01, 60: 1, 85-96.
10. Barbeau, H, Marchand, Pauvert, V., Meunier, S., Nicolas, G., Pierrot, Deseilligny, E. (2000). Posture-related changes in heteronymous recurrent inhibition from quadriceps to ankle muscles in humans. Experimental Brain Research, 02, 130: 3, 345-61.

11. Carter, SA, Birkhead, NC, Wood, EH (1959) Intracardiac Shunts Effect Of Valsalva Maneuver On Oxygen Saturation In Patients with Intracardiac Shunts Circulation 20;574-586.

12. Basaranoglu, G, M Basaranoglu, V Erden, H Delatioglu, A F Pekel and L Saitoglu (2006) The effects of Valsalva manoeuvres on venepuncture pain European Journal of Anaesthesiology 23: 591-593.

13. Sahni, T, Singh, P, John, M.J. (2003) Hyperbaric oxygen therapy: current trends and applications. Journal of the Association of Physicians of India 51:, 280-4.

14. Cholewicki J, Panjabi MM, Khachatryan A, (1997). Stabilizing function of trunk flexor-extensor muscles around a neutral spine posture. 19, 2207-12.

15. Cholewicki J, Juluru K, McGill SM, (1999). Intra-abdominal pressure mechanism for stabilizing the lumbar spine. 1, 13-7.

16. Hodges PW, Gandevia SC. (2000) Changes in intra-abdominal pressure during postural and respiratory activation of the human diaphragm. Journal of Applied Physiology. 89(3):967-76.

17. Borg-Olivier, S.A. and Machliss B.E. (2005) Applied Anatomy and Physiology of *Yoga*. *Yoga* Synergy, Sydney.

18. Yogeshwarananda, S. (1970). 'Bahiranga *Yoga* - First Steps to Higher *Yoga*'. *Yoga* Niketan Trust, Bharat India.

19. Corrigan GE (1969). Fatal air embolism after *Yoga* breathing exercises JAMA 210 (10): 1923.

20. Hanus SH, Homer TD, Harter DH (1977). Vertebral artery occlusion complicating *yoga* exercises. Archives of Neurology 34 (9): 574-5.

21. Fong KY, Cheung RT, Yu YL, Lai CW, Chang CM (1993) Basilar artery occlusion following *yoga* exercise: a case report. Clinical and experimental neurology 30: 104-109.

22. Iyengar, B.K.S. (1966). Light on *Yoga*. Schocken Books, New York.

23. Liu, D. (1991). Taoist Health Exercise Book. Paragon House New York.

24. Sat Chuen Hon (2003) Taoist Qigong for Health and Vitality: A Complete Program of Movement, Meditation, and Healing Sounds. Shambhala. Also available at http://users.erols.com/dantao/breath.html.

25. Karambelkar, P.V., Deshpande, R.R., Bhole, M.V. (1982). Oxygen consumption during Ujjayi *pranayama*. *Yoga* Mimamsa, Volume XXI: 3 & 4.

26. Desikachar, T.K.V. (2000). *Yoga*-yajnavalkya Samhita. Krishnamacharya *Yoga* Mandiram.

27. Wolkove N, Kreisman H, Darragh D, Cohen C, Frank H, (1984). Effect of transcendental meditation on breathing and respiratory control., Journal of Applied Physiology: Respiratory, Environmental and Exercise Physiology 56: 3, 607-12.

28. Sudsuang R, Chentanez V, Veluvan K. (1991).Effect of Buddhist meditation on serum cortisol and total protein levels, blood pressure, pulse rate, lung volume and reaction time. Physiology and Behavior 50: 3, 543-8.

29. Peng CK, Mietus JE, Liu Y, Khalsa G, Douglas PS, Benson H, Goldberger AL, (1999). Exaggerated heart rate oscillations during two meditation techniques., International Journal of Cardiology 70: 2, 101-7.

30. Badawi K, Wallace RK, Orme-Johnson D, Rouzere AM, (1984). Electrophysiologic characteristics of respiratory suspension periods occurring during the practice of the Transcendental Meditation Program., Psychosomatic Medicine 46: 3, 267-76.

31. Arambula P, Peper E, Kawakami M, Gibney KH, (2001). The physiological correlates of Kundalini *Yoga* meditation: a study of a *yoga* master., Applied psychophysiology and biofeedback 26: 2, 147-53.

32. Travis, F.T. & Pearson, C. (2000). Distinct Phenomenological and Physiological Correlates of 'Consciousness Itself.' International Journal of Neuroscience, 100, 77-89.

33. Travis F, (2001). Autonomic and EEG patterns distinguish transcending from other experiences during Transcendental Meditation practice. International Journal of Psychophysiology. 42: 1, 1-9.

34. Hewitt J. (1983).The *yoga* of breathing posture and meditation. London: Random House, 89-91.

35. Iyengar, B.K.S. (1993). Light on the *Yoga* Sutras of Patanjali. Aquarian Press, London.

36. Vishnu-Devananda, S. (1987). *Hatha Yoga* Pradipika of Swatmarama: The Classic Guide for the Advanced Practice of *Hatha Yoga*, with 1897 commentary of Brahmananda, and 1987 commentary of Vishnu-Devandana. OM Lotus Publishing Company, New York.

37. Corby JC, Roth WT, Zarcone VP Jr, Kopell BS, (1978). Psychophysiological correlates of the practice of Tantric *Yoga* meditation., Archives of General Psychiatry 35: 5, 571-7.

38. Aftanas LI, Golocheikine SA, (2001). Human anterior and frontal midline theta and lower alpha reflect emotionally positive state and internalized attention: high-resolution EEG investigation of meditation.,

Neuroscience letters 310: 1, 57-60.

39. Farrow JT, Hebert JR, (1982). Breath suspension during the transcendental meditation technique., Psychosomatic Medicine 44: 2, 133-53.

40. Gallois P, (1984). [Neurophysiologic and respiratory changes during the practice of relaxation technics], (Modifications neurophysiologiques et respiratoires lors de la pratique des techniques de relaxation.), L'Encephale. 10: 3, 139-44.

41. Travis F, Wallace RK, (1997). Autonomic patterns during respiratory suspensions: possible markers of Transcendental Consciousness., Psychophysiology 34: 1, 39-46.

42. Stanescu DC, Nemery B, Veriter C, Marechal C (1981). Pattern of breathing and ventilatory response to C02 in subjects practising *hatha-yoga*. Journal of Applied Physiology. 51: 1625-29.

43. Miyamura M, Nishimura K, Ishida K, Katayama K, Shimaoka M, Hiruta S, (2002). Is man able to breathe once a minute for an hour?: the effect of *yoga* respiration on blood gases., Japanese journal of physiology 52: 3, 313-6.

44. Hebert, R, Lehmann, D. (1977). Theta bursts: an EEG pattern in normal subjects practising the transcendental meditation technique. Electroencephalography and clinical neurophysiology *42*(3), 397-405.

45. Stancak A Jr, Pfeffer D, Hrudova L, Sovka P, Dostalek C, (1993). Electroencephalographic correlates of paced breathing., Neuroreport 4: 6, 723-6.

46. Guyton, A.C. (1991). A Textbook of Medical Physiology. W.B. Saunders, Co, Philadelphia. USA.

47. Heuser, G. (2002) in Proceedings of the 2nd International Symposium on Hyperbaric Oxygenation for Cerebral Palsy and the Brain-Injured Child (Hardcover) by James T. Joiner (Editor).

48. Borg-Olivier, SA, Machliss, BE (1997). *Hatha yoga* stretching & muscle strengthening A Guide for Physiotherapists. The Australian Physiotherapy Association 1997 Conference for Alternative Therapies,

49. Borg-Olivier, SA, Machliss, BE (1998). Integrating *yoga* and physiotherapy. Proceedings of the Australian Physiotherapy Association 1998 in 'Physiotherapy: Balancing the Art with the Science Sydney Australia.

50. Ewing DJ, Kerr F, Leggett R, Murray A (1976) Interaction between cardiovascular responses to sustained handgrip and Valsalva manoeuvre. British Heart Journal, Vol 38, 483-490.

51. Niinikoski, JH, (2004) Clinical hyperbaric oxygen therapy, wound perfusion, and transcutaneous oximetry., World Journal of Surgery 28:3, 307-11.

52. Zamboni, WA, Browder, L,K., Martinez, J. (2003) Hyperbaric oxygen and wound healing., Clinics in Plastic Surgery 30: 1, 67-75.

Figures

Figure 3a: Practical example: Hip extensor stretch - 'The cross-legged forward bend':

In the cross-legged forward bend, which can stretch the hip extensors (and the muscles around the buttocks), the agonist muscles are the hip flexors (muscles at the front of the groins) and the antagonist muscles are the hip extensors. Hatha yoga can work with these opposing hip muscle groups in four distinct ways. Each of these four states of activation/ relaxation of the muscles around the hip joint complex has distinct advantages and disadvantages and is useful in various situations:

State 1: Relaxed agonist and antagonist: Relax both hip flexors and hip extensors
Advantages:
- does not involve any effort physically
- allows the joint to be easily moved with no restriction from active muscle tension
Disadvantages:
- usually causes resistance from stretch reflex muscle tension in the antagonist
- does not offer any additional stabilisation to the joint complex

State 2: Agonist activation: Generates hip flexor (agonist) activity by 'trying to lift the inner thighs off the floor' and keep hip extensors relaxed
Advantages:
- helps to strengthen the hip flexors (muscles at the front of the groins) in a shortened position
- stimulates the reciprocal reflex, causing reciprocal relaxation and easier lengthening of the hip extensors (antagonist)
Disadvantages:
- uses muscle effort
- only strengthens one side (the front) of the hip joint complex

State 3: Antagonist activation: Generates hip extensor (antagonist) muscle group activity by 'pressing the feet into the floor' or by 'tensing the buttock muscles' and keep hip flexors relaxed
Advantages:
- helps to strengthen the hip extensors (antagonist) in a lengthened state
- stimulates the inverse myotatic reflex, leading to an increase in the stretch and subsequent increase in the ability of the hip extensors (antagonist) to relax
Disadvantages:
- uses muscle effort
- only strengthens one side (the rear) of the hip joint complex

State 4: Co-activation of opposing muscle groups (bandha): Simultaneously generates hip flexor (agonist) and hip extensor (antagonist) muscle group activity (co-activation):
Advantages:
- helps to give stability to the hip joint complex
- helps to regulate circulation around the hip joint complex
- helps to improve strength, flexibility and the ability to relax in the muscles of the hip joint complex
Disadvantages:
- uses muscle effort
- makes it harder to freely move the hip joint complex

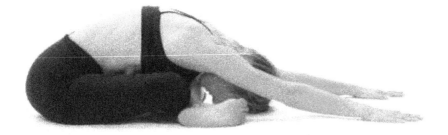

Figure 3b: Advanced hip extensor stretching – 'the balancing lotus forward bend': This advanced *yoga* posture also requires tremendous neuromuscular control and a balance between strength and flexibility around the hip joint and the whole body. However, for the hip joint complex it is basically the same exercise as shown in figure 1 (the cross-legged forward bend) and exactly the same principles are used in terms of activation, relaxation and co-activation of agonist and antagonist muscles around the hip as well as the other main joint complexes in the body.

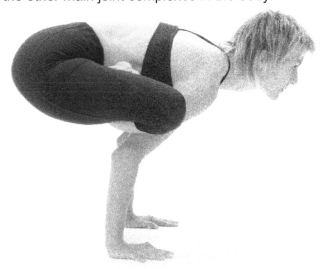

Figure 4a: Practical example: Hip flexor stretch - 'the standing lunge':
In the lunge which can stretch the hip flexors (the front of the groin), the agonist muscles are the hip extensors (muscles around the buttocks) and the antagonist muscles are the hip flexors. *Hatha yoga* can work with these opposing hip muscle groups in four distinct ways. Each of these four states of activation/ relaxation of the muscles around the hip joint complex has distinct advantages and disadvantages and is useful in various situations:

State 1: Relaxed agonist and antagonist: Relax both hip flexors and hip extensors
Advantages:
• does not involve any effort physically
• allows the joint to be easily moved with no restriction from active muscle tension
Disadvantages:
• usually causes resistance from stretch reflex muscle tension in the antagonist
• does not offer any additional stabilisation to the hip joint complex

State 2: Agonist activation: Generates hip extensor (agonist) activity by 'squeezing the buttocks' and keep hip flexors relaxed
Advantages:
• helps to strengthen the hip extensors ('buttocks muscles') in a shortened state
• stimulates the reciprocal reflex, causing reciprocal relaxation and easier lengthening of the hip flexors (antagonist)
Disadvantages:
• uses muscle effort
• only strengthens one side (the rear) of the hip joint complex

State 3: Antagonist activation: Generates hip flexor (antagonist) muscle group activity 'pressing the feet into the floor as if trying to bring the feet together' and keep hip extensors relaxed
Advantages:
• helps to strengthen the hip flexors (antagonist) in a lengthened position
• stimulates the inverse myotatic reflex, leading to an increase in the stretch and subsequent increase in the ability of the hip flexors (antagonist) to relax
Disadvantages:
• uses muscle effort
• only strengthens one side (the front) of the hip joint complex

State 4: Co-activation of opposing muscle groups: Simultaneously generates hip extensor (agonist) and hip flexor (antagonist) muscle group activity (co-activation):

Advantages:
- helps to give stability to the hip joint complex
- helps to regulate circulation around the hip joint complex
- helps to improve strength, flexibility and the ability to relax in the muscles of the hip joint complex

Disadvantages:
- uses muscle effort
- makes it harder to freely move the hip joint complex

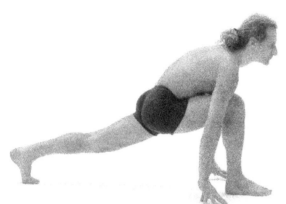

Figure 4b: Advanced hip flexor stretching – 'the balancing deep lunge': this advanced *yoga* posture requires tremendous neuromuscular control and a balance between strength and flexibility around the hip joint and the whole body. However, around the hip joint complex it is basically the same exercise as shown in Figure 4a (the lunge) and exactly the same principles are used in terms of activation, relaxation and co-activation of agonist and antagonist muscles around the hip as well as the other main joint complexes in the body.

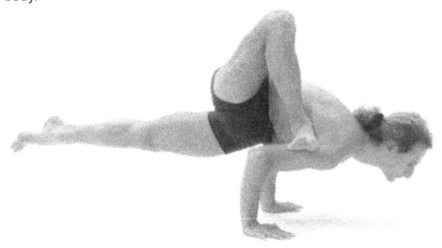

Figures 6abc: Advanced spinal muscular co-activation and breath-control for the regulation of internal energy and the manipulation of joints and internal organs: These advanced *yoga kriyas* (cleansing processes) are performed without any air in the lungs and thus requires the ability to hypoventilate and tolerate higher than normal levels of carbon dioxide in the body which can only be maintained if an adequate (alkaline) diet is also maintained.

Figures 6a and 6b: This advanced *yoga kriya* (cleansing process) involves using an expansive circumferential muscular co-activation around the thoracic spine joint complex (*tha-uddiyana bandha*) and an expansive flexor-extensor co-activation around the lumbar spine joint complex (*tha-mula bandha*). This is commonly known as *nauli*. The expansive flexor-extensor co-activation can also be performed with a compressive circumferential muscular co-activation around the thoracic spine joint complex (*ha-uddiyana bandha*) while doing diaphragmatic breathing. In that case the spine can become mobile and lengthened yet remain stable and strong as the diaphragm causes an increase in intra-abdominal pressure.

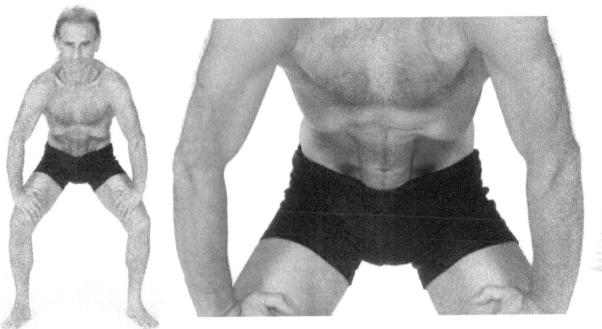

Figure 6c: This advanced *yoga kriya* (cleansing process) involves using an expansive circumferential muscular co-activation around the thoracic spine joint complex (*tha-uddiyana bandha*) and a compressive circumferential co-activation around the lumbar spine joint complex (*ha-mula bandha*). Here the external oblique abdominal muscles are defined. With time and practice this *ha-mula bandha* can be performed with a compressive circumferential muscular co-activation around the thoracic spine joint complex (*ha-uddiyana bandha*) while doing diaphragmatic breathing. In that case tremendous physical power is generated as the diaphragm causes an increase in intra-abdominal pressure.

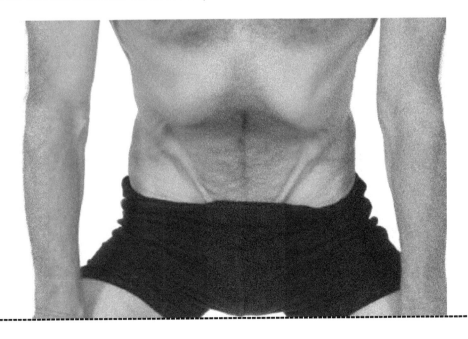

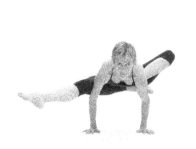
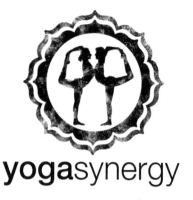
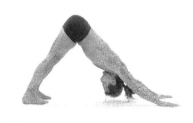

yogasynergy

Yoga Synergy offers a range of practice DVDs designed for beginner to advanced students.
Each Yoga Synergy elemental sequence features variations of each pose that are easy to follow.

Practice any time, any place.

Original series

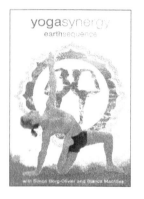
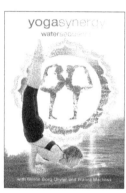
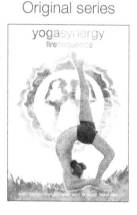
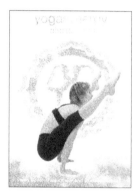
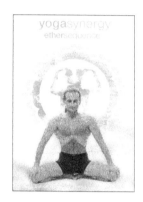

Beginner series

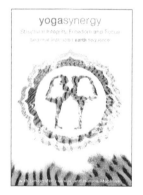
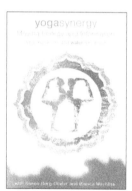
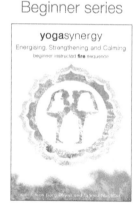
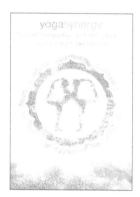
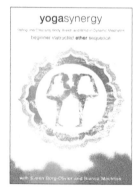

Complete 5 DVD set, Prenatal and Nutrition

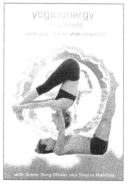
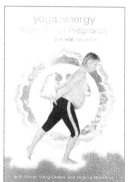
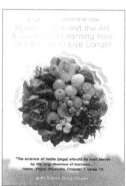